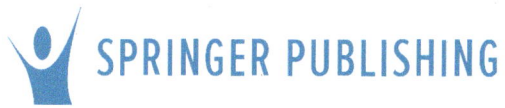

GET THE MOST FROM YOUR BOOK

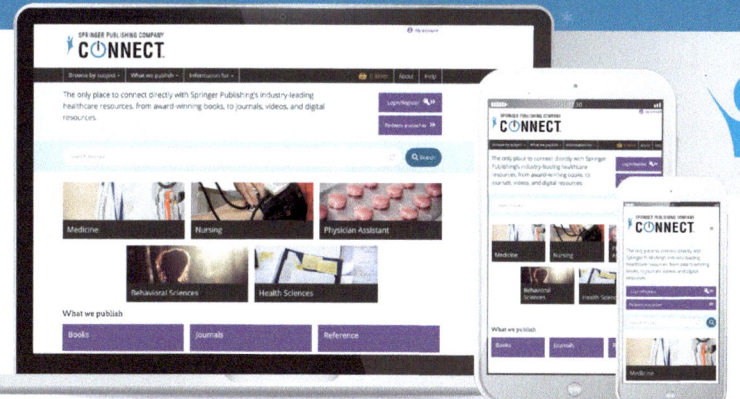

VOUCHER CODE:

V3ED65J4

Online Access

Your print purchase of *Teaching in Nursing and Role of the Educator: The Complete Guide to Best Practice in Teaching, Evaluation, and Curriculum Development,* Fourth Edition, includes **online access via Springer Publishing Connect**™ to increase accessibility, portability, and searchability.

Insert the code at http://connect.springerpub.com/content/book/978-0-8261-8892-2 or scan the QR code and insert the voucher code today!

Having trouble? Contact our customer service department at **cs@springerpub.com**

Instructor Resource Access for Adopters

Let us do some of the heavy lifting to create an engaging classroom experience with a variety of instructor resources included in most textbooks SUCH AS:

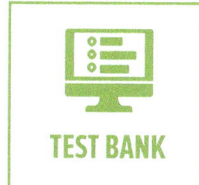

Visit **https://connect.springerpub.com/** and look for the **"Show Supplementary"** button on your **book homepage** to see what is available to instructors! First time using Springer Publishing Connect?

Email **textbook@springerpub.com** to create an account and start unlocking valuable resources.

Teaching in Nursing and Role of the Educator

The Complete Guide to Best Practice in Teaching, Evaluation, and Curriculum Development

Jennie C. De Gagne, PhD, DNP, RN, NPD-BC, CNE, ANEF, FAAN, is a professor of nursing and director of the nursing education specialty at Duke University School of Nursing. With extensive experience in nursing education, she has provided consultation to nursing schools worldwide, including in South Korea, Ghana, India, Tanzania, Saudi Arabia, Oman, and Lebanon, focusing on curriculum and faculty development. Dr. De Gagne is an expert in educational technology and online education, particularly in the effective use of instructional technology and cybercivility across the curriculum. She has authored or coauthored over 200 publications, including more than 120 peer-reviewed journal articles, and has presented at nearly 150 national and international conferences, establishing herself as a thought leader in the nursing education community.

Marilyn H. Oermann, PhD, RN, ANEF, FAAN, is the Thelma M. Ingles Professor of Nursing at Duke University School of Nursing. She is the author or coauthor of 35 books and many articles on evaluation, teaching in nursing, and studies of the nursing literature. She is the editor-in-chief of *Nurse Educator*. Dr. Oermann received the National League for Nursing (NLN) Award for Excellence in Nursing Education Research, the Sigma Theta Tau International Elizabeth Russell Belford Award for Excellence in Education, the American Association of Colleges of Nursing Scholarship of Teaching and Learning Excellence Award, the Margaret Comerford Freda Award for Editorial Leadership in Nursing from the International Academy of Nursing Editors, and the NLN President's Award. The NLN established an award in her honor, the Marilyn H. Oermann Award for Distinguished Research in Nursing Education, to recognize an individual or team who has generated an evidentiary base for the science of nursing education.

Teaching in Nursing and Role of the Educator

The Complete Guide to Best Practice in Teaching, Evaluation, and Curriculum Development

Fourth Edition

Jennie C. De Gagne, PhD, DNP, RN, NPD-BC, CNE, ANEF, FAAN

Marilyn H. Oermann, PhD, RN, ANEF, FAAN

Editors

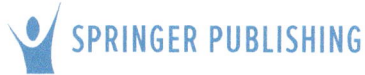

Copyright © 2025 Springer Publishing Company, LLC
All rights reserved.
First Springer Publishing edition 978-0-8261-9553-1 (2013); subsequent editions 2017, 2021

No part of this publication may be reproduced, stored in a retrieval system, or transmitted in any form or by any means, electronic, mechanical, photocopying, recording, or otherwise, without the prior permission of Springer Publishing Company, LLC, or authorization through payment of the appropriate fees to the Copyright Clearance Center, Inc., 222 Rosewood Drive, Danvers, MA 01923, 978-750-8400, fax 978-646-8600, info@copyright.com or at www.copyright.com.

Springer Publishing Company, LLC
902 Carnegie Center, Princeton, NJ 08540
www.springerpub.com
connect.springerpub.com

Acquisitions Editor: Joseph Morita
Compositor: Amnet
Production Manager: Kris Parrish

ISBN: 978-0-8261-8891-5
ebook ISBN: 978-0-8261-8892-2
DOI: 10.1891/9780826188922

SUPPLEMENTS:

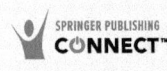

A robust set of instructor resources designed to supplement this text is located at http://connect.springerpub.com/content/book/978-0-8261-8892-2. Qualifying instructors may request access by emailing textbook@springerpub.com.

Instructor Materials:
LMS Common Cartridge With All Instructor Resources ISBN: 978-0-8261-8893-9
Instructor Manual ISBN: 978-0-8261-8897-7
Instructor PowerPoints ISBN: 978-0-8261-8896-0
Mapping to AACN Essentials: 978-0-8261-8894-6
Transition Guide to the Fourth Edition ISBN: 978-0-8261-8895-3

24 25 26 27 / 5 4 3 2 1

The author and the publisher of this Work have made every effort to use sources believed to be reliable to provide information that is accurate and compatible with the standards generally accepted at the time of publication. Because medical science is continually advancing, our knowledge base continues to expand. Therefore, as new information becomes available, changes in procedures become necessary. We recommend that the reader always consult current research and specific institutional policies before performing any clinical procedure or delivering any medication. The author and publisher shall not be liable for any special, consequential, or exemplary damages resulting, in whole or in part, from the readers' use of, or reliance on, the information contained in this book. The publisher has no responsibility for the persistence or accuracy of URLs for external or third-party Internet websites referred to in this publication and does not guarantee that any content on such websites is, or will remain, accurate or appropriate.

Library of Congress Control Number: 2024950665

Contact sales@springerpub.com to receive discount rates on bulk purchases.

Publisher's Note: **New and used products purchased from third-party sellers are not guaranteed for quality, authenticity, or access to any included digital components.**

Printed in the United States of America by Gasch Printing.

Contents

Contributors to the Fourth Edition   ix
Contributors to Earlier Editions   xi
Preface   xiii
Instructor Resources   xix

SECTION I: NURSING EDUCATION: ROLES OF TEACHER

1. Role of the Nurse Educator   3
   Marilyn H. Oermann

2. The Transition From Clinician to Educator   19
   Anne M. Schoening and Lorraine M. Rusch

3. Contemporary Learning Theories   35
   Paula D. Koppel

4. Understanding the Diverse Learner   53
   Stephanie A. Gedzyk-Nieman and Mark C. Hand

SECTION II: TEACHING IN NURSING

5. Teaching Methods   75
   Debra Hagler and Brenda Morris

6. Ethical, Legal, and Social Challenges in Academic Nursing   107
   Mary Ellen Smith Glasgow

7. Integrating Technology in Education   123
   Jennie C. De Gagne

8. Teaching in Online Learning Environments   143
   Jennie C. De Gagne

9. Incorporating Simulation in Nursing Education: Overview, Essentials, and the Evidence   163
   Kristina T. Dreifuerst, Pamela R. Jeffries, Katie A. Haerling, and Michelle Aebersold

SECTION III: TEACHING IN A CLINICAL AND INTERPROFESSIONAL EDUCATION SETTING

10. Clinical Teaching in Nursing   189
    Lisa K. Woodley and Leslie M. Sharpe

11. Weaving Interprofessional Education Into Nursing Curricula   215
    Karen T. Pardue, Shelley Cohen Konrad, and Dawn-Marie Dunbar

12. Academic–Practice Partnerships   237
    Elizabeth Gatewood

SECTION IV: CURRICULUM DEVELOPMENT

13. Competency-Based Education in Nursing   257
    Gerry Altmiller

14. Curriculum Development and Course Design in Nursing Education   273
    Stephanie Stimac DeBoor

SECTION V: EVALUATION OF LEARNER AND PROGRAM

15. Assessment Methods   295
    Marilyn H. Oermann

16. Developing and Using Tests   315
    Desirée Hensel

17. Clinical Evaluation   345
    Marilyn H. Oermann

18. Program Evaluation and Accreditation   359
    Marilyn H. Oermann

SECTION VI: SCHOLARSHIP, SERVICE, AND LEADERSHIP

19. Evidence-Based Teaching in Nursing   377
    Marilyn H. Oermann

20. Becoming a Scholar in Nursing Education   389
    Marilyn H. Oermann

21. Mentorship, Service, Leading, and Learner Success   401
    Richard L. Pullen Jr.

22. Nursing Professional Development Practitioner in a Clinical Practice Setting   423
    Joan Such Lockhart and Denise M. Petras

APPENDICES

A. Nursing and Higher Education Organizations   447
*B. Worksheets to Align End-of-Program and Course Outcomes
   to AACN Essentials   453*
*C. Selected Organizations, Journals, and Educational Conferences
   of Interest for Nursing Professional Development Practitioners   457*

Mapping Grids of Chapters and Certified Nurse Educator Examination Blueprints   461
Index   493

Contributors to the Fourth Edition

Michelle Aebersold, PhD, RN, CHSE, FSSH, FAAN Clinical Professor, School of Nursing, University of Michigan, Ann Arbor, Michigan

Gerry Altmiller, EdD, APRN, ACNS-BC, ANEF, FAAN Professor Emeritus, School of Nursing and Health Sciences, The College of New Jersey, Ewing, New Jersey;, Clinical Nurse Specialist, Jefferson Einstein Health System, Philadelphia, Pennsylvania

Stephanie Stimac DeBoor, PhD, APRN, ACNS-BC, CCRN Associate Dean for Graduate Programs and Professor, Orvis School of Nursing, University of Nevada, Reno, Reno, Nevada

Jennie C. De Gagne, PhD, DNP, RN, NPD-BC, CNE, ANEF, FAAN Professor, School of Nursing, Duke University, Durham, North Carolina

Kristina T. Dreifuerst, PhD, RN, CNE, ANEF, FAAN Director of PhD Program and Professor, College of Nursing, Marquette University, Milwaukee, Wisconsin

Dawn-Marie Dunbar, MSN/ED, RN, CHSE, CNE Clinical Product Manager, Oxford Medical Simulation, Boston, Massachusetts

Elizabeth Gatewood, DNP, FNP-C, CNE, FAANP, FAAN Assistant Dean of Education, Technology, and Innovation; Clinical Professor, University of California San Francisco, San Francisco, California

Stephanie A. Gedzyk-Nieman, DNP, RNC-MNN Assistant Dean of Pre-Licensure Programs and Assistant Professor, School of Nursing, Duke University, Durham, North Carolina

Mary Ellen Smith Glasgow, PhD, RN, ACNS-BC, ANEF, FNAP, FAAN Dean and Professor, School of Nursing, Duquesne University, Pittsburgh, Pennsylvania

Katie A. Haerling, PhD, RN, CHSE Graduate Program Coordinator and Professor, School of Nursing and Healthcare Leadership, University of Washington Tacoma, Tacoma, Washington,

Debra Hagler, PhD, RN, ACNS-BC, CNE, CHSE, ANEF, FAAN Clinical Professor, Edson College of Nursing and Health Innovation, Arizona State University, Phoenix, Arizona

Mark C. Hand, PhD, RN, CNE Clinical Professor, College of Nursing, East Carolina University, Greenville, North Carolina

Desirée Hensel, PhD, RN, PCNS-BC, CNE, ANEF, CHSE Visiting Professor, Teachers College, Columbia University, New York, New York

Pamela R. Jeffries, PhD, RN, ANEF, FSSH, FAAN Dean and Valere Potter Distinguished Professor of Nursing, Vanderbilt University School of Nursing, Nashville, Tennessee

Shelley Cohen Konrad, PhD, LCSW, FNAP Director, Center to Advance Interprofessional Education and Practice, University of New England, Portland, Maine

Paula D. Koppel, PhD, RN, GNP-BC, AHN-BC, NBC-HWC Founder/CEO and Integrative Nurse Consultant, Age Well Be Well, LLC, Brewster, Massachusetts

Joan Such Lockhart, PhD, RN, CNE, ANEF, FAAN Professor Emerita, School of Nursing, Duquesne University, Pittsburgh, Pennsylvania

Brenda Morris, EdD, RN, CNE Clinical Professor, Edson College of Nursing and Health Innovation, Arizona State University, Phoenix, Arizona

Marilyn H. Oermann, PhD, RN, ANEF, FAAN Thelma M. Ingles Professor of Nursing, School of Nursing, Duke University, Durham, North Carolina

Karen T. Pardue, PhD, RN, ANEF, FNAP Associate Provost, Strategic Initiatives and Professor, University of New England, Biddeford and Portland, Maine

Denise M. Petras, DNP, RN, NPD-BC Director, Professional Practice and Education, Allegheny General Hospital, Pittsburgh, Pennsylvania

Richard L. Pullen Jr., EdD, MSN, RN, CNE, CNE-cl, ANEF, FAAN RN to BSN Program Director and Professor, Texas Tech University Health Sciences Center, Lubbock, Texas

Lorraine M. Rusch, PhD, RN, CNE Associate Professor, College of Nursing, Creighton University, Omaha, Nebraska

Anne M. Schoening, PhD, RN, CNE Nursing Practice Coordinator, Creighton University Medical Center-Bergan Mercy, CHI Health, Omaha, Nebraska

Leslie M. Sharpe, DNP, FNP-BC Program Director, FNP Program and Clinical Associate Professor, School of Nursing, University of North Carolina at Chapel Hill, Chapel Hill, North Carolina

Lisa K. Woodley, PhD, MSN, RN, CNE, CHPN Clinical Professor, School of Nursing, University of North Carolina at Chapel Hill, Chapel Hill, North Carolina

Contributors to Earlier Editions

Darlene E. Baker, MSN, RN, CNE, CHSE

Donna L. Boland, PhD, RN, ANEF

Jamie L. Conklin, MSLIS

Helen B. Connors, PhD, RN, FAAN, ANEF

Sabreen A. Darwish, PhD, MSN, RN

Martha A. Dawson, DNP, RN, FACHE

Carol F. Durham, EdD, RN, ANEF, FAAN

Katherine Foss, MSN, RN

Betsy Frank, PhD, RN, ANEF

Kathleen B. Gaberson, PhD, RN, CNOR, CNE, ANEF

C. Ann Gakumo, PhD, RN

Karen L. Gorton, PhD, MS, FNP, RN

Sarah B. Keating, EdD, RN, FAAN

Amy C. Pettigrew, PhD, RN, CNE, ANEF

Beth Cusatis Phillips, PhD, RN, CNE, CHSE

JoAn M. Stanek, DNP, RN, ANP

Kathy Tally, MS

Theresa M. Valiga, EdD, RN, CNE, ANEF, FAAN

Lynda Wilson, PhD, RN

Preface

There is a critical need to prepare nurses for roles as educators in schools of nursing and healthcare settings. This book, in its fourth edition, is written to meet that need: It is a comprehensive text that provides, within one volume, essential concepts for effective teaching in nursing and carrying out other dimensions of the educator role. The book begins with a description of the role of a faculty member in a school of nursing and nurse educator in other settings. A chapter examines the transition from clinician to educator, barriers and facilitators to the transition process, and strategies to facilitate this transition. Other chapters describe contemporary learning theories and understanding the diverse learner; teaching methods, including integrating technology in teaching; teaching in online courses, simulation, and clinical settings; interprofessional education; and developing partnerships with clinical agencies.

Teachers in nursing should understand the curriculum and how it is developed, course design, and preparing a syllabus for a course. There is a new chapter in this edition on competency-based education. This chapter compares competency-based education principles with traditional teaching and learning structures, describes backward design, and explains how to implement competency-focused teaching and assessment.

Nurse educators also need to evaluate learning and performance, and for this reason the book includes chapters on assessment, testing including test and item analysis, clinical evaluation, and program evaluation and accreditation of nursing programs. It is important that nurse educators use evidence to guide their educational practices and develop their own scholarship; those areas are addressed in the last section of the book. This section also explores the roles of the nurse educator in service, as an advisor and mentor and as a leader. Nurse educators also are employed in healthcare settings. A chapter describes the roles and responsibilities of nursing professional development practitioners who help employees to become and remain competent.

The book was written for students in master's, doctor of nursing practice (DNP), doctor of philosophy (PhD), and certificate programs who are preparing themselves for a role as a nurse educator; for nurses who are transitioning into educator roles or are teaching students in addition to their practice positions; and for novice and experienced teachers who want to expand their knowledge and gain new ideas for their courses. If students are taking only one or two nursing education courses in their graduate program, this book will be of particular value because of its comprehensiveness.

The content in this book will be helpful in preparing for certification as a Certified Nurse Educator (CNE®), Certified Academic Clinical Nurse Educator (CNE®cl), and Certified Novice Nurse Educator (CNE®n). We have mapped the content in each chapter with the test blueprint for these three certification examinations. These mapping grids are provided following the appendix.

Nurse educators are employed in academic institutions and in healthcare and other types of settings. They educate nursing students at all levels, and in healthcare settings, they are responsible for providing continuing education and training. Many clinicians also teach nursing students in the clinical setting as part of their role, serving as preceptors and clinical nurse educators. Chapter 1 discusses trends supporting careers in nursing education, the role and responsibilities of nurse educators, ranks or academic titles of faculty, tracks (tenure track and nontenure track), and the educational preparation needed for a faculty role and for educator roles in healthcare settings. As nurse educators develop their knowledge and expertise, they can pursue certification as a nurse educator, which is also discussed in Chapter 1. A later chapter (22) examines the role and responsibilities of educators in nursing professional development.

The transition from clinician to nurse educator is rarely easy. Most novice educators assume an academic or a professional development role without formal preparation in nursing education. Chapter 2 examines the transition from clinician to educator, describes barriers and facilitators to the nurse educator transition process, and provides resources to help novice educators gain competence in their new role. The core competencies for academic nurse educators are discussed in this chapter. The Nurse Educator Transition Model and core competencies of nurse educators provide a framework for understanding the process that occurs during the role transition from nurse to nurse educator.

Understanding how students learn is essential for effective teaching. Theories explain the learning process and direct the selection of teaching methods. Nurse educators need to be grounded in a teaching philosophy that they can embody, using methods based on the best evidence of teaching and learning. They should understand theories of learning to ensure that their students receive a high-quality education. Chapter 3 examines foundational learning theories as well as some recent transformative theories and frameworks. Examples are provided of teaching methods guided by different learning theories. This chapter illustrates how learning theories can guide the development of course curriculum and teaching philosophy.

Nurse educators play a pivotal role in shaping the future healthcare workforce, but to do so effectively, they need to possess an understanding of the diverse attributes, such as age, gender, race, and social determinants of health, which influence student learning processes and outcomes. By tailoring teaching approaches to accommodate diversity, nurse educators can create an inclusive and supportive learning environment that nurtures the unique strengths of each student and contributes to the development of well-rounded and culturally sensitive nursing professionals. Chapter 4 examines how the diverse attributes of nursing students shape their learning and presents multiple strategies that nurse educators can use to meet the needs of diverse learners.

Chapter 5 describes the teacher's role in developing a supportive learning environment and in using a variety of teaching methods, with guidance for selecting methods to fit the intended learning outcomes, learner characteristics, and available resources. This chapter describes teaching methods for use in nursing education. Teaching methods are considered in relation to supporting learner development in the cognitive, affective, and psychomotor learning domains. Strategies are described for incorporating active learning and for promoting critical thinking.

Nursing faculty are expected to possess knowledge not only of theory, practice, and teaching but also of ethical, legal, and social issues within academic settings. Chapter 6 addresses the challenges facing higher education, with a specific focus on nurse educators, administrators, and their students. It assists nursing faculty and administrators in learning strategies to prevent academic misconduct and use social media appropriately. The chapter also discusses the importance of addressing interpersonal incivility, conflicts of interest, and adhering to academic policies within academic settings. Emphasizing a practical approach, this chapter incorporates case studies to illustrate the identification and management of ethical, legal, and social dilemmas prevalent in academic nursing today.

The rapid advances and constant pace of change in technology create challenges and opportunities for teaching and learning. Successful integration of technology in the nursing curriculum requires new competencies for the teacher as the technology continues to evolve. Chapter 7 focuses on technology integration that supports achievement of learning outcomes with attention to curriculum and classroom alignment. The chapter guides nurse educators in exploring and embracing technology tools, such as artificial intelligence, that support good teaching practices.

Teaching online is not the same as teaching in a classroom. Chapter 8 focuses on the differences between teaching in the traditional classroom and teaching online. The roles of the facilitator and the student are discussed in relation to pedagogy, course content, teaching strategies including cybercivility and cyberethics. This chapter also addresses reconceptualizing and designing online learning environments, interacting online, and using technology to teach and learn.

Traditionally, simulations have been used to provide opportunities for learners to practice patient care in a safe environment before going into the clinical setting. However, in the current environment of increasing patient acuity and limited clinical placements, simulation serves a broader role as an adjunct or replacement for traditional clinical hours and as an environment to assess learner competency. Chapter 9 provides an overview of types of clinical simulations in nursing including advances in augmented reality, virtual reality, and immersive virtual reality. The chapter presents implementation of simulations into a nursing curriculum, debriefing models, and evaluation processes to use when developing and implementing clinical simulations. Finally, it highlights the evidence regarding the use of clinical simulations and corresponding advances in regulation and credentialing.

Students' clinical practice in a nursing program is a cornerstone of nursing education. Students gain hands-on experience in real-world healthcare environments where they apply theory to practice and learn professional norms, values, and ethical standards by interacting with patients, families, healthcare teams, and educators. Principles of clinical teaching and various models of clinical teaching are addressed in Chapter 10. The clinical teaching process, including learner needs assessments and outcomes, planning of clinical activities, faculty and student organization, site visits, and the effective use of feedback are described. Challenges in clinical teaching are included along with strategies to mitigate these challenges. Specific attention is paid to considerations when working with nurse practitioner and other advanced practice students.

There is growing evidence to support interprofessional education (IPE) as an essential pedagogy to improve team-based collaborative practice. Over the last decade, many universities have integrated IPE competencies into the curriculum.

Most health professions accrediting bodies, including all three in nursing, advance standards that mandate incorporation of collaborative team-based competencies as part of the program of study. Chapter 11 explores the content, pedagogical theories, and processes for weaving IPE and collaborative learning into nursing curricula. Foundational frameworks are provided, along with examination of in-person and virtual didactic, simulation, and clinical experiences that promote collaborative practice capabilities across the continuum of care.

Academic–practice partnerships exist at several levels to prepare the nursing workforce to meet nursing practice realities and to address contemporary healthcare challenges. Chapter 12 provides guidelines for establishing meaningful partnerships across institutions and describes the roles and responsibilities of nurse educators in collaboration with practice partners in establishing and sustaining effective partnerships. Specific examples are provided to illustrate concepts and strategies to improve the educational preparation of nurses and ultimately the quality and safety of patient care. Different models of clinical training within academic–practice partnerships are described including faculty practice models.

National nursing organizations are calling for and supporting the transition of nursing education to a competency-based framework to better prepare the nursing workforce and promote practice-readiness. The transition to competency-based education (CBE) is challenging for faculty as the focus of nursing education has been traditionally on content and knowledge development. With CBE, the focus is on the outputs of education demonstrated by the learner as competencies. Chapter 13 explains CBE, compares CBE principles with traditional teaching and learning structures, uses the American Association of Colleges of Nursing *Essentials* as a framework for designing CBE and assessment, and presents a wealth of strategies for implementing competency-focused teaching and assessment.

It is vital that nurse educators take into account the context in which teaching takes place. Often, both new and experienced teachers focus on the specific content of the classes they teach and lose sight of the outcomes and how they relate to the overall program. Chapter 14 describes the components and processes for curriculum development or revision in schools of nursing and for programs related to professional education in healthcare settings; reviews the factors that influence educational programs and curricula; and provides educators with guidelines for collecting and analyzing data to make informed decisions about the curriculum. This chapter also provides an example of course design based on the framework of using backward design.

Through the process of assessment, the educator collects information about student learning and performance. Assessment reveals gaps in learning and performance and the need for further instruction, and provides the data on which the grade is based. Chapter 15 explains assessment, evaluation, and grading in nursing education. The chapter compares formative and summative evaluation, norm- and criterion-referenced interpretations of data, and assessing competencies. Methods are described for assessing learning and performance, with examples of these methods.

A test is a measurement instrument designed to assess learners' knowledge and cognitive abilities. Like every measurement instrument, a test must produce relevant and consistent results to form the basis for sound inferences about what learners know and can do. Good planning, careful test construction, proper administration, accurate scoring, and sound interpretation of scores are essential for producing useful test results. Chapter 16 describes the process of planning, constructing, administering, scoring, and analyzing tests and items. Different types of test items are presented with examples: true–false, matching, multiple-choice, multiple-response, matrix, drop-down, drag-and-drop, highlight, short answer, essay, context dependent item sets, case studies, and stand alone (bow-tie and trend). The chapter also discusses the Next Generation NCLEX® and explains test and item analysis.

As students learn about nursing, they develop their knowledge base, higher level thinking skills, and a wide range of competencies essential for patient care. Clinical nurse educators and preceptors guide student learning in the clinical setting and evaluate their performance in practice. Chapter 17 describes the clinical evaluation process; the importance of giving prompt, specific, and instructional feedback to students as they are learning; principles that are important when observing and rating performance; and grading clinical practice.

Program evaluation provides data to judge the quality of a nursing program and evidence on its outcomes. Through program evaluation, faculty, administrators, and other stakeholders collect the data needed to make informed decisions and determine the effectiveness of the program in meeting its goals and achieving important outcomes. Chapter 18 describes program evaluation in nursing and the development of a systematic program evaluation plan for a school of nursing. Discussion is included on accreditation of nursing programs, the three accrediting agencies in nursing education, types of and standards for accreditation, and student evaluation of courses and teachers.

Evidence-based teaching is the use of research findings and other evidence to guide educational decisions and practices. Available evidence should be used when developing the curriculum and courses, selecting teaching methods and approaches to use with students, and planning learning activities for students. Chapter 19 describes evidence-based teaching in nursing, the need for more rigorous research in nursing education, and a process for engaging in evidence-based teaching.

The role of the nurse educator includes more than teaching, assessing learning, and developing courses: It also includes scholarship and contributing to the development of nursing education as a science. Scholars in nursing education question and search for new ideas; they debate and think beyond how it has always been done. For the teacher's work to be considered as scholarship, it needs to be public, peer-reviewed, and critiqued, and shared with others so they can build on that work. Chapter 20 examines scholarship in nursing education and developing one's role as a scholar. Given the importance of dissemination to scholarship, the chapter includes a description of the process of writing for publication and other strategies for dissemination.

Nurse educators engage in service and leadership activities to develop a scholarly persona and influence learners, colleagues, and the nursing profession. Chapter 21, a new chapter in this edition, discusses the professional development of the nurse educator to promote learner success. It emphasizes nurse educator mentorship and explores various opportunities for educators to actively engage in service activities within their educational institutions and the broader community. This includes active participation in committees, professional organizations, and community initiatives that significantly contribute to the advancement of nursing education. This chapter also addresses the role of the nurse educator as a leader, the effective advisement of learners, and strategies for fostering success, addressing challenges, and promoting personal and professional growth of students.

Nurse educators employed in clinical practice settings, such as hospitals and healthcare systems, are referred to as nursing professional development (NPD) practitioners. These nurse educators help employees to become and remain competent in their roles. Similar to academic educators, NPD practitioners follow a set of core competencies. Their targeted learners vary depending on their role, but most often are nursing professionals. Chapter 22 describes the role and responsibilities of NPD practitioners, their scope and standards of practice, the importance of their role in clinical practice settings, and suggested pathways to prepare for, transition to, and develop in the NPD practitioner role.

In addition to this book, we have provided Instructor Resources that include a sample course syllabus; chapter-based PowerPoint presentations; and ready-to-use modules for an online course (with chapter summaries, student learning activities, discussion forum questions, online resources, and assessment strategies). Our editor at Springer Publishing, Joseph Morita, deserves a special acknowledgment for his continued support, enthusiasm, and commitment to nursing education.

Jennie C. De Gagne
Marilyn H. Oermann

Instructor Resources

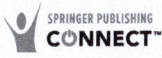 A robust set of instructor resources designed to supplement this text is located at http://connect.springerpub.com/content/book/978-0-8261-8892-2. Qualifying instructors may request access by emailing **textbook@springerpub.com**.

Available resources include:
- LMS Common Cartridge—All Instructor Resources
- PowerPoint Presentations for Lecture
- Instructor Manual:
  - Each of 22 Modules Include:
    - Chapter Summaries
    - Student Learning Activities
    - Discussion Questions
    - Online Resources
    - Assessment Strategies
  - Sample Course Syllabus
- Mapping to AACN Essentials: Core Competencies for Professional Nursing Education
- Transition Guide: Third Edition to Fourth Edition

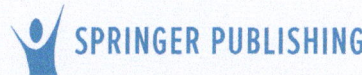

Visit https://connect.springerpub.com/ and look for the "**Show Supplementary**" button on the **book homepage**.

Teaching in Nursing and Role of the Educator

The Complete Guide to Best Practice in Teaching, Evaluation, and Curriculum Development

Nursing Education: Roles of Teacher   I

Role of the Nurse Educator

Marilyn H. Oermann

OBJECTIVES

1. Describe the roles and responsibilities of nurse educators in academic and healthcare settings
2. Compare educational requirements for nurse educators in different employment settings
3. Describe the competencies of nurse educators for effective teaching

INTRODUCTION

Many reports have highlighted the need for more nurse educators. Nurse educators teach in academic institutions and in a variety of healthcare agencies. They educate nursing students at all levels, from certified nursing assistants (CNAs) to doctorally prepared current and future nurse educators, clinicians, and researchers. Nursing professional development practitioners teach in healthcare settings and are responsible for providing nurses and other healthcare professionals with orientation and continuing education and training. This chapter describes the role of the nurse educator, educational preparation, nurse educator competencies and responsibilities, and certification.

TRENDS SUPPORTING CAREERS IN NURSING EDUCATION

Nursing shortages are cyclical and affected by economic conditions, population growth, the aging of the population, retirement of nurses, and other factors. In some healthcare settings and geographic regions, there is a high turnover of nurses, which adds to the shortage. The U.S. Department of Labor (2023) projects a 6% growth of RNs through 2032, but it is not enough to meet the need for nurses, particularly with older nurses retiring. At the national level, shortages are projected for RNs and LPN/LVNs through 2036. The Health Resources and Services Administration (HRSA) estimates that the demand for RNs in 2036 will exceed supply by 9%, a shortage of 337,970 full-time equivalent RNs (U.S. Department of Health and Human Services [DHHS], HRSA, 2024a). Although the number of nurses younger than 30 has increased, the mean age of RNs is 47.9 years (DHHS, HRSA, 2024b). About one third (34%) of RNs are over 55 years old: The retirement of these nurses will not only result in the loss of experienced RNs in the workforce but also will have an impact on the supply of nurses in future years.

To maintain an adequate supply of nurses, schools of nursing need qualified faculty to teach those students. One current issue, which is projected to worsen in future years, is the aging of the nursing faculty workforce. The average ages of doctorally prepared nurse faculty were 62.5 years, professor rank; 56.7 years, associate professor; and 50.6 years, assistant professor. Nurse faculty with master's degrees ranged from an average age of 55.0 years (professor) to 48.6 years (assistant professor; American Association of Colleges of Nursing [AACN], 2022). Retirements of these faculty combined with a nurse faculty shortage will continue to have a significant impact on schools of nursing. Thousands of qualified applicants to nursing programs are turned away each year because of a lack of faculty, classroom space, funding to hire more educators, and clinical sites. However, one positive sign in the nurse faculty shortage has been an increase in the recruitment of younger nurses into faculty positions. Fang et al. (2024) documented an increase in the number of younger nurses with a DNP degree entering academia and recommended schools implement innovative strategies to mentor these new educators.

Nursing faculty are not the only educators needed to meet the demands of the healthcare system. Nursing professional development practitioners, who provide training and education for nurses and other providers in healthcare settings, are also vital. A rapidly changing healthcare system requires those in the workforce to keep abreast of new knowledge and skills, changing standards of practice, technologies, and regulatory requirements. Educators in healthcare settings play a key role in helping nursing and other staff members keep up to date with these changes. Chapter 22 explores the role of the nurse educator in professional development.

Prospects of long-term employment for nurse educators across all education and practice settings are excellent. By choosing a career as a nurse educator, one has the opportunity to teach learners across varied types of nursing programs from short-term training for nursing assistants to teaching students at the doctoral level, orienting and onboarding new nurses, and keeping nurses and other healthcare providers up to date and competent for care of patients.

EDUCATIONAL PREPARATION FOR ACADEMIC EMPLOYMENT

In the United States, preparation as an RN occurs in community colleges at the associate degree level, in bachelor's and direct entry master's programs in colleges and universities, and in a small number of diploma programs in hospitals. RNs from these programs work across a range of healthcare agencies. Increasingly, however, healthcare systems are requiring their staff to be baccalaureate prepared or working on a bachelor of science in nursing (BSN) degree. The Institute of Medicine's (IOM) *Future of Nursing* report had called for 80% of the nursing workforce to be prepared at the baccalaureate degree level or higher by the year 2020 (IOM, 2011). Although this goal was not met, barriers for achieving a BSN are being removed, and nurses with associate degrees are returning to school in greater numbers than in years past.

Most practical nursing programs, referred to as vocational nursing programs in a few states, and some CNA programs take place in community colleges. Many of these occur in career ladder education programs leading to an associate degree in nursing.

Academic credentials for nurse educators employed in postsecondary institutions are set by state boards of nursing and accreditation agencies. For example, the Commission on Collegiate Nursing Education (CCNE), an agency that accredits baccalaureate and higher degree nursing programs, requires that faculty are academically prepared for the courses and areas in which they teach (CCNE, 2018, 2023). The Accreditation Commission for Education in Nursing (ACEN) provides accreditation for all levels of nursing education programs, including doctor of nursing practice (DNP), master's/postmaster's certificate, baccalaureate, associate, diploma, and practical nursing programs. The 2023 accreditation standards indicate that nursing faculty should have the educational qualifications and experience required by the governing organization and regulatory agencies, should be experientially qualified for their roles and responsibilities, and should be sufficient in number (ACEN, 2023). The National League for Nursing (NLN) Commission for Nursing Education Accreditation (CNEA), the third accrediting agency in nursing education, indicates that nursing faculty should be qualified by education, professional credentials, and experience for their assigned teaching responsibilities and meet qualifications of the state, other relevant regulatory agencies, and professional nursing organizations (NLN CNEA, 2021).

Faculty Ranks

Ranks or academic titles of faculty positions include instructor, assistant professor, associate professor, and professor. Beginning faculty are hired as instructors or assistant professors depending on the institution. As faculty meet the criteria of the school of nursing for promotion to a higher rank, they progress in the order seen in Figure 1.1. If faculty are in the tenure track, promotion to associate professor may include tenure. However, in some schools, faculty can be promoted first to associate professor without tenure and then to associate professor with tenure. The highest academic rank is professor. For nontenure tracks, faculty have the same academic titles and progression.

Tenure and Nontenure Tracks

Schools of nursing and universities generally have two academic tracks: tenure track and nontenure track. Each of these tracks has its own expectations for faculty performance and criteria for promotion.

Tenure track positions provide job security. In the tenure track, once a faculty member meets certain requirements, they are granted tenure, which is a permanent position in the school and college or university. Tenured faculty have lifetime appointments; however, tenure can be revoked for financial exigencies (a financial crisis that may result in the termination of tenured faculty) and for ethical reasons. In schools of nursing with a research mission, tenure track faculty are hired to conduct research and engage in scholarship. They also teach students and participate in service, but conducting research, obtaining grants, and publishing are of prime importance. In schools with a research mission, appointment to the tenure track generally requires a PhD in nursing. PhD in nursing programs prepare nurses as scientists with the knowledge and competencies to conduct research.

Most colleges and universities also have clinical or teaching tracks, which are nontenure tracks and have different requirements for faculty. With nontenure tracks, faculty may have yearly or multiyear contracts for employment versus a permanent

Instructor ⟹ Assistant Professor ⟹ Associate Professor ⟹ Professor

Figure 1.1 Faculty ranks.

position that accompanies tenure. Typically, their role focuses on teaching, clinical practice, and service, with some scholarship.

Colleges and universities that do not have research missions will have tenure track appointments that focus on teaching, clinical practice, and service. Although faculty also may have some requirements for scholarship, this generally includes conducting evaluations of teaching innovations, developing new guidelines for practice, presenting at conferences or publishing articles and chapters, among others. In these schools, faculty can be employed in the tenure track with PhDs, DNPs, EdDs, and other degrees. The focus is not on research, and faculty do not need to be prepared as nurse scientists. Table 1.1 compares tenure and nontenure tracks.

TABLE 1.1 COMPARISON OF TENURE AND NONTENURE TRACKS FOR FACULTY

Tenure	Nontenure
Permanent position awarded after probationary period	Not permanent, by contract
Job security	No job security, contract might not be renewed Continued employment based on teaching needs in the school; affected by low enrollment in courses or program and institution's financial situation
Probationary period (usually 7 or 10 years depending on the university). Includes pretenure review at 3 or 5 years	Annual or multiyear (e.g., 3 to 5 year) contracts
Protects academic freedom (faculty can share own views and opinions and can engage in intellectual debate with students without fear of retaliation)	No protection of academic freedom
Need to demonstrate contributions to research, teaching, and service	Need to demonstrate contributions to teaching and service, with some scholarship
Criteria for tenure (and promotion), policies, and procedures determined by school of nursing consistent with university/college guidelines	Criteria for nontenure reappointments (and promotion), policies, and procedures determined by school of nursing consistent with university/college guidelines
Time allotted in workload for research	No time allotted for research Higher teaching load than tenure track
Number of tenure track positions is limited	Number of nontenure track positions fluctuates based on teaching needs of school

Types of Appointments and Educational Credentials

The educational degrees and credentials needed for employment as faculty members in schools of nursing vary widely based on the mission of the school and track (tenure vs. nontenure). Colleges and universities are classified based on their research activities and missions by the Carnegie Classification of Institutions of Higher Education® (American Council on Education, 2024). There are six classifications defined in Table 1.2.

TABLE 1.2 CARNEGIE CLASSIFICATION OF INSTITUTIONS OF HIGHER EDUCATION®

Classification	Definition
Doctoral Universities: - R1: Doctoral Universities– Very high research activity - R2: Doctoral Universities– High research activity - D/PU: Doctoral/Professional Universities	Institutions that awarded at least 20 research/scholarship doctoral degrees or fewer than 20 doctoral degrees but awarded 30 or more professional practice doctoral degrees in at least 2 programs. R1 and R2 also had at least $5 million in total research expenditures.
Master's Colleges and Universities: - M1: Master's Colleges and Universities – Larger programs - M2: Master's Colleges and Universities – Medium programs - M3: Master's Colleges and Universities – Small programs	Institutions that awarded at least 50 master's degrees and fewer than 20 doctoral degrees.
Baccalaureate Colleges: - Arts and Science Focused - Diverse Fields	Institutions with 50 percent of degrees that are baccalaureate or higher and fewer than 50 master's or 20 doctoral degrees.
Baccalaureate/Associate Colleges: - Mixed Baccalaureate/ Associate Colleges - Associate Dominant	4-year colleges that award at least one baccalaureate degree program and more than 50 percent of associate degrees and other combinations of both baccalaureate and associate degrees.
Associates Colleges	Institutions at which the highest level of degree is an associate degree. Institutions are sorted into nine categories based on disciplinary focus (transfer, career and technical or mixed) and dominant student type (traditional, nontraditional, or mixed).

(continued)

TABLE 1.2 CARNEGIE CLASSIFICATION OF INSTITUTIONS OF HIGHER EDUCATION® *(continued)*

Classification	Definition
Special Focus Institutions	Institutions where a high concentration of degrees is in a single field or set of related fields (e.g., health professions).

Source: American Council on Education. (2024). Carnegie Classification of Institutions of Higher Education®. https://carnegieclassifications.acenet.edu/carnegie-classification/classification-methodology/basic-classification/

Carnegie Classification of Institutions of Higher Education® is licensed under a Creative Commons Attribution-NonCommercial-ShareAlike 4.0 International License. Based on a work at https://carnegieclassifications.acenet.edu

Full- or part-time clinical teaching positions require a BSN or master's degree depending on the nursing program. In associate degree and LPN programs, a BSN may be needed. Clinical teaching positions in a baccalaureate program typically require a master of science in nursing (MSN) or other master's in nursing degree. When teaching in an advanced practice nursing program, there are additional requirements to be met; for example, the faculty member needs to be doctorally prepared, currently licensed or authorized to practice, and nationally board certified as a nurse practitioner in the population focus of the major (National Task Force, 2022). The type of degree required for a faculty position varies across schools of nursing because of differences in the missions of the schools and requirements for faculty positions.

When considering a faculty position, it is important to clarify the track (tenure versus nontenure) and the expectations for faculty in that track. By clarifying these criteria, one can better match career goals to institutional expectations. Table 1.3 summarizes the types of academic appointments and the educational preparation required.

EDUCATIONAL PREPARATION FOR EMPLOYMENT IN HEALTHCARE SETTINGS

Educators in nursing professional development teach in acute care, long-term care, and community settings. Their role is to facilitate the professional development and growth of nurses and other healthcare personnel (Harper & Maloney, 2022). Most of these positions require a master's degree. The role and responsibilities of the nurse educator in professional development and their educational preparation are described in Chapter 22.

PREPARATION FOR TEACHING

Nurses need to be prepared for their role as educator, regardless of the type of program in which they are teaching (Hansbrough et al., 2023; Oermann, 2017; Oermann & Kardong-Edgren, 2018; Young-Brice et al., 2022). This preparation can be gained

TABLE 1.3 EDUCATIONAL REQUIREMENTS FOR EMPLOYMENT AS A NURSE EDUCATOR

Employment Setting	Education Required
Hospitals and other healthcare agencies	BSN or MSN
Community colleges: CNA and practical nursing programs	BSN or MSN
Community colleges: Associate degree programs	BSN or MSN for clinical teaching; MSN for teaching in the classroom or online (doctoral degree may be preferred in some schools)
Colleges and universities: Baccalaureate and master's programs	MSN for clinical teaching Doctoral for classroom, online
Colleges and universities: Doctoral programs	Doctoral degree

CNA, certified nursing assistant.

by completing a master's program or track in nursing education, a postmaster's certificate program in nursing education, education courses, or through continuing education. In some DNP and PhD programs, students have an option to take nursing education courses as electives. There are varied strategies to gain essential knowledge and competencies to transition into a faculty role, but some type of preparation is essential.

RESPONSIBILITIES OF NURSE EDUCATORS

Responsibilities of nurse educators differ according to type of institution. Prior to deciding on a career in nursing education, job shadowing a nurse faculty member or an educator in a clinical setting can provide a realistic view of the role and responsibilities.

In academic institutions, faculty teach, conduct research (depending on the mission of the school) or have some form of scholarly activity, and perform service to the institution and the profession. How one's overall duties are allotted depends on the institutional type. Nurse educators who are employed in community colleges will spend most of their time teaching in the classroom, simulation and skills laboratories, and clinical setting, with some time allotted for service and scholarship. Faculty in prelicensure and graduate programs in colleges and universities will also teach, but will have greater expectations for scholarly productivity, including supporting research through funded grants if in a tenure track position in a school with a research mission. Faculty with doctoral degrees in nontenure-track positions will be expected to engage in some scholarly activities in most schools of nursing.

Across all schools of nursing, an expectation of nurse faculty is that they participate in service—for example, as a member of committees—to the school of nursing, college or university, and nursing profession.

When considering employment in an academic setting, one should be clear about the job expectations. Is the position tenure track, or with a renewable yearly or multiyear contract? If the position is tenure track, what are the responsibilities for research and scholarship, teaching, and service? If the position is full time, but on the clinical or teaching track (nontenure), what kind of scholarship is expected? What are the teaching and service expectations?

Teaching Responsibilities

Teaching involves more than transmitting knowledge through lectures and guiding students in simulation and clinical practice. Faculty must have evidence-based knowledge of student learning styles or preferences, teaching methods, and methods for assessing and evaluating student learning and performance. Facilitating students' application of theory to practice is key. Some nursing education programs employ full-time clinical faculty whose primary role is teaching in the clinical setting and sometimes also in the simulation and skills laboratories. All full- and part-time nurse educators teaching in those settings need to have knowledge of the curriculum, expected learning outcomes, and competencies to be developed by students.

Aside from teaching, faculty also have the responsibility of formulating a curriculum that not only meets contemporary standards of practice, but also prepares students for future nursing roles. A curriculum is not static, but constantly needs revision to meet the needs of patients and populations and changes in healthcare. Providing leadership and promoting curriculum change involves ensuring that the curriculum is based on the most current educational standards and competencies, including the core competencies needed by all healthcare professionals:

- Patient-centered care
- Teamwork and collaboration
- Evidence-based practice
- Quality improvement
- Safety
- Informatics (Quality and Safety Education for Nurses [QSEN], 2022)

Committee work is essential to the process of developing and revising the curriculum, including leading committees and task forces in the nursing program and sometimes in the larger institution to develop and shepherd the revised curriculum through the approval process. Nurse educators have an important role in curriculum development and revision in the school of nursing and carrying out other activities to provide a quality education for students. Educators develop innovative learning activities for students, assessment strategies, and tests in their courses; serve on committees to make decisions about admissions and progression in the nursing program; evaluate their courses and nursing program; advise students and support them in their education; and serve in other roles that are essential to offering a quality educational experience for students.

Scholarship Responsibilities

Scholarship includes research, obtaining grant funding, publishing in peer-reviewed journals, and presenting at professional conferences, but scholarship is more than these traditional research activities. Evaluations of educational innovations and programs and their impact on student learning, reviews of research to provide evidence to guide teaching, application of theories to generate new approaches to teaching, development and evaluation of educational innovations and new initiatives, and implementation of educational evidence and studies of the implementation process are all forms of scholarship in nursing education (Oermann, 2017). For these types of activities to be considered as scholarship, however, they need to be disseminated for others to critique. This dissemination also is critical because sharing innovations and outcomes spreads new ideas and builds evidence for teaching in nursing. Scholarship is a "spirit of inquiry"—reflecting on teaching practices, asking if there are better ways of helping students learn, and searching for evidence to improve teaching. A spirit of inquiry involves the ability to search the literature for evidence and work with colleagues to understand their educational practices in the classroom, online environment, and clinical setting. Becoming a scholar in nursing education is described in Chapter 20.

Boyer's seminal work, *Scholarship Reconsidered: Priorities of the Professoriate*, broadened the definition of scholarship from only viewing scholarship as generating new knowledge to also include the scholarship of teaching (Boyer, 1990). This original work included the scholarship of discovery, integration, application, and teaching. Later, Boyer added the scholarship of engagement, which includes the work of nursing faculty in solving community-based problems, engaging with the community, and developing partnerships that lead to improved health (Boyer, 1996). Table 1.4 lists the forms of scholarship and their definitions, with examples of each form of scholarship.

Service Responsibilities

The role of nurse educators in providing service to the school of nursing is critical to the work and functioning of the school. Full-time nursing faculty are expected to participate in committees in the nursing program and the larger institution. Committees include those concerned with faculty issues; student admission, progression, and retention issues; curriculum development; and program evaluation, among others.

Professional service includes leadership in professional nursing and nursing education organizations and other activities such as reviewing manuscripts for journals. Other forms of professional service may include partnerships with healthcare settings and in the community. Faculty may be called on to participate in research and quality improvement studies in the healthcare system.

TABLE 1.4 SUMMARY OF BOYER'S TYPES OF SCHOLARSHIP

Type of Scholarship	Definition	Evidence
Scholarship of Discovery	Conducting original research to gain knowledge about nursing	Grants, peer-reviewed publications, presentations
Scholarship of Integration	Syntheses of research done by others, making connections across disciplines	Systematic, integrative, scoping, narrative, and other types of reviews of research; peer-reviewed publications of those reviews; articles, books, other products resulting from interprofessional activities
Scholarship of Application	Development of clinical knowledge, applying evidence to practice to solve clinical problems, service to profession, and scholarship of engagement	Consultations, outcomes of clinical practice, presentations and publications about practice, practice partnerships
Scholarship of Teaching	Inquiry that focuses on learning and teaching, developing and evaluating educational innovations, new approaches to teaching, and courses	Peer-reviewed publications, presentations about educational innovations, chapters, books

Source: Boyer, E. L. (1990). *Scholarship reconsidered: Priorities of the professoriate.* The Carnegie Foundation for the Advancement of Teaching; Oermann, M. H. (2014). Defining and assessing the scholarship of teaching in nursing. *Journal of Professional Nursing, 30*(5), 370–375. https://doi.org/10.1016/j.profnurs.2014.03.001

One of the competencies of nurse educators is functioning as a change agent and leader. This leadership role is critical to improve quality and advance nursing and nursing education. Through their leadership, nurse educators also contribute to shaping policies and legislation that affect nurses and patient care. As leaders, nurse educators motivate and support others to achieve common goals.

Leaders in academic settings are role models for students and colleagues. They strive to promote a positive and supportive work environment in the school—a healthy work environment for faculty, students, staff, and others. A healthy work environment supports and empowers others; is characterized by collaborative and collegial relationships and respect for others and their ideas; and is a caring environment, leading to higher levels of satisfaction among faculty and others in the school (Saunders et al., 2021).

PROFESSIONAL DEVELOPMENT PRACTITIONERS

Educators in nursing professional development also have teaching, scholarship, and service responsibilities. Although typically the curriculum process is thought of as occurring in the academic setting, educators in healthcare settings formulate, implement, and evaluate various curricula. For example, these educators design and evaluate nurse residency and orientation programs, as well as programs for ensuring continuing competency of staff. The educator in this setting has an important role in providing interprofessional education. Knowledge of standards of practice, healthcare trends, and competencies to be developed by staff are critical for practice in nursing professional development. These educators also have an important role in promoting evidence-based practice in their setting and preparing nurses to access and use evidence in their patient care.

Although scholarship and research in nursing are often thought of as responsibilities of only nursing faculty, educators in nursing professional development also participate in and facilitate scholarly activities. These include conducting clinical research and other studies that generate new knowledge, developing and evaluating practice and educational innovations, and promoting evidence-based practice and quality improvement. Nursing professional development practitioners play a key role in creating programs that help nurses and others to engage in these scholarly activities.

Educators in nursing professional development are change agents and leaders in their clinical setting and the larger healthcare delivery system. Through their education of nurses and other healthcare providers and their leadership, they work toward improving the quality and safety of care. Nurses in professional development may provide education for the community and promote increased access to healthcare through their community and professional service efforts. They also may assume a leadership role in a professional organization. Nursing professional development practitioners are guided by their standards for practice (Harper & Maloney, 2022). The role of the educator in nursing professional development is discussed in depth in Chapter 22.

BALANCING ROLE RESPONSIBILITIES

Satisfaction in one's role as a faculty member and nurse educator in other settings depends on balancing all dimensions of the role. Whereas nursing professional development practitioners have some autonomy in how to organize responsibilities, they generally have more regular work hours as compared to faculty. Aside from assigned times for teaching and posted office hours, most nurse educators in schools of nursing can decide when and where work is done. They can typically prepare classes, evaluate assignments, and complete scholarship activities from home. Many nursing faculty teach online courses, which provides for flexibility in preparing classes and interacting with students.

Clinical expertise is essential for teaching clinical courses in nursing programs, and educators need to be up to date on technologies, new medications and treatments, and changes in practice. For faculty teaching in nurse practitioner and other advanced practice nursing programs, maintaining clinical expertise is critical for effectiveness as an educator. In some schools of nursing, faculty practice as part of their faculty role; in other schools they might maintain a clinical practice in addition to their role as a full-time faculty member. When faculty teach full time in a school of nursing and in addition practice as a clinician, even if part time, they are at risk for burnout. As new nurse educators plan their career trajectory, they should consider the dimensions of their role and priorities. Securing a faculty position in which clinical practice can be part of that full-time role might be preferable to teaching full time and practicing on a part-time basis. Not taking on too many role responsibilities is important not only for faculty but also for clinicians who teach in addition to their clinical practice.

One particular challenge for those teaching in schools of nursing is salary levels. Nurses in practice have higher salaries than faculty in schools of nursing. Some faculty members who teach 9 or 10 months during the academic year practice over the summer to keep current in their clinical skills and earn extra income.

FACULTY DEVELOPMENT

As clinicians transition to the nurse educator role, they need to be well oriented to the position and supported as they move into their new role. Chapter 2 examines this transition process from clinician to educator. All full- and part-time faculty and nurse educators in other settings need continuing education to maintain their competency as educators and keep up to date with research findings and other evidence to guide their teaching. Although continuing education related to one's clinical specialty is important, so too is continuing education related to the educator competencies. Organizations such as the NLN, AACN, Organization for Associate Degree Nursing, and Association for Nursing Professional Development offer conferences and webinars for faculty and educators in other settings. Like any specialty, nursing education changes, and attending professional meetings and reading the literature help educators stay abreast of new trends and best practices. Appendix A provides a list of nursing and higher education organizations that provide continuing education and offer other resources for nurse educators to keep current in their role.

CERTIFICATION FOR NURSE EDUCATORS

As nurse educators develop their knowledge and expertise, they can pursue certification as a nurse educator. This certification, offered by the NLN, provides a way for educators to demonstrate their specialized knowledge, skills, and expertise and also contributes to their professional and career development (NLN, 2024). There are three certifications for nurse educators: Certified Nurse Educator (CNE®), Certified Academic Clinical Nurse Educator (CNE®cl), and Certified Novice Nurse Educator (CNE®n).

Eligibility for initial certification as a CNE includes two options. In addition to licensure, one option requires the educator to have a master's or doctoral degree in nursing with a major emphasis in nursing education, a postmaster's certificate in nursing education, or nine or more credits of graduate-level education courses. The second option is for nurse educators who have a master's or doctoral degree in nursing in a role other than nursing education and at least 2 years of employment in an academic nursing program within the last 5 years (NLN, 2023b).

Certification is also available for clinical nurse educators who teach nursing students as part of an academic program and are guided by faculty from the program. Eligibility for certification as a CNEcl, is (a) licensure, a graduate degree with a focus in nursing education, and 3 years of practice experience, or (b) licensure, a baccalaureate degree or higher in nursing, 3 years of practice experience, and 2 years of teaching experience in an academic nursing program within the last 5 years (NLN, 2023a).

The third certification as a CNEn validates the knowledge of nurse educators who have less than 3 years of teaching experience. Eligibility for this certification includes licensure; a graduate degree in nursing with a major in nursing education, a postmaster's certificate in nursing education, nine or more credits of graduate-level education courses, or a postbaccalaureate certificate in nursing education; and being within the first 3 years of practice as an academic nurse educator (NLN, 2023c).

For all of these certifications, nurse educators need to pass an examination validating their knowledge. Exhibit 1.1 lists the percent of items on the test for each of the competency areas assessed on these examinations.

EXHIBIT 1.1 Competency Areas and Percent of Test Items

Certified Nurse Educator[a] (CNE®)
- Facilitate Learning, 47 items, 36%
- Facilitate Learner Development and Socialization, 18 items, 14%
- Use Assessment and Evaluation Strategies, 18 items, 14%
- Participate in Curriculum Design and Evaluation of Program Outcomes, 13 items, 10%
- Function as a Change Agent and Leader, 9 items, 7%
- Pursue Continuous Quality Improvement in the Academic Nurse Educator Role, 9 items, 7%
- Engage in Scholarship, 7 items, 5%
- Function within the Organizational Environment and Academic Community, 9 items, 7%

Certified Academic Clinical Nurse Educator (CNE®cl)
- Function Within the Education and Healthcare Environments, 15%
- Facilitate Learning in the Healthcare Environment, 26%
- Demonstrate Effective Interpersonal Communication and Collaborative Interprofessional Relationships, 15%
- Apply Clinical Expertise in the Healthcare Environment, 15%
- Facilitate Learner Development and Socialization, 13%
- Implement Effective Clinical Assessment and Evaluation Strategies, 16%

Certified Novice Nurse Educator (CNE®n)
- Facilitate Learning, 39%
- Facilitate Learner Development and Socialization, 11%
- Use Assessment and Evaluation Strategies, 15%
- Participate in Curriculum Design and Evaluation of Program Outcomes, 5%
- Function as a Change Agent and Leader, 7%
- Pursue Continuous Quality Improvement in the Role of Nurse Educator, 8%
- Engage in Scholarship, 4%
- Function within the Educational Environment, 11%

[a] Examination contains 150 items including 20 unscored items being pretested for future use.
Sources: National League for Nursing. (2023a). *Certified Academic Clinical Nurse Educator (CNE®cl) 2023 candidate handbook*. https://www.nln.org/awards-recognition/certification-for-nurse-educators-overview/cne-cl/Certification-for-Nurse-Educatorscnecl/cne-cl-handbook; National League for Nursing. (2023b). *Certified Nurse Educator (CNE®) 2023 candidate handbook.* https://www.nln.org/awards-recognition/cne/Certification-for-Nurse-Educatorscne/cne-handbook; National League for Nursing. (2023c). *Certified Nurse Educator Novice (CNE®n) 2023 candidate handbook*. https://www.nln.org/certification/Certification-for-Nurse-Educatorscne-n/cne-n-handbook

Nurse educators in professional development also can be certified. For this certification, through the American Nurses Credentialing Center (ANCC), nurses need licensure, to have a bachelor's or higher degree in nursing, to have at least 2 years full-time practice as a RN, to have a minimum of 2,000 hours of clinical practice in nursing professional development within the last 3 years, and to complete 30 hours of continuing education in nursing professional development within the last 3 years (ANCC, n.d.).

SUMMARY

Prospects of long-term employment for nurse educators across all education and practice settings are excellent. By choosing a career as a nurse educator, one has the opportunity to teach learners in varied types of nursing programs from short-term training for nursing assistants to teaching students at the prelicensure through the doctoral levels, orienting and onboarding new nurses, and keeping nurses and other healthcare providers up to date and competent for care of patients. Choosing a career as a nurse educator provides many rewards. Nurse educators can have a profound influence on how the current and next generation of nurses function within the healthcare system.

Academic credentials for nurse educators employed in postsecondary institutions are set by state boards of nursing and accreditation agencies. Standards related to faculty qualifications from each of the three accrediting agencies in nursing were described in this chapter. Ranks or academic titles of faculty positions include instructor, assistant professor, associate professor, and professor. As faculty meet the criteria of the school of nursing for promotion to a higher rank, they progress in rank in that order.

Schools of nursing and universities generally have two academic tracks: tenure track and nontenure track. Each of these tracks has its own expectations for faculty performance and criteria for promotion. These were examined in this chapter with a table comparing the two tracks.

The educational degrees and credentials needed for employment as faculty members in schools of nursing vary widely based on the mission of the school and track (tenure versus nontenure). The chapter examined these differences and also presented the Carnegie Classification of Institutions of Higher Education®. Regardless of the type of program in which nurses teach, they need to be prepared for their role as an educator. This preparation can be gained by completing a master's program or track in nursing education, a postmaster's certificate program in nursing education, education courses, or through continuing education. There are varied strategies to gain essential knowledge and competencies to transition into a faculty role, but some type of preparation is essential.

Responsibilities of nurse educators differ according to type of institution. In academic institutions, faculty teach, conduct research (depending on the mission of the school) or have some form of scholarly activity, and perform service to the institution and the profession. How one's overall duties are allotted depends on the institutional type. As nurse educators develop their knowledge and expertise, they can pursue certification as a nurse educator. This certification, offered by the NLN, provides a way for educators to demonstrate their specialized knowledge, skills, and expertise and also contributes to their career development. There are three certifications for nurse educators: CNE, CNEcl, and CNEn.

The nurse educator role is complex. Each succeeding chapter in this book presents an in-depth discussion of the specific role competencies that are necessary for functioning as a nurse educator across varied settings.

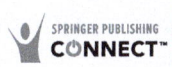

A robust set of instructor resources designed to supplement this text is located at http://connect.springerpub.com/content/book/978-0-8261-8892-2. Qualifying instructors may request access by emailing textbook@springerpub.com.

REFERENCES

Accreditation Commission for Education in Nursing. (2023). *ACEN standards and criteria. Standard 2 - Faculty.* https://resources.acenursing.org/space/SAC/1825603701/STANDARD+2+-+Faculty

American Association of Colleges of Nursing. (2022). *Fact sheet: Nursing faculty shortage.* https://www.aacnnursing.org/Portals/0/PDFs/Fact-Sheets/Faculty-Shortage-Factsheet.pdf

American Council on Education. (2024). *Carnegie Classification of Institutions of Higher Education®.* https://carnegieclassifications.acenet.edu/carnegie-classification/classification-methodology/basic-classification/

American Nurses Credentialing Center. (n.d.). *Nursing professional development certification (NPD-BC).* Retrieved March 25, 2024, from https://www.nursingworld.org/our-certifications/nursing-professional-development/

Boyer, E. L. (1990). *Scholarship reconsidered: Priorities of the professoriate.* The Carnegie Foundation for the Advancement of Teaching.

Boyer, E. L. (1996). The scholarship of engagement. *Journal of Public Service and Outreach, 1*(1), 11–20.

Commission on Collegiate Nursing Education. (2018). *Standards for accreditation of baccalaureate and graduate degree nursing programs.* https://www.aacnnursing.org/Portals/42/CCNE/PDF/Standards-Final-2018.pdf

Commission on Collegiate Nursing Education. (2023). *Standards for accreditation of baccalaureate and graduate nursing programs proposed revisions for public comment fall 2023.* https://www.aacnnursing.org/Portals/0/PDFs/CCNE/Clean-2018-Standards.pdf

Fang, D., Zangaro, G. A., & Kesten, K. (2024). Assessment of nursing faculty retirement projections. *Nursing Outlook, 72*(2), 102135. Advance online publication. https://doi.org/10.1016/j.outlook.2024.102135

Hansbrough, W., Dunker, K., Duprey, M., & Lawrence, A. (2023). Descriptive analysis of newly hired academic nurse educator onboarding practices. *Nurse Educator, 48*(4), 192–196. https://doi.org/10.1097/NNE.0000000000001402

Harper, M. G., & Maloney, P. (Eds.). (2022). *Nursing professional development: Scope and standards of practice* (4th ed.). Association for Nursing Professional Development.

Institute of Medicine. (2011). *The future of nursing: Leading change, advancing health.* National Academies Press.

National League for Nursing. (2023a). *Certified Academic Clinical Nurse Educator (CNE®cl) 2023 candidate handbook.* https://www.nln.org/awards-recognition/certification-for-nurse-educators-overview/cne-cl/Certification-for-Nurse-Educatorscnecl/cne-cl-handbook

National League for Nursing. (2023b). *Certified Nurse Educator (CNE®) 2023 candidate handbook.* https://www.nln.org/awards-recognition/cne/Certification-for-Nurse-Educatorscne/cne-handbook

National League for Nursing. (2023c). *Certified Nurse Educator Novice (CNE®n) 2023 candidate handbook.* https://www.nln.org/certification/Certification-for-Nurse-Educatorscne-n/cne-n-handbook

National League for Nursing. (2024). *Certification for nurse educators.* https://www.nln.org/awards-recognition/certification-for-nurse-educators-overview

National League for Nursing Commission for Nursing Education Accreditation. (2021). *Accreditation standards for nursing education programs.* https://irp.cdn-website.com/cc12ee87/files/uploaded/CNEA%20Standards%20October%202021-4b271cb2.pdf

National Task Force. (2022). *Standards for quality nurse practitioner education, A report of the national task force on quality nurse practitioner education, 6th Edition.* https://www.nonpf.org/page/NTFStandards

Oermann, M. H. (2017). Preparing nurse faculty: It's for everyone. *Nurse Educator, 42*(1), 1. https://doi.org/10.1097/NNE.0000000000000345

Oermann, M. H., & Kardong-Edgren, S. K. (2018). Changing the conversation about doctoral education in nursing: What about research in nursing education? *Nursing Outlook, 66*(6), 523–525. https://doi.org/10.1016/j.outlook.2018.10.001

Quality and Safety Education for Nurses Institute. (2022). *Competencies.* https://www.qsen.org/competencies

Saunders, J., Sridaromont, K., & Gallegos, B. (2021). Steps to establish a healthy work environment in an academic nursing setting. *Nurse Educator, 46*(1), 2–4. https://doi.org/10.1097/NNE.0000000000000829

U.S. Department of Labor. Bureau of Labor Statistics. (2023). *Occupational outlook handbook.* https://www.bls.gov/ooh/healthcare/registered-nurses.htm

U.S. Department of Health and Human Services, Health Resources and Services Administration. (2024a). *2022 National sample survey of Registered Nurses snapshot.* https://bhw.hrsa.gov/sites/default/files/bureau-health-workforce/Nurse-Survey-Fact-Sheet-2024.pdf

U.S. Department of Health and Human Services. Health Resources and Services Administration. (2024b). *National sample survey of Registered Nurses (NSSRN).* https://bhw.hrsa.gov/data-research/access-data-tools/national-sample-survey-registered-nurses

Young-Brice, A., Farrar-Stern, K., & Malin, M. (2022). Comprehensive onboarding and orientation to support newly hired faculty in a nursing program. *Nurse Educator, 47*(6), 347–351. https://doi.org/10.1097/NNE.0000000000001242

The Transition from Clinician to Educator

Anne M. Schoening and Lorraine M. Rusch

OBJECTIVES

1. Describe the role transition from clinician to novice nurse educator
2. Examine barriers and facilitators in the transition from clinician to educator
3. Identify evidence-based elements of new faculty orientation programs to assist in the transition from clinician to educator
4. Identify resources available for clinicians making the transition from clinician to educator

INTRODUCTION

The transition from bedside to classroom is rarely easy. Most novice nurse educators assume an academic or professional development role without formal preparation. While they may be expert clinicians, novice nurse educators often lack the foundational knowledge necessary for success in the nurse educator role. This chapter examines barriers and facilitators to the nurse educator transition (NET) process and provides resources to help novice educators gain competence in their new role.

HISTORICAL PERSPECTIVES

Preparing Nurse Educators

Decades ago, graduate nursing programs focused heavily on role preparation in nursing education or nursing administration; however, in the early 1970s, there was a call for graduate programs to focus on clinical specialization and advanced nursing practice (American Nurses' Association Commission on Nursing Education, 1969). This resulted in decreased enrollment in graduate programs to prepare nurse educators. By the 1990s, only 4% of nurses enrolled in master's programs were pursuing degrees that specifically prepared them for a nursing faculty role (National League for Nursing [NLN], 2002).

This trend continues today. Though doctoral preparation for advanced practice nurses with clinical expertise is critical, these programs rarely intentionally prepare graduates for a career in academia. Since 2007, doctor of nursing practice (DNP) programs, which are generally focused on clinical nursing for improving patient outcomes and translating research into practice, have expanded in scope and focus so rapidly that they now outnumber nursing PhD programs (American Association of Colleges of Nursing [AACN], 2023). A 2014 survey of nursing deans and department heads revealed that few newly hired DNP- and PhD-prepared faculty were adequately prepared for teaching in an academic setting (Agger et al., 2014). Later work by Dreifuerst et al. (2016) and McNelis et al. (2019) revealed that doctorally prepared nurse educators feel unprepared to teach and are dissatisfied with how their doctoral programs prepared them for the faculty role.

Although a degree in nursing education is not required to teach in an academic nursing program or in professional development, knowledge of principles of teaching and learning, assessment, curriculum design, and administrative issues is necessary for success in the role. The absence of formal preparation for teaching creates challenges for novice educators as they transition to new roles. Since 2002, the NLN has advocated for specialized preparation at the graduate level for the nurse educator role (NLN, 2017). The NLN's advocacy is consistent with the groundbreaking work from the Carnegie Foundation for the Advancement of Teaching, which suggested that graduate-level preparation is imperative to "better prepare future nursing faculty for teaching" (Benner et al., 2010, p. 224). In addition to clinical and research expertise, skill in the specialty of nursing education is critical to ensure the development of new pedagogical strategies to prepare the future nursing workforce to provide safe, quality care (NLN, 2017). The *Essentials: Core Competencies for Professional Nursing Education* (AACN, 2021) suggest that nurses may be prepared for education roles through optional electives offered during advanced practice graduate programs.

Nurse educators must be equipped to manage not only what future nurses must know and be able to do, but educators must also navigate the diverse and complex needs of the learner and the educational environment. The COVID-19 pandemic resulted in changes to the cognitive and social development and the learning needs of younger people who are growing and joining the workforce (Di Pietro, 2023). Nurse educators need to be able to "embrace the changing landscape in education and learn how faculty can best facilitate student competency development" (Wells-Beede et al., 2023, p. 235) through innovative active learning strategies and ever-developing technologies.

Transition to the Educator Role

As nurses make the transition into an educator role, not only must they learn skills related to classroom and clinical teaching, but they must also learn how to function within the educational setting, be it a college, university, or clinical practice environment. Included in this transition is learning how to balance new and often foreign requirements of the position and to navigate a professional environment that is notably different from their previous experience.

The transition experience of novice nurse educators has been examined by numerous authors over the past four decades. As early as 1989, Locasto and Kochanek (1989) used the theory of "reality shock" to describe the role transition experienced by those entering the academic work setting. Throughout the early 21st century, research about the transition experience described it as a time of role confusion and ambiguity. Common themes in this research are a lack of formal preparation for the role and a lack of intentional orientation, mentorship, and guidance. Scanlan (2001) described the novice period of a nurse educator's career as a time of learning by trial and error. Anderson (2009) depicted the work-role transition in the form of a metaphor, describing it as "treading water" in a vast sea (p. 206).

More recent inquiries into the transition experience note similar challenges. In a qualitative study of nurse faculty, Hoffman (2019) found that one of the most consistent struggles faced by new faculty was feeling like a "perpetual novice" from constantly starting over when assigned to new courses or clinical rotations. In this study, in the absence of formal preparation and structured orientation, inexperienced faculty relied on their past nursing experiences to guide them through unfamiliar situations with students, often considering "student as patient" (p. 263). Shapiro (2018) found similar results when examining the transition of novice faculty teaching in associate degree programs. In this study, participants described the transition as "chaotic, challenging, emotional" and "overwhelming" (p. 217). They were also unprepared for the complexity and workload of the academic educator role.

THE NURSE EDUCATOR TRANSITION MODEL

The NET model provides a framework for understanding the social process that occurs during the role transition from nurse to nurse educator (Schoening, 2013). Although this model was developed through grounded theory research with nurse educators in baccalaureate nursing programs, it can be applied to educators in a variety of roles. Since its publication, the NET model has been validated in small studies of part-time clinical faculty and faculty teaching in associate degree programs and community college settings (Shapiro, 2018; Wenner et al., 2020). This model is widely referenced in the literature as a framework or validation of other transition-related studies.

The NET model describes the transition from nurse to nurse educator as a four-phase process (Figure 2.1). The first phase is one of *anticipation/expectation* and begins once a decision is made to enter academia. This is a generally positive time in which the nurse educator looks forward to the benefits of their new career choice, such as a more flexible schedule and advancing scholarly interests. There is also the hope of making a difference in the lives of students and having a positive influence on the future of the profession.

The second phase of the transition is a period of *disorientation* that starts when the nurse begins work in the educational setting. This stage is characterized by an absence of structure and mentorship. Because there is often inadequate orientation and socialization to the role, the novice educator may feel confused about role expectations and may lack an understanding of the organizational structure in their new setting. Nurse educators experiencing this transitional phase often refer to it as being left to "sink or swim" and "flying by the seat of my pants" (Schoening, 2013, p. 169). Disorientation also results from becoming a novice after having previously been an expert in another nursing role. Those without formal preparation for the educator role may find this phase particularly challenging. The disorientation phase is compounded by the realization that the student–teacher relationship is different from the nurse–patient relationship and not every encounter with students is positive.

The third phase of transition is characterized by *information seeking* as the novice educator actively, and sometimes independently, works to fill gaps in their knowledge. This phase often involves multiple self-directed strategies for learning how to teach, such as fact-finding and seeking out peer mentors to support them in their new role. Because novice educators are often unsure of their learners' current level of knowledge and skill, they tend to over prepare for learner encounters and express fear of failing as a teacher. Because they lack experience in the educational role, novice educators tend to draw on their past experiences as nurses with patients, which allows them to slowly acquire confidence in their new roles.

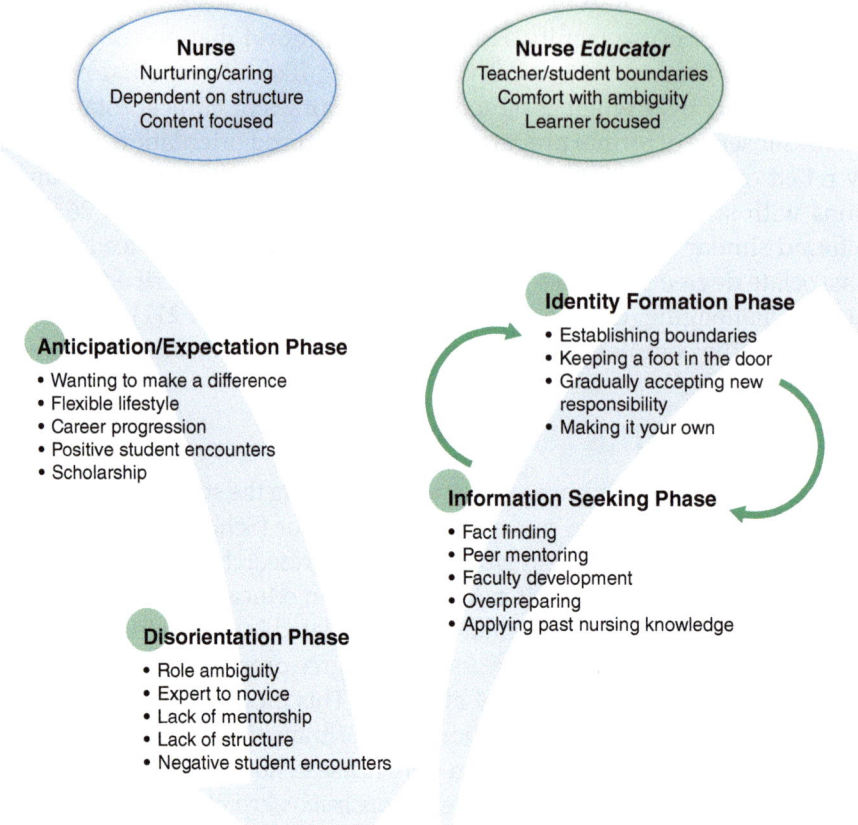

Figure 2.1 The Nurse Educator Transition Model.
Source: Copyright by Schoening, A. M. (2013). From bedside to classroom: The nurse educator transition model. *Nursing Education Perspectives, 34*(3), 167–172. https://doi.org/10.5480/1536-5026-34.3.167; reprinted with permission of Schoening (2024).

The final phase of the NET model is a period of *identity formation* in which a new professional identity as nurse *educator* emerges. Successful role transition is characterized by learning how to negotiate the differences between the nurse–patient and teacher–learner relationship by establishing boundaries with learners. The nurse educator also identifies strategies to maintain their nursing knowledge and skills through clinical practice or research while continuing to develop their knowledge and skills as an educator. They develop their own teaching style and voice by individualizing learning experiences and making it "their own" (Schoening, 2013, p. 170). This final phase of development is facilitated if their employer allows gradual acceptance of responsibility during the first year of teaching.

BARRIERS AND FACILITATORS TO A SUCCESSFUL TRANSITION

Both the NET model and the nursing education literature identify several common barriers and facilitators to a successful transition experience in both academic and clinical practice settings. To support and retain novice educators during their early employment, leaders must be aware of and implement strategies to support them in their new role.

Barriers to a Successful Transition

Integrative literature reviews by Summers (2017), Fritz (2018), and Wells-Beede et al. (2023) identified several common barriers to a successful role transition. These include unrealistic or unclear expectations and responsibilities, role ambiguity, poor orientation, lack of mentoring, and inadequate knowledge of educator skills. Almost universally across all settings, participants in the studies reviewed by these authors described orientation programs of inadequate length or missing essential information related to the nurse educator role. A lack of formal preparation for the educator role was also identified as a major barrier. Fritz (2018) described several specific educational needs of novice educators, such as knowledge of adult learning principles, learning styles, teaching techniques, learner evaluation, giving feedback, and professional communication with students. Summers (2017) reported similar needs for novices but added curriculum design and classroom management to the list of essential learning needs. Wells-Beede et al. (2023) also highlight a lack of clear and consistent guidance for preparing faculty as well as a lack of measurable outcomes that define nurse educator competency in preparing the future workforce.

Facilitators for a Successful Transition

Multiple facilitators for a successful transition are evident in the literature and apply to both academic and clinical practice settings. Such facilitators include formal structured orientation, effective mentoring, intentional development of educator skills, clear and consistent expectations, and frequent communication (Cox et al., 2021; Fritz, 2018; Hoffman, 2019; McPherson, 2019; McPherson & Candela, 2019; Ross & Kerrigan, 2020; Summers, 2017). McPherson and Candela (2019) affirmed that novice educators with formal coursework in nursing education at the graduate level had a better understanding of the roles and responsibilities of the clinical educator role. Hoffman (2019) stated that consistent course assignment during the first years of employment also supports building expertise and comfort during the time of transition.

Effective mentorship has been identified by many as a critical facilitator for attaining competence in the nurse educator role, yet there is a lack of consensus in the literature about the best model for new faculty mentorship (Cox et al., 2021; Jeffers & Mariani, 2017; Nowell et al., 2017; Rogers et al., 2020; Ross & Dunker, 2019; Wells-Beede et al., 2023). Jeffers and Mariani (2017) found no significant differences in career satisfaction between faculty who were formally mentored and those who were not; however, participants reported that being assigned a mentor helped them feel more supported as they learned the complexity of the faculty role. They also pointed out that assigned mentors were not always helpful and, in some cases, even engaged in incivility and bullying. Nowell et al. (2017) recommend including mentors and mentees in the matching process and in developing orientation plans due to the importance of the relationship on mentorship outcomes.

Multiple studies show that novice educators reported success when seeking out their own mentors among peers (Hoffman, 2019; Jeffers & Mariani, 2017; McPherson & Candela, 2019; Rogers et al., 2020; Schoening, 2013; Shapiro, 2018). These studies also support a combination of formal and informal mentoring or seeking more than one mentor as effective strategies for facilitating the transition from nurse to nurse educator. For example, while a teaching mentor may be formally assigned to guide

TABLE 2.1 BARRIERS AND FACILITATORS FOR A SUCCESSFUL ROLE TRANSITION

Barriers	Facilitators
Unrealistic or unclear expectations (role ambiguity)	Clear expectations Consistency of assignment during early years of career
Lack of or inadequate orientation	Structured orientation over at least 1 year Gradual assignment of new responsibilities over first year (committee work, advising) Co-creation of orientation agendas
Lack of formal preparation for teaching	Graduate-level coursework in preparation for teaching Faculty development
Lack of mentoring	Formal and informal mentoring Multiple mentors assigned based on purpose (teaching, scholarship) Including mentee and mentors in the matching process
Inadequate communication	Frequent, role development–focused communication Clear performance expectations (scholarship, professional service)

the novice through course planning, providing student feedback, and orienting to clinical teaching, a different mentor may be sought to provide guidance on scholarship or service expectations of the new role. Novice educators may also want to self-select mentors to help them navigate the stresses and complexities of the political and social culture of the organization as well as learn how to function in the educational setting (Nowell et al., 2017; Ross & Kerrigan, 2020).

In their study about mentoring new doctorally prepared faculty, Agger et al. (2017) conclude that mentorship should be designed to incorporate the novice's professional background, academic preparation, and anticipated new role. With the variety of pathways available for nurses to become educators, expectations for teaching and scholarly productivity may differ, thus role-specific peer mentorship may be beneficial (Agger et al., 2017). Ross and Kerrigan (2020) also propose that support from mentors at various stages of their careers may facilitate the novice educator's navigation of new responsibilities and expectations.

Table 2.1 summarizes the barriers and facilitators for a successful role transition. These are applicable when transitioning to an educator role in an academic or a clinical practice setting.

NEW FACULTY ORIENTATION

The need for structured orientation has been identified as one of the most important facilitators of a successful transition to the nurse educator role; however, orientation programs are often inadequate to meet the needs of novices (Brower et al., 2022; Cox et al., 2021; Rogers et al., 2020; Ross & Dunker, 2019; Seaman, 2021). Both full-time and part-time educators should receive a comprehensive orientation to their roles and responsibilities. Because part-time clinical educators may feel isolated from the larger academic program, knowing expectations and how clinical experiences align with the curriculum may ease feelings of isolation (McPherson, 2019). Although formal preparation as a nurse educator has been identified as facilitating the transition, it should not be assumed that this preparation leads to immediate competency (Hoffman, 2019). Orientation time and activities should not be shortened or abbreviated for those with degrees in nursing education.

Orientation programs should be of sufficient length with mentors available for ongoing support as needed. An orientation period of 1 to 2 years has been suggested for full-time nursing faculty (Hoffman, 2019; Schoening, 2013). This is particularly important for those faculty members practicing in the full scope of the academic nurse educator role; however, the literature does not provide conclusive guidance on this. Orientation programs may be delivered in a face-to-face or a hybrid manner, combining online modules with in-person meetings, but there is no consensus on the most effective model (Ross & Dunker, 2019). Due to the complex nature of the nurse educator role and the identified obstacles novices face during their transition period, administrators in schools of nursing should designate an individual to coordinate orientation activities and ongoing faculty development needs. This should be a formally appointed administrative role, with the appropriate workload to support all stages of career development for faculty.

The content included in novice educator orientation may vary depending on the role of the educator and the academic or clinical setting. In a study of new faculty orientation programs, Cox et al. (2021) found the top three most important aspects were orientation to the academic environment (teaching, scholarship, and service expectations and resources); the educational environment (courses, content, curriculum, student evaluation, and clinical placement); and the social milieu of the academic setting and program (history, structure, and student and faculty organizations). Other important inclusions for the new faculty orientation were political aspects of the institution, campus support systems, the local community, and the local professional milieu.

The NLN's Core Competencies for Academic Nurse Educators (Christensen & Simmons, 2020) provide a useful framework for planning a comprehensive new faculty orientation program. The NLN's Core Competencies for Academic Clinical Nurse Educators are a separate and distinct set of competencies that focus on facilitating learning in the healthcare environment. Table 2.2 outlines key components of a new faculty orientation program that meets the NLN's Core Competencies for Academic Nurse Educators functioning in the full scope of the role.

COMPONENTS OF NEW FACULTY ORIENTATION

Facilitate Learning

All nurse educators should be provided with information on the institution's mission, vision, and values and how these inform the educational philosophy of the school or clinical practice setting. Those teaching in the classroom or laboratory should be provided with instructional objectives for assigned course content and coached on using active learning strategies to engage students. If teaching in the

TABLE 2.2 COMPONENTS OF A NEW FACULTY ORIENTATION PROGRAM

NLN Core Competency	Key Components
Facilitate Learning	- Institutional mission, vision, and values - Instructional objectives for assigned courses - Education/coaching on active learning strategies - Observation of experienced faculty in clinical and classroom - Access to textbooks and course resources - Clinical agency orientation - Online teaching mentor if appropriate
Facilitate Learner Development and Socialization	- Demographics of learners - Education on teaching–learning theories - Americans with Disabilities Act and reasonable accommodations - Referrals for students with mental health concerns
Use Assessment and Evaluation Strategies	- Education on exam writing and item analysis - Orientation to exam item banks and software - Exam item writing mentor if appropriate - Agency policies on exam administration and security - Orientation to clinical evaluation instrument - Education on providing objective feedback to learners - Course or program progression policies
Participate in Curriculum Design and Evaluation of Program Outcomes	- Curricular model - Course alignment with program outcomes and institutional mission - Systematic evaluation plan
Function as Change Agent and Leader	- Service to school or department and college or university - Development opportunities on evidence-based teaching
Pursue Continuous Quality Improvement in the Role	- Short-term and long-term career goals - Expectations for scholarship, service, and teaching - Rank and tenure procedures if on tenure track - Mentor for tenure process; mid tenure review - Policies for conduct, attendance, and clinical incidents - Family Educational Rights and Privacy Act and student information
Engage in Scholarship	- Scholarship expectations for current position - Resources for scholarship - Existing scholarship teams - Mentor for scholarship - Balancing teaching and service demands with scholarship
Function Within the Educational Environment	- Culture and work environment - Service expectations at the college department or university level - Education on forces influencing higher education

clinical learning environment, new faculty should receive guidance on how to ask questions that promote the development of clinical judgment in learners and how to facilitate meaningful clinical conferences. Providing new faculty with the opportunity to observe experienced educators in the clinical and classroom setting as well as the opportunity to be observed themselves may help them develop skill as educators (Shapiro, 2018). All faculty should have access to textbooks, supplemental resources used to teach nursing skills, and online learning management systems.

Faculty teaching in the clinical setting must be provided with adequate time to orient to their assigned clinical agency and to complete necessary compliance requirements. Gaining knowledge of an agency's policies and procedures and building a trusting relationship with clinical partners are critical in facilitating student learning in the clinical environment. It is also necessary for the educator to develop confidence and skill within that setting; thus, it is recommended that novice educators be consistently assigned to a clinical unit or community agency throughout their early years in the role.

Faculty who are teaching online should be assigned a mentor for online course design to ensure that they follow best practices for engaging online learners and are able to navigate the learning management system. Novice educators teaching online may face a steep learning curve if they do not consider themselves adept with technology. Even if teaching in a face-to-face program, all nursing faculty should gain skills in navigating electronic platforms for virtual clinical experiences and learning management systems. Support from instructional designers, information technology departments, and a school's teaching and learning center, if available, may facilitate development in this area.

Facilitate Learner Development and Socialization

All educators must know their learners. It is important for novice educators to understand the characteristics of their learners with respect to cultural and spiritual diversity, age, gender, socio economic background, and educational preparation. For example, teaching in a 4-year traditional university setting in which most of the students are 18 to 22 years old requires a different approach than teaching in a community college setting or accelerated nursing program in which the students are often older and considered adult learners. Those without formal educational preparation may need development on teaching and learning theories and how these inform the choice of instructional strategies for diverse learners. Nurse educators will also encounter an increasing number of students with disabilities, so they should receive information on how qualified students with disabilities request and receive reasonable accommodations in a nursing program under the Americans with Disabilities Act. They should also be provided with information on how and where to refer students with mental health concerns.

Use Assessment and Evaluation Strategies

If teaching in the classroom setting, novice nurse educators should receive instruction on methods used to assess and evaluate student learning. Because nursing programs often evaluate achievement of outcomes through administration of exams, new faculty should have instruction on writing exam items, analyzing and interpreting exam results, developing assessment strategies, and grading. New faculty should be assigned a mentor for exam item selection, item writing, and item analysis throughout their first semester of classroom instruction. Development in this area should also include information on agency policies related to exam administration, security, scheduling, and absences.

Faculty teaching in the clinical setting should receive information on providing feedback in real-time to students at the point of care, as well as how to provide both formative and summative evaluation of clinical performance. This includes strategies for communicating learner strengths and areas for needed improvement. Faculty should be provided with one-to-one instruction on the use of clinical evaluation tools and how to provide objective feedback to students. The importance of timely feedback should be part of this discussion, as should strategies for providing feedback to students on clinical assignments that encourage growth of their clinical reasoning skills. All faculty should receive guidance and support if they are working with a student who is not meeting instructional objectives and is in danger of failing a course. McPherson and Candela (2019) suggest simulation as a tool to help new faculty learn to navigate difficult conversations with students.

Participate in Curriculum Design and Evaluation of Program Outcomes

Although new faculty will not immediately engage in curriculum planning and design, they should receive information on the structure and design of the curriculum, and how the course to which they are assigned fits within that structure. Novice educators without formal preparation for the role will also need additional information on how course objectives map to program objectives and how program objectives align with the institutional mission. Full-time faculty and those practicing in the full scope of the academic role should receive a brief overview of the school's systematic evaluation plan and how assessment data are gathered at the course level. If teaching in a concept or theory-based curriculum model, additional information should be provided about how relevant concepts and theories are operationalized in course assignments and learning experiences.

Function as Change Agent and Leader

It may be difficult at first for a novice nurse educator to view themselves as a leader. However, it is critical that those beginning their career understand how they can affect change within their workplace. For nurse educators in the academic setting, this can be accomplished through service on school, department, and eventually university or college level committees. Nurse educators working in professional development should understand their service role on educational, practice, and policy committees within their institution. Nurse educators in all settings should be encouraged to cultivate leadership roles within their community and professional organizations.

Pursue Continuous Quality Improvement in the Nurse Educator Role

Even though they are just beginning their role as nurse educators, novices should be encouraged to develop short- and long-term career goals as part of a faculty development or career development plan. This is particularly important for academic nurse educators who are on a tenure track and must meet more rigorous expectations for teaching, scholarship, and service. New faculty should be oriented to the expectations for their rank at the time of initial employment as well as the standards for promotion to a higher rank. If not already in place at their institution, faculty on a tenure track should be assigned a mentor for this process and counseled yearly on their progress toward this goal. A mid-tenure review conducted halfway through the tenure timeline may also be helpful.

Faculty also should understand the potential legal and ethical issues they may face as nurse educators in an academic setting. At the time of initial employment, new faculty should be provided with an orientation to relevant student policies, such as those related to conduct, attendance, grading, and course progression. Faculty teaching in the clinical setting should be aware of institutional policies related to student incidents, such as blood and body fluid exposure and student errors. They also should have access to the clinical setting's policies on student practice, including any restrictions.

All faculty in the academic setting must receive instruction on the Family Educational Rights and Privacy Act (FERPA). This act ensures student privacy and provides students with the right to inspect their educational record and request corrections to inaccuracies. It also limits access to student records and assessment information to those who have a need to know (U.S. Department of Education, 2021). Faculty should understand how to manage student requests for job references and inquiries from parents regarding student performance, as these require the student's written authorization. They should also be counseled on how to keep student work secure in both hard copy as well as in electronic form.

Engage in Scholarship

Novice nurse educators in a university setting should receive clear guidance on performance standards related to scholarship, and how these impact contract renewal, promotion, and tenure. New faculty who are beginning a research trajectory should be assigned a mentor for research and scholarly work. It is also important that they are oriented to resources that are available for scholarship at their institution, such as grant-writing assistance and processes associated with the institutional review board. New faculty should be aware of any existing faculty research groups to identify potential areas for collaboration. An important part of new faculty mentorship in this area is guidance on how to balance one's time so that scholarly goals can be achieved. Balancing teaching, scholarship, and service expectations may cause role stress if the scholarship expectations are higher than what was required in prior settings.

Nurses in professional development roles should also be encouraged to pursue scholarly work, whether that includes collaboration on original research or leading quality improvement efforts. They should be aware of potential sources for mentorship and collaboration, such as joining a research committee within a healthcare organization or working directly with an academic partner.

Function Within the Educational Environment

Nurse educators in the academic setting need guidance on how to function as a "good citizen" of the academy (Christensen & Simmons, 2020). Although educators who have been full-time clinicians are familiar with a healthcare agency's culture and role expectations, becoming socialized to higher education presents additional challenges. The academic work setting is vastly different from the clinical work setting, with far less structure and sometimes ambiguous expectations. This new-found autonomy may be unsettling to a clinician who is accustomed to rigid schedules, policies, and procedures, resulting in role confusion (Schoening, 2013). Development of a new professional self-identity as a nurse educator is a component of the transition from nurse to nurse educator which can be supported through intentional mentorship that highlights the educator's impact on the profession and society (Brower et al., 2022; Schoening, 2013). Nurse educators also need to understand current trends and issues in higher education and how those influence the academic workplace and their students. Functioning within the educational environment requires participation in professional service and leadership at the university or college level and developing relationships that advance the nursing department's standing within the wider academic community (Christensen & Simmons, 2020).

Table 2.3 provides resources to facilitate the transition from clinician to educator. In addition to this table, many of the organizations in Appendix A provide continuing education and other resources for novice educators.

TABLE 2.3 RESOURCES FOR NOVICE NURSE EDUCATORS

Resource	Organization	Website/Source
Toolkit: Transitioning From Clinical Nursing to Nurse Faculty	American Association of Colleges of Nursing	https://www.aacnnursing.org/our-initiatives/education-practice/faculty-tool-kits/transitioning-from-clinical-nursing-to-nursing-faculty
Toolkit: Accommodating Students With Disabilities	American Association of Colleges of Nursing	https://www.aacnnursing.org/our-initiatives/education-practice/faculty-tool-kits/accommodating-students-with-disabilities
Vision Series: Graduate Preparation for Academic Nurse Educators	National League for Nursing	https://www.nln.org/docs/default-source/uploadedfiles/about/nln-vision-series-position-statements/vision-graduate-preparation2.pdf
Healthful Work Environment Toolkit	National League for Nursing	https://www.nln.org/docs/default-source/uploadedfiles/professional-development-programs/healthful-work-environment-toolkit.pdf?sfvrsn=87d8da0d_0
Policies: Family Educational Rights and Privacy Act (FERPA)	U.S. Department of Education	https://www2.ed.gov/policy/gen/guid/fpco/ferpa/index.html

(continued)

TABLE 2.3 RESOURCES FOR NOVICE NURSE EDUCATORS (continued)

Resource	Organization	Website/Source
Policies: Americans with Disabilities Act (ADA)	U.S. Department of Justice, Civil Rights Division	https://www.ada.gov/
Documentary film: "Open the Door, Get 'Em a Locker"	National Organization of Nurses with Disabilities	https://youtu.be/q3WQtR7yUpI?si=s5JYYR0KLwAcD8eo

CHOOSING THE RIGHT WORK SETTING

Choosing the right work setting is critical in making the transition from clinician to educator. In deciding on the setting in which to teach, the goals and mission of the school should be examined in relation to one's own career goals. Expectations vary by school and the type of institution. Schools with a research mission emphasize scholarship more so than schools with a mission that focuses only on education. Furthermore, understanding institutional culture is an important factor in acclimating to the values and norms of the academic setting. Exhibit 2.1 suggests some questions for reflection when considering full- or part-time employment as a nurse educator in an academic or health setting.

SUMMARY

Although the transition from clinician to educator presents many challenges, there are several strategies that may facilitate this transition in the academic or professional development setting. These strategies include formal, structured orientation, effective mentoring, and development of instructional skills. Novice educators, particularly those practicing in the full scope of the academic nurse educator role, may

---

EXHIBIT 2.1 Questions to Consider Prior to Seeking Employment as a Nurse Educator

Do I want to work in an academic environment or healthcare setting?
What are the academic credentials needed for employment?
What kind of flexibility do I want and need in setting my work hours?
Do I want to work full- or part-time as a nurse educator?
Do I want to combine academic and clinical practice responsibilities?
In my career, do I want to spend the majority of my time teaching or combining research and teaching?
What service activities are expected in the role of an educator?
If I seek employment in an academic setting, what level of students and types of courses do I want to teach?
If I work in an academic setting, do I want to maintain some practice as a staff nurse, nurse practitioner, or clinical specialist?

need more than one mentor as they adjust to teaching, scholarship, and service expectations in their new role. They should also be encouraged to seek out their own informal mentors among their peers. Orientation programs for full-time faculty should be structured, robust, and last for at least 1 year.

The NET model and NLN's Core Competencies provide useful frameworks for designing a new faculty orientation program. A designated administrative position should be dedicated to faculty development. This individual will need to work collaboratively with other departments within the university to ensure novice faculty receive the necessary support and guidance they need for a successful transition from clinician to educator.

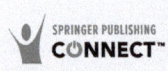 A robust set of instructor resources designed to supplement this text is located at http://connect.springerpub.com/content/book/978-0-8261-8892-2. Qualifying instructors may request access by emailing textbook@springerpub.com.

REFERENCES

Agger, C., Oermann, M., & Lynn, M. (2014). Hiring and incorporating doctor of nursing practice-prepared nurse faculty into academic nursing programs. *Journal of Nursing Education, 53*(8), 439–446. https://doi.org/10.3928/01484834-20140724-03

Agger, C., Oermann, M., & Lynn, M. (2017). Mentoring and development resources available to new doctorally prepared faculty in nursing. *Nursing Education Perspectives, 38*(4), 189–192. https://doi.org/10.1097/01.NEP.0000000000000180

American Association of Colleges of Nursing. (2021). *The essentials: Core competencies for professional nursing education*. https://www.aacnnursing.org/Portals/42/AcademicNursing/pdf/Essentials-2021.pdf

American Association of Colleges of Nursing. (2023). *Fact sheet: The Doctor of Nursing Practice (DNP)*. https://www.aacnnursing.org/news-data/fact-sheets/dnp-fact-sheet

American Nurses' Association Commission on Nursing Education. (1969). *Statement on graduate education in nursing*. American Nurses' Association.

Anderson, J. (2009). The work-role transition of expert clinician to novice academic educator. *Journal of Nursing Education, 48*(4), 203–208. https://doi.org/10.3928/01484834-20090401-02

Benner, P., Sutphen, M., Leonard, V., & Day, L. (2010). *Educating nurses: A call for radical transformation*. Jossey-Bass.

Brower, E., Nemec, R., Ritchie, H., & Nicastro, O. (2022). A qualitative exploration of self-identity during role transition to a nurse educator. *Nurse Education Today, 112*, 105331. https://doi.org/10.1016/j.nedt.2022.105331

Christensen, L., & Simmons, L. E. (2020). *The scope of practice for academic nurse educators and academic clinical nurse educators* (3rd ed.). National League for Nursing.

Cox, C. W., Jordan, E. T., Valiga, T. M., & Zhou, Q. (2021). New faculty orientation for nurse educators: Offerings and needs. *Journal of Nursing Education, 60*(5), 273–276. https://doi.org/10.3928/01484834-20210420-06

Di Pietro, G. (2023). The impact of Covid-19 on student achievement: Evidence from a recent meta-analysis. *Educational Research Review, 39*, 100530. https://doi.org/10.1016/j.edurev.2023.100530

Dreifuerst, K., McNelis, A., Weaver, M., Broome, M., Draucker, C., & Fedko, A. (2016). Exploring the pursuit of doctoral education by nurses seeking or intending to stay in faculty roles. *Journal of Professional Nursing, 32*(3), 202–212. https://doi.org/10.1016/j.profnurs.2016.01.014

Fritz, E. (2018). Transition from clinical to educator roles in nursing: An integrative review. *Journal for Nurses in Professional Development, 34*(2), 67–77. https://doi.org/10.1097/NND.0000000000000436

Hoffman, D. (2019). Transitional experiences: From clinical nurse to nurse faculty. *Journal of Nursing Education, 58*(5), 260–265. https://doi.org/10.3928/01484834-20190422-03

Jeffers, S. & Mariani, B. (2017). The effect of a formal mentoring program on career satisfaction and intent to stay in the faculty role for novice nurse faculty. *Nursing Education Perspectives, 38*(1), 18–22. https://doi.org/10.1097/01.NEP.0000000000000104

Locasto, L. W., & Kochanek, D. (1989). Reality shock in the nurse educator. *Journal of Nursing Education, 28*(2), 79–81. https://doi.org/10.3928/0148-4834-19890201-10

McNelis, A. M., Dreifuerst, K. T., & Schwindt, R. (2019). Doctoral education and preparation for nursing faculty roles. *Nurse Educator, 44*(4), 202–206. https://doi.org/10.1097/NNE.0000000000000597

McPherson, S. (2019). Part-time clinical nursing faculty needs: An integrated review. *Journal of Nursing Education, 58*(4), 201–206. https://doi.org/10.3928/01484834-20190321-03

McPherson, S., & Candela, L. (2019). A Delphi study to understand clinical nursing faculty preparation and support needs. *Journal of Nursing Education, 58*(10), 583–590. https://doi.org/10.3928/01484834-20190923-05

National League for Nursing. (2002). *Position statement: The preparation of nurse educators*. https://www.nln.org/docs/default-source/uploadedfiles/about/archived-position-statements/the-preparation-of-nurse-educators-pdf.pdf?sfvrsn=b84cdc0d_0

National League for Nursing. (2017). *Graduate preparation for academic nurse educators: A living document from the National League for Nursing*. https://www.nln.org/docs/default-source/uploadedfiles/about/nln-vision-series-position-statements/vision-graduate-preparation2.pdf

Nowell, L., Norris, J. M., Mrklas, K., & White, D. E. (2017). A literature review of mentorship programs in academic nursing. *Journal of Professional Nursing, 33*(5), 334–344. https://doi.org/10.1016/j.profnurs.2017.02.007

Rogers, J., Ludwig-Beymer, P., & Baker, M. (2020). Nurse faculty orientation: An integrative review. *Nurse Educator, 45*(6), 343–346. https://doi.org/10.1097/NNE.0000000000000802

Ross, B., & Kerrigan, M. R. (2020). Addressing the faculty shortage through connections: Stories of becoming a nurse educator. *Journal of Nursing Education, 59*(10), 545–550. https://doi.org/10.3928/01484834-20200921-02

Ross, J. G., & Dunker, K. S. (2019). New clinical nurse faculty orientation: A review of the literature. *Nursing Education Perspectives, 40*(4), 210–215. https://doi.org/10.1097.01.NEP.0000000000000470

Scanlan, J. M. (2001). Learning clinical teaching: Is it magic? *Nursing & Healthcare Perspectives, 22*(5), 241–246.

Schoening, A. M. (2013). From bedside to classroom: The nurse educator transition model. *Nursing Education Perspectives, 34*(3), 167–172. https://doi.org/10.5480/1536-5026-34.3.167

Seaman, R. A. (2021). *The relationship of transition on job satisfaction and intent to stay among novice nurse educators in baccalaureate degree nursing programs*. [Unpublished doctoral dissertation]. Immaculata University. https://library.immaculata.edu/Dissertation/digitalB/Doc894SeamanR2021.pdf

Shapiro, S. (2018). An exploration of the transition to the full-time faculty role among associate degree nurse educators. *Nursing Education Perspectives, 39*(4), 215–220. https://doi.org/10.1097/01.NEP.0000000000000306

Summers, J. (2017). Developing competencies in the novice nurse educator: An integrative review. *Teaching and Learning in Nursing, 12*(4), 263–276. https://doi.org/10.1016/j.teln.2017.05.001

U.S. Department of Education. (2021). *Family educational rights and privacy act*. https://www2.ed.gov/policy/gen/guid/fpco/ferpa/index.html

Wells-Beede, E., Sharpnack, P., Gruben, D., Klenke-Borgmann, L., Goliat, L., & Yeager, C. (2023). A scoping review of nurse educator competencies: Mind the gap. *Nurse Educator, 48*(5), 234–239. https://doi.org/10.1097/NNE.0000000000001376

Wenner, T. A., Hakim, A. C., & Schoening, A. M. (2020). The work-role transition of part-time clinical faculty: Seeking to validate the nurse educator transition model. *Nurse Educator, 45*(2), 102–105. https://doi.org/10.1097/NNE.0000000000000704

Contemporary Learning Theories

Paula D. Koppel

3

OBJECTIVES

1. Describe foundational theories of learning as well as recent transformative theories and frameworks
2. Explain how learning theories can be used to create a teaching philosophy and select teaching methods

INTRODUCTION

Nurse educators play a key role in the teaching and learning processes, not only in the classroom and online but in nursing skills laboratories, clinical areas, simulations, and student advisement sessions. Understanding how students learn in each of these settings is paramount to good instruction. Theories explain the learning process and direct the selection of learning methods. Nurse educators need to be grounded in a teaching philosophy that they can embody, using methods based on the best evidence of teaching and learning. They must examine and understand theories of learning to ensure that their students receive a high-quality education. This chapter examines foundational learning theories as well as some recent transformative theories and frameworks. Additionally, this chapter illustrates how learning theories can guide the development of a course curriculum and teaching philosophy.

THE BEGINNING OF LEARNING THEORIES

The first known writing about teaching and learning dates back to 2100 BCE: The Babylonian Code of Hammurabi briefly addressed teaching as an apprenticeship model of learning by practical experience (King, n.d.). As early as 300 BCE, the Greeks were employing what is now recognized as the Socratic method, a question-and-answer form of teaching that encourages students to develop their thoughts and ideas (Fabio, 2019). Over the past 150 years, scientists and philosophers have developed theoretical and conceptual models representing the learning process, yet they have struggled to fully understand how learning occurs.

Current neuroscience research has fundamentally altered the theory and practice of education. Never before have we had the capability to observe learning occurring within the brain. Through the use of PET scans and functional MRIs, we can now witness the brain's components in action as information is processed. From this research, the concept of brain plasticity has emerged—the notion that experiences can actually alter both the brain's anatomy and physiology (Boyle, 2010). Research into neurotransmitters in the brain has provided insights into structuring learning processes effectively. For example, Pi et al. (2019) studied changes in brain plasticity and found that motor skill learning can improve the brain's ability to control behavior, make decisions more effectively, and switch the focus of attention more accurately. Such findings are significant to nursing education, which seeks to instill and cultivate essential decision-making and psychomotor skills. Moreover, educators need an understanding of the role of technology in the learning process, as learning through technology and on technological platforms has increased exponentially in the past few years (Bower, 2019).

WHAT IS LEARNING?

Learning is a fundamental aspect of human existence, and much of our learning journey relies on the guidance of teachers. The puzzle of explaining how we learn, and consequently how to teach effectively, has been at the forefront of education discussions since the mid-19th century. There exist numerous definitions of learning; one contemporary perspective comes from Schunk (2020) who states, "Learning is an enduring change in behavior, or in the capacity to behave in a given fashion, which results from practice or other forms of experience" (p. 3).

THEORIES OF LEARNING

Theories can explain phenomena, including assumptions, and provide guidelines for actions. Many theories of teaching and learning have evolved over time to improve pedagogical decisions and enhance our ability to predict and achieve favorable outcomes (Knowles et al., 2020). Before modern tools allowed us to visualize the learning process in the brain, theorists had to hypothesize how learning worked in order to provide a rationale for an event (learning) that they could not otherwise explain. Early theories based on direct observation were elaborated upon by later schools of thought. This section and Table 3.1 provide a general overview of major foundational schools of thought. Over the past few decades, new theories and frameworks have transformed teaching and learning in traditional and virtual classrooms. Table 3.2 summarizes some of these theories as well as related resources. Additionally, helpful web-based resources with overviews of teaching and learning theories are listed at the end of this chapter.

Behaviorism

Behaviorism emerged at a time when scientists lacked the ability to directly observe the inner workings of the brain during the learning process, leading early educators and researchers to speculate on the mechanisms of learning. From the latter half of the 19th century through the early 20th century, scientists sought methods to modify fundamental behaviors. Behavioral theories conceptualized learning as the alteration in the method or frequency of a behavior resulting from interactions with the external environment. Within these theories, the interaction with the environment was deemed paramount, with conditioning playing a central role in behavior modification. The seminal works of renowned scientists such as Pavlov, Skinner,

TABLE 3.1 FOUNDATIONAL LEARNING THEORIES

Schools of Thought	Major Tenets	Major Theorists and Contributors
Behaviorism	Learning is a change in behavior, shaped by responses to the external environment; the educator transmits information to student	- Pavlov (classical conditioning) - Thorndike (connectionism) - Skinner (operant conditioning)
Cognitivism	Learning is internal, the result of processing and organizing information	- Bruner (cognitive growth theory) - Gagne (information processing theory) - Bloom (cognitive taxonomy)
Sociological	Social processes and the environment play a role in learning	- Vygotsky (social cognitivism) - Bandura (social learning theory) - Lave and Wenger (situated learning theory)
Constructivism	Learning is an internal process built on previous knowledge and experiences	- Dewey - Piaget (theory of cognitive development) - Kolb and Fry (experiential learning model)
Humanism	People intentionally act based on perceived needs and are capable of self-improvement and growth	- Maslow (hierarchy of needs) - Rogers
Feminist pedagogy	Shared learning environments featuring respectful discussion and reflection support critical thinking and empowerment	- Gilligan - Shrewsbury

and Thorndike exemplify this behaviorist perspective, which views learning as the acquisition of new behaviors through external conditioning and reinforcement (Schunk, 2020).

Ivan Pavlov (1839–1946) is known for his work with *classical conditioning*, a multistep process of introducing an unconditioned stimulus that would bring about an unconditioned response. Pavlov's best-known experiment entailed presenting a dog

TABLE 3.2 TRANSFORMATIVE THEORIES AND FRAMEWORKS

School of Thought	Helpful Resources
Brain-based learning	- Jensen, E. (n.d.). *Principles of Brain-Based Learning.* Jensen Learning Corporation. https://www.jensenlearning.com/what-is-brain-based-research/principles/
Motivational learning - Growth mindset	- Mindset Works, Inc. (2017). *Decades of scientific research that started a growth mindset revolution.* https://www.mindsetworks.com/science/
Learning style - Adult learning theory - Multiple intelligence theory	- Harvard Medical School. (2022, April 20). *Unlocking effective medical education through Adult Learning Theory.* https://postgraduateeducation.hms.harvard.edu/trends-medicine/unlocking-effective-medical-education-through-adult-learning-theory - Marenus, M. (2024, February 2). *Howard Gardner's Theory of Multiple Intelligences.* https://www.simplypsychology.org/multiple-intelligences.html
Technological and virtual learning - Technology-mediated learning - Community of inquiry	- The Community of Inquiry. (n.d.). *The Community of Inquiry.* https://www.thecommunityofinquiry.org/
Inclusive pedagogy - Universal design learning	- Chicago Center for Teaching. (2020). *Inclusive pedagogy.* The University of Chicago. https://inclusivepedagogy.uchicago.edu/ - Duke Learning Innovation & Lifetime Education. (2024). *Inclusive Teaching Quick Start Guide.* https://learninginnovation.duke.edu/resources/art-and-science-of-teaching/creating-an-inclusive-and-equitable-course/inclusive-teaching-quick-start-guide/ - CAST, Inc. (2024). *About universal design for learning.* https://www.cast.org/impact/universal-design-for-learning-udl/ - Pacansky-Brock, M. (2020). *How to humanize your online class, version 2.0* [Infographic]. https://brocansky.com/humanizing/infographic2

with meat while a metronome ticked in the background. Over time, the dog became conditioned to the metronome and would salivate when it ticked (Pavlov, 1927).

Edward Thorndike (1874–1949) is known for developing psychological *connectionism* based on his work on learning, individual differences, intelligence, and transfer of knowledge (Hilgard, 1996). Thorndike hypothesized that learning describes a formulation of connections between sensory stimuli and neural impulses which is identified through behavior. He also believed that learning often occurs by trial and error. Thorndike noted that teachers must help students form good habits, and that teaching should contextualize content so that students can understand how to apply what they have learned. He further proposed that information should be presented when the student is ready to learn or just before the information can be used in a serviceable way (Thorndike & Gates, 1929).

B. F. Skinner (1904–1990) formulated the theory of *operant conditioning* in the 1930s. Based on the work of Thorndike, Skinner believed that the best way to understand behavior was to examine the causes of an action and its consequences (Skinner, 1953). Skinner created the term "operant conditioning," which describes changing behavior by using reinforcement that follows a desired response. Skinner identified three types of responses that can follow behavior: (a) neutral operants, or responses from the environment which neither increase nor decrease the probability of a behavior being repeated; (b) reinforcers, or responses from the environment which increase the probability of a behavior being repeated; and (c) punishers, or responses from the environment which decrease the likelihood of a behavior being repeated.

Positive reinforcement strengthens a behavior by providing a reward or positive consequence (Skinner, 1953). Behavior can also be strengthened by negative reinforcement, or the removal of an adverse stimulus. Negative reinforcement strengthens behavior because it stops or removes an unpleasant experience. Punishment is the opposite of reinforcement as it is designed to inhibit behavior by directly applying an unpleasant stimulus or removing a potentially rewarding stimulus following a response (McLeod, 2024a).

Although popular through much of the 20th century, behaviorism is no longer a predominant educational perspective. However, the concepts of positive and negative reinforcement retain their usefulness today. Behavioral objectives, learning contracts, and programmed learning are based on behaviorism. Exhibit 3.1 provides examples of teaching methods influenced by this educational perspective.

EXHIBIT 3.1 Examples of Teaching Methods Based on Behaviorism

Classroom norm-setting to ensure consistency
Behavioral course objectives
Grades for class participation
Guided practice
Lecture without discussion
Rewards for performance
Repetition
Reward systems
Skill exercises

Cognitivism

Cognitivism encompasses a collection of theories influenced by the work of scholars such as Bruner, Gagne, and Bloom. The cognitive aspects of learning gained recognition in the 1960s, as the behaviorist perspective struggled to elucidate why individuals organize and make sense of the information they acquire. Cognitive theory defines learning as a semipermanent change in mental processes or associations. Unlike behaviorists, cognitivists do not necessarily require outward demonstrations of learning; instead, they focus on the internal processes and connections that occur during learning.

Cognitivists view learning as a mental construct that serves as a foundation for organizing and expanding knowledge. Since learning entails a transformation in mental structures rather than a change in behavior, any observable behavioral changes are attributed to alterations in cognition. According to cognitivism, the locus of control for learning resides within the learner rather than the external environment (Utley, 2011).

Jerome Bruner's (1915–2016) *cognitive growth theory* examined intellectual growth in children. Bruner proposed that as children grow, they depend on a widening array of modes of understanding: Infants rely on enactive responses (action) to process and represent information, children 1 to 4 years of age rely on images to process information, and children over the age of 4 begin to use language to shape and augment information processing (Bruner, 1964).

Cognitive psychology places significant emphasis on memory, a topic that has been scrutinized for millennia. The *information processing theory* elucidates the acquisition of knowledge through a systematic approach. Scholars such as **Robert Gagne** (1919–2002), proponents of the information processing perspective, prioritize mental processes occurring between stimuli and responses over external influences (Schunk, 2020). These theorists propose that individuals selectively attend to environmental cues, convert data into information, and engage in rehearsal, linking new information with existing knowledge (Aubrey & Riley, 2022). Within this model, Gagne (1985) delineated four key processes: (a) encoding, where environmental information is sensed or attended to (resulting in neural impulses), (b) processing of information (filtering out irrelevant details), (c) storage postencoding (potentially in short-term or long-term memory), and (d) retrieval when the information is needed for a task (prompting action).

Bloom's *Taxonomy of the Cognitive Domain* is a notable application of cognitive theory. Initially formulated in 1956 and subsequently revised in 2001, this framework categorizes educational objectives into six cognitive domains, spanning from basic to advanced levels of complexity (Aubrey & Riley, 2022). The taxonomy serves as a valuable tool for structuring educational goals and objectives within a

---

EXHIBIT 3.2 Examples of Teaching Methods Based on Cognitivism

Problem-solving
Linking new knowledge with that already learned
Reciprocal teaching: dialogues about segments of text to understand its meaning
Scaffolding: supportive resources and guides to promote a deeper level of learning
Organizing curriculum goals and objectives basic to higher levels of cognitive thinking

curriculum, facilitating the progression of cognitive thinking from foundational to more advanced levels. Additional examples of teaching methods based on cognitivism are illustrated in Exhibit 3.2.

Sociological Learning Theories

Vygotsky's (1896–1934) *social cognitivism* expanded Piaget's basic developmental theory of cognitive abilities of the individual to include the concept of social–cultural cognition, the idea that all learning occurs in a cultural context and involves social interactions (Schunk, 2020). He emphasized the role that culture and language play in developing students' thinking and the ways in which teachers and peers assist learners in developing new ideas and skills. Vygotsky proposed the concept of the zone of proximal development, which suggested that students learn subjects best just beyond their range of existing experience with assistance from the teacher or another classmate. Assistance from others bridges the distance from what students know or can do independently to what they can know or do with assistance.

Social learning theory also emphasizes the importance of social context. Based on the work of **Albert Bandura** (1925–), this theory conceives that much of human learning occurs in the environment (Schunk, 2020). Social learning theory is built on the importance of observational learning, imitation, and modeling. Bandura's theory hypothesizes that there is continuous interaction among behaviors, cognitions, and the environment. The learner and environment are in a reciprocal relationship in which one influences the other, and human behavior is learned visually through modeling based on observing others (Bandura, 1977, 1986). For a student to learn, three internal processes must occur: attention, or observation; retention, or processing in memory; and motivation, or having a reason to replicate another's behavior.

Learning in an environment that reflects the skills that will eventually be applied is the focus of **Lave and Wenger's** (1991) *situated learning theory*. This theory proposes that learning is more than just a reception of knowledge. Rather, knowledge is presented in as authentic a context as possible, with social interaction and collaboration among community members considered imperative to learning. Apprenticeship experiences enable the learner to engage with the real environment in order to learn. Because nursing education involves social interaction and collaboration, and emphasizes the real practice of nurses, an authentic context is critical; therefore, selecting teaching strategies that best prepare learners to acquire and retain knowledge is important. Exhibit 3.3 provides examples of teaching methods based on sociological learning theories.

EXHIBIT 3.3 Examples of Teaching Methods Based on Sociological Learning Theories

Apprenticeships in authentic contexts (preceptorships)
Demonstration/return demonstration
Interprofessional groupwork
Observational learning
Role modeling
Socratic questioning
Self-evaluation of learning

Constructivism

Constructivism, emerging as a reaction to didactic approaches like behaviorism and programmed instruction, asserts that learning is not merely about acquiring knowledge but rather involves an active, contextualized process of constructing knowledge through experiencing and reflecting upon experiences (Bruning et al., 2010). Knowledge is built upon personal experiences and hypotheses that learners continually test through social interaction. Each learner is not a "blank slate" but an active participant who brings past experiences and cultural influences to the learning process, resulting in a unique interpretation and construction of knowledge.

John Dewey (1859–1952), one of the most influential educators of the 20th century, championed the idea of experiential education, emphasizing meaningful learning activities and student participation in the classroom (Schunk, 2020). Unlike traditional teacher-centered approaches focused on rote learning, Dewey's concept of progressive education emphasized student engagement and relevance of the curriculum to students' lives. He viewed experiential learning of practical life skills as integral to education.

Jean Piaget (1896–1980) pioneered the notion that learning is a developmental process and that children actively construct knowledge rather than passively absorbing it from teachers (Hilgard & Bower, 1975; Huitt & Hummel, 2003). His cognitive constructivist theory of learning bridged cognitive and constructionist schools of thought. Piaget recognized that children construct knowledge based on practice, which is related to biological and developmental maturation. He observed young children and mapped out four stages of growth: sensorimotor (birth to about 2 years), preoperational (ages 2–7), concrete operations (ages 7–14), and formal operations (beginning around ages 11–15 and extending into adulthood). While recognizing the importance of some rote learning, Piaget emphasized the significance of activities that support student exploration.

In the early 1970s, **David Kolb and Roger Fry** developed the *experiential learning model* composed of four key elements: concrete experience, reflective observation, abstract conceptualization, and active experimentation (Aubrey & Riley, 2022). These elements form a cyclical process of learning, which can commence with any one of the four components but typically begins with a concrete experience. Although initially developed for adult education, the model has had far-reaching implications in higher education pedagogy. Kolb (1984) further elucidated the model with a graphical representation featuring two perpendicular continua—one pertaining to the learning process and the other to perception. Exhibit 3.4 provides examples of teaching methods grounded in constructivism.

Humanism

Rooted in humanistic psychology, *humanistic learning theory*, although largely constructivist, emphasizes both cognitive and affective learning. Learners are viewed as inherently good, with basic needs that should be met in order for them to learn well. Within this paradigm, learning is viewed as a personal act to fulfill one's potential (Schunk, 2020).

The humanistic learning theory was developed by **Abraham Maslow** (1908–1970) and **Carl Rogers** (1902–1987). Maslow's *hierarchy of needs*, first described in

EXHIBIT 3.4 Examples of Teaching Methods Based on Constructivism

Case-based learning
Class discussions and debates
Collaborative learning
Discovery learning
Field trips
Flipped classroom
Guided experimentation
Mind mapping
Peer tutoring
Problem and inquiry-based learning
Reflective logs
Project-based learning
Research projects
Scaffolded assignments
Simulation

1943, posits that all human actions are directed toward goal attainment. According to Maslow's hierarchy, individuals prioritize their needs in a hierarchical manner, with lower-order needs taking precedence over higher-order ones (Maslow, 1968). Physiological needs, such as food and water, form the foundation, followed by safety needs in response to environmental threats. Love and belonging needs become salient once basic physiological and safety needs are met, followed by esteem needs, which revolve around acceptance, achievement, and respect from others. At the pinnacle is the need for self-actualization, which entails personal growth and fulfillment (Maslow, 1943).

Notably, Maslow categorized the first four needs as deficiency needs, motivating individuals to address them in order to progress toward self-actualization. Encouraging learners to fulfill their deficiency needs empowers them to strive toward realizing their full potential (McLeod, 2024c). Maslow conceptualized self-actualization as a state of growth achievable only by individuals who have satisfied all lower-level needs, enabling them to "become everything that one is capable of becoming" (Maslow, 1943, p. 382). In 1970, Maslow expanded his hierarchy to include cognitive, aesthetic (1970a), and transcendence needs (1970b).

In recent years, there has been discussion about the relevance of the hierarchal order of Maslow's needs. Tay and Diener (2011) found that the order in which needs are met may vary based on socioeconomic status and ability to meet lower-level needs. Hopper (2020) has noted, however, that many researchers have built on Maslow's theory and still find relevance and use in it. For example, Carl Rogers extended and endorsed Maslow's work, emphasizing the importance of an environment characterized by genuineness, acceptance, and empathy to foster individual growth. Rogers asserted that individuals have the capacity to achieve their aspirations and goals, with self-actualization realized through this process (McLeod, 2024b). He advocated for student-centered classrooms and teacher facilitation of learning, rather than the mere dissemination of knowledge (Knowles et al., 2020). Examples of teaching methods based on humanism are displayed in Exhibit 3.5.

> **EXHIBIT 3.5 Examples of Teaching Methods Based on Humanism**
>
> Ensuring safe learning environments in which basic needs are met
> Allowing students to create personal learning goals and select opportunities
> Using participatory and discovery teaching methods to facilitate engagement
> Providing diverse resources
> Journaling to facilitate self-discovery and self-evaluation
> Checking in with students to establish a supportive student-teacher relationship

Feminist Pedagogy

Feminist pedagogy is described as engaged teaching and learning. Learners are self-reflective and engage with content within their learning community to enhance knowledge and envision social change (Shrewsbury, 1987). This educational practice, rooted in the works of scholars such as **Shrewsbury** (1987) and **Gilligan** (1982), emphasizes the importance of creating a space where critical thinking, empowerment, and growth are facilitated. The educator, in this setting, maintains a respectful learning environment, encourages open dialogue, and prompts reflection on diverse perspectives and assumptions. By adopting methods that allow students and teachers to co-construct knowledge through mutual learning, feminist pedagogy highlights the intrinsic connection between power and knowledge. It often brings issues of social justice and intersectionality to the forefront of the learning experience (Bostow et al., 2015). Additionally, the approach advocates for the educator's receptiveness to student input and flexibility in adjusting course content and activities to meet the evolving needs of the class (Yates, 2018). Exhibit 3.6 provides examples of teaching methods based on feminist pedagogy.

Other Transformative Theories and Frameworks

Other theorists and educators have developed useful models that build upon or align with the foundational schools of thought. Some of these are highlighted in the following.

Brain-Based Learning

In light of the rapid advancements in brain research over the past two decades, a new educational paradigm has emerged with educators like **Eric Jensen** (2020)

> **EXHIBIT 3.6 Examples of Teaching Methods Based on Feminist Pedagogy**
>
> Creation of safe and empowering environment where all voices are heard
> Discussion-based learning
> Critical thinking assignments
> Collaborative assignments and assessments
> Consciousness-raising exercises, activities, and resources
> Course materials examined to ensure that minoritized groups, voices are represented
> Role modeling, reflective dialogue, inclusive behaviors, embodiment of action, and leadership
> Receptivity to changing activities and content based on student input

synthesizing findings from neuroscience with pedagogical practices. *Brain-based learning* entails the deliberate utilization of purposeful strategies rooted in principles derived from an understanding of the brain (Jensen, 2020). According to cognitive neuroscientists, learning induces structural changes in the brain. Enhanced neuronal signaling leads to the proliferation of dendritic branches in the neocortex, thereby augmenting cellular density and fostering connections with neighboring neurons (resulting in increased synapses). Notably, these changes occur selectively in brain regions that are stimulated during learning. The amplification of synapses is facilitated by the repetitive activation of neurons specifically engaged in learning, under the influence of emotional neurotransmitters such as adrenaline and serotonin. The durability of learning correlates with the extent of engagement in these neocortical regions (Sousa, 2022). Jensen delineated seven core principles guiding brain-based learning, which hold significant implications for nurse educators. Exhibit 3.7 illustrates these brain-based principles and some implications for teaching.

Motivational Learning

Carol Dweck's research on self-beliefs about learning and intelligence exemplifies motivational learning theory (Mindset Works, Inc., 2017). Her work provided the terms *fixed mindset* and *growth mindset* and a theory on motivation, personality, and development. Building on recent research on brain plasticity, Dweck discovered that when individuals believe that their brain can grow, they act differently, which results in a change in mindset and associated increases in motivation and achievement. Her research has shown that teacher feedback impacts the mindset of students; for example, praising intelligence encourages a fixed mindset, whereas recognizing effort promotes a growth mindset.

Teaching Adults and Multiple Intelligences

Malcolm Knowles (1913–1997) coined the word *andragogy* to differentiate the learning needs of adults from children, thus identifying unique characteristics of adult learners in his *adult learning theory* (Knowles et al., 2020). For example, adult learners

---

EXHIBIT 3.7 Guiding Principles for Brain-Based Learning and Implications for Teaching

Brains are dynamic, not static: Remember that the brain changes every day.

Human brains are unique: Provide a variety and choice of teaching methods.

Brains use active construction of learning: Provide opportunities to use knowledge to do things.

Human brains are social brains: Intentionally foster relationships between students and with students.

Physical–cognitive connectivity: Engage students kinesthetically, provide breaks, and reduce stress.

Brains are designed for "gist" processing: Teach in small chunks and allow time for processing.

The arts boost attention, working memory, and visual spatial skills: Incorporate arts when feasible.

Humans are emotional by nature: Read and manage emotional states in the classroom.

Memory is malleable: Use multiple strategies to strengthen memory over time.

Source: Adapted from Jensen, E. (2020). *Brain-based learning* (3rd ed.). Corwin Press.

are internally motivated and need to be approached as capable, self-directed, and valued for their previous experiences. Adult learners value knowledge that is relevant to their specific learning goals and related to current life challenges. See Exhibit 3.8 for other characteristics and implications for teaching.

Howard Gardner (1943–present) argued that learning occurs in a variety of ways based on eight different intelligences. His *theory of multiple intelligences* suggests that human beings have a number of relatively discrete intellectual capacities (Gardner, 2011). This theory postulates that all humans possess the capacity to develop several intelligences, each of which has a unique and distinct profile. From the educator's perspective, this theory implies that all people are individuals, and each person should be taught in a way that best fits their intellectual profile. In addition, this theory lends itself well to the idea that teaching should use multiple methods in order to reach more students. Gardner's eight intelligences are as follows: spatial, bodily–kinesthetic, musical, linguistic, logical–mathematical, interpersonal, intrapersonal, and naturalistic.

Technology and Virtual Learning

It is important that educators consider the relationship between technology and learning. The questions of whether to integrate digital technology into teaching have been replaced by questions regarding which pedagogies take the newest technological and social contexts fully into account.

Matt Bower (2019) has proposed a *theory of technology-mediated learning* in which educators maintain power and agency over the technology used. This theory operates under the premise that technology should aid in conveying meaning to students, enhancing their learning experience. Through an integrated review of theory and research in the learning technology field, several premises of technology-mediated learning have emerged (Exhibit 3.9). These premises assert that educators must possess the knowledge and skills to understand, use, evaluate, and control technology, rather than allowing it to dictate the learning process.

Recent research has explored how technology-mediated learning specifically impacts experiential learning in a virtual environment (Mayer & Schwemmle, 2023), requiring educators to extend their roles. For example, educators must become both subject matter experts and digital experts able to translate a virtual setting into a clinical environment. Exhibit 3.10 provides examples of teaching methods consistent with technology-mediated learning theory.

EXHIBIT 3.8 Knowles's Core Adult Learning Principles

Adult students need to know why, what, and how.

Adult students are autonomous and self-directed.

Adult students come with prior experiences, resources, and mental models.

Adult students are motivated to learn in depth about problems related to real-life situations.

Adult students are problem-oriented rather than subject-oriented learners.

Although responsive to some external motivators, adult students are motivated most by internal factors (e.g., job satisfaction and self-esteem).

Source: Knowles, M. S., Holton, E. F., Swanson, R. A., & Robinson, P. A. (2020). *The adult learner: The definitive classic in adult education and human resource development* (9th ed.). Routledge.

EXHIBIT 3.9 Premises of Technology-Mediated Learning

Premise 1: Digital technologies can perform a mediating role for participants in their attempts to achieve learning goals.

Premise 2: In technology-mediated learning contexts, participant beliefs, knowledge, practices, and the environment all mutually influence one another.

Premise 3: In technology-mediated learning settings, the role of teachers is to help optimize student learning outcomes and experiences through the purposeful deployment of learning technologies.

Premise 4: The affordances of technologies, including their recognition and use, influences the sorts of representation, interaction, production, and learning that can take place.

Premise 5: The way in which modalities are used and combined influences the way in which meaning is processed, interpreted, created, and interrelated.

Premise 6: The way in which technology is used to mediate interaction patterns and possibilities between networks of participants influences the learning that takes place.

Premise 7: Arrangements of technologies and the way in which they are used can influence the sense of presence and community experienced.

Source: Bower, M. (2019). Technology-mediated learning theory. *British Journal of Educational Technology, 50*(3), 1035–1048. https://doi.org/10.1111/bjet.12771 Reprinted with permission of John Wiley & Sons, Inc.

EXHIBIT 3.10 Examples of Teaching Methods for Technology-Mediated Learning

Augmented reality programs
Immersive learning experiences
Live video discussion/class/demonstration
Participative learning online live forums, breakout groups
Virtual reality programs

The *community of inquiry framework,* developed by **Garrison et al.** (1999), is a learner-centered approach that underscores the active and collaborative nature of learning. Rooted in constructivism, this framework posits that knowledge is constructed through personal experience and continuous hypothesis testing via social interaction. It provides guidance on how communities of learners and educators can effectively engage in online environments to foster meaningful learning experiences.

The framework emphasizes three interdependent elements: social presence, cognitive presence, and teaching presence. Cognitive presence allows learners to "construct and confirm meaning through sustained reflection and discourse" (Garrison, et al., 2001, p. 11). Social presence develops when individuals can authentically express themselves in the online environment, fostering a sense of community. Teaching presence encompasses the intentional design, facilitation, and direction of both cognitive and social processes by the educator. Examples of teaching methods grounded in this framework are provided in Exhibit 3.11.

EXHIBIT 3.11 Examples of Teaching Methods Guided by the Community of Inquiry Framework

Planning course content
Supporting discourse
Establishing a course climate that facilitates social presence
Modeling caring behaviors
Providing opportunities for students to get to know one another
Connecting with students during the week through announcements
Creating smaller learning circles for discussion posts
Acknowledging when students post something interesting before adding new ideas
Ending posts with questions that encourage further dialogue in forums

Inclusive Pedagogy

Inclusive pedagogy aims to humanize the learning experience for all students by prioritizing flexibility, accessibility, sustainability, and sensitivity to diversity and inclusivity (Cotan et al., 2021). Key aspects of inclusive pedagogy include fostering a classroom environment where every student feels a sense of belonging and designing course activities and assessments with inclusivity and accessibility in mind (Chicago Center for Teaching, 2020). Exhibit 3.12 provides examples of specific teaching strategies using inclusive pedagogy.

Universal design for learning (UDL) is a framework that assists educators in designing curricula that offer equal learning opportunities to all students. Grounded in the provision of multiple means of engagement, representation, and action (CAST, 2024), UDL is particularly relevant as learning increasingly transitions to virtual environments. In these settings, students with limited broadband access may encounter challenges navigating digital platforms and video technologies (Stamler & Upvall, 2021). Pacansky-Brock and colleagues (2020) demonstrate how to integrate the theoretical foundations of UDL, culturally responsive teaching, social presence, and validation theory using humanizing strategies to cultivate instructor–student relationships and foster community in online teaching.

EXHIBIT 3.12 Examples of Teaching Methods Guided by Inclusive Pedagogy

Avoiding scheduling examinations or projects on religious or cultural holidays
Encouraging different perspectives and participation from all students
Sharing resources useful for students with different levels of accessibility or financial resources
Integrating course content and assessments that accommodate different learning styles
Encouraging cooperative learning

> **EXHIBIT 3.13 Resources for Developing a Teaching Philosophy**
>
> Center for Educational Innovation. (2024). *Writing your teaching philosophy*. University of Minnesota. https://cei.umn.edu/teaching-resources/writing-your-teaching-philosophy
>
> Center for Teaching and Learning. (2024). *Writing a teaching philosophy statement*. Western University. https://teaching.uwo.ca/awardsdossiers/teachingphilosophy.html
>
> Rao, A. (2020). *Writing a teaching philosophy or a teaching statement*. Indiana University Center for Teaching and Learning. https://ctl.iupui.edu/Resources/Documenting-Your-Teaching/Tips-for-Writing-a-Statement-of-Teaching-Philosophy

USING THEORIES AND FRAMEWORKS IN PRACTICE

Teaching Philosophy

As Palmer (2017) describes in *The Courage to Teach*, although good teaching can take many forms, a good educator is always authentically present and connected with their self, their students, and their subject. Understanding of teaching and learning theories can provide a foundation for exploring your personal teaching philosophy or philosophy of education. Your teaching philosophy may evolve, supported by intentional reflection on your teaching and learning experiences in addition to theories, methods, and outcomes. This reflective practice should include cultivating awareness of how your personal values, beliefs, and experiences resonate with various schools of thought and theories, specific student populations, and the subjects that you teach.

As you begin your journey as a nurse educator, consider writing a teaching philosophy to demonstrate the purposefulness of your course development, teaching strategies, and methods of assessing teaching and learning. Academic organizations often request a statement of teaching philosophy during the application process. Your teaching philosophy statement should (a) explain your teaching methods; (b) include your view of the purpose and goals of education and of the roles of the educator and learner; and (c) provide a picture of how your learning environment looks and feels. Your teaching philosophy can be shared with students and should be evidenced throughout your course materials, starting with your syllabus. Exhibit 3.13 provides a few helpful resources for writing a teaching philosophy.

SUMMARY

Nurse educators play a pivotal role in shaping the teaching and learning landscape, extending their influence beyond the traditional classroom to nursing skills laboratories, clinical settings, simulations, and student advisement sessions. Understanding the nuances of how students learn in these diverse environments is crucial for effective instruction. Foundational and transformative theories provide frameworks to elucidate the learning process and inform the selection of appropriate teaching methodologies. It is imperative for nurse educators to cultivate a robust teaching philosophy rooted in evidence-based practices and grounded in a comprehensive understanding of learning theories. While this chapter provides an overview of foundational and transformative learning theories, readers are encouraged to delve deeper into the subject matter through web-based resources such as Simply Psychology (https://www.simplypsychology.org/theories/learning-theories), Education Corner (https://www.educationcorner.com/learning-theories-in-education), and The Helpful Professor (https://helpfulprofessor.com/learning-theories). These resources serve as valuable guides for nurse educators seeking to enhance their pedagogical practices and optimize student learning outcomes.

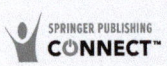 A robust set of instructor resources designed to supplement this text is located at http://connect.springerpub.com/content/book/978-0-8261-8892-2. Qualifying instructors may request access by emailing textbook@springerpub.com.

REFERENCES

Aubrey, K., & Riley, A. (2022). *Understanding and using educational theories*. SAGE.

Bandura, A. (1977). *Social learning theory*. General Learning Press.

Bandura, A. (1986). *Social foundations of thought and action: A social cognitive theory*. Prentice Hall.

Bostow, R., Brewer, S., Chick, N., Galina, B., McGrath, Al., Mendoza, K., Navarro, K., & Valle-Ruiz, L. (2015, March). *A guide to feminist pedagogy*. Vanderbilt University Center for Teaching. https://my.vanderbilt.edu/femped

Bower, M. (2019). Technology-mediated learning theory. *British Journal of Educational Technology, 50*(3), 1035–1048. https://doi.org/10.1111/bjet.12771

Boyle, T. (2010). *The brain: Changing the adult mind through the power of plasticity*. https://www.brainhq.com/news/latest-news/the-brain-changing-the-adult-mind-through-the-power-of-plasticity

Bruner, J. (1964). The course of cognitive growth. *American Psychologist, 19*(1), 1–15. https://doi.org/10.1037/h0044160

CAST (2024). Universal Design for Learning Guidelines version 3.0. https://udlguidelines.cast.org

Chicago Center for Teaching. (2020). *Inclusive pedagogy*. The University of Chicago. https://inclusivepedagogy.uchicago.edu

Cotán, A., Aguirre, A., Morgado, B., & Melero, N. (2021). Methodological strategies of faculty members: Moving toward inclusive pedagogy in higher education. *Sustainability, 13*(6), 3031. https://doi.org/10.3390/su13063031

Fabio, M. (2019). *How the Socratic method works and why is it used in law school*. ThoughtCo. https://www.thoughtco.com/what-is-the-socratic-method-2154875

Gagne, R. M. (1985). *The conditions of learning and theory of instruction* (4th ed.). Holt, Rinehart, and Winston.

Gardner, H. (2011). *Frames of mind: The theory of multiple intelligences*. Basic Books.

Garrison, D. R., Anderson, T., & Archer, W. (1999). Critical inquiry in a text-based environment: Computer conferencing in higher education. *The Internet and Higher Education, 2*(2–3), 87–105. https://doi.org/10.1016/S1096-7516(00)00016-6

Garrison, D., Anderson, T., & Archer, W. (2001). Critical thinking, cognitive presence, and computer conferencing in distance education. *American Journal of Distance Education, 15*, 7–23. https://doi.org/10.1080/08923640109527071

Gilligan, C. (1982). *In a different voice: Psychological theory and women's development*. Harvard University Press.

Hilgard, E. R. (1996). Perspectives on educational psychology. *Educational Psychology Review, 8*(4), 419–431. https://doi.org/10.1007/BF01463942

Hilgard, E. R., & Bower, G. H. (1975). *Theories of learning*. Prentice-Hall.

Hopper, E. (2020, February 24). *Maslow's hierarchy of needs explained*. https://www.thoughtco.com/maslows-hierarchy-of-needs-4582571

Huitt, W., & Hummel, J. (2003). Piaget's theory of cognitive development. In *Educational psychology interactive*. Valdosta State University. https://www.edpsycinteractive.org/topics/cognition/piaget.html

Jensen, E. (2020). *Brain-based learning* (3rd ed.). Corwin Press.

King, L. (n.d.). *Ancient history sourcebook: Code of Hammurabi*. http://www.fordham.edu/halsall/ancient/hamcode.asp

Knowles, M. S., Holton, E. F., Swanson, R. A., & Robinson, P. A. (2020). *The adult learner: The definitive classic in adult education and human resource development* (9th ed.). Routledge.

Kolb, D. A. (1984). *Experiential learning as the source of learning and development*. Prentice Hall.

Lave, J., & Wenger, E. (1991). *Situated learning: Legitimate peripheral participation*. Cambridge University Press.

Maslow, A. (1943). A theory of human motivation. *Psychological Review, 50*(4), 370–396. https://doi.org/10.1037/h0054346

Maslow, A. H. (1968). *Toward a psychology of being* (2nd ed.). Van Nostrand Reinhold.

Maslow, A. H. (1970a). *Motivation and personality*. Harper & Row.

Maslow, A. H. (1970b). *Religions, values, and peak experiences*. Penguin.

Mayer, S., & Schwemmle, M. (2023). Teaching university students through technology-mediated experiential learning: Educators' perspectives and roles. *Computers & Education, 207*, 104923. https://doi.org/10.1016/j.compedu.2023.104923

McLeod, S. A. (2024a, February 2). *B.F. Skinner operant conditioning*. http://www.simplypsychology.org/operant-conditioning.html

McLeod, S. A. (2024b, January 29). *Carl Rogers*. https://www.simplypsychology.org/carl-rogers.html

McLeod, S. A. (2024c, January 24). *Maslow's hierarchy of needs*. www.simplypsychology.org/maslow.html

Mindset Works, Inc. (2017). *Decades of scientific research that started a growth mindset revolution*. https://www.mindsetworks.com/science

Pacansky-Brock, M., Smedshammer, M., & Vincent-Layton, K. (2020). Humanizing online teaching to equitize higher education. *Current Issues in Education, 21*(2), 1–21. https://cie.asu.edu/ojs/index.php/cieatasu/article/view/1905

Palmer, P. J. (2017). *The courage to teach: Exploring the inner landscape of a teacher's life* (Twentieth anniversary edition). Jossey-Bass.

Pavlov, I. (1927). *Conditioned reflexes*. Oxford University Press.

Pi, Y. L., Wu, X. H., Wang, F. J., Liu, K., Wu, Y., Zhu, H., & Zhang, J. (2019). Motor skill learning induces brain network plasticity: A diffusion-tensor imaging study. *PLoS One, 14*(2), e0210015. https://doi.org/10.1371/journal.pone.0210015

Schunk, D. H. (2020). *Learning theories: An educational perspective* (8th ed.). Pearson.

Shrewsbury, C. M. (1987). What is feminist pedagogy? *Women's Studies Quarterly, 15*(3/4), 6–14.

Skinner, B. F. (1953). *Science and human behavior*. Free Press.

Sousa, D. (2022). *How the brain learns* (6th ed.). Corwin Press.

Stamler, L. L., & Upvall, M. J. (2021). Global inequity in nursing education: A call to action. *International Journal of Nursing Education Scholarship, 18*(1), 20210131. https://doi.org/10.1515/ijnes-2021-0131

Tay, L., & Diener, E. (2011). Needs and subjective well-being around the world. *Journal of Personality and Social Psychology, 101*(2), 354–365. https://doi.org/10.1037/a0023779

Thorndike, E. L., & Gates A. I. (1929). *Elementary principles of education*. MacMillan.

Utley, R. (2011). *Theory and research for academic nurse educators*. Jones and Bartlett.

Yates, H. T., & Rai, A. (2018). A scoping review of feminism in U.S. social work education: Strategies and implications for the contemporary classroom. *Journal of Evidence Based Social Work, 16*(2), 1–13. https://doi.org/10.1080/23761407.2018.1555070

Understanding the Diverse Learner

4

Stephanie A. Gedzyk-Nieman and Mark C. Hand

OBJECTIVES

1. Examine the diverse attributes that learners bring to a nursing program
2. Analyze learner differences that can influence teaching methods and student engagement
3. Explore effective strategies for inclusive pedagogy

INTRODUCTION

Nurse educators play a pivotal role in shaping the future healthcare workforce, but to do so effectively, they must possess a profound understanding of the diverse attributes such as age, gender, race, and social determinants of health (SDOH) which influence student learning processes and outcomes. By tailoring teaching approaches to accommodate diversity, nurse educators can create an inclusive and supportive learning environment that nurtures the unique strengths of each student and contributes to the development of well-rounded and culturally sensitive nursing professionals. This chapter examines how the diverse attributes of nursing students shape their learning and presents multiple strategies that nurse educators can use to meet the needs of diverse learners.

LEARNER ATTRIBUTES

As the population of the United States becomes increasingly diverse, nursing education programs must strive to prepare future nursing professionals whose diversity reflects that of the broader population and who can provide knowledgeable and respectful care to all people. Traditionally, most nursing students have been White, non-Hispanic, and female. However, in 2022, underrepresented student enrollment increased to 41.5% (from 30.9% in 2020), and male enrollment increased to 13.3% (National League for Nursing [NLN], 2023a). To foster diversity beyond gender and ethnicity, many nursing programs have begun using a holistic approach to their admissions process. Applicants are still required to meet minimum educational standards, such as GPA requirements and prerequisite coursework, to ensure that they have the foundational knowledge necessary for success in the program; however, schools are considering additional factors to select candidates who demonstrate a significant potential to thrive in the program and contribute positively to the profession (Dawkins et al., 2022).

A holistic admissions approach assesses applicants' experiences, attributes, and personal characteristics, including leadership skills, resilience, empathy, communication abilities, cultural competence, and ethical values. These qualities are essential for nursing professionals who must interact effectively with diverse patients and provide compassionate, patient-centered care. Applicants' involvement in extracurricular activities, volunteer work, healthcare-related experiences, research projects, internships, or employment in healthcare settings may also be considered (Jung et al., 2021), as these experiences provide insights into applicants' interests, passions, service dedication, and healthcare field exposure. Consideration of applicants' socioeconomic status, race, ethnicity, gender, sexual orientation, and cultural background serves to create a more diverse learning environment and enhances the diversity of the nursing workforce (Lewis et al., 2021).

As a result of holistic admissions, learners are coming to nursing education programs with varied backgrounds, perspectives, life experiences, preferences, capabilities, and resources. Nurse educators must recognize how these various attributes influence student learning in order to implement effective teaching strategies. However, even if an attribute can be identified in a learner, the educator must always be mindful of the danger of generalizing.

Culture

Rapid globalization is creating unprecedented diversity in higher education and providing intercultural learning environments in which students learn from and with one another (Markey et al., 2020). Nurse educators are tasked with understanding the unique learning needs of students from diverse linguistic, cultural, and ethnic backgrounds, and they need to be familiar with multiple teaching methods to accommodate this range of needs.

Nursing education requires the use and understanding of rigorous academic language and terminology, so nursing students from diverse linguistic backgrounds face an additional challenge. According to the U.S. Department of Education, National Center for Education Statistics (2023a), the number of non-English speaking public school students continues to rise, with an estimated 5 million students in 2020 learning English as their additional language. This reality suggests that students for whom English is not a primary language may experience a lower level of verbal fluency in English (Tigert & Golnar, 2022), often finding reading and writing in English more accessible than verbal communicate. Teaching strategies to help such students include (a) making digitally archived video and audio class sessions available for access outside the classroom; (b) providing content in a written format for access before class; (c) being mindful of the use of colloquialisms and idioms; and (d) using activities such as simulation to provide kinesthetic as well as auditory and visual cues to meaning.

In North America, Western perspectives of learning and knowing are ubiquitous. Such perspectives value the individual learner over the collective and promote autonomy and independence of thought and action, whereas Eastern perspectives tend to place a primary value on communal connections (Layman, 2018). Similarly, Western cultural norms are based on an ideology of individualism (i.e., focus

> **EXHIBIT 4.1 Teaching Strategies for Inclusion in Multicultural Classrooms**
>
> Become aware of your own cultural biases.
> Treat each student as a unique individual.
> Maintain a culturally neutral classroom.
> Emphasize cooperation instead of competition.
> Recognize the complexity of diversity.
> Foster intergroup relations.
> Be concrete and explicit.
> Monitor your use of idioms, abbreviations, and slang.
> Be accessible, with clear times of availability.
> Digitally archive videos or audio files of classes for students to review.
> Use diverse examples, pictures, case studies, etc., but avoid stereotypes.
> Encourage sharing of culturally diverse life experiences.
> Provide discussion questions in advance to allow non-native English speakers an opportunity to process them.

primarily on the intrinsic worth of the individual), whereas certain Asian, African, Latin American, and Native American cultures are based on collectivism (i.e., place a higher value on the whole than on the individual; Layman, 2018). Both Western and Eastern perspectives have produced valuable lessons in education (Chang, 2021); therefore, nurse educators should recognize ethnocentrism and develop courses with multicultural perspectives. Examples of teaching strategies for use in multicultural classrooms are provided in Exhibit 4.1.

RACE

Racial diversity in nursing programs mirrors the growing racial diversity of the U.S. population. Racially diverse students include those who are Black, Latinx, Native American, and Asian. The proportion of racially diverse RN students grew from 10% in 2020 to 42% in 2022 (NLN, 2023b). However, because 76% of nurse educators are White (NLN, 2023b), some nursing students are at risk for experiencing bias and microaggressions which could negatively impact their success and well-being.

Microaggressions are repeated subtle verbal and nonverbal derogatory exchanges that target individuals based on their identification of belonging to a minority group (Sue, 2010). A national study found that racially diverse nursing students experienced significantly higher rates of microaggressions than their White counterparts, with Black students experiencing the highest rate (Ackerman-Barger et al., 2022). Such experiences can result in dissatisfaction with school; lead to disengagement, decreased sense of belonging, or depression; or manifest in academic difficulties or leaving nursing school.

Nurse educators have a responsibility to identify and mitigate microaggressions, which often arise from unconscious or conscious biases including those of the nurse educator. Nurse educators should explore unconscious and conscious biases that might damage efforts to enhance diversity, inclusion, and belonging (American Association of Colleges of Nursing [AACN], 2017) and should practice micro-affirmation strategies such as active listening, affirming emotions, and validating experiences. Exhibit 4.2 provides additional methods of avoiding microaggressions.

> **EXHIBIT 4.2 Strategies to Avoid and Mitigate Microaggressions**
>
> Learn the names of all students and pronounce them correctly.
> Ask questions of all students.
> Do not allow a few students to dominate discussions.
> Assess how you respond to students.
> Avoid interrupting student responses.
> Use group activities to foster student confidence and inclusivity.
> Create affinity groups for students around a shared identity or common interests.
> Provide all students with feedback and encouragement.
> Promote respectful classroom and online environments that are accepting of differences.
> Use diverse examples that do not assume a specific background or experience.
> Ensure that all students are held to the same academic standards.
> If a microaggression occurs, do not be afraid to talk about it. Own and apologize for the incident and explore how it can be avoided in the future.

AGE

The age composition of the student population in higher education has changed significantly over the past decades. Since the end of World War II, when many returning veterans enrolled in programs, colleges have seen rapid increases in the number of adult learners. Adult learners are considered "nontraditional" college students, a term that describes any student who delays starting college, attends college on a part-time basis, works full time, has dependents, is a single parent, is financially independent, or does not have a high school diploma (U.S. Department of Education, National Center for Education Statistics, n.d.).

Although students often have competing demands, the demands of nontraditional learners can be more difficult to manage and increase their likelihood of attrition (U.S. Department of Education, National Center for Education Statistics, n.d.). In one study, nontraditional nursing students indicated that encouragement from friends, both internal and external to their programs, had the most influence on their success (Priode et al., 2020). To promote peer encouragement, nurse educators should create opportunities for students to connect and share a sense of community; such opportunities can be achieved through peer mentorship programs, small study groups, and social events.

It is important to recognize and accommodate adult learners' unique learning needs. In 1973, Malcolm Knowles outlined differences between children and adult learners, introducing the term "andragogy" in reference to the learning needs of adult learners. Knowles identified six assumptions about adult learning (Knowles et al., 2015):

1. Need to Know: Adults prefer to know why they are learning particular content at the outset of learning. Teachers should assist adults to contextualize the learning to recognize its importance.

2. Learner's Self-Concept: Adult self-concept is dependent on progress toward self-direction. Adults need to be approached as capable and self-directed learners.

3. Role of the Learner's Experiences: Adults enter into education with prior experiences that provide them with additional valuable resources; therefore, developing active learning strategies that build on adults' experiences is beneficial.

4. Readiness to Learn: Adults become ready to learn when they can use their learning to deal with real-life situations or perform a task. They want to learn what they can apply to current situations.

5. Orientation to Learning: Adults are life-centered (task-centered, problem-centered) in their orientation to learning. They want to learn what will help them perform tasks or deal with problems they confront in everyday situations and those presented in the context of application to real life.

6. Motivation: Adults are responsive to some external motivators (e.g., better job, higher salary), but the most potent motivators are internal (e.g., desire for increased job satisfaction and self-esteem)

Adult learners, although often classified as one large age group, comprise several age groups based on the year (or generation) in which they were born (Table 4.1). Millennials currently comprise the largest generation in America (Fry, 2020). Much has been published about learning, values, motivation, and delivery method preferences for each generation; it is important to note that age, formative life experiences such as world events or major shifts, and life cycle can affect how individuals approach learning and education.

Nurse educators must accommodate intergenerational classrooms and clinical settings, the needs of traditional and adult learners, and generational differences between themselves and their learners. In the 2021 to 2022 academic year, 54% of students in RN programs were under the age of 25, yet 41% of nurse educators were between 46 and 60 years old (NLN, 2023b), and the average age of RNs was 46 years old (National Council State Boards of Nursing, 2022). Baby boomer and Gen X educators and nurses who teach Gen Z students may rely on learning strategies, educational tools, and norms used in their own educational attainment, which can lead to misunderstanding and frustration. For example, educators may become frustrated if students do not complete assigned textbook readings to prepare for class. Similarly, nursing staff could misinterpret students' use of cell phones in a clinical as disrespectful, not realizing that they are accessing online videos to prepare for a nursing procedure. Exhibit 4.3 lists helpful teaching strategies for use in multigenerational classrooms.

GENDER AND SEXUALLY DIVERSE GROUPS

Although historically dominated by women, the nursing profession is experiencing a significant transformation that challenges traditional gender stereotypes and enriches the diversity of the healthcare workforce. Nationally, 11.2% of the RN workforce is male (National Council State Boards of Nursing, 2022), and only 8% of full-time faculty who teach in baccalaureate and higher degree programs are men (NLN, 2022). However, in nursing programs, male students comprise 13% of enrollees in associate degree or BSN programs, 13% in RN-BSN programs, 12% in MSN programs, and 11% in doctoral nursing programs (AACN, 2022). Despite the increasing number of men pursuing careers in nursing, male nurses may face

TABLE 4.1 GENERATIONAL DIFFERENCES IN VALUES, LEARNING, AND TEACHING METHODS

Generation and Ages	Values	Learning Motivation	Delivery Methods	Feedback
Baby Boomers 1946–1964	Optimistic, involved, hard working	Self-directed learners, public and peer recognition, relevance to career goals	Traditional lecture and textbooks, face-to-face interactions, independent work, small group discussion	Well-documented feedback all at once
Generation X 1965–1980	Informal, skeptical, self-reliant	Relevance to career goals, recognition by faculty	Flexible learning environment, mix of traditional and non-traditional teaching methods, hands-on learning, e-learning, independent work	Regular ongoing feedback
Millennial/ Gen Y 1981–1996	Realists, confident, frequent use of social networking	Fast track to success, use of technology is an expectation, structured assignments with clear deadlines, short attention span	e-learning, blogs, wikis, podcasts, mobile apps, gamification, hands-on learning, socialization assignments, visuals and images	Frequent, immediate feedback
Generation Z, iGen, Centennials 1997–2012	Ethnically diverse, globally aware, socially minded, value self-care, concerned about their mental health	Digital natives, technology-dependent and adaptive, collaborative, instant gratification	Dislike traditional classroom format and textbooks, multitaskers, gamification, online polling, videos, microlearning, high-level of interaction	Instant feedback

> **EXHIBIT 4.3 Examples of Teaching Strategies for Multigenerational Classrooms**
>
> Provide study or reading guides and terminology worksheets.
> Create group, cooperative learning, and hands-on learning opportunities.
> Incorporate class time devoted to clarifying difficult concepts and answering questions.
> Utilize mini-lectures and problem-based learning.
> Provide multiple modalities and opportunities for students to engage with the educator.
> Incorporate examples that resonate with all generations.

Source: Schnell-Peskin, L., Riley, G., Hodnett, K., Gryta, V., & Kisamore, A. (2024). Meeting the needs of students in higher education multigenerational classrooms: What can educators do? *International Journal of Information and Learning Technology, 41*(1), 73–85. https://doi.org/10.1108/IJILT-04-2023-0057

challenges related to negative perceptions of their abilities, motivations, or suitability for certain roles, creating the need for continuous efforts to break down such barriers (Mulkey, 2023).

Men in nursing often confront stereotypes and societal expectations regarding caregiving roles predominantly associated with women (Bordelon et al., 2023), which can lead to bias, discrimination, and the perpetuation of gender norms within the healthcare sector, yet men contribute valuable diverse perspectives and strengths to problem-solving, teamwork, and communication within the nursing profession. Their unique experiences and backgrounds enhance the multidimensional nature of patient care and contribute to more holistic and patient-centered healthcare (Bayuo et al., 2022). The increasing representation of men in nursing also broadens the diversity of role models for aspiring healthcare professionals, inspiring future generations to pursue careers based on passion and aptitude rather than on traditional gender expectations.

An inclusive environment in nursing education is vital to ensuring that male students feel respected and valued. Educators must challenge gender biases and stereotypes, promote diversity within educational curricula, and establish policies that prohibit discrimination based on gender (Bordelon et al., 2023). Gender-associated incivility in nursing schools is influenced by stereotypes related to touch and masculinity, insufficient social support during school and transition to practice, and gender bias in recruitment and retention and in clinical rotations, particularly in obstetrics (Smallheer et al., 2021). Educational institutions should actively work to address male nursing students' specific needs and experiences, recognizing that fostering an inclusive environment benefits all student learners.

LGBTQ+ nursing students may face unique challenges in their educational journey due to societal prejudices, discrimination, and a lack of inclusive policies within academic institutions (Jaekel, 2021). In order to foster a supportive and equitable learning environment, educators must understand and address the potential for discrimination or bias, both subtle and overt, which can create a hostile atmosphere for LGBTQ+ students. Instances include inappropriate comments, microaggressions, or exclusionary behaviors that can negatively impact mental health or hinder academic performance (Miller et al., 2021). Another challenge for

LGBTQ+ nursing students entails their lack of representation and visibility within the curriculum. Limited inclusion of LGBTQ+ health topics in nursing education can result in a gap in knowledge related to the specific healthcare needs and disparities experienced by LGBTQ+ individuals (Hand & Gedzyk-Nieman, 2022). Additionally, the absence of LGBTQ+ role models in the nursing field can contribute to a sense of isolation and hinder the formation of professional identity. LGBTQ+ students also face challenges related to the disclosure of their identities, as fear of stigma or discrimination may lead to hesitancy in expressing their true selves. In some instances, this fear can impact their ability to engage fully in the learning process or hinder their development of trusting relationships with faculty and peers.

To address these challenges, nursing education programs should strive to create an inclusive and affirming environment by (a) implementing policies that explicitly prohibit discrimination based on sexual orientation and gender identity, (b) incorporating LGBTQ+ health content into the curriculum, and (c) promoting diverse role models (Beasy et al., 2023; MacDaniel, 2020). All nurse educators should receive training in LGBTQ+ cultural competency to foster understanding of LGBTQ+ nursing students' unique needs and experiences. Additionally, the establishment of support networks, mentorship programs, and mental health resources specific to LGBTQ+ students can promote inclusivity in the learning environment and help all nursing students to thrive (Cox et al., 2023). Exhibit 4.4 provides some strategies for creating a gender-inclusive teaching situation.

EXHIBIT 4.4 Teaching Strategies to Create a Gender-Inclusive Learning Environment

- Use inclusive language that avoids assumptions about gender. Instead of "he" or "she," use "they" when referring to an individual in a hypothetical context.
- Be sure examples include both male, female, and nonbinary references.
- Encourage students to share their pronouns, and model this practice by including your pronouns in introductions.
- Incorporate diverse examples and case studies that feature individuals from various gender identities, backgrounds, and experiences.
- Ensure that educational resources, including textbooks, reading materials, and visual aids, avoid reinforcing gender stereotypes.
- Use gender-neutral language in case studies, examples, and exam questions.
- Highlight the achievements and contributions of diverse role models within the subject matter, showcasing a range of gender identities.
- Avoid gender-based grouping whenever possible. Instead, use various criteria such as interest, skills, or randomly assigned groups to encourage diverse interaction
- Be mindful of implicit bias when forming groups and ensure equitable opportunities for participation.
- Provide feedback and recognition based on individual achievements and efforts, rather than focusing on gender.
- Acknowledge and celebrate the diverse talents and contributions of all students.

Source: Iduye, D., Vukic, A., Waldron, I., Price, S., Sheffer, C., McKibbon, S., Dorey, R., & Yu, Z. (2021). Educators' strategies for engaging diverse students in undergraduate nursing education programs: A scoping review protocol. *JBI Evidence Synthesis, 19*(5), 1178–1185. https://doi.org/10.11124/JBIES-20-00039

Social Determinants of Health

Nursing education is increasingly recognizing the importance of teaching students about the impact of SDOH on patient-centered care delivery, health equity, and patient outcomes. SDOH are "conditions in the environments where people are born, live, learn, work, play, worship, and age that affect a wide range of health, functioning, and quality-of-life outcomes and risks" (Healthy People 2030, n.d.). Exhibit 4.5 lists the five critical domains of SDOH listed in Healthy People 2030 (n.d.). The World Health Organization (n.d.) also includes economic policies and systems, and social policies and norms, as elements of the environment. This approach to exploring health outcomes considers the impact of external forces rather than focusing solely on individual biological factors. Nurse educators should consider incorporating exploration of the elements of SDOH into their curriculum to increase student success and education equity.

Building upon the health concepts in the SDOH model, Levinson and Cohen (2023) developed the *Social Determinates of Learning* (SDOL) model (Figure 4.1) to identify "social and structural factors outside the individual learner, often beyond

---

EXHIBIT 4.5 Five Social Determinants of Health

Economic Stability
- Poverty
- Employment
- Food security
- Housing stability

Education Access and Quality
- High school graduation
- Enrollment in higher education
- Language, literacy, and mathematics
- Early childhood education and development
- Addressing disabilities

Social and Community Context
- Social cohesion and inclusion
- Civic participation
- Discrimination
- Incarceration

Healthcare Access and Quality
- Access to primary and dental care
- Health literacy and communication

Neighborhood and Built Environment
- Access to healthy foods
- Access to the internet
- Access to transportation
- Quality of housing and neighborhoods
- Crime and violence
- Environmental conditions

Source: Healthy People 2030. U.S. Department of Health and Human Services, Office of Disease Prevention and Health Promotion. (n.d.). *Social determinants of health.* https://health.gov/healthypeople/priority-areas/social-determinants-health

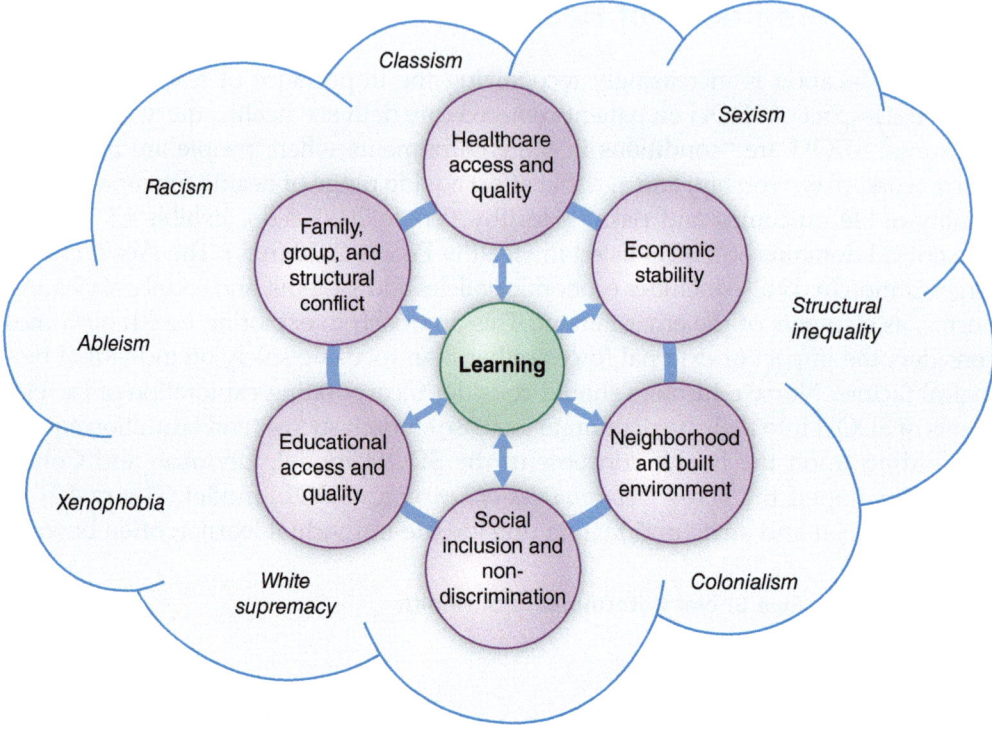

Figure 4.1 Social determinants of learning model.
Source: Levinson, M., & Cohen, A. K. (2023). Social determinants of learning: Implications for research, policy, and practice. *American Educational Research Association, 9,*(1–8). https://doi.org/10.1177/23328584231206087 This article is distributed under the terms of the Creative Commons Attribution-NonCommercial 4.0 License (https://creativecommons.org/licenses/by-nc/4.0/).

EXHIBIT 4.6 Strategies to Address Social Determinants of Learning

Create a freely accessible student food pantry.
Provide healthy snacks in class and/or office.
Confidentially solicit student class and clinical schedule needs when semester planning.
Encourage the creation of student carpools.
Become aware of school and community housing and healthcare resources.
Offer school-funded or volunteer tutoring and/or writing assistance.
Create a student emergency fund.
Offer extended building hours to increase access to safe spaces and the internet.
Create a uniform and/or textbook exchange program.
Create student community-building opportunities.
Offer loaner laptops.

---

the traditional reach of teachers and schools, that can affect learning" (p. 2). Similar to Maslow's hierarchy of needs, discussed in Chapter 3, this model posits that basic need attainment allows increased cognitive processing and achievement of growth and development. For example, a nursing student who is unable to afford adequate nutrition or housing may not process information as quickly or as well as others due to hunger and fatigue. Furthermore, the SDOL moves beyond basic human needs and encourages consideration of other factors that can impact student success. For instance, a nursing student who does not have access to a vehicle may face challenges related to attending class and clinical; similarly, a student without access to reliable internet may be unable to complete assignments. It is essential to recognize that students may feel reluctant to share their experiences of challenges; therefore, nurse educators should examine classroom and institutional policies and resources to ensure that students can have their needs addressed without having to share information about their personal circumstances and request assistance directly. Exhibit 4.6 provides strategies for nurse educators to address SDOL.

STRATEGIC LEARNING AND GROWTH MINDSET

There are cognitive and motivational models available to inform nurse educators' development of instructional strategies that promote a sense of autonomy and agency, thus allowing students to become strategic learners. Strategic learners are active and persistent learners; their self-determined goals for learning are reasonable and attainable, which motivate them to continue studying (Schunk, 2020). They recognize that learning is under their own control and know when to seek out resources to facilitate meeting their learning goals (Schunk, 2020).

It is important to realize that the goals of strategic learners are learning based rather than performance based: These learners focus not on how well they learn compared to others but on the value of learning and the acquisition of new knowledge (Wolcott et al., 2021). The growth mindset model offers one method of helping students become strategic learners. According to Dweck's mindset model (2006), learners either believe that intelligence is fixed and success is based on talent (i.e., fixed mindset) or that intelligence is malleable and success is based on effort (i.e., growth mindset). Subscribing to a fixed mindset can limit learning; however, subscribing to a growth mindset can make learning limitless. Table 4.2 compares characteristics of these two mindsets.

TABLE 4.2 FIXED AND GROWTH MINDSET FEATURES

Features	Fixed Mindset	Growth Mindset
Goals/focus	"I have to get an A, or they will think I am not smart enough to be here."	"I want to be able to understand and apply these concepts."
Perception of effort	"I am having a hard time with this. There is something wrong with me."	"I am having a hard time with this. I had better ask for help."
Response to criticism	"They do not know what they are talking about."	"This is helpful for me moving forward."
Response to failure/obstacles	"I'll never learn this."	"I have not learned this, yet."

> **EXHIBIT 4.7 Strategies to Promote Growth Mindset**
>
> Formally introduce the growth mindset approach early in the course and then reinforce it throughout.
>
> Have students write letters to themselves about how what they are learning will impact their future practice.
>
> Have students write letters to future or new students about how they belong, and encourage help-seeking behaviors.
>
> Consider replacing the customary rubric heading "Does Not Meet Expectations" with a "Not Yet" heading.
>
> Encourage collaboration, not competition.
>
> Create a safe learning environment.
>
> Avoid making premature assumptions regarding student likelihood of success (e.g., based on the score of the course's first exam).
>
> Call on all students, not just those perceived as successful in the course.
>
> Focus on building student competence and personal growth over time.
>
> Praise students for effort, persistence, acceptance of challenges, and personal growth.

Changing to a growth mindset approach is challenging due to higher education's practice of ranking learners and its historical focus on competition and high performers; however, there are documented benefits to its use. For students, these include improved resiliency and psychological well-being, greater openness to failure and feedback, and improved academic performance (Schunk, 2020; Wolcott et al., 2021). For educators, these include improved relationships with students, self-esteem, and confidence (Wolcott et al., 2021). There are several strategies that nurse educators can use to foster a growth mindset (Exhibit 4.7). At the core of these strategies are three key concepts: praise for process and effort, not talent; creating a sense of belonging; and reinforcing how the belief in brain growth when learning new things can positively influence academic success (Williams, 2020).

Learning Style Preferences

Learning styles, also described in the literature as learning preferences, have been studied for more than 50 years. Boland and Amonoo (2021) explained that learning styles are "how learners collect, assimilate, organize, and store information" (p. 142). A *learning style preference* is the learner's tendency to utilize a particular style of learning. This preference does remain constant over time, but there is mixed evidence that students learn better using their preferred learning style (Boland & Amonoo, 2021). The value for educators in understanding learning styles is to improve students' learning experiences via the creation of multiple approaches to teaching a topic. Identification of learning style preferences encourages greater engagement and deeper learning; it is also useful for students to examine their preferences to develop better study methods and identify ways to improve their learning outcomes.

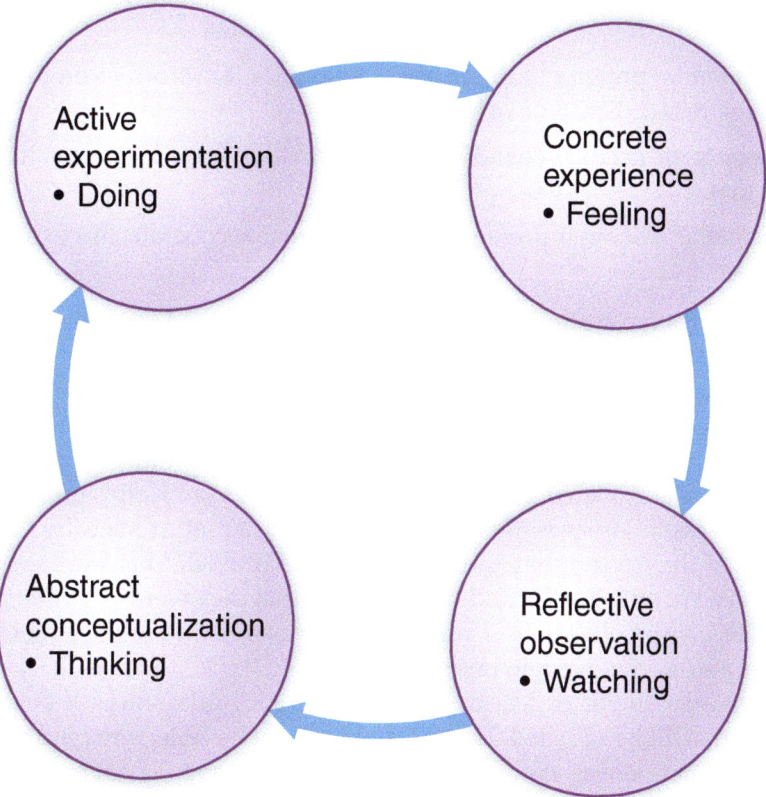

FIGURE 4.2 Kolb's learning cycle and learning styles.
Source: Adapted from Kolb, D. (1984). *Experiential learning: Experience as the source of learning and development*. Prentice-Hall.

There are many models of learning style preferences. Popular theorists such as Kolb (1975, 1984) and Fleming and Mills (1992) described learning styles and learner preferences from different theoretical and physiological perspectives. Based on the concepts of his experiential learning model, Kolb hypothesized that the four quadrants of the perceiving and processing continua could be interpreted as four preferred learning preferences: *Divergers* (concrete and reflective) view concrete experiences from multiple perspectives and adapt by thinking rather than doing; *convergers* (abstract and active) prefer the practical application of problem-solving and technical tasks over personal issues; *assimilators* (abstract and reflective) focus more on ideas than on people and integrate multiple ideas into a conceptual whole; and *accommodators* (concrete and active) are comfortable with people and tend to use trial and error in problem-solving (Kolb, 1984; Figure 4.2).

In 1992, Fleming and Mills introduced the VARK learning preference model, which consists of four learning modality preferences: **v**isual, **a**uditory, **r**ead/write, and **k**inesthetic (VARK). The authors suggested that these learning modalities relate to only one component of learning—how to take in and give out information. Each modality can be measured using the VARK tool (Fleming, 2012). Details of the four learning modality preferences are as follows:

- A *visual* preference provides information in graphic formats such as maps, charts, and flow charts rather than in text format.
- An *auditory* preference describes a preference for information that is language-based (heard or spoken).
- A *read/write* preference indicates an inclination for information in text format.
- A *kinesthetic* learner prefers information that is concrete and experience based.

Several studies have attempted to identify the preferred learning style of nursing students, but the results have been inconsistent. A systematic review conducted by Shumba and Lipinge (2019) found nine studies that had used the VARK model and six that had used Kolb's model: Those that used the VARK model identified the dominant learning preference of nursing students as multimodal, followed (in order) by kinesthetic, visual, and auditory. Those that used Kolb's model identified divergers and assimilators as most prevalent. In a systematic review by Childs-Kean et al. (2020), of the studies that had used the VARK model, four reported that nursing students were multimodal and two reported that they were kinesthetic learners; in the studies using Kolb's model, nursing students were identified as convergers in two studies and as divergers in one study.

No single assessment of learning style preference guarantees that a student's learning needs will be satisfied. Educators can begin by reflecting on their personal learning style preferences. Although these preferences should not negate the use of multiple approaches, they can be shared and role modeled to illustrate that learning can be strengthened by using different modes. For example, teachers who are auditory learners could share that they challenge themselves by practicing learning kinesthetically to strengthen their knowledge base and skills. Exposure to different learning modalities may help students to identify methods that best align with their learning style.

The educator should create learning environments that address the content and concepts to be learned using a multitude of methods rather than trying to match instruction to each student's learning style preference. Ezzeddine et al. (2023) recommend an approach that begins with identifying the desired student outcome or skillset, followed by deciding which learning styles are most conducive to achieving this outcome or skillset, and finally, creating related lesson goals, teaching strategies, and methods of evaluation. This approach facilitates the achievement of educational outcomes and the acquisition of diverse learning styles. Additionally, the use of a variety of methods to present material helps to keep students engaged with the content and learning. Exhibit 4.8 provides examples of teaching strategies for diverse learning style preferences.

TEACHER–STUDENT RELATIONSHIPS

Student engagement is a strong predictor of success in higher education. The teacher–student relationship is a fundamental aspect of the educational experience which impacts academic achievement, social development, and overall well-being. Because positive relationships are built on trust and respect, teachers

> **EXHIBIT 4.8 Examples of Teaching Strategies for Diverse Learning Style Preferences**
>
> Vary teaching methods, assignments, and learning activities in class and laboratory.
> Encourage learners to accept the challenge of exploring multiple learning preferences.
> Do not teach solely by using your personal learning style preference.
> Create mnemonics or acrostics; make the most of rhythm, rhymes, jingles, and songs.
> Use color, charts, diagrams, and graphics in presentations.
> Include individual and group activities.
> Use discussion in the classroom and/or online environment.
> Use role-play and simulations.
> Provide opportunities to learn by doing.

must create safe and supportive environments in which students feel valued and respected for their unique abilities and perspectives. Students, in turn, need to trust teachers to guide and support their learning journey. Effective communication is essential for fostering a strong teacher–student relationship. Teachers should actively listen to students, encourage open dialogue, and provide constructive feedback to support academic growth and personal development (Han, 2021).

Teachers play a crucial role in providing emotional support and encouragement to students. By showing empathy, understanding individual needs, and offering encouragement, teachers can create a nurturing environment in which students feel comfortable taking risks, and making and learning from mistakes. To build meaningful connections, educators must recognize each student's unique strengths, interests, and learning style, as well as strive to provide individualized attention, personalized learning experiences, and differentiated instruction to meet their diverse needs.

Teachers serve as role models for students, demonstrating positive attitudes, values, and behaviors inside and outside the classroom. By exemplifying integrity, resilience, and a commitment to lifelong learning, they inspire their students to strive for excellence and become responsible members of society (Berg & Lepp, 2023). A supportive teacher–student relationship empowers students to take ownership of their learning and confidently pursue their goals. Truly competent teachers encourage autonomy, initiative, and self-reflection, thus empowering students to overcome challenges, set meaningful objectives, and celebrate their achievements (Heilporn et al., 2021).

In competency-based education, the role of the teacher as a coach is crucial in facilitating student learning, assessing competency attainment, and providing personalized support (Teal et al., 2023). The teacher–coach role in competency-based education emphasizes personalized instruction, formative assessment, frequent and constructive feedback, and support to help students develop essential competencies and succeed in their educational goals. By adopting a coaching mindset, teachers can empower students to become self-directed learners, critical thinkers, and lifelong problem-solvers. Exhibit 4.9 provides strategies to promote student engagement.

EXHIBIT 4.9 Strategies to Promote Student Engagement

Create an environment that is primed for student participation.

Use varied teaching methods and types of assessments.

Divide students into small groups to foster collaboration, peer learning, and teamwork.

Incorporate opportunities for peer teaching and peer feedback into the learning process

Provide visual, auditory, and kinesthetic opportunities to learn when possible.

Flip the classroom to ensure student-centered learning.

Find appropriate ways to use technology in the classroom (e.g., polling, audience-response systems).

Include writing exercises such as 1-minute papers, muddiest points, best part of class.

Set expectations and norms for class early.

Integrate curricular topics with other connected disciplines when possible.

Use real-world examples and stories that are relevant to the topic.

Establish work teams and partners for pursuing and achieving learning goals.

Incorporate appropriate use of social media.

Use preclass assignments/quizzes to increase familiarity with the material.

Add frequent, formative assessments versus heavily weighted summative assessments only.

Include realistic simulations.

Source: Han, F. (2021). The relations between teaching strategies, students' engagement in learning, and teachers' self-concept. *Sustainability, 13*(9), 5020. https://doi.org/10.3390/su13095020

STUDENTS WITH DISABILITIES

More students with disabilities are entering college. Twenty-one percent of undergraduate college students who enrolled in the 2019 to 2020 school year reported having a disability (U.S. Department of Education, National Center for Education Statistics, 2023b). Nursing students with disabilities bring unique perspectives, experiences, and strengths to nursing, but may face challenges regarding accessibility, accommodation, and stigma (Englund & Lancaster, 2022).

Nurse educators must ensure that students with disabilities have physical accessibility to classrooms, labs, and clinical settings as well as accessibility to instructional materials, technology, and other resources. Often, the specific needs of the student with disabilities will be documented in an accommodation plan and coordinated with the school's disability services office. Such accommodations may include assistive technology, alternative formats of classroom materials and exams, flexible seating arrangements, extended time for exams, note-taking support, sign language interpreters, or mobility assistance. It is expected that all documented accommodations will be provided; any inability to do so should be discussed with the disability services office. Educators should encourage peer-to-peer collaboration, mentoring relationships, and mutual support among students with disabilities and their peers (Englund & Lancaster, 2022). Peer mentors can provide valuable guidance, encouragement, and practical assistance to help students navigate academic and clinical challenges. In addition to regularly evaluating the effectiveness of support services and accommodations, educators should empower students with disabilities to advocate effectively for their needs and rights.

AMERICAN ASSOCIATION OF COLLEGES OF NURSING DIVERSITY, EQUITY, AND INCLUSION FACULTY TOOL KIT

AACN Diversity, Equity, and Inclusion (DEI) Faculty Tool Kit is designed to align the dimensions of the Inclusive Excellence Ecosystem for Academic Nursing (AACN, 2023). It serves as a strategic approach to assist nursing schools in organizing and guiding DEI efforts and provides evidence-based, exemplary practices for promoting DEI and fostering inclusive initiatives in academic nursing.

The AACN DEI Faculty Tool Kit has four components: Institutional Visibility and Capacity, Access and Success, Climate and Culture, and Education and Scholarship (AACN, 2023). The Education and Scholarship section is designed to provide tools, strategies, and in-depth readings to support nurse educators in advancing DEI initiatives in academic nursing. It offers resources for preparing educators to guide schools on DEI efforts and inform them of promising practices, including creating a welcoming environment, challenging students to achieve academically, and addressing cultural differences to achieve inclusive excellence. This component aims to assist nurse educators in developing knowledge, skills, and attitudes for advancing DEI, and provides exemplary practices to inform diversity and inclusion initiated at nursing schools.

SUMMARY

Nurse educators are in an ideal position to significantly impact student learning in a myriad of ways. The diversity of our classrooms no longer allows a "one-size-fits-all" approach to teaching. To effectively engage students in the learning process, nurse educators need to understand multiple factors; culture, race, age, gender, social determinants of learning, learning preference, and disabilities are only a few of the significant differences among students. Teachers should first assess the diversity of their program and consider striving for a holistic admissions process. Next, each teacher should assess the content of their courses and the outcomes to be met. What is the goal of the learning? How best will students learn the concepts and other types of material in each course? What do the students already know about the subject? How can the teacher best connect the new content to material the students have already learned? Understanding the learner encourages growth and learning by all and creates an open and welcoming environment in which to learn.

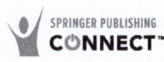

A robust set of instructor resources designed to supplement this text is located at http://connect.springerpub.com/content/book/978-0-8261-8892-2. Qualifying instructors may request access by emailing textbook@springerpub.com.

REFERENCES

Ackerman-Barger, K., Goldin, P., Draughon-Moret, J., London, M., & Boatright, D. (2022). Microaggressions, school satisfaction and depression: A national survey of nursing students, *Nursing Outlook, 70*(3), 496–505. https://doi.org/10.1016/j.outlook.2022.02.002

American Association of Colleges of Nursing. (2017). *Diversity, equity, and inclusion in academic nursing.* https://www.aacnnursing.org/Portals/0/PDFs/Position-Statements/Diversity-Inclusion.pdf

American Association of Colleges of Nursing. (2022). *Enrolment and graduation in baccalaureate and graduate programs in nursing.* https://www.aacnnursing.org/store/product-info/productcd/idsr_23enrollbacc

American Association of Colleges of Nursing. (2023). *Diversity, equity, & inclusion: An AACN faculty tool kit.* https://www.aacnnursing.org/diversity-tool-kit

Bayuo, J., Wong, K. C., Abu-Odah., & Wong, F. K. (2022). Becoming and overcoming: A qualitative synthesis of the experience of men in nursing academia. *Journal of Professional Nursing, 43*, 83–106. https://doi.org/10.1016/j.profnurs.2022.07.022

Beasy, K., Grant, R., & Emery, S. (2023). Multiple dimensions of safe space for LGBTQ students: School staff perceptions. *Sex Education, 23*(1), 35–48. https://doi.org/10.1080/14681811.2021.2018677

Berg, E., & Lepp, M. (2023). The meaning and application of student-centered learning in nursing education: An integrative review of the literature. *Nurse Education in Practice, 69*, 103622. https://doi.org/10.1016/j.nepr.2023.103622

Boland, R. J., & Amonoo, H. L. (2021). Types of Learners. *The Psychiatric clinics of North America, 44*(2), 141–148. https://doi.org/10.1016/j.psc.2020.12.001

Bordelon, C. J., Mott, J., McArthur, E., & MacWilliams, B. (2023). Men in female-dominated nursing specialties. *Nursing Clinics of North America, 58*(4), 617–625. https://doi.org/10.1016/j.cnur.2023.06.005

Chang, B. (2021). Incorporating eastern and western learning perspectives into a western learning environment. *Journal of Interdisciplinary Studies in Education, 10*(1), 16–40. http://ojed.org/jise

Childs-Kean, L., Edwards, M., & Smith, M. D. (2020). Use of learning style frameworks in health science education. *American Journal of Pharmaceutical Education, 84*(7), 919–927. https://doi.org/10.5688/ajpe7885

Cox, R., Bernstein, S., & Roy, K. (2023). A guide to application of diversity, equity, and inclusion for (DEI) principles for prelicensure nursing education. *Journal of Professional Nursing, 46*, 146–154. https://doi.org/10.1016/j.profnurs.2023.03.002

Dawkins, D., Sheri, R. P., Onglengco, R., Stobbe, B., Kaufman, S., Hampton, C. A., & Palazzo, C. (2022). Holistic admissions review integration in nursing programs. *Journal of Nursing Education, 61*(7), 361–366. https://doi.org/10.3928/01484834-20220610-01

Dweck, C. S. (2006). *Mindset: The new psychology of success. How we can learn to fulfil our potential.* Ballantine Books.

Englund, H. M., & Lancaster, R. J. (2022). Differences in marginality between nursing students with and without disabilities. *Journal of Nursing Education, 61*(8), 429–438. http://doi.org/10.3928/01484834-20220602-03

Ezzeddine, N., Hughes, J., Kaulback, S., Houk, S., Mikhael, J., & Vickery, A. (2023). Implications of understanding the undergraduate nursing students' learning styles: A discussion paper. *Journal of Professional Nursing, 49*, 95–101. https://doi.org/10.1016/j.profnurs.2023.09.006

Fleming, N. (2012). *VARK: A guide to learning styles.* http://www.vark-learn.com/21nglish/index.asp

Fleming, N., & Mills, C. (1992). Not another inventory, rather a catalyst for reflection. *To Improve the Academy, 11*(1), 137. https://onlinelibrary.wiley.com/doi/abs/10.1002/j.2334-4822.1992.tb00213.x

Fry, R. (2020). *Millennials overtake baby boomers as America's largest generation.* Pew Research Center. http://pewrsr.ch/2FgVPwv

Han, F. (2021). The relations between teaching strategies, students' engagement in learning, and teachers' self-concept. *Sustainability, 13*(9), 5020. https://doi.org/10.3390/su13095020

Hand, M., & Gedzyk-Nieman, S. A. (2022). Graduating nursing students' preparedness and comfort levels in caring for LGBTQ+ patients. *Journal of Professional Nursing, 41*, 75–80. https://doi.org/10.1016/j.profnurs.2022.04.011

Healthy People 2030. (n.d.). *Social determinants of health*. U.S. Department of Health and Human Services, Office of Disease Prevention and Health Promotion. Accessed January 15, 2024, from https://health.gov/healthypeople/priority-areas/social-determinants-health

Heilporn, G., Lakhal, S., & Belisle, M. (2021). An examination of teachers' strategies to foster student engagement in blended learning in higher education. *International Journal of Educational Technology in Higher Education, 18*(25), 1–25. https://doi.org/10.1186/s41239-021-00260-3

Iduye, D., Vukic, A., Waldron, I., Price, S., Sheffer, C., McKibbon, S., Dorey, R., & Yu, Z. (2021). Educators' strategies for engaging diverse students in undergraduate nursing education programs: A scoping review protocol. *JBI Evidence Synthesis, 19*(5), 1178–1185. https://doi.org/10.11124/JBIES-20-00039

Jaekel, K. S. (2021). Supporting LGBTQ students through precarity: Policies and practices for inclusion. *New Directions for Community Colleges, 2021*(196), 33–42. https://doi.org/10.1002/cc.20481

Jung, D., Latham, C., Fortes, K., & Schwartz, M. (2021). Using holistic admissions in prelicensure programs to diversify the nursing workforce. *Journal of Professional Nursing, 37*(2), 359–365. https://doi.org/10.1016/j.profnurs.2020.04.006

Knowles, M. S. (1973). *The adult learner: A neglected species*. Gulf Publishing Company.

Knowles, M. S., Holton, E. F., & Swanson, R. A. (2015). *The adult learner: The definitive classic in adult education and human resource development* (8th ed.). Routledge.

Kolb, D. (1984). *Experiential learning: Experience as the source of learning and development*. Prentice-Hall.

Kolb, D. A., & Fry, R. (1975). Toward an applied theory of experiential learning. In C. Cooper (Ed.), *Theories of group process*. John Wiley.

Layman, E. (2018). MIXED: Educational perspectives from families of mixed east and westeducational background. *Global Education Review, 5*(1), 52–73.

Levinson, M., & Cohen, A. K. (2023). Social determinants of learning: Implications for research, policy, and practice. *American Educational Research Association, 9*, 1–8. https://doi.org/10.1177/23328584231206087

Lewis, L., Biederman, D., Hatch, D., Li, A., Turner, K., & Molloy, M. A. (2021). Outcomes of a holistic admissions process in an accelerated baccalaureate nursing program. *Journal of Professional Nursing, 37*(4), 714–720. https://doi.org/10.1016/j.profnurs.2021.05.006

MacDaniel, T. E. (2020). Enhancing learning in diverse classrooms to improve nursing practice. *Teaching and Learning in Nursing, 15*, 245–247. https://doi.org/10.1016/j.teln.2020.05.004

Markey, K., Sackey, M. E., & Oppong-Gyan, R. (2020). Maximising intercultural learning opportunities: Learning with, from and about students from different cultures. *British Journal of Nursing, 29*(18), 1074–1077. https://doi.org/10.12968/bjon.2020.29.18.1074

Miller, R. A., Dika, S. L., Nguyen, D. J., Woodford, M., & Renn, K. A. (2021). LGBTQ+ college students with disabilities: Demographic profile and perceptions of well-being. *Journal of LGBTQ Youth, 18*(1), 60–77. https://doi.org/10.1080/19361653.2019.1706686

Mulkey, D. (2023). The history of men in nursing: Pioneers of the profession. *Journal of Christian Nursing, 40*, 96–101. https://doi.org/10.1097/CNJ.0000000000001040

National Council State Boards of Nursing. (2022). *NCSBN & the forum of state nursing workforce centers 2022 national workforce survey of RNs*. https://www.ncsbn.org/research/recent-research/workforce.page

National League for Nursing. (2022). *NLN annual survey of schools of nursing*. https://www.nln.org/news/research-statistics/nln-annual-survey-2021-2022

National League for Nursing. (2023a). *NLN annual survey of schools of nursing academic year 2021–2022: Executive summary.* https://www.nln.org/docs/default-source/research-statistics/nln-annual-survey-2022/headlineseditedgfm_8_15_2023_publication-.pdf?sfvrsn=2c6f050a_3

National League for Nursing. (2023b). *NLN national survey of schools of nursing 2021–2022: Infographics highlights.* https://www.nln.org/docs/default-source/research-statistics/nln-annual-survey-infographic-2021-2022.pdf?sfvrsn=fb2c3d52_3

Priode, K. S., Dail, R. B., & Swanson, M. (2020). Nonacademic factors that influence nontraditional nursing student retention. *Nursing education perspectives, 41*(4), 246–248. https://doi.org/10.1097/01.NEP.0000000000000577

Schnell-Peskin, L., Riley, G., Hodnett, K., Gryta, V., & Kisamore, A. (2024). Meeting the needs of students in higher education multigenerational classrooms: What can educators do? *International Journal of Information and Learning Technology, 41*(1), 73–85. https://doi.org/10.1108/IJILT-04-2023-0057

Schunk, D. H. (2020). *Learning theories: An educational perspective.* Pearson.

Shumba, T. W., & Lipinge, S. N. (2019). Learning style preferences of undergraduate nursing students: A systematic review. *Africa Journal of Nursing and Midwifery, 21*(1), 1–25. https://doi.org/10.25159/2520-5293/5758

Smallheer, B., Gedzyk-Nieman, S. A., Molloy, M. A., Clark, C. M., Gordon, H., & Morgan, B. (2021). Faculty development workshop on gender-associated incivility in nursing education. *Nursing Forum, 56,* 1044–1051. https://doi.org/10.111/nuf.12615

Sue, D. W. (2010). *Microaggressions in everyday life: Race, gender, and sexual orientation.* John Wiley & Sons.

Teal, J. S., Vaughn, S., & Fortes, K. (2023). The nurse coach's role in supporting students well-being. *Teaching and Learning in Nursing, 18*(4), 508–511. https://doi.org/10.1016/j.teln.2023.06.016

Tigert, J., & Fotouhi, G. (2022). "Sometimes my tongue stucks with fluency": International Students' English needs at a higher education institution. *NERA Conference Proceedings, 1.* https://opencommons.uconn.edu/nera-2022/1

U.S. Department of Education, National Center for Education Statistics. (n.d.). *Nontraditional graduates: Definitions and data.* https://nces.ed.gov/pubs/web/97578e.asp

U.S. Department of Education, National Center for Education Statistics. (2023a). *The condition of education.* English learners in public schools. https://nces.ed.gov/programs/coe/indicator/cgf

U.S. Department of Education, National Center for Education Statistics. (2023b). *2019–20 National Postsecondary Student Aid Study (NPSAS:20).* Number and percentage distribution of students enrolled in postsecondary institutions, by level, disability status, and selected student characteristics: Academic year 2019–20. https://nces.ed.gov/programs/digest/d22/tables/dt22_311.10.asp

Williams, C. A. (2020). Nursing students' mindsets matter: Cultivating a growth mindset. *Nurse educator, 45*(5), 252–256. https://doi.org/10.1097/NNE.0000000000000798

Wolcott, M. D., McLaughlin, J. E., Hann, A., Miklavec, A., Beck Dallaghan, G. L., Rhoney, D. H., & Zomorodi, M. (2021). A review to characterise and map the growth mindset theory in health professions education. *Medical education, 55*(4), 430–440. https://doi.org/10.1111/medu.14381

World Health Organization. (n.d.). *Health topics: Social determinants of health.* Accessed January 15, 2024, from https://www.who.int/health-topics/social-determinants-of-health#tab=tab_1

Teaching in Nursing   II

Teaching Methods

Debra Hagler and Brenda Morris

5

OBJECTIVES

1. Describe characteristics of a supportive learning environment
2. Select teaching/learning activities to support cognitive, affective, and psychomotor learning
3. Describe a variety of teaching methods suitable for nursing education

INTRODUCTION

This chapter describes the teacher's role in developing a supportive learning environment and using a variety of teaching methods, with guidance for selecting methods to fit the intended outcomes, learner characteristics, and available resources. Teaching methods are considered in relation to supporting learner development in the cognitive, affective, and psychomotor learning domains. Strategies are described for incorporating active learning and for promoting critical thinking.

DEVELOPING A LEARNING ENVIRONMENT

Teaching is a professional nursing role that takes place in formal and informal settings. A nurse educator may be guiding a student in caring for an individual who is acutely ill, teaching healthy behaviors in a community setting, organizing group work in a classroom, facilitating a reflection session after a high-fidelity simulation, leading a discussion via webinar, or responding to learners asynchronously. Regardless of the setting and context, teachers can demonstrate a supportive presence and help their learners construct knowledge.

Recent changes in educational policy, progressing from emphasis on the teacher's actions to focusing more on students' learning outcomes, mirror healthcare systems' progress from emphasizing care provision to a focus on patient outcomes. In education and healthcare, there is still much work to be done in prioritizing learner and patient outcomes.

Students face significant stresses in their personal and academic roles, but teachers can make a positive difference by establishing a supportive learning environment. Prelicensure nursing students have identified aspects of supportive student–faculty relationships to include building connections inside and outside of the classroom, modeling attributes of caring, practicing mutual respect, and viewing diversity in broad terms (Ingraham et al., 2018).

> **EXHIBIT 5.1 Elements of Teaching That Promote Safety in Learning**
>
> **Communication**
>   Sharing your philosophy of teaching and learning
>   Setting clear expectations for assignments
> **Shared vulnerability**
>   Allowing for shared connectedness
>   Maintaining appropriate boundaries
> **Transparency**
>   Providing honest and respectful responses
>   Modeling evidence-based decisions
> **Intentionality**
>   Planning purposefully for students to meet learning outcomes
>   Providing explanations for the meaning of assigned coursework

Source: Adapted from Patterson, B. J., & Forneris, S. (2023). Faculty as learners: Neuroscience in action. *Journal of Nursing Education, 62*(5), 291–297. https://doi.org/10.3928/01484834-20230306-02

The connections that students make with other students can also support learning outcomes. While the teacher may role model and encourage respectful communication, the support and validation of peers are additional powerful sources of motivation for learners to participate in activities and accept the risks of contributing diverse viewpoints (Addy et al., 2021). Establishing shared expectations for respectful civil interaction from the beginning helps a group of learners focus on learning together. Research-based strategies such as those in Exhibit 5.1 are useful in facilitating a classroom climate that feels safe for learning.

SELECTING TEACHING METHODS

Start with the end in mind: Before choosing teaching methods or planning learning activities, pay careful attention to the purpose of the educational session and the evidence that will determine whether students have reached the expected outcomes (Cline & Rinaldi, 2023; Wiggins & McTighe, 2005). This process, known as backward design, may feel awkward because teachers often want to begin planning by choosing a favorite teaching method. However, taking the time to consider the broad purpose, expected outcomes, and learner characteristics, as well as the ways the learners will demonstrate competency, supports instructional alignment. That alignment across objectives, evaluation strategies, and teaching methods is powerful in support of learning.

The most important question to ask about a teaching method is whether it is a good fit for the specific learning objectives, learners, teachers, and available resources. If the goal is to support students in mastering key competencies, then the same teaching method will not work equally well for all situations. Nurse educators who would be appalled at the idea of treating each patient with identical interventions regardless of patients' individual needs might not appear as concerned about using identical teaching methods for all learners and instructional purposes. Yet, choosing teaching methods congruent with specific learner needs and desired educational outcomes is critical for effective instruction. The single most important factor in choosing a teaching method is whether that method will help students meet the intended learning outcomes and/or competencies.

It is unreasonable to expect that a teacher will become skilled in using every teaching method. However, reflecting on assumptions about learning can lead to becoming more comfortable in trying out new teaching methods. There is more than one way to teach any topic.

Domains of Learning

Learning can be described as development in one or more of three knowledge domains: cognitive, affective, and psychomotor. Cognitive development, which involves thinking, cannot be directly observed but is seen through behaviors or the products of thinking. Affective development, which involves values and beliefs, cannot be directly observed either, so it is seen through attitudes, behaviors, and choices that express values. Psychomotor development, which involves skilled movement, is directly observable in physical action. Program outcomes, course objectives (also referred to as expected learning outcomes), and module or daily objectives are written to reflect expected development across the three domains of learning. Nurse educators need to design instruction, teach, and assess for student development in all three domains because nurses in practice rely on all three domains to provide care and perform other nursing roles (Oermann et al., 2025).

Patients see the physical care that nurses provide (psychomotor skills) and recognize that nurses have high ethical standards (Gallup, 2023) reflecting nursing values and beliefs (affective comportment). Patients, however, may not be aware of the intense thinking and planning that nurses engage in to promote health and prevent harm (cognitive knowledge). Despite the hidden nature of the thinking process, the cognitive domain is often the easiest domain to address in writing objectives and in choosing teaching methods. In some teaching/learning situations, the affective and psychomotor aspects of learning are ignored or expected to develop without much attention, but educators who plan only for cognitive development should not be surprised when learners' beliefs and physical skills do not change with accumulation of information alone. Development in affective values and physical skills is needed in concert with cognition in order to change behavior.

Some teaching strategies support learning in all three domains, whereas other strategies are more specific to learning in only one or two of the domains. Strategies chosen for a single class meeting do not need to represent each of the domains, but all domains should be included regularly for integrative experiences. It is important to note the hierarchical nature of each domain and to align the levels of learning objectives, teaching strategies, and evaluation methods. Descriptions of the levels within each learning domain and examples of activities that might be used for teaching in that domain are in Tables 5.1 to 5.3.

Coaching students practicing tracheal suctioning on task trainer manikins in the learning laboratory might support psychomotor skill development, but the activity lacks the context of care for a valued individual. Listening to an audio-recorded interview with a patient who has a debilitating disease with ineffective airway clearance might work well for supporting the affective objectives of valuing the patient perspective and cognitive objectives related to disease management, but not

TABLE 5.1 ACTIVITIES TO SUPPORT LEARNING IN THE COGNITIVE DOMAIN

Level	Definition	Examples of Teaching Strategies/Learning Activities
Remembering	Recall previous information.	Practice definitions with online flash cards, matching games.
Understanding	Comprehend the meaning.	Draw an image to represent a specific concept.
Applying	Use a concept in a new situation; carry out a procedure.	Calculate an equivalent dose of a different narcotic.
Analyzing	Distinguish between facts and inferences.	Discuss what is known based on laboratory results versus what can be inferred about a patient's health situation.
Evaluating	Make judgments about the value of ideas or materials.	Compare a patient's activity level with the collaborative goals for activity set by the patient and healthcare team.
Creating	Build a structure or pattern from diverse elements.	Develop self-care learning materials for a specific patient or group of patients.

Source: Anderson, L. W., Krathwohl, D. R., Airasian, P., Cruikshank, K. A., Mayer, R. E., Pintrich, P., Raths, J., & Wittrock, M. (2001). *A taxonomy for learning, teaching, and assessing: A revision of Bloom's taxonomy of educational objectives.* Longman.

for psychomotor skill development. However, a carefully planned experience of providing care for an authentic patient in the clinical environment, a standardized patient in the clinical laboratory, or a simulated patient in the simulation laboratory can support development across all three domains.

Learner Characteristics

The characteristics of the intended learners, including their social and cognitive cultures, are important to consider in choosing teaching methods. Students who are not comfortable interacting with peers or learning in cooperation with peers need support to develop knowledge, skills, and attitudes for professional-level communication and collaboration. Disagreeing in a way that remains respectful and still furthers the discussion is a complex communication skill to develop, yet planning

TABLE 5.2 ACTIVITIES TO SUPPORT LEARNING IN THE AFFECTIVE DOMAIN

Level	Definition	Examples of Teaching Strategies/Learning Activities
Receiving	Open to experience; willing to hear.	Listen to a lecture or story, watch a film.
Responding	React and participate actively.	Participate in discussions, ask questions, suggest interpretations.
Valuing	Attach values and express personal opinions.	Develop a plan for incorporating a new professional behavior.
Organization or integration of different values	Reconcile internal conflicts; develop value system.	Explain your philosophy of nursing including examples of your current behaviors that reflect your philosophy.
Characterization by a value	Adopt belief system and philosophy.	Carry out a plan for personal health improvement and reflect on the process

Source: Krathwohl, D. R., Bloom, B. S., & Masia, B. B. (1964). *Taxonomy of educational objectives: The classification of educational goals. Handbook II: Affective domain.* David McKay.

for that development may be ignored, based on an assumption that students enter higher education with such skills.

Beginning clinical students often express high levels of anxiety. Vo et al. (2023) found from their meta-analysis that most nursing students reported a moderate level of stress (42.1%) and mild to moderate levels of anxiety (19.4% vs. 25.1%). However, upper division nursing students were at higher risk for severe stress levels. Teachers can anticipate and plan for additional attention to helping students learn to manage their anxiety, rather than being surprised when learners' anxieties overtake the scheduled learning session.

When teaching strategies do not fit well with the characteristics of the learners, there is a greater need for resources to help students reach learning goals. When learners have not developed the prerequisite knowledge and skills to support them toward a later learning goal, the need for other resources, such as instructional time, increases. For example, if students admitted to an online program are familiar and comfortable with online technology, then orientation and learning related to the technology do not require as much instructional time or focused attention. However, when students admitted to an online program have little previous experience with online learning, teachers need to plan for extra time and effort to support the learners in developing skills as new technologies are introduced.

TABLE 5.3 ACTIVITIES TO SUPPORT LEARNING IN THE PSYCHOMOTOR DOMAIN

Level	Definition	Examples of Teaching Strategies/Learning Activities
Imitation	Copy action of another; observe and replicate.	Watch a demonstration of how to safely position a patient and repeat the action.
Manipulation	Reproduce activity from instruction or memory.	Practice positioning a patient with verbal coaching or written instructions for reference.
Precision	Execute skill reliably, independent of help.	Practice giving an intramuscular injection independently on an injection model.
Articulation	Adapt and integrate expertise to satisfy a nonstandard objective.	Practice transferring patients who have a variety of mobility challenges from beds to chairs.
Naturalization	Automated, unconscious mastery of activity and related skills at strategic level.	Practice taking blood pressures until simultaneously able to accurately hear the pulse, watch the dial, manipulate the equipment, and remember the readings.

Source: Dave, R. H. (1970). Developing and writing educational objectives (psychomotor levels). In R. J. Armstrong (Ed.), *Developing and writing behavioral objectives.* Educational Innovators Press.

Resources

Teaching method choices are sustainable when they are realistic for the reasonably available resources. Resources to consider in choosing teaching methods include time, space, support staff, technology, and materials.

Time is a most precious resource for teachers and learners. The teacher's time plan for using a particular teaching method should include the time in preparation, direct instruction, and providing formative feedback/coaching students. The students' time to be considered includes accessing the materials needed, preparatory assignments, instructional time, and any follow-up assignments. An experience that requires extensive instructional time should be considered only for the most important course and program goals.

Physical spaces and course enrollment can facilitate interaction or constrain teaching methods and activities. Large classes and lecture rooms make group interaction challenging, but not impossible. Even in lecture halls with unmovable desks, students can interact in pairs or clusters. Students in large online classes that are arranged in smaller work groups may not even realize that they are in a large enrollment course.

Availability and access to *support staff* can make the difference in the outcomes of some learning activities. Librarians can be amazing resource persons for students and faculty struggling to search for clinical evidence. Writing-center staff can be helpful for students learning to write in the discipline of nursing and for faculty developing writing assignments. Technology experts can help ensure that classroom plans for new software use or online resources go smoothly. In settings without support staff, the teacher should plan learning activities with the understanding that troubleshooting library database searches, coaching students to use new software, or managing other technical challenges will add to the teacher's responsibilities.

Technology is a resource and a means to an end. When students are learning to manipulate a stethoscope, it is reasonable to focus both on developing auscultation skills and on the stethoscope as a tool, because nurses can expect to use stethoscopes throughout their careers for obtaining assessment data that will support clinical decisions. At times, however, technology that is not the direct focus of a learning objective becomes the focus of a misguided instructional effort. For example, leadership students learning the important skill of realistically budgeting for a clinical project might be directed to use a specific format or software for an assignment. If the format or software that learners are directed to use will require live instruction or tutorials and extensive practice, the teacher should consider whether learning to use the tool is a reasonable investment of student time. A larger investment in time and effort might be appropriate when learners will use the software program or other technology in the future workplace; however, a high level of investment in learning a new technology is generally not worthwhile for a single assignment.

Availability of *materials* for learning may impact decisions about instructional methods. Attention to the physical realism of the learning situation is important, but simple and inexpensive materials often are sufficient for supporting a particular objective. When students are practicing integrating their assessments, judgments, and interventions in complex situations, interacting with a simulated patient may add a level of realism that engages the student and improves the overall learning experience.

PLANNING FOR ACTIVE LEARNING

Higher education has often been associated with a type of lecture learning where students passively listen (or maybe only appear to listen) to their teachers' wise thoughts. Promoting more active learning requires student engagement far beyond mere attendance. A focus on learner engagement and active learning is aligned with a general trend away from teacher-centered strategies and toward strategies focused on what helps students learn.

Lecture, a frequently used teaching method in higher education, may call to mind an image of a teacher on the auditorium stage talking at an audience of students while the students doze off to sleep. Many nurse educators continue to rely on lecture quite heavily. Lectures can be insidious in settings outside the classroom as well: When the post clinical conference, the laboratory session, or the simulation debriefing/reflection time involves the teacher doing most of the talking, those sessions have been subtly converted to lectures. The students slip from their intended roles as active participants back to being more passive recipients.

When teaching consists only of delivering a lecture or assigning readings from a textbook, educators seem to expect that students can transform the words directly into the students' authentic nursing actions. However, telling a student to remember a list of airway clearance measures is very different from asking the student to actively determine what types of airway clearance measures might be suitable for a specific patient with an abdominal incision who is unable to sit up or walk. Applying principles and concepts to new situations requires practice and coaching.

Action and Reflection

Two processes are important for active learning: action and reflection. Taking part in meaningful activity followed by reflecting on the learning processes and outcomes transforms the learner from a passive recipient of someone else's thoughts to an active constructor of knowledge and meaning. This does not mean that all passive strategies should be abandoned. Interposing active and passive strategies can create a rich opportunity for students to actively participate. For instance, a class session on substance abuse might be changed from continuous lecture to a series of activities: students completing a classroom survey of attitudes, pairing for brief discussion, participating in a large group discussion, viewing a related film clip, analyzing a short case study in a small group, synthesizing recommendations from the case analysis, and summarizing key learning points.

The passive activities of reading textbook chapters or watching a film can be shifted to more active learning by pairing those activities with specific reflection activities and expectations. Simple instructions can help the student become a more active participant: "While you read this passage (or watch this film clip) about a recent news event, identify at least three specific opportunities for health promotion at the individual, family, and community level. Bring your list for discussion to the next class session." Rather than the teacher identifying extensive lists of examples for new concepts, asking the learners to identify and share additional examples of the concept in the environment tests their understanding of the concept and helps them find individual meanings for a concept.

Reflection and debriefing strategies gained attention through educational simulation, but debriefing also is effective in the classroom and during post clinical conferences. After a complex experience such as service learning, the strategy of guided reflection helps learners construct knowledge and establish meaning for the experience (Steven et al., 2020).

DEVELOPING HIGHER LEVEL THINKING

Educators aim to foster the development of critical thinking abilities among their graduates. Terms that have similar meanings to critical thinking and are occasionally used interchangeably include higher order or higher level thinking, metacognition, critical reflection, and reflective thinking.

There are two aspects of critical thinking: ability and disposition. *Critical thinking ability* involves using higher level thinking skills such as conceptualizing, applying, analyzing, interpreting, inferring, explaining, evaluating, and synthesizing. *Critical thinking disposition* defines the characteristics of the ideal critical thinker: being habitually inquisitive, open-minded, mindful of alternatives, well-informed, fair-minded, and honest in facing personal biases. Critical thinking incorporates the elements of thought and applies the universal intellectual standards (Foundation for Critical Thinking, 2019).

The context in which critical thinking is applied may be discipline specific. For example, how a nursing graduate applies critical thinking to nursing practice is very different from how an engineering graduate applies critical thinking to engineering practice. Both of these graduates may use similar higher order thinking skills; however, the context in which these thinking skills are applied will be different.

Teaching Methods to Promote Critical Thinking

There are many teaching methods that promote the development of critical thinking, including case studies, concept mapping, collaborative learning, problem-based learning (PBL), gaming, and service learning. Teachers can structure learning activities to develop critical thinking by focusing attention on reflection, providing reasons, and developing alternatives.

Questioning is a key strategy for facilitating critical thinking. Teachers may support learners by posing questions or structuring a written assignment to include reflection. Posing questions such as "How do you know?" and "What evidence supports this conclusion?" help learners identify the reasons for their views and remind them to seek reasons for others' views. To encourage learners to develop alternative hypotheses and evaluate alternate points of view, the teacher can prompt the learner to explain from a different perspective.

Learners who are becoming critical thinkers will ask difficult questions of their teachers. As educators, in which contexts do we consider student questions to be reasonable? Are there situations where educators tend to receive questions with irritation rather than generosity? Are there changes in teacher responses to questions that might promote a more thoughtful discourse?

TEACHING METHODS

Nursing programs are most often organized using curriculum models including a traditional model organized by care of specific populations (pediatrics, behavioral health); a concept-based model organized by categories of information (grief, tissue perfusion); a competency-based model organized around achievement of specific behaviors; or a combination of the previous models (Ignatavicius, 2019). The educator's choices of teaching methods are not dependent on the curricular model. The same teaching/learning method may be used across each of the models as long as the method is aligned with the expected learning outcomes or objectives.

In the next section, a variety of teaching methods are described in categories such as independent learning methods, small-group methods, and large-class methods. However, each of the methods can be used in more than one way. For instance, reading is described as an independent learning activity, but there may be times that reading aloud in the classroom suits the instructional purpose. Discussion can take place in pairs, small groups of three to four, or with the entire class.

INDEPENDENT LEARNING METHODS

Reading

Assigning passages for students to read in a textbook or scholarly journal is a simple instructional plan, but many students find that reading is a difficult way to learn.

Learning through reading requires understanding, then interpreting and synthesizing the text into useful application.

Students often report that they begin the assigned reading for the week, completing part of the assignment each day, but never finishing a week's reading before the next week's assigned chapters are due. By default, the chapters at the end of each week's list are the least likely to have been read. Two simple instructional strategies can improve the reading-to-learn experience: limiting the assignment to the most pertinent readings, and identifying the recommended sections by priority order rather than sequential order. Rather than assigning 10 chapters totaling 800 pages each week, assigning only the most important passages from each chapter or the most important chapters improves the likelihood that students might be able to finish a week's reading assignment. Prioritizing the passages among the assigned readings that are required versus those recommended for enrichment or review helps students make informed choices and use their time efficiently.

Teachers also help students improve reading effectiveness by suggesting specific comprehension strategies. Levels of support for comprehension increase as the teacher introduces reading strategies, provides the rationale for a particular strategy, and even models the strategy. Recommendations that students may find useful include reading slowly and carefully, taking notes while reading, paraphrasing/summarizing text, and attending to the purpose and context for the reading.

The increasing availability of electronic books (e-books) that are read on a screen may offer students savings over traditional textbooks. Students are able to access e-books rapidly, rent them short term, perform automated searches for specific content, and return them online. However, students may experience frustration with complex sign-on processes, publisher restrictions, and incompatibility of the e-book with some reading devices (Casselden & Pears, 2020). Students adjusting to the transition from printed books to e-books may need assistance to develop or adapt previously effective reading strategies. Educators can incorporate intentional strategies to help students take advantage of the ability to bookmark, search, and make extensive notes in e-books. Incorporating modeling and practice with critical reading during the transition can improve students' attitudes about reading text on the screen.

Strategies that teachers can recommend or model for improving reading comprehension in higher education are listed in Table 5.4. Many of the strategies can be incorporated in both classroom and online activities.

TABLE 5.4 TEACHING STRATEGIES FOR IMPROVING READING COMPREHENSION

Strategy	Rationale	Activities to Recommend and Model
Develop and activate prior knowledge	Connecting learners' existing information and experiences to a new topic improves understanding and memory.	Provide experiential learning activities. Preview headings or key concepts; make predictions.

(continued)

TABLE 5.4 TEACHING STRATEGIES FOR IMPROVING READING COMPREHENSION (continued)

Strategy	Rationale	Activities to Recommend and Model
Communicate reading goals	Help students understand the purpose and intended scope of the reading assignment.	Align the assigned readings with the intended learning outcomes. Discuss the author's purpose. Narrow down the reading assignment to the most pertinent chapters of a technical text.
Use graphic organizers	Using visual representations helps students identify, organize, and remember important ideas.	Create timelines, framed outlines, concept maps, story maps, and Venn diagrams.
Teach comprehension monitoring strategies	Students should keep track of their understanding as they read and implement "fix-up" strategies when identifying breakdown.	Note confusing or difficult words and concepts, create images, stop after each paragraph to summarize, and generate questions. When understanding breaks down: reread, re-state, use context to figure out unknown words or ideas.
Teach note-taking and summarization skills	Consolidate large amounts of information (several paragraphs or passages) into key ideas.	Identify topic sentences, identify words or concepts that represent a list of related terms, practice summarizing, and use graphic organizers to summarize.
Teach students to ask and answer questions	Asking questions before, during, and after reading supports engagement and understanding.	Ask explicit and inferential questions, identify whether the answers to the teacher's questions are likely to be found in text or require an inference.
Model multicomponent comprehension strategies	Combine several comprehension strategies into an organizational system for reading.	Teach students to independently use strategies. Support students in generalizing strategy use across contexts and courses. Actively engage students in using comprehension strategies and applying what was read through cooperative learning, group discussions, and other interactions.

Source: Fisher, D., & Frey, N. (2019). Best practices in adolescent literacy instruction. In L. Morrow, L. Gambrell, & H. Casey (Eds.), *Best practices in literacy instruction* (6th ed.). Guilford Publications; Ritchey, K. A., & List, A. (2022). Task-oriented reading: A framework for improving college students' reading compliance and comprehension. *College Teaching, 70*(3), 280–295. https://doi.org/10.1080/87567555.2021.1924607

Writing

Clear writing is important for communicating with patients and colleagues in many nursing roles and settings. Writing effectively is also a means for career progression: synthesizing complex ideas into a coherent written message is a critical leadership skill. The task of writing requires a number of competencies including organizing a logical argument, addressing a specific audience, conceptualizing and critiquing ideas, and ethically citing sources.

However, communicating effectively in writing is not easy. The basic writing skills that students attain in secondary schools do not extend to the types of writing needed for professionals. Even students with strong basic writing skills need instruction and practice to develop as skilled writers in the context of nursing or healthcare. Examples of common writing assignments used in higher education to prepare nurses for professional writing are provided in Exhibit 5.2.

Students are admitted to nursing programs with a wide range of writing skills. Nursing faculty members can expect to teach students how to write using vocabulary and formatting requirements specific to health professions as well as to support students in remediating basic writing skills. Many schools have student support services available for writing development and remediation, but those services do not take the place of nursing faculty emphasizing written communication consistently throughout the curriculum.

There are a number of strategies for helping students develop effective writing skills, including the use of assignment rubrics, exemplars, successive drafts, and feedback from peers and instructors. Table 5.5 indicates teaching strategies that support students' writing skills development.

Reflection

Benner et al. (2009) describe the process of helping students learn to identify what is important in a given situation as *teaching for salience*. One of the key strategies they

---

EXHIBIT 5.2 Types of Writing Assignments

Appraisal	Memo
Book report	Narrative
Blog	Pamphlet
Care plan	Patient instructions
Case analysis	Poetry
Critique	Policy/procedure
Dramatic script	Process reflection
Editorial	Project proposal
Evidence synthesis	Research paper
Film report	Summary
Journal	Technical description
Legislative policy brief	Tweet
Letter	Wiki

TABLE 5.5 STRATEGIES FOR IMPROVING WRITING AND STRUCTURING WRITING ASSIGNMENTS

Strategy	Teacher's Action	Rationale
Detailed rubrics	Provide specific criteria for content and quality.	Communicate expectations.
Exemplar papers in the discipline	Share excellent papers written by previous students (with their permission) as examples. Share well-written papers addressing a range of nursing audiences.	Clarify intended level and scope of assignment. Promote awareness of the publication genres and different audiences for scholarly writing in nursing.
Drafts with feedback	Provide feedback on successive versions of the work.	Expect revision of the initial draft.
Sequential section writing	Provide feedback and guidance on one section or aspect of a larger project before the next section is written.	Redirect efforts early.
Peer coaching	Facilitate student peers in providing feedback to one another and revising their own work before they submit for teacher feedback.	Learn from how others conceptualize. Learn to give and receive effective feedback about writing.

Source: Lipnevich, A. A., Panadero, E., & Calistro, T. (2023). Unraveling the effects of rubrics and exemplars on student writing performance. *Journal of Experimental Psychology: Applied, 29*(1), 136–148. https://doi.org/10.1037/xap0000434; Panadero, E., García-Pérez, D., Fernández Ruiz, J., Fraile, J., Sánchez-Iglesias, I., & Brown, G. T. L. (2023). Feedback and year level effects on university students' self-efficacy and emotions during self-assessment: Positive impact of rubrics vs. instructor feedback. *Educational Psychology (Dorchester-on-Thames), 43*(7), 756–779. https://doi.org/10.1080/01443410.2023.2254015

describe as an exemplar of good teaching is that of helping learners reflect on practice. Reflecting on clinical practice allows students to examine clinical experiences and determine which actions were effective and were not effective. The process of reflection facilitates increased self-awareness and enhances learning. The focus of the reflection should be on the learning outcomes rather than the reflecting (Steven et al., 2020).

Coaching for reflection requires active engagement of the teacher, whereas reflecting requires active engagement of the learner. Strategies such as incorporating regular opportunities for reflective discussion, using structured reflection, providing individual student feedback on the reflection, and providing clear guidelines on the reflective activity will assist students to engage in reflective learning practices. Exhibit 5.3 provides suggested questions to frame reflection in a dialogue or in a writing activity such as journaling or blogging.

Contract Learning

Contract learning is based on the principles of adult learning which places emphasis on the desire of adult learners to be self-directed and have learning individualized to style, time, place, and pace (Knowles et al., 2020). The steps in contract learning include diagnosing a learning need, creating learning objectives, identifying learning resources and strategies, determining performance criteria and expectations (Knowles et al., 2020). There are several variations to contract learning, depending on the format of the course, the level of learners, and the purpose. Common examples of how contract learning is used in education include a team learning contract, a course learning contract, a clinical learning contract, or an individual learning contract with a student. The terms contract learning and learning contract are frequently used interchangeably.

Team Learning Contract

Teachers may use a team learning contract to specify performance behaviors for members completing a group assignment. A team learning contract is helpful because the learners define what behaviors and outcomes are acceptable to the team, and the team is accountable for enforcing the contract standards among members (Mertz et al., 2023). For example, a team learning contract may identify assignments, responsibilities, and due dates for team members. This type of approach is useful with adult learners who want to set performance parameters and team behavior expectations.

Course Learning Contract

Educators may use a contract learning approach to managing a course. Using this approach, the teacher provides the learner with a menu of options available to demonstrate course learning outcomes and establishes the minimum standards for satisfactory performance. The learner contracts with the teacher for the number

---

EXHIBIT 5.3 Questions to Frame Reflection

What did you know or assume about this topic?
What new information have you gained?
What credible evidence supports confirming or changing your belief?
What questions have not been answered?

and types of learning assignments that will be completed to achieve the desired level of performance. This approach allows the motivated, self-directed learner the ability to guide their learning experience by contracting with the teacher to complete a series of learning assignments that demonstrate the desired level of course performance. One drawback to this approach is that it may be challenging for learners who are less motivated, not self-directed, or unable to articulate learning needs.

Clinical Learning Contract

A clinical learning contract provides a structured approach for field or practicum experiences where a precepted clinical education model is used. The purpose of this contract is to provide a consistent framework for the application of didactic content with practice experiences (Chicca & Shellenbarger, 2021). The faculty, preceptor, and learner establish mutually agreed upon learning outcomes that facilitate the transfer of didactic knowledge to the practice setting. Additionally, the clinical learning contract facilitates evaluation of learning and attainment of competencies by defining the learning objectives and the evaluation parameters for the student's field experience.

Individual Learning Contract

An individual learning contract specifies what the learner must accomplish to meet the course outcomes. This contract will specify individual student learning objectives, learning assignments, evaluation methods, and deadlines. The teacher may initiate the learning contract, or the learner may initiate it, depending on the structure of the course and the purpose of the learning contract. Teachers may initiate the individual learning contract as a tool to clarify requirements with a student who is not meeting course expectations. In contrast, a student initiated learning contract allows the self-directed student to individualize a learning experience. Learning contracts are frequently used to guide directed or independent study courses, graduate courses, and fieldwork. Oh et al. (2019) found that the use of individual learning contracts with undergraduate nursing students in the clinical setting increased problem-solving skills, self-directed learning capabilities, and communication self-efficacy.

The principles of andragogy support the use of learning contracts to help facilitate adult learning. A well-written learning contract includes the following items: measurable learning objectives; learning activities and resources required to meet the objectives; deliverables or evidence to demonstrate that the outcomes have been met; and the specific criteria for evaluation.

Concept Mapping

Concept mapping is commonly used as an instructional method to facilitate the development of critical thinking by allowing the learner to integrate new concepts into an existing cognitive structure, fostering meaningful learning. A concept map provides a visual representation of a concept and the interrelationships between the central concept and subconcepts. A commonly used structure for concept mapping involves placing the major concept in the center of the map and locating the subconcepts around the major concept, then connecting the subconcepts and major concept to show interrelationships. Figure 15.1 in Chapter 15 is an example of a concept map. Concept mapping encourages learners to build upon previous knowledge, integrate new concepts, and explore the interconnections between concepts. It is important to note that each learner's concept map will be different because learners construct knowledge based upon their previous knowledge.

Concept maps may be unstructured or highly structured. The educator should match the amount of structure for the concept map to the purpose of the concept map. In some circumstances, it may be desirable to use a highly structured approach to concept mapping, whereas it may be preferable to use an unstructured approach when the goal of the teaching method is for the learners to construct their own knowledge. The concept map helps the educator assess a student's understanding of the concept and the connections among subconcepts. Concept mapping is an appropriate teaching strategy when the faculty member is teaching cognitive information and wants to facilitate active learner participation.

In nursing education, concept mapping may be used to help students organize assessment data, integrate interventions and the nursing process, and understand the interrelationships among data (Eisenmann, 2021). Some advantages of concept mapping are helping students who are visual learners see inter relationships between concepts and subconcepts, and allowing students to build on prior knowledge and assimilate new information in a way that is meaningful to the student. Other advantages include facilitation of active engagement with content, increased knowledge, and enhanced learner satisfaction (Yarmohammadi et al., 2023), increased clinical judgment in nursing students (Eisenmann, 2021), and increased critical thinking (Barta et al., 2022).

Variations of concept mapping include mind mapping and argument mapping. Mind maps use lines and associative words to link pictures, words, and diagrams to form a map of the connections between ideas (Wu & Wu, 2020). Argument maps have a low level of abstraction and use boxes, lines, and linking words to show the inferences between claims and supporting evidence, helping students develop reasoning skills (Uçar & Çevik, 2021). These different forms of knowledge mapping help foster meaningful learning, allow learners to scaffold or build upon previous learning, and facilitate critical thinking.

Self-Paced Modules/Reusable Learning Objects

A reusable learning object (RLO) is a small, self-contained educational unit that may include objectives, content, interactive learning activities, animations, narrated text, visual images, self-assessments, and feedback tools. RLOs may be used to introduce new content, reinforce or clarify existing content, or provide demonstrations (Zakrajsek & Nilson, 2023). They may be used independently or combined with other RLOs to teach larger content areas. Some teachers use RLOs when they "flip" the classroom by having the learners review the RLO prior to coming to class, then use class time for more active learning activities.

When developing and designing an RLO, it is important for the teacher to keep the RLO focused on a small area of content, clearly define the scope of the RLO, and incorporate strategies that facilitate ease of navigation and interactivity. Some teachers use a storyboard approach to help facilitate the development of RLOs. Most RLOs are between 2 and 15 minutes in length.

RLOs developed by publishing companies are available for purchase or may be included when students purchase textbook packages. The role of the teacher in using RLOs developed by others is to ensure that the RLO is congruent with the course objectives, is of sufficient quality to meet students' learning needs, and is used in compliance with copyright restrictions.

The benefits of RLOs include the ability of the student to engage in self-paced learning, actively engage with content, review content, and perform self-assessment to identify learning needs. RLOs promote knowledge-based and performance-based learning (Zakrajsek & Nilson, 2023). For these reasons, RLOs can be more effective than traditional lecture.

SMALL GROUP METHODS

Discussion

Discussion is the most commonly used teaching method in graduate education (Vinette et al., 2023). A good discussion is engaging, explores diverse ideas, and helps participants clarify their own thinking in the face of colleagues' alternative ideas. However, poorly planned discussions can take up a large amount of time with little learning impact. Even after a well-focused discussion, students may not understand what points in the discussion are important to remember or apply in future work. Periodic restatements and summaries by group members can help everyone stay on track and remember key points. During discussion, some students focus on the comments their instructor makes, but not the comments that their peers make, which detracts from students learning from each other (Brookfield et al., 2023).

To facilitate effective discussion, clear learning objectives and agreed-upon ground rules are essential. For example, clarify how students will participate in the discussion. Will students raise their hands, speak out at will, or indicate in some other way that they would like to have the floor? Is participation required or optional? It's also important to clarify how the group will manage those who dominate the discussion, avoid participation, move off topic, or show disrespectful behavior to other group members. The process of setting group discussion norms collaboratively creates a good starting point for a respectful and scholarly discussion. Examples of teacher responses that enhance discussion are in Table 5.6.

Experiential Learning

Activities that engage the senses help learners understand and recall concepts. Trying to breathe through a straw for several minutes evokes both physical sensations to

TABLE 5.6 TEACHER RESPONSES THAT FACILITATE DISCUSSION

If the Student Contribution Is...	Possible Teacher's Response to Facilitate Discussion
Accurate and complete	Provide some reinforcement or praise such as a nod or brief affirming statement.
Correct, and there could be many other correct responses as well	Ask another student to add to the response; avoid implying that there is only one correct answer.
Incomplete	Ask a question that encourages the student to include more information.
Not clear	Ask the student to rephrase it, or try to rephrase the response and ask if this is what the student means.
Seemingly incorrect	Invite the student to explain, clarify, or elaborate. Use gentle Socratic questions to lead the student to understand and clarify the error.

Source: Zakrajsek, T. D., & Nilson, L. B. (2023). *Teaching at its best: A research-based resource for college instructors* (5th ed.). Jossey-Bass.

remember and a beginning sense of understanding how arduous and frightening it can be to feel short of breath. Taking part in a group exercise, such as building a bridge with dry spaghetti or assembling a puzzle, can open frank discussion about the dynamics of working in groups to complete tasks. Sorting a collection of items in three different ways helps promote understanding of competing classification systems or nomenclatures. Although doing kinesthetic activities in class takes time, the additional understanding that learners develop through the activity and facilitated reflection promotes lasting learning.

Case Study

A case study is a description of a person, event, or situation. Case studies are often created or adapted based upon life experiences. Case studies may be included in a lecture, discussion, or small group learning activity in classroom, online, or simulation environments. Case studies actively engage learners by providing opportunities to apply concepts or content to real or simulated scenarios, facilitating knowledge retention and deep learning (Mechtel et al., 2024). Effective case studies are relevant, are realistic, promote student engagement, and provide a cognitive challenge for the learners. Case studies provide the experiential context for authentic practice which facilitates development of clinical judgment in competency-based education (Dugan & Altmiller, 2023).

Case studies may present a one-time snapshot of the situation or a continuous, unfolding story over time. Some case studies use a sequential-interactive approach where the learners move through the case study by making decisions or narrowing down solutions and requesting additional information from the teacher to ultimately solve the case (Zakrajsek & Nilson, 2023). Whatever approach is used for the case study, it is important for the teacher to debrief the learners by discussing the problems and solutions identified through the case study. In larger classes, educators can use an audience response system to engage learners and increase interaction around case decisions.

In nursing education, case studies can provide practice opportunities in assessing situations and making decisions. Case studies vary in length from short two- to three-sentence descriptions of a situation to extensive, multipage cases. The length of the case study is determined by the educational purpose for using the approach. Teachers may purchase or create the case studies; frequently, nurse educators develop their own case studies based on prior clinical practice experiences. When creating a case study, the teacher develops objectives and questions that correspond with the case study to engage the learner and foster the development of higher level thinking abilities (analysis, synthesis, evaluation).

Collaborative Learning

The terms cooperative learning and collaborative learning are frequently used interchangeably. However, collaborative learning is the broader term, which is inclusive of cooperative learning. Collaborative learning encourages students to work interdependently to answer questions or solve problems, while still maintaining individual accountability for learning. Collaborative learning increases knowledge retention, engages learners, and facilitates problem-solving and critical thinking disposition (Flott et al., 2022; Zhang & Chen, 2021). Collaborative learning strategies may be used in multiple settings, including classroom, clinical, and online learning environments.

Teachers create a collaborative learning environment by providing opportunities for learner interaction and group collaboration by creating assignments that require small groups of students to work together. Educators build individual accountability into collaborative learning activities by having learners complete self, peer, and group evaluation of contributions to the group's project and functioning. Learners who participate in collaborative learning activities learn group processing skills such as managing group dynamics, ensuring participation by all group members, treating each group member's contributions with respect, and arriving at group consensus.

The teacher's role in collaborative learning is to provide a structure that facilitates problem-solving, assists learners in managing the group process, and helps learners to synthesize and apply their learning (Zakrajsek & Nilson, 2023). It is important for the teacher to clearly articulate the purpose of the collaborative learning activity, help the learners understand the value of the learning activity, provide clear instructions, and facilitate closure on completion of the learning activity. Ideally, small groups of two to four students work best for collaborative learning activities. It is important for the teacher to intentionally incorporate heterogeneity into collaborative learning by forming groups with diversity in characteristics such as individual ability, perspective, gender, academic major, or age. Group heterogeneity provides the opportunity to work with and learn from others who are different.

Team learning agreements may be used to define how the collaborative learning group will work together, thereby encouraging students to be more responsible for their own learning and to actively engage in the learning process because they participated in the creation of the learning environment structure. Collaborative learning groups also need to work together long enough to form effective working relationships. Teaching methods that promote collaborative learning can be used in traditional classroom or online learning environments, including think-write-pair-share, group investigations, three-step interviews, wikis, blogs, threaded discussions, and the use of clickers for interactive academic gaming.

Team-Based Learning

Team-based learning (TBL) is a collaborative learning, that is, an instructor-led, learner-centered approach that facilitates active learning (Yeung et al., 2023). It is comprised of three phases: preparation, readiness assurance, and application of concepts. During the first phase, preparation, students are assigned to review course materials prior to class. In the second phase, assessment of individual and group readiness to participate in the TBL activities is completed. This is frequently accomplished through the use of multiple-choice questions directed toward assessing student readiness. During the third phase, the learners work together to apply course concepts to case-based scenarios and respond to questions as a team. The teams then share their answers and discuss how they reached their conclusions with the whole class. TBL has been found to increase critical thinking skills and problem-solving abilities (Yeung et al., 2023). Additionally, TBL facilitates the development of communication skills, interprofessional collaboration, and active participation in learning (Tatterton & Fisher, 2022).

Problem-Based Learning

PBL is a student-centered learning method that allows learners to be actively engaged in their learning, acquire new information in the context they will use, and create a link between theory and practice. Benefits of PBL include increased critical thinking, knowledge retention, and student satisfaction (Ren et al., 2023; Sharma et al., 2023). Some programs use PBL as a learning method to deliver the entire curriculum, whereas other programs use PBL techniques to deliver selected learning experiences. PBL has been used as a teaching/learning method in traditional theory-based, online, and clinical practice courses. The many different approaches to PBL share common attributes, including that (a) problems are used as the central focus to initiate or motivate learning, (b) students collaborate in small groups and work over a period of time to solve problems, (c) the teacher serves as a facilitator of learning instead of a disseminator of content, (d) the teacher coaches teams for managing group processes, and (e) students initiate and direct learning.

There are four basic stages in implementing a PBL method. The first stage is problem analysis, where introductory information is given to the students, and the group identifies what is known and unknown about the situation. The second stage is brainstorming, where the group identifies resources to meet learning needs. During this stage, the group may also pose questions to the facilitator or their peers to clarify the situation. The third stage is self-directed learning, where each group member researches and gathers information to share. The final stage is solution testing, which is an iterative process where group members share resources and information to test solutions by applying new knowledge to solve the situation.

PBL requires the teacher to actively facilitate group learning rather than deliver content. Because PBL relies on students building upon prior content knowledge, PBL may not be the most effective teaching method for entirely new content. It can take students time to adapt to active teaching methods, such as PBL, if they have been previously socialized to more passive teaching methods. To help students transition, the teacher can introduce PBL gradually and explain how the roles of educator and student are different in PBL.

Simulation, Standardized Patients, Role-Play, and Drama

Simulation-based education is a form of experiential learning that provides a safe environment for learning. It is based on the learning theories of constructivism and Kolb's experiential learning theory. the National League for Nursing's Jeffries simulation theory, comprised of five components (context, background, design, simulation experience, and outcomes), is frequently used to guide the development of simulation-based education (Bowden et al., 2022). The range of fidelity, or faithfulness, to reality in simulation is wide. At the low-fidelity end, learners practice injecting a medication into a practice pad or even a piece of fruit to feel the sense of puncturing through a barrier, while at the high end of simulation fidelity, learners provide care to standardized patients enacting health conditions or manikins programmed with realistic physiological responses.

Simulation can support learning in the cognitive, affective, and psychomotor domains. Simulation is a powerful teaching method and is usually integrated throughout most undergraduate nursing curricula. The use of simulation may increase clinical judgment, deductive reasoning, critical thinking, and student self-confidence (Brown et al., 2023; Strauch et al., 2024). Teaching with clinical simulation is described in detail in Chapter 9.

Standardized patients (i.e., individuals who are specially trained to act as patients for the instruction) are used in nursing education to provide students with simulated patient experiences to practice skills such as performing assessments, communicating with families, interviewing patients, and teaching patients (Taylor & Coulter, 2023). The use of clinical experiences with standardized patients provides the faculty with an opportunity to assess student learning and evaluate student preparation for live clinical patient encounters. Formative and summative evaluation of student clinical performance may also be conducted with the assistance of standardized patients. Many advanced practice nursing programs use objective structured clinical examinations (OSCEs) staffed with standardized patients to evaluate learner competencies.

Role-play is a teaching method that allows the learner to portray the role of another individual, anticipating how that individual will respond in a given situation. In nursing education, role-play may be used to teach therapeutic communication, conflict resolution skills, and other competencies. It is important for the teacher to create a safe environment to help learners feel comfortable engaging in role-play. Role-play helps the learner anticipate and respond to what an individual might say or do in a situation. Role-playing promotes the development of clinical judgment, empathy, reflection, and self-efficacy (Huang et al., 2023; Kim et al., 2022). It is challenging to use role-play as a teaching method in large enrollment classes because only a few learners will have the opportunity to actively participate in the role-play activity, whereas the majority of learners may observe as members of the audience.

Participating in a scripted *drama* or theatrical presentation is a specific type of role-play that has been used to help nursing students learn about communication, conflict management, end-of-life care, social justice, and ethical or legal issues. Students may participate in the drama as actors or they may watch the drama as observers. The use of drama as a teaching method allows the learner to acquire new knowledge by experiencing a situation and relating to the characters in the situation. Drama increases awareness and empathy, promotes understanding of diverse perspectives, and changes attitudes (Kesgin & Tok, 2023; Khanlou et al., 2022). Role-playing and drama are most effective for learning experiences when followed by thoughtful debriefing and reflection. The use of drama as a teaching method is an effective approach for providing experiential learning around situations that are difficult to arrange in the clinical environment.

Teaching Others and Making Presentations

There is nothing like developing a presentation to encourage immersion in a topic. Through preparing and giving presentations, students have the opportunity to learn the same way that many teachers have learned unfamiliar content. Organizing a presentation forces thinking about what information is needed, what the audience already knows, and how to explain a complex topic. Presentations focus on information in a chosen or assigned content area but have the additional advantage of providing real practice in the authentic workplace skill of teaching or explaining a concept to others.

Although the student presenter has an active role in learning through the preparation and delivery of a presentation, the other students observing the presentation stay in the positions of passive learners unless their roles are restructured. Assigning the audience members to some of the roles traditionally held by the teacher, such as moderator, timekeeper, provider of positive feedback, and provider of suggestions for further improvement changes the experience of the audience members to active participants in the learning. Engaging each of the students in some role helps adjust the experience to be more collegial and improves the learning potential for both the student presenter and the student audience.

Recording their presentations provides students the opportunity to see how they look and sound as presenters, and it allows for repeated or asynchronous viewing. Class members can provide feedback live or through online interactive video software programs.

Service Learning

Service learning is a form of experiential education, which provides students with the opportunity to apply theory to practice while meeting an identified community or organization need (Baker et al., 2021). Student participation in service learning increases engagement in learning, promotes a positive attitude toward civic involvement, enhances cultural humility, and improves students' abilities to apply course concepts to the real world (Baker et al., 2021). Service learning is distinguished from volunteer work by the primary goal of learning through providing service.

To effectively implement service learning, the teacher facilitates discovery learning and critical reflection to ensure that new knowledge, concepts, and skills are meaningfully linked to the learner's personal experiences. Characteristics of effective service-learning experiences include joint planning between the academic institution and community partner, reciprocity between partners, clearly defined roles and responsibilities, effective communication among all parties, and a comprehensive student orientation to the service-learning project.

LARGE CLASS METHODS

Lecture

A well-organized and enthusiastic lecture can be an inspiring event, while a lecture in which the presenter reads the slides aloud can lead to learners daydreaming. Some advantages of lecturing include that it is an efficient method for delivering content to large groups of students and that students receive the same information. Additionally, lecturing provides the teacher with a sense of control over the learning environment. Lectures may also be used to supplement other learning materials.

Lecture may be delivered live or video recorded. Teachers prefer synchronous live lectures to engage learners whereas students report preferring asynchronous video-recorded lectures because they are accessible, convenient, flexible and allow for repeat viewing of the content (Watson et al., 2023). Teachers may be concerned about knowledge retention with asynchronous video-recorded lectures; however, Alharbi et al. (2022) found that immediate knowledge retention among nursing students was equivalent in live lectures and video-recorded lectures.

Teachers organizing and preparing lectures may learn about the intended content through their own active engagement in the process; however, the students attending a lecture often remain passive, which may result in decreased engagement and knowledge retention. The key to keeping students engaged is to divide a longer lecture into several minilectures and stop talking every few minutes while students participate in active thinking tasks. Tasks that help students understand what they are hearing might be generating examples of the concept under discussion, taking part in a kinesthetic activity related to the concept, or applying the concept to solve a problem. For lectures to be effective, it is important to integrate active learning techniques, summarize critical information, and clarify any information that is unclear to the students. Exhibit 5.4 describes teacher actions that improve the effectiveness of lectures.

EXHIBIT 5.4 Suggestions for an Effective Lecture

- Determine intended learning outcomes.
- Budget extra time for questions and interaction.
- Subdivide content in 15-minute or shorter segments of content.
- Intersperse lecture with learning activities.
- Use attention grabbers to engage learners.
- Incorporate visuals, examples, and restatements.
- Engage students in recapping and summarizing key points.

Source: Zakrajsek, T. D., & Nilson, L. B. (2023). *Teaching at its best: A research-based resource for college instructors* (5th ed.). Jossey-Bass.

QUESTIONING

Questions are a powerful tool for understanding what learners are thinking and helping learners organize and expand their thinking. However, a teacher's question can strike fear into the heart of a learner who is overly worried about what answer the teacher expects. It is important for the teacher to create a safe learning environment built on mutual respect between the teacher and students, and to convey a nonjudgmental, supportive attitude to effectively use questioning strategies as a teaching/learning method (Gonzalez et al., 2021).

Brookfield et al. (2023) describe supporting development of critical thinking through asking learners first about the general ideas or concepts being presented, then later asking more direct questions about the learner's own ideas. They suggest a process of asking learners questions related to identifying their assumptions, checking their assumptions, seeing multiple viewpoints, and taking informed actions. Another approach is to ask learners open-ended questions that promote higher order thinking (Gonzalez et al., 2021).

A Socratic inquiry approach may be used across educational settings (didactic, clinical, experiential, and online). The purpose of Socratic inquiry is to help the student or group uncover their knowledge, make connections among concepts, evaluate assumptions, appraise evidence, and reflect upon their thinking through a series of exploratory questions. When using this approach, the teacher asks the learner different types of questions to clarify, conclude, connect, define, explore, justify, or probe (Dinkins & Cangelosi, 2019; Makhene, 2019). It can be intimidating for learners to be asked a series of direct questions, thus the teacher can ask some questions indirectly in the form of a request that begins with "please share" or "tell me more." Socratic questioning increases critical thinking, enhances moral reasoning, develops problem-solving, and promotes self-reflection (Dinkins & Cangelosi, 2019; Makhene, 2019; Torabizadeh et al., 2018). Table 5.7 lists types of questions and sample Socratic questions for each type.

Educational Games

Educational games are effective in reinforcing knowledge, motivating effort, engaging learners, enhancing collaboration, improving communication, developing teamwork, and creating a relaxed atmosphere that facilitates comprehension of content (Chang et al., 2022; Tavares, 2022; Zehler & Musallam, 2021). Many students perceive games as positive and motivational; however, some learners experience anxiety, embarrassment, and intimidation with the peer competition aspect of gaming (Tavares, 2022). Educational games provide immediate formative feedback to the learners and allow the teacher to assess the amount of learning that has occurred (Chang et al., 2022; Tavares, 2022; Zehler & Musallam, 2021).

Educational games can be high or low technology and are classified by genre such as adventure, music, puzzle, racing, role-play, simulation, sports, and strategy. Learners playing high-tech simulation or strategy games may use virtual reality or interactive video gaming to experience real-life situations or events that facilitate learning and decision-making. Low-tech games such as question-and-answer board games, team quizzes, card games, and tossing the ball to answer the question on-the-spot are effective in reinforcing learning.

TABLE 5.7 SAMPLE SOCRATIC QUESTIONS

Type of Question	Purpose	Sample questions/probes
Analogy	Help learner draw comparisons between concepts	How is concept "x" similar to concept "y"? How is concept "x" different than concept "y"? What are the similarities between "x" concept and "y" concept? What are the differences between "x" concept and "y" concept?
Clarifying	Help learner refine beliefs	What is your belief about "x"? Tell me why you believe that. Share the information you have that supports your belief. What information do you have that does not support your belief?
Connecting	Help learner discuss connections or relationships between concepts	How are these concepts connected? How is concept "x" related to concept "y"?
Concluding	Help learner arrive at conclusions or judgments	How did you arrive at this conclusion? Share the evidence you used to reach this conclusion. What evidence supports this conclusion? What evidence does not support this conclusion?
Defining	Help learner define concepts or foundational knowledge	Share your understanding of "x" concept. Tell me why "x" situation/problem is occurring.
Probing	Help learner develop a deeper understanding	Tell me more about . . . What other information do you know about . . . that you have not already shared? Is there any additional information that you'd like to gather to help you understand this concept?

Source: Dinkins, C., & Cangelosi, P. (2019). Putting Socrates back in Socratic method: Theory-based debriefing in the nursing classroom. *Nursing Philosophy, 20*(2), e12240. https://doi.org/10.1111/nup.12240; Makhene, A. (2019). The use of the Socratic inquiry to facilitate critical thinking in nursing education. *Health SA Gesondheid, 24*, a1224. https://doi.org/10.4102/hsag.v24i0.1224

The teacher should assess and match the fit between the goal for the education session (i.e., delivering new content or reinforcing information) and the readiness of the learners to participate in the game. To effectively use gaming, teachers should be confident in their ability to lead the gaming session and be able to adjust it, dependent on the learners' responses. Logistical factors such as the amount of time, class size, and the teaching environment might be constraints to implementing gaming.

Film

Cinemeducation or digital storytelling is the use of movies or film clips to teach concepts, facilitate discussion, encourage affective learning, and foster deeper thinking (Rueb et al., 2024; Wiles & Enslein, 2021). Movies are effective in promoting reflective thinking, perspective taking, and emotional narratives which facilitate empathy, changes in attitudes, and knowledge acquisition (Rueb et al., 2024). Movies create a controlled learning environment and an opportunity to experience new situations. One drawback of using movies is that learners may make unsupported inferences about what they observe, and they may not have the opportunity to ask questions as they would in a live practice situation. The teacher can ask specific questions to guide learners in identifying inferences from the movie and considering additional information they would obtain if they could interact with the characters.

The teacher should preview the film and ensure that it supports the desired concept, then provide learners with objectives to guide the experience and reflective questions to stimulate critical thinking. The students might submit responses to the teacher for evaluation or discuss responses with peers. Another approach is to have them write about specific concepts seen in the movie. Wiles and Enslein (2021) used this type of approach to teach critical thinking concepts.

Debate

Debate helps learners develop collaboration, communication, and critical thinking skills; structure logical arguments; and engage in rebuttals (Chen et al., 2022). Teachers can use debate with small or large groups of learners. A common format for debate involves assigning groups of learners opposing positions on a controversial topic. The teacher provides the structure, facilitates learners' argument development, poses logical questions, manages group dynamics and interpersonal communications, and facilitates learners' reflection. Nurse educators frequently use debate to facilitate thinking about ethical issues. Debate encourages learners to develop logical arguments and impromptu fact-based responses about controversial issues.

Narrative Pedagogy/Storytelling

The use of stories for teaching and learning purposes facilitates awareness through connection with the characters in the story, engagement in the learning process, and application to the clinical context (Nash-Patel et al., 2023; Padden-Denmead et al., 2023). Storytelling formats can range from a simple face-to-face verbal or audio recording recounting an experience to a polished multimedia production. Narratives provide a strategy to expose students to experiences of other people and cultures.

The same experience can be told as a story from different perspectives and with different themes in mind. For example, stories told on a nursing unit to newly hired staff may have the purpose of a cautionary tale, an orientation to the unit culture, establishment of a hierarchy, or providing other information. Although storytelling is common to many purposes, educators have systematically investigated the use of narrative in nursing. Narrative pedagogy is a unique approach that calls upon teachers to "create opportunities to talk with students about their thinking, how they understand (interpret) the situations they encounter, and what this means to their emerging nursing practice" (Ironside, 2015, p. 85).

The wide availability of digital media has provided many options for narratives, including videos and podcasts. A simple recording of a story in the patient's own voice could provide the prompt for an engaging class discussion or other assignment. Teachers need to obtain written permission from the storyteller before recording and sharing narratives.

SUMMARY

Teachers can make a significant difference in outcomes for learners by establishing a supportive learning environment. Encouraging a positive class climate and respectful interactions among peers promotes the development of an effective environment for learning. The educator selecting a teaching method should consider the fit of that method with the learning objectives, learner and teacher characteristics, and available resources. Of these factors, the single most critical aspect in choosing a teaching method is judging the fit of that method with the intended learning outcomes or objectives.

Learning can be described as development in one or more of three different domains: cognitive, affective, and psychomotor. Some teaching strategies support learning in all three domains, whereas other strategies are more specific to learning in only one or two of the domains.

The characteristics of the intended learners, including their social and cognitive cultures, are important to consider in choosing teaching methods. A teacher does not have to be skilled in using every method. It is important for the teacher to be comfortable with the methods chosen so that the focus of attention stays on learners and the learning process. Choices of teaching method are sustainable when they are realistic for the reasonably available resources. Resources to consider in choosing teaching methods include time, space, support staff, technology, and materials.

A focus on learner engagement and active learning is aligned with a general trend away from teacher-centered strategies and toward strategies focused on what students learn. Two processes are important for active learning: action and reflection. Taking part in some meaningful activity followed by reflecting on the learning processes and outcomes transforms the learner from a passive recipient of someone else's thoughts to a constructor of knowledge and meaning. There are many teaching methods for active learning that promote the development of critical thinking. These include case studies, concept mapping, collaborative or team learning, PBL, service learning, and gaming.

Teaching methods were categorized in this chapter as independent learning, small group methods, and large class methods. However, each of the methods can be used in more than one way. Independent learning methods include reading; writing;

reflection; contract learning (including a team learning contract, contract learning approach to a course, and an individual learning contract); concept mapping; and RLOs. Small group methods presented in the chapter were discussion; experiential methods; case study; collaborative learning; PBL; simulation (including standardized patients, role-play, imagined script writing, and drama); presentations; and service learning. Large class methods include lecture, questioning, demonstration, educational games, film (and other media), debate, and narrative pedagogy/storytelling. Each of these teaching methods was discussed in the chapter.

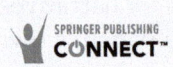

A robust set of instructor resources designed to supplement this text is located at http://connect.springerpub.com/content/book/978-0-8261-8892-2. Qualifying instructors may request access by emailing textbook@springerpub.com.

REFERENCES

Addy, T. M., Dube, D., Mitchell, K. A., & SoRelle, M. (2021). *What inclusive instructors do: Principles and practices for excellence in college teaching*. Routledge. https://doi.org/10.4324/9781003448655

Alharbi, H. A., Shehadeh, F., & Awaji, N. Y. (2022). Immediate knowledge retention among nursing students in live lecture and video-recorded lecture: A quasi-experimental study. *Nurse Education in Practice, 60*, 103307. https://doi.org/10.1016/j.nepr.2022.103307

Anderson, L. W., Krathwohl, D. R., Airasian, P., Cruikshank, K. A., Mayer, R. E., Pintrich, P., Raths, J., & Wittrock, M. (2001). *A taxonomy for learning, teaching, and assessing: A revision of Bloom's taxonomy of educational objectives*. Longman.

Baker, H., Pfeiffer, K., Field, M., Nasatir-Hilty, S., Doiev, J., Worland, B. J., Clark-Youngblood, M., Harrell, K., & Mascorro, A. (2021). A substance use disorder service-learning immersion experience for prelicensure nursing students. *Nurse Educator, 46*(5), 273–275. https://doi.org/10.1097/NNE.0000000000000952

Barta, A., Fodor, L. A., Tamas, B., & Szamoskozi, I. (2022). The development of students critical thinking abilities and dispositions through the concept mapping learning method – a meta-analysis. *Educational Research Review, 37*, 100481. https://doi.org/10.1016/j.edurev.2022.100481

Benner, P., Sutphen, M., Leonard, V., & Day, L. (2009). *Educating nurses: A call for radical transformation*. Jossey-Bass.

Bowden, A., Traynor, V., Chang, H. (Rita), & Wilson, V. (2022). Beyond the technology: Applying the NLN Jeffries Simulation Theory in the context of aging simulation. *Nursing Forum, 57*(3), 473–479. https://doi.org/10.1111/nuf.12687

Brookfield, S., Rudolph, J., & Tan, S. (2023). *Teaching well: Understanding key dynamics of learning-centered classrooms*. Routledge. https://doi.org/10.4324/9781003447467

Brown, K. M., Swoboda, S. M., Gilbert, G. E., Horvath, C., & Sullivan, N. (2023). Curricular integration of virtual reality in nursing education. *The Journal of Nursing Education, 62*(6), 364–373. https://doi.org/10.3928/01484834-20230110-01

Casselden, B., & Pears, R. (2020). Higher education student pathways to ebook usage and engagement, and understanding: Highways and cul de sacs. *Journal of Librarianship and Information Science, 52*(2), 601–619. https://doi.org/10.1177/0961000619841429

Chang, Y.-S., Hu, S. H., Kuo, S.-W., Chang, K.-M., Kuo, C.-L., Nguyen, T. V., & Chuang, Y.-H. (2022). Effects of board game play on nursing students' medication knowledge: A randomized controlled trial. *Nurse Education in Practice, 63*, 103412. https://doi.org/10.1016/j.nepr.2022.103412

Chen, X., Wang, L., Zhai, X., & Li, Y. (2022) Exploring the effects of argument map-supported online group debate activities on college students' critical thinking. *Frontiers in Psychology, 13*, 856462. https://doi.org/10.3389/fpsyg.2022.856462

Chicca, J., & Shellenbarger, T. (2021). Preparing, maintaining, and evaluating remote preceptorships: Considerations for nurse educators. *Teaching and Learning in Nursing, 16*(4), 396–400. https://doi.org/10.1016/j.teln.2021.04.006

Cline, G., & Rinaldi, K. (2023). A compelling case for the use of backward design to advance competency-based nursing education. *Nurse Educator, 48*(5), E168–E169. https://doi.org/10.1097/NNE.0000000000001388

Dave, R. H. (1970). Developing and writing educational objectives (psychomotor levels). In R. J. Armstrong (Ed.), *Developing and writing behavioral objectives*. Educational Innovators Press.

Dinkins, C., & Cangelosi, P. (2019). Putting Socrates back in Socratic method: Theory-based debriefing in the nursing classroom. *Nursing Philosophy, 20*(2), e12240. https://doi.org/10.1111/nup.12240

Dugan, M., & Altmiller, G. (2023). AACN Essentials and nurse practitioner education: Competency-based case studies grounded in authentic practice. *Journal of Professional Nursing, 46,* 59–64. https://doi.org/10.1016/j.profnurs.2023.02.003

Eisenmann, N. (2021). An innovative clinical concept map to promote clinical judgment in nursing students. *Journal of Nursing Education, 60* (3), 143–149. https://doi.org/10.3928/01484834-20210222-04

Fisher, D., & Frey, N. (2019). Best practices in adolescent literacy instruction. In L. Morrow, L. Gambrell, & H. Casey (Eds.), *Best practices in literacy instruction* (6th ed.). Guilford Publications.

Flott, E., Ball, S., Hanks, J., Minnich, M., Kirkpatrick, A., Rusch, L., Koziol, D., Laughlin, A., & Williams, J. (2022). Fostering collaborative learning and leadership through near-peer mentorship among undergraduate nursing students. *Nursing Forum (Hillsdale), 57*(5), 750–755. https://doi.org/10.1111/nuf.12755

Foundation for Critical Thinking. (2019). *Using intellectual standards to assess student reasoning.* https://www.criticalthinking.org/pages/using-intellectual-standards-to-assess-student-reasoning/602

Gallup. (2023). *Honesty/ethics in professions.* http://www.gallup.com/poll/1654/-honesty-ethics-professions.aspx

Gonzalez, L., Nielsen, A., & Lasater, K. (2021). Developing students clinical reasoning skills: A faculty guide. *Journal of Nursing Education, 60*(9), 485–493. https://doi.org/10.3928/01484834-20210708-01

Huang, S.-M., Fang, S.-C., Lee, S.-Y., Yu, P.-J., Chen, C.-J., & Lin, Y.-S. (2023). Effects of video-recorded role-play and guided reflection on nursing student empathy, caring behavior and competence: A two-group pretest-posttest study. *Nurse Education in Practice, 67,* 103560. https://doi.org/10.1016/j.nepr.2023.103560

Ignatavicius, D. (2019). *Teaching and learning in a concept-based nursing curriculum: A how-to best practice approach.* Jones & Bartlett.

Ingraham, K., Davidson, S., & Yonge, O. (2018). Student-faculty relationships and its impact on academic outcomes. *Nurse Education Today, 71*(12), 17–21. https://doi.org/10.1016/j.nedt.2018.08.021

Ironside, P. M. (2015). Narrative pedagogy: Transforming nursing education through 15 years of research in nursing education. *Nursing Education Perspectives, 36*(2), 83–88. https://doi.org/10.5480/13-1102

Kesgin, M. T., & Tok, H. H. (2023). The impact of drama education and in-class education on nursing students' attitudes toward violence against women: A randomized controlled study. *Nurse Education Today, 125,* 105779. https://doi.org/10.1016/j.nedt.2023.105779

Khanlou, N., Vazquez, L. M., Khan, A., Orazietti, B., & Ross, G. (2022). Readers Theatre as an arts-based approach to education: A scoping review on experiences of adult learners and educators. *Nurse Education Today, 116,* 105440. https://doi.org/10.1016/j.nedt.2022.105440

Kim, J. H., Lim, J. M., & Kim, E. M. (2022). Patient handover education programme based on situated learning theory for nursing students in clinical practice. *International Journal of Nursing Practice, 28*(1), e13005. https://doi.org/10.1111/ijn.13005

Knowles, M. S., Holton, E. F., Stanson, R. A., & Robinson, P. A. (2020). *The adult learner: The definitive classic adult education and human resource development* (9th ed.). Routledge.

Krathwohl, D. R., Bloom, B. S., & Masia, B. B. (1964). *Taxonomy of educational objectives: The classification of educational goals. Handbook II: Affective domain.* David McKay.

Lipnevich, A. A., Panadero, E., & Calistro, T. (2023). Unraveling the effects of rubrics and exemplars on student writing performance. *Journal of Experimental Psychology: Applied, 29*(1), 136–148. https://doi.org/10.1037/xap0000434

Makhene, A. (2019). The use of the Socratic inquiry to facilitate critical thinking in nursing education. *Health SA Gesondheid, 24*, a1224. https://doi.org/10.4102/hsag.v24i0.1224

Mechtel, M., Kitt-Lewis, E., Reaves, C., Sinacori, B., O'Brien, T., Logan, P., Rimbey, P., Streiff, K., & Phillips, K. (2024). Durable learning strategies in nursing education: State-of-the-evidence review. *Journal of Nursing Education, 63*(1), 24–31. https://doi.org/10.3928/01484834-20231112-05

Mertz, P. S., Sherrer, S. M., & Bowers, G. M. (2023). Teaching and assessing undergraduate collaboration skills scaffolded through the biochemistry curriculum using collaboration rubrics and student learning contracts. *Biochemistry and Molecular Biology Education, 51*(5), 499–507. https://doi.org/10.1002/bmb.21760

Nash-Patel, T., Anderson, E., O'Donoghue, B., Paliokosta, P., & Morrow, E. (2023). StoryAid: Nursing students' relational learning for adolescents with intellectual learning disabilities. *Journal of Nursing Education, 62*(1), 51–57. https://doi.org/10.3928/01484834-20220912-12

Oermann, M. H., Gaberson, K. B., & De Gagne, J. C. (2025). *Evaluation and testing in nursing education* (7th ed.). Springer Publishing Company.

Oh, J.-W., Huh, B., & Kim, M.-R. (2019). Effect of learning contracts in clinical pediatric nursing education on students' outcomes: A research article. *Nurse Education Today, 83*(12), 104191. https://doi.org/10.1016/j.nedt.2019.08.009

Padden-Denmead, M. L., Adelung, M., Arnone, J., Ludan, L., Ruffin, L., & Scaffidi, R. M. (2023). Nursing students' perceptions of racism in nursing and health care. *Journal of Nursing Education, 62*(10), 563–569. https://doi.org/10.3928/01484834-20230815-07

Panadero, E., García-Pérez, D., Fernández Ruiz, J., Fraile, J., Sánchez-Iglesias, I., & Brown, G. T. L. (2023). Feedback and year level effects on university students' self-efficacy and emotions during self-assessment: Positive impact of rubrics vs. instructor feedback. *Educational Psychology (Dorchester-on-Thames), 43*(7), 756–779. https://doi.org/10.1080/01443410.2023.2254015

Patterson, B. J., & Forneris, S. (2023). Faculty as learners: Neuroscience in action. *Journal of Nursing Education, 62*(5), 291–297. https://doi.org/10.3928/01484834-20230306-02

Ren, S., Li, Y., Pu, L., & Feng, Y. (2023). Effects of problem-based learning on delivering medical and nursing education: A systematic review and meta-analysis of randomized controlled trials. *Worldviews on Evidence-Based Nursing, 20*(5), 500–512. https://doi.org/10.1111/wvn.12663

Ritchey, K. A., & List, A. (2022). Task-oriented reading: A framework for improving college students' reading compliance and comprehension. *College Teaching, 70*(3), 280–295. https://doi.org/10.1080/87567555.2021.1924607

Rueb, M., Rehfuess, E. A., Siebeck, M., & Pfadenhauer, L. M. (2024). Cinemeducation: A mixed methods study on learning through reflective thinking, perspective taking and emotional narratives. *Medical Education, 58*(1), 63–92. https://doi.org/10.1111/medu.15166

Sharma, S., Saragih, I. D., Tarihoran, D. E. T. A. U., & Chou, F.-H. (2023). Outcomes of problem-based learning in nurse education: A systematic review and meta-analysis. *Nurse Education Today, 120*, 105631. https://doi.org/10.1016/j.nedt.2022.105631

Steven, A., Wilson, G., Turunen, H., Vizcaya-Moreno, M., Azimirad, M., Kakurel, J., Porras, J., Tella, S., Pérez-Cañaveras, R., Sasso, L., Aleo, G., Myhre, K., Ringstad, Ø., Sara-Aho, A., Scott, M., & Pearson, P. (2020). Critical incident techniques and reflection in nursing and health professions education. *Nurse Educator, 45*(6), E57–E61. https://doi.org/10.1097/NNE.0000000000000796

Strauch, K. A., Renz, S. M., DeMutis, K. O., & Sochalski, J. (2024). Use of simulation to integrate behavioral health into primary care nurse practitioner programs. *Journal of Nursing Education, 63*(2), 128–133. https://doi.org/10.3928/01484834-20230815-03

Tatterton, M. J., & Fisher, M. J. (2022). Team-based learning and nurse education. *Evidence Based Journals, 25*(4), 117–118. https://doi.org/10.1136/ebnurs-2022-103595

Tavares, N. (2022). The use and impact of game-based learning on the learning experience and knowledge retention of nursing undergraduate students: A systematic literature review. *Nurse Education Today, 117*, 105484. https://doi.org/10.1016/j.nedt.2022.105484

Taylor, P. H., & Coulter, K. (2023). Exploring the effectiveness of telehealth simulation in a standardized patient scenario. *Journal of Nursing Education, 62*(3), 162–166. https://doi.org/10.3928/01484834-20230109-06

Torabizadeh, C., Homayuni, L., Moattari, M., Monteverde, S., & Defilippis, T. (2018). Impacts of Socratic questioning on moral reasoning of nursing students. *Nursing Ethics, 25*(2), 174–185. https://doi.org/10.1177/0969733016667775

Uçar, B., & Çevik, Y. D. (2021). The effect of argument mapping supported with peer feedback on pre-service teachers' argumentation skills. *Journal of Digital Learning in Teacher Education, 37*(1), 6–29. https://doi.org/10.1080/21532974.2020.1815107

Vinette, B., Lapierre, A., Lavoie, A., Leclerc-Loiselle, J., Charette, M., & Deschênes, M.-F. (2023). Educational strategies used in master's and doctoral nursing education: A scoping review. *Journal of Professional Nursing, 48*, 84–92. https://doi.org/10.1016/j.profnurs.2023.06.006

Vo, T. N., Chiu, H.-Y., Chuang, Y.-H., & Huang, H.-C. (2023). Prevalence of stress and anxiety among nursing students a systematic review and meta-analysis. *Nurse Educator, 48*(3), E90–E95. https://doi.org/10.1097/NNE.0000000000001343

Watson, C., Templet, T., Leigh, G., Broussard, L., & Gillis, L. (2023). Student and faculty perceptions of effectiveness of online teaching modalities. *Nurse Education Today, 120*, 105651–105651. https://doi.org/10.1016/j.nedt.2022.105651

Wiggins, G., & McTighe, J. (2005). *Understanding by design* (2nd ed.). Pearson Education

Wiles, B., & Enslein, T. (2021). From sully to nightingale: Critical thinking through esthetic learning. *Journal of Nursing Education, 60*(5), 281–285. https://doi.org/10.3928/01484834-20210420-08

Wu, H.-Z., & Wu, Q.-T. (2020). Impact of mind mapping on the critical thinking ability of clinical nursing students and teaching application. *Journal of International Medical Research, 48*(3), 300060519893225. https://doi.org/10.1177/0300060519893225

Yarmohammadi, A., Mostafazadeh, F., & Shahbazzadegan, S. (2023). Comparison lecture and concept map methods on the level of learning and satisfaction in puerperal sepsis education of midwifery students: A quasi-experimental study. *BMC Medical Education, 23*(1), 251. https://doi.org/10.1186/s12909-023-04247-8

Yeung, M. M.-Y., Yuen, J. W.-M., Chen, J. M.-T., & Lam, K. K.-L. (2023). The efficacy of team-based learning in developing the generic capability of problem-solving ability and critical thinking skills in nursing education: A systematic review. *Nurse Education Today, 122*, 105704. https://doi.org/10.1016/j.nedt.2022.105704

Zakrajsek, T. D., & Nilson, L. B. (2023). *Teaching at its best: A research-based resource for college instructors* (5th ed.). Jossey-Bass

Zehler, A., & Musallam, E. (2021). Game-based learning and nursing students' clinical judgment in postpartum hemorrhage: A Pilot Study. *The Journal of Nursing Education, 60*(3), 159–164. https://doi.org/10.3928/01484834-20210222-07

Zhang, J., & Chen, B. (2021). The effect of cooperative learning on critical thinking of nursing students in clinical practicum: A quasi-experimental study. *Journal of Professional Nursing, 37*(1), 177–183. https://doi.org/10.1016/j.profnurs.2020.05.008

Ethical, Legal, and Social Challenges in Academic Nursing

6

Mary Ellen Smith Glasgow

OBJECTIVES

1. Discuss the array of ethical, legal, and social matters confronting nursing faculty in the academic setting
2. Describe practical recommendations for handling current ethical, legal, and social challenges in nursing education

INTRODUCTION

Competent nursing faculty are expected to possess knowledge not only of theory, practice, and teaching but also of ethical, legal, and social issues within academic settings. This chapter addresses the challenges facing higher education, with a specific focus on nurse educators, administrators, and their students. It aims to assist nursing faculty and administrators in learning strategies to prevent academic misconduct and use social media appropriately. The chapter also discusses the importance of addressing interpersonal incivility, conflicts of interest, and adhering to academic policies within academic settings. Emphasizing a practical approach, this chapter incorporates case studies to illustrate the identification and management of ethical, legal, and social dilemmas prevalent in academic nursing today. By exploring these critical issues, the chapter provides nurse educators and administrators with the necessary tools to cultivate an environment characterized by integrity, responsibility, and ethical conduct within the academic setting.

ROLE OF UNIVERSITY LEGAL COUNSEL

It is essential for nursing faculty to navigate ethical and legal challenges effectively within academic settings. When faculty members encounter questions or concerns regarding the ethical or legal implications of behaviors exhibited by students, staff, or colleagues, they should first consult the faculty and student handbooks and then share these concerns with their team leader or department chair to seek guidance. They should not discuss the issue with students, staff, or other faculty members due to privacy issues. The first-line nursing administrator may be able to offer helpful advice to resolve the problem.

In instances where complexities arise or issues have been previously reported, escalation to the academic dean becomes necessary. If concerns extend beyond the

> **EXHIBIT 6.1 When to Contact University Legal Counsel**
>
> A faculty member can typically contact the university legal counsel's office through human resources, the department chairs, or other administrators in the case of student infractions. The university counsel's role is to represent the university; this is their ethical and professional obligation.
>
> If the university's redress is insufficient, it might be wise to speak with a private attorney in extreme cases. Consequently, if there are disagreements with an institutional policy, the university counsel will not be able to represent a specific faculty member or group of faculty members. If a member of a protected class experiences bullying, harassment, or discrimination at the hands of a faculty or staff member, they have the right to file a complaint with the office of equality.

Source: Adapted from Smith Glasgow, M. E., Dreher, H. M., Dahnke, M., & Gyllenhammer, J. (2020). *Legal and ethical issues in nursing education: An essential guide.* Springer Publishing Company. Reprinted by permission.

department or school of nursing, collaboration with higher administration levels such as the provost, human resources department, or university's legal office is vital to ensure a comprehensive resolution. Today, most universities and colleges have legal offices (Exhibit 6.1).

Attorneys and paralegal personnel advise their colleagues in academics, student life, and the physical plant on policies, contracts, public safety concerns, financial aid, grant management, academic affairs, and state and federal regulations. Most of the work performed by the university legal counsel's office is preventive, aimed at avoiding lawsuits, negative publicity, and low morale. The legal office cannot assume that university colleagues are well informed about legal issues; therefore, staff in the university counsel's office can help inform the academic community through webinars and personal meetings.

Legal issues are often complex; however, what happens if the faculty concern relates to the legal implications of administrator or organizational behavior (Hunter et al., 2020; Smith Glasgow et al., 2020)? To whom is university counsel loyal—the administrator, dean, student, academic staff member, or the nursing faculty member who raised the concern? Whose confidence, rights, and privacy will they protect? When there is a lawsuit brought against the faculty member, claiming that they injured a student or other third party, the educator's interests align with the institution, and it is critical for all involved to be aware of the situation. However, what if the faculty member's disagreement is with the dean or head of the department? Does it make a difference if the faculty member's concern is organizational (i.e., they believe their supervisor is violating university policy) or personal (i.e., they believe they were treated unfairly)? These are some of the most difficult issues university counsel must contend with, and if the lawyer exercises poor judgment, there may be serious legal repercussions. If the university is directly involved in the legal issue, an attorney outside the university or school may be engaged. It may be advisable for the faculty member to seek their own external legal counsel if they perceive there is a conflict of interest with the institution (Smith Glasgow et al., 2020).

University legal counsel can advise deans and chairs about a range of concerns encompassing hiring decisions, discriminatory behavior, student relations, employee management, and other issues. Facts are critical, and even a slight alteration in the facts can have significant legal ramifications. Therefore, careful documentation and good record keeping is key. It is generally advisable to involve legal affairs early in the process rather than later (Smith Glasgow et al., 2020). If the issue is internal to the university, the assistance provided may be more practical than legal.

ROLE OF THE UNIVERSITY OMBUDSPERSON

Alcover (2009) observed, "Universities and academia are the ideal breeding grounds for conflicts, disputes, problems, and grievances because of their nature, structure, and internal relationships. One popular dispute resolution procedure in these circumstances is mediation" (p. 275). A faculty or staff ombudsperson is another option used to resolve internal complaints, in addition to other conflict resolution and problem-solving strategies. An organizational ombudsperson employs diplomacy, informal mediation, facilitation, and conflict coaching to offer people discreet, unofficial, and unbiased assistance (Howard, 2013). An organizational ombudsperson also serves as a resource to help faculty figure out how to raise concerns they may have about potential misconduct. In addition to handling complaints and disputes raised by guests, the organizational ombudsperson may confidentially report organizational issues, systemic issues, and trends to executives and senior administrators. Rather than standing up for specific people, organizations, or things, in the ideal scenario, they defend the principles of justice and equity (Spitalniak, 2022).

ACADEMIC POLICIES

Academic policies and procedures are integral components of any university or academic program. They reflect the ideals of the institutions and faculty at the departmental, school, or university level. When combined, policies and procedures offer a roadmap for daily operations including guidelines for specific situations. They are intended to ensure adherence to legal and regulatory requirements, provide direction for making decisions, and optimize internal operations.

Academic policies and procedures should be just, transparent, and disseminated. They should address the question, "What problem are we trying to prevent or solve?" The university or school may be held liable for breach of contract if established policies and procedures are unfair, unclear, or not disseminated, or disregarded.

It is critical for faculty and students to follow consistent policy and procedures. Everyone should be aware of the standards and what is expected from different constituents (e.g., students, faculty, chairs, deans). Liability is also reduced with clear policies and procedures. When students believe they are not receiving fair treatment, they may become litigious. Faculty also object to not being treated in an equitable manner (Gasior, 2019). Effective policies protect students, faculty, and their patients, making them vital elements of nursing education.

ETHICAL BEHAVIOR

Academic policies and/or ethical standards can raise conflict among those who have competing interests (Smith Glasgow et al., 2020). The American Nurses Association's (ANA) Code and Standards also state that ethical behavior between nurses and nursing students benefits patients and enhances patient safety. Nursing schools need to establish and reinforce a culture of civility, professional responsibility, patient safety, and ethical practice among faculty, staff, and students (Anselmi et al., 2014; Clark et al., 2022).

Nursing faculty and the entire healthcare team are responsible for protecting and promoting the health, safety, and dignity of patients. This involves recognizing bias and prejudice, upholding patient autonomy, protecting privacy and confidentiality, and promoting "professional, respectful, and caring relationships with colleagues" (ANA, 2015, p. 4). Nurses must respect professional boundaries, avoid conflicts of interest, and prioritize patient needs. Claiming one's own moral and professional authority, taking responsibility, upholding moral integrity, taking care of one's own health and well-being, and continuing one's own personal and professional development are all examples of duties to oneself (Storaker et al., 2022).

Regardless of practice levels, healthcare professionals are required to have the essential competencies to identify ethical challenges in clinical settings, thoughtfully deliberate to find resolutions to ethical dilemmas, and implement ethical principles in their practice (Deem et al., 2020). Similarly, administrators and faculty within nursing education are tasked with confronting the ethical issues that arise. Ethics imbues health professionals with a moral mindset, crucial for providing high-quality care and facilitating critical reflection among students (Andersson et al., 2022). Ethically oriented academic institutions play a key role in creating, expanding, and sharing nursing science—it is vital for both the general public and healthcare professionals to be informed about the latest in nursing education and practice (Kim et al., 2022).

CLINICAL PRACTICE AND THE FACULTY ROLE

Nursing is a practice discipline. Nursing faculty have a professional obligation to stay up to date and retain a high standard of competence in their clinical specialty. Keeping up with current clinical practice to inform curricula and professional preparation has become a necessity rather than a preference in today's dynamic healthcare environment. For that reason, nursing schools must create a deliberate strategy to make sure that faculty members are equipped to take on the urgent problems that the nursing profession is currently experiencing. These concerns include educating future nurses to support public and population healthcare delivery systems, implementing cutting-edge technologies, and paying attention to health inequities (American Association of Colleges of Nursing [AACN], 2021). Both the National Organization of Nurse Practitioner Faculty (NONPF) and AACN advocate that academic nurses involved in clinical education must be proficient clinicians, which includes regular engagement in clinical practice (AACN, 2016; NONPF, 2016).

Faculty practice refers to the clinical practice in which nursing faculty members engage. Practically speaking, maintaining a dual role in clinical practice can significantly influence a faculty member's work–life balance. Faculty employed by two different organizations describe problems with calendar alignment, where vacation time and officially observed holidays can vary, requests for paid time off or sick leave need to be submitted to both entities, and human resource policies might not match. When administrative requirements like competency training and credentialing documentation need to be completed for two different employers, they are frequently redundant and ineffective. Additionally, part-time employment for two organizations can adversely affect retirement planning and benefits. A viable solution is the academic–clinical partnership faculty practice model, which offers protected time to manage patient care and educational responsibilities within one's workload, thereby enhancing work–life balance (Moss et al., 2022). Numerous examples of successful academic–clinical partnerships highlight the benefits of such collaborations (Smith Glasgow & Colbert, 2022). For nursing faculty at universities without formal practice arrangements, negotiating scheduling with their chair or supervisor and securing a written agreement for clinical practice is critical. Generally, university faculty handbooks contain policies regarding consultation and clinical practice, which typically restrict clinical practice to 1 day per week.

CONFLICTS OF INTEREST

An ethical dilemma emerges when there is a clash between a faculty member's professional obligations to the university and their personal interests. Questions arise about whether a faculty member's motivations align with the university's best interests. For instance, a conflict of interest may occur when a faculty member prefers certain vendors for educational materials or technologies, from which they receive personal benefits, thereby potentially compromising the impartiality of their teaching resources selection. Such conflicts can undermine the credibility of educational decisions.

This issue extends to scenarios involving the employment of married couples, first-degree relatives, or parents and children within the same department or office. Spouses or first-degree relatives of university senior administrators pose a unique challenge if an issue arises. Often the relative is not held to the same standards as other employees. Faculty should not teach or evaluate their spouses, children, or first-degree relatives. Applications for employment should specifically inquire if any first-degree relatives work or attend the university. If, over time, relationships change, the human resources department and the department head should be notified. Administrators are tasked with navigating interpersonal conflicts and allegations of favoritism, as these issues adversely affect employee morale and productivity (Smith Glasgow et al., 2020). All of these situations become more complex if the university's policies on conflicts of interest are either non existent or ambiguous. Exhibit 6.2 identifies elements to consider with conflicts of interest.

EXHIBIT 6.2 Critical Elements to Consider With Conflicts of Interest

- Refer to the university's conflict-of-interest policy.
- Put procedures in place to manage any potential or real conflicts of interest.
- Report any potential conflicts to your supervisor and those noted in the conflict-of-interest policy.
- If you are an administrator, treat all direct reports equitably, regardless of "special" relationships.
- Maintain professional boundaries with students.
- Maintain academic standards for nursing majors as published in the syllabus and in the student handbook.
- Maintain confidentiality of faculty, staff, and students.
- Administrators should not have any decision-making or approval authority over spouses or first-degree relatives
- Report episodes of student, staff, or faculty misconduct to the appropriate administrator per policy and procedure.

Source: Adapted from Smith Glasgow, M. E., Dreher, H. M., Dahnke, M., & Gyllenhammar, J. (2020). *Legal and ethical issues in nursing education: An essential guide*. Springer Publishing Company. Reprinted by permission.

ACADEMIC INTEGRITY

Academic dishonesty puts the public, faculty members, and higher education institutions at risk because it erodes trust among constituents. Universities have an obligation to ensure that curriculum plans and transcripts accurately reflect the students' work. Awarding a degree or giving a certificate to someone who has not earned it deceives the public and casts doubt about the credibility of the institution (Smith Glasgow et al., 2020).

Academic dishonesty encompasses a broad spectrum of fraudulent academic misconduct, including collusion, fabrication, falsification, plagiarism, and false information or misrepresentation. This malpractice also involves the theft of published or unpublished intellectual property. Technological advancements have significantly increased the efficiency, complexity, and sophistication of cheating, thereby facilitating academic misconduct with greater ease (Alguacil et al., 2023). Academic dishonesty, however, is not solely characterized by deliberate wrongdoing. It also includes less serious mistakes, such as the inadvertent failure to attribute an idea to its originator or acknowledge assistance in writing an article. The focal point of concern is the integrity of the act itself, irrespective of the intentions or mental state of the student or faculty member involved (Abbott et al., 2021).

One common area where academic integrity can be threatened is plagiarism and cheating. All articles must be original and carefully referenced, even those that expand upon another person's work. Publishing an article that is flawed by inaccurate collection or reporting of data or the undocumented use of the work of others are common forms of academic dishonesty. Student cheating is not uncommon. Educators always have a professional obligation to identify deviant behavior, address unethical circumstances, and create policies and procedures that either prevent or correct academic misconduct. Unfortunately, it is often the case that faculty members develop strategies for deterring misbehavior through a process of trial and error. This approach underscores the need for more formalized training and resources to equip educators with effective tools for maintaining academic integrity.

Dishonesty in clinical practice can lead to the loss of human life. As gatekeepers to the profession, nursing faculty should take their legal and ethical duties seriously in light of the consequences of cheating. Taking proactive measures to prevent academic dishonesty, teaching and upholding ethical standards, responding swiftly and seriously to infractions, and enforcing suitable sanctions to hold students accountable for academic misconduct are some strategies to reduce cheating (Exhibit 6.3). It is important to establish a connection with patient safety. Faculty should illustrate the detrimental effects of unethical behavior on patient safety and outcomes during their clinical conferences as well as in the classroom. When a nursing student cheats, practices without a firm grasp of the plan of care, or neglects patients, there should be consequences. To protect patient safety, nursing faculty must uphold policies pertaining to academic and clinical integrity even to the point of student dismissal.

SOCIAL MEDIA

As nursing students shape their professional identities, they are significantly influenced by social media platforms such as blogs, X (formerly Twitter), YouTube, Facebook, Instagram, TikTok, podcasts, and LinkedIn. These platforms meet

> **EXHIBIT 6.3 Critical Elements to Consider With Academic Integrity**
>
> Develop an academic integrity policy.
>
> Consult university counsel in the development and management of academic honesty or academic misconduct policies; include instances of academic honesty or misconduct that overlap with issues regarding academic performance or evaluations.
>
> Conduct faculty development sessions related to managing and documenting acts of academic dishonesty.
>
> Develop a rubric on the management of specific academic dishonesty violations to ensure that students are treated consistently and fairly.
>
> Establish a student conduct committee to investigate cases of academic dishonesty.
>
> Develop a testing/proctoring policy for faculty.
>
> To prevent cheating during a test, faculty members can:
> - use testing software to prevent cheating;
> - offer different course examinations to different sections;
> - prohibit laptops, cell phones, books, notes, and personal items from the testing area;
> - require academic honesty tutorials and discussions early in the students' academic program;
> - require that students sign an academic honesty statement before each examination; and
> - assign seats to students during tests.
>
> Develop testing, test review, and test appeal policies; make sure that students are aware of the appeal process for examination; discuss with students the program's policy on audiotaping test reviews, note taking, etc.
>
> Consider the use of a software program to detect plagiarism.
>
> Include the due process policy in the student handbook.
>
> Develop an academic policy with respect to the use of artificial intelligence (AI) so students are informed about the responsible and ethical use of AI.

Source: Adapted from Smith Glasgow, M. E., Dreher, H. M., Dahnke, M., & Gyllenhammer, J. (2020). *Legal and ethical issues in nursing education: An essential guide*. Springer Publishing Company. Reprinted by permission.

technologically adept students' desire for connection, highlighting the importance for faculty to establish clear policies that delineate professional expectations for students' conduct on social media (De Gagne et al., 2018). Social media behavior should mirror the ethical and professional standards of nursing, emphasizing cyber etiquette, patient privacy, prudent sharing of personal information, and the delineation of personal and professional boundaries. The benefits of social media include professional networking and personal expression, yet faculty play a crucial role in guiding students on appropriate usage (De Gagne et al., 2019).

The development of explicit academic social media policies is critical because inappropriate use of social media may put students and their universities in legal jeopardy (Exhibit 6.4). The Health Insurance Portability and Accountability Act (HIPAA) reinforces patients' privacy rights, highlighting the legal consequences of breaches in confidentiality. As future healthcare professionals, nursing students bear a legal responsibility to protect patient privacy. Recent research underscores

> **EXHIBIT 6.4 Critical Elements to Consider With Social Media**
>
> Develop a code of professional conduct for nursing students' use of social media.
>
> Include web etiquette in new student and clinical orientations.
>
> Educate nursing students about the importance of following hospital privacy policies and Health Insurance Portability and Accountability Act and other guidelines.

the necessity of educating nursing students on safeguarding patient privacy and the various factors that influence their practices (Chan et al., 2022). The impact of nursing professionalism on the perception of patient privacy protection among nursing students, mediated by nursing informatics competency, suggests a need for curricula that enhance both professionalism and informatics skills to improve privacy protection awareness (Park & Jeong, 2021).

INCIVILITY

Disruptive behavior that materially or regularly impedes teaching and learning is referred to as academic incivility (Clark et al., 2021). The well-being of every member of the educational community is at risk because of incivility on college campuses and in academic settings (Small et al., 2024). Many nursing students reported having either engaged in or witnessed rudeness; consistent tardiness of students; students talking in class, leaving early, taunting, or showing disrespect for faculty; texting and using cell phones and computers in class; and openly expressing disapproval of faculty. Nurse educators are concerned about these scenarios because uncivil students can become uncivil nurses, endangering patient safety and the work environment (Small et al., 2024).

At the beginning of each semester, faculty should set expectations for appropriate classroom and clinical behavior. The syllabus is a good place to include these guidelines in addition to the section in the student handbook. Guidelines for civil conduct include refraining from using cell phones and laptops in class, texting during lectures, and engaging in unrelated distracting side conversations. It is important for the teacher to record the incident and refer the student to the appropriate body such as the Office of Judicial Affairs or Student Conduct Committee. If the student's incivility does not improve after being counseled, the faculty member should follow the university policy. Reporting of incivility to public safety is very important if the student's actions or threats make the faculty feel threatened.

Although student incivility has received more attention in the literature, faculty incivility cannot be ignored. In uncivil environments, few nursing faculty aspire to or have any desire to become chairs or deans. Everyone has encountered gossip, egocentric faculty members focused on their careers or teaching schedules, passive–aggressive behavior, and hurtful and disparaging remarks made about administrators.

Toxic leadership is an extreme expression of incivility. Toxic administrators put themselves first before students or faculty or the organization. Their accomplishments and financial well-being are more important than that of the faculty or staff. Toxic leaders discourage innovation, autonomy, and creativity; this type of destructive leadership is known as the "silent killer" (Hudgins et al., 2022). The detrimental impact of toxic leadership on faculty work environments is profound. Individuals who dissent against such leaders may fear reprisal, while those who align with them may receive preferential treatment in terms of career progression. Examples of toxic leadership behaviors include bullying, authoritarianism, manipulation, rankism, intimidation, micromanagement, narcissism, microaggressions, and incivility (Labrague, 2020). These behaviors need to be addressed in schools of nursing (Exhibit 6.5).

The culture of the academic work environment plays a pivotal role in shaping morale, productivity, and the quality of patient care. The decision to teach in a specific university or department is a critical personal and professional choice, making the assessment of the culture within a school of nursing or department a crucial part of the job interview process. Recent studies continue to highlight the prevalence of bullying within academic settings, affecting not only the well-being of faculty members but also their productivity and the learning environment for students.

For instance, a study by Hudgins et al. (2022) emphasized the negative impact of academic nurse leaders' toxic behaviors on job satisfaction and anticipated turnover among nursing faculty, suggesting a need for increased awareness and accountability to address these behaviors effectively. Furthermore, research on the mental health, burnout, and perceived wellness culture among nursing faculty revealed significant concerns regarding depression, anxiety, and burnout, underscoring the

---

EXHIBIT 6.5 Critical Elements to Consider Related to Academic Incivility

- Academic leaders should address bullying and incivility on an individual and organizational level.
- Victims of bullying or of academic incivility should document these events.
- If attempts to resolve these issues with the offender fail, consult the university policy and notify the department chair in writing.
- If the offender is in violation of human resource policies, consider reporting them to the appropriate officer of the university.
- If the normal chain of command is not working, go to the dean, provost, or another administrator and file a written complaint that also explains the actions that have been taken.
- For faculty disputes that cannot be resolved at the departmental level, consult the campus ombudsperson, human resources, or dean.
- A faculty witness to bullying behavior of a faculty colleague toward students should initially speak to that individual directly if they are comfortable doing so. If the violation observed is severe or unethical, it should be reported through normal administrative channels.
- Some universities have anonymous ethics hotlines that can be used to report abuse.
- Be aware that simply because an activity is reported to a department chair or other administrator, it does not perpetually guarantee the anonymity of the reporter.
- Consult human resources or the Title IX Office if you feel threatened, harassed, or discriminated against.
- Consult public safety if you feel physically threatened.

Source: Adapted from Smith Glasgow, M. E., Dreher, H. M., Dahnke, M., & Gyllenhammer, J. (2020). *Legal and ethical issues in nursing education: An essential guide.* Springer Publishing Company. Reprinted by permission.

importance of fostering a supportive and inclusive work environment (Melnyk et al., 2023). In light of these findings, it is clear that academic culture plays a critical role in either perpetuating or mitigating incivility and toxic behaviors. Exhibit 6.6 provides a case study that applies these concepts.

EXHIBIT 6.6 Case Study: Associate Dean's Incivility and Ethical Violation

You are the new department chair, Dr. Kelly. The senior associate dean for academic affairs is Dr. Johnson. He rose through the faculty ranks and has over 20 years of experience. However, he exhibits a coercive leadership style and is controlling, allowing little faculty autonomy. Spiteful, he abruptly dismisses faculty members' ideas that do not fit his agenda or plan. His superior, Dean Swift, has received formal and informal complaints about Dr. Johnson's behavior from a number of faculty members. The faculty see no action in response to their complaints. If faculty disagree with Dr. Johnson's viewpoint, they are essentially silenced. Known for being Dean Swift's confidant, Dr. Johnson's ongoing toxic behavior is not addressed, which is negatively affecting faculty morale.

Dr. Kelly recently took over Dr. Johnson's position in the graduate nursing program and now reports to Dr. Johnson. She found in reviewing the *US News & World Report* rankings and accreditation surveys inconsistencies that gave the graduate program a higher ranking. Dr. Kelly informs Dr. Johnson that the data are erroneous and do not correspond with the program outcomes from the prior year. Dr. Johnson loudly chastises Dr. Kelly, claiming that she does not understand the data. Dr. Kelly knows that she cannot approve the report and believes Dr. Johnson is attempting to intimidate her.

Questions
- How should Dr. Kelly proceed?
- Should the dean or another administrator investigate the situation?
- How can Dr. Kelly protect herself from retaliation?

Discussion of Case Study
Dr. Kelly emails the Office of Institutional Research (IR) to request that they examine the data summarized in the report, pointing out the consequences of providing false information. The Director of IR responds with corrections based on university data. Dr. Kelly forwards IR's email to Dean Swift and Dr. Johnson. Later that afternoon, Dr. Johnson walks by Dr. Kelly's office and says harshly, "You do not want to mess me with me; do you understand?" Dr. Kelly, who is worried, records and summarizes the event. She then requests protection from Dr. Johnson in an email to Dean Swift and the university's Title IX Officer. Dr. Kelly questions whether she went too far in alerting Dean Swift and the University Title IX Officer, asking for protection from Dr. Johnson, but she considered his remark as threatening.

Susan Preston, the Title IX Officer, contacts Dr. Kelly to arrange a meeting. To look into the complaint, she also meets with Dean Swift, Dr. Johnson, and the Director of IR. Ms. Preston mentions that during the past year, there have been multiple complaints made about Dr. Johnson's intimidating behavior that were reported to Human Resources and the Ethics Hotline and subsequently reported to Dean Swift. Ms. Preston provides the provost, Dean Swift, and legal counsel with a synopsis of her findings. Because of the results, Dr. Johnson must seek counseling from the Employee Assistance Program and is explicitly forbidden to use intimidation or retaliation.

(continued)

> **EXHIBIT 6.6 Case Study: Associate Dean's Incivility and Ethical Violation** (*continued*)
>
> Dr. Johnson received a formal disciplinary warning letter about advising Dr. Kelly to submit false data to the *US News & World Report*. He was advised that any further incidents of serious misconduct would result in termination.
>
> *Case Summary*
> This case is troubling for a number of reasons. The associate dean appears to be fabricating data for *US News & World Report* and wants the new department chair to submit the report. It would be unethical for Dr. Kelly to knowingly submit inaccurate data.
>
> Dr. Johnson exhibits toxic leadership behaviors. Leading by example and instituting a zero-tolerance policy for incivility are important leadership behaviors in healthy work environments. Toxic leadership styles not only erode trust and morale but are also detrimental to the overall health of the organizational culture, potentially leading to increased instances of burnout, disengagement among faculty, and a toxic workplace atmosphere. The importance of leading by example and enforcing a zero-tolerance stance on incivility cannot be overstated in fostering a work environment that values respect, integrity, and ethical conduct. The repercussions of toxic leadership extend beyond individual interactions, affecting the broader institutional ecosystem and underscoring the critical need for vigilance, accountability, and corrective measures to uphold ethical standards and promote a healthy, supportive work environment (Hudgins et al., 2022).

Healthy Academic Work Environments

Faculty and deans would be well served to endorse a culture consistent with a healthy work environment. In academic settings, faculty and staff support are needed to implement a healthy work environment, the standards of which are described in Table 6.1.

TABLE 6.1 HEALTHY WORK ENVIRONMENT STANDARDS FOR THE ACADEMIC WORKPLACE

HWE Standard	Academic Workplace Standard
1. Skilled Communication	Faculty and staff are as proficient in using and role modeling communication skills as they are in their respective academic duties and skills.
2. True Collaboration	Faculty and staff are relentless in pursuing, fostering, and role-modeling collaboration within and beyond the university.
3. Effective Decision-Making	Faculty and staff are valued and committed partners in implementing shared governance within the school and university setting.

(continued)

TABLE 6.1 HEALTHY WORK ENVIRONMENT STANDARDS FOR THE ACADEMIC WORKPLACE (continued)

HWE Standard	Academic Workplace Standard
4. Appropriate Staffing	Faculty and staff ensure the effective match between the mission of the school and designated employee competencies.
5. Meaningful Recognition	Faculty and staff are recognized and recognize others for the value each brings to the work of the organization.
6. Authentic Leadership	Faculty and staff leaders fully embrace the imperative of a healthy work environment, authentically live it, and engage others in its achievement.
7. Self-Care	Faculty and staff engage and are supported in developing self-care as foundational to the creation of a healthy work and learning environment in which all members of the academic community can thrive.

HWE, healthy work environment.

Source: Adapted from American Association of Critical-Care Nurses (AACN). (2016). *American Association of Critical-Care Nurses' standards for establishing and sustaining healthy work environments: A journey to excellence (2nd ed.).* AACN. https://www.aacn.org/WD/HWE/Docs/HWEStandards.pdf; Fontaine, D., Koh, E. H., & Carroll, T. (2012). Promoting a healthy workplace for nursing faculty and staff. *Nursing Clinics of North America, 47*(4), 557–566. https://doi.org/10.1016/j.cnur.2012.07.008

Another Example of Incivility: Grade Disputes

Student grade disputes often create stressful situations for students, faculty, and administrators. These situations, in turn, can lead to uncivil behaviors not only from students but in some cases also by parents. Exhibit 6.7 provides a second case study that includes the impact of the Family Educational Rights and Privacy Act (FERPA) on faculty responses.

ACADEMIC DECISIONS

Both federal and state courts respect the institution's and faculty's rightful academic decisions, whether the challenger is a faculty member contesting tenure denial or student contesting an academic dismissal. Courts accord this deference for a variety of reasons. For example, the dismissal of two medical students was at issue in the two landmark U.S. Supreme Court cases, *Regents of the University of Michigan v. Ewing* (474 U.S. 214, 106 S.Ct. 507; 1985) and *Board of Curators of the University of Missouri v. Horowitz* (435 U.S. 78, 98 S.Ct. 948; 1978), where the courts upheld the faculty's evaluation of the student's academic performance. Federal courts and the

EXHIBIT 6.7 Case Study: Graduate Student Parent Incivility and Grade Dispute

You are Dr. Gallagher, a nursing faculty member in the nurse practitioner program. A graduate student Mallory Franks is enrolled in the family nurse practitioner program. She is in her second term of school. Mallory received a grade of C in the advanced physical assessment course. To pass the course, a B grade is required. Mallory is a traveling nurse and is requesting accommodations. Every week, she makes the trip from Florida to Pennsylvania to finish her laboratory and clinical hours for the course. It is also noted that she did not pass two of the four examinations. Mallory files an appeal of her final grade, which you deny.

In your final grade appeal, you respond: *Final grade appeals shall be based on problems of process and not on differences in judgment or opinion concerning academic performance. The acceptable grounds for a final grade appeal as outlined in your Graduate Nursing Student Handbook are:*

An error was made in grade computation.

The grade assignment was capricious or arbitrary; that is, the grade assigned was based on criteria other than the student's performance in the course; was based on standards different than those applied to other students registered in the same course at the same time; or constitutes a substantial departure from the published or announced grading standards for the course.

In your academic circumstances, these conditions were met. Your grade did not deviate from the published grading standards for NURS xxx: Advanced Physical Assessment as per the course syllabus.

In your meeting with Mallory, you clarify that the advanced physical assessment course is a prerequisite for the more intellectually demanding clinical courses and that she has not mastered the content based on her exam results. You also inform Mallory that her work schedule does not meet the criteria for an accommodation.

Later that evening, Mallory's father, Mr. Franks, e-mails you multiple times. Because of his daughter's hectic work schedule, he demands to speak with you to save her time and stress. He discloses that his daughter works more than 40 hours a week most weeks while upholding a strong work ethic to finish her graduate program. You clarify that before you can talk to him about his daughter's academic situation, you inform him that Mallory must complete the Student Authorization to Discuss and Disclose an Education Record Form, in accordance with the FERPA. You also clarify that it is preferable for Mallory to speak for herself in this circumstance because she is an adult and a practicing registered nurse. Angry, Mr. Franks yells at you and addresses you by your first name.

Mr. Franks continues to yell so you politely tell him that he should call back when you have FERPA release, and both of you can engage in a calm, civil conversation. Subsequently, you are copied on derogatory emails from Mr. Franks to the dean, provost, and university president, in which he labels you as unreasonable and difficult. Additionally, he posts a comment about you on the university parents' Facebook page.

Questions
- Is FERPA relevant in this case?
- Does the student have a legitimate appeal?
- How should you and the dean proceed?
- What policies should be in place?

(continued)

> **EXHIBIT 6.7 Case Study: Graduate Student Parent Incivility and Grade Dispute** *(continued)*
>
> *Discussion of Case Study*
> In this case, Dr. Gallagher acted appropriately requesting a FERPA release before agreeing to speak to Mr. Franks about his daughter's grades. FERPA is a federal law that protects the privacy of students' education records. The law applies to all schools that receive funds under an applicable program of the U.S. Department of Education. FERPA gives parents certain rights with respect to their children's education records. These rights transfer to the student when they reach the age of 18 or attend a school beyond the high school level. Students to whom the rights have transferred are eligible students (U.S. Department of Education, 2021).
>
> The professor cannot capitulate to student or parental external pressure to pass the graduate student when the student has not passed the course based on the evaluation methods published in the syllabus. Further, the student has not met the grounds for a final grade appeal. As such, Dr. Gallagher was well within her rights to deny the appeal. The final grade appeal policy is clear and applies to all students. Lastly, graduate students should be informed that, as adults, faculty and administrators will only communicate with parents in extreme cases involving issues pertaining to their health.
>
> *Case Summary*
> There is no doubt that Mr. Franks, the parent of the graduate student, treated Dr. Gallagher poorly. Demand and consumer-driven higher education has contributed to a rise in aggressive behavior by students, spouses, and parents. Dr. Gallagher was respectful yet firm with Mr. Franks despite his uncivil behavior. The professor also has an ethical duty to graduate knowledgeable, safe clinicians, therefore, requiring additional course work when the student has not mastered the course content according to the course syllabus. The professor also has a duty to follow applicable student privacy laws, such as FERPA. If Mr. Franks's behavior had escalated beyond these e-mails and one Facebook post, Dr. Gallagher should consult her dean, legal counsel, and public safety to obtain advice.

Federal courts and the state courts that are subordinate to them regularly refer to the principles stated in these two decisions, which set a precedent for the broad deference that courts accord in academic decision-making as long as the faculty have followed their own policies related to academic matters (Smith Glasgow et al., 2020). Courts are particularly ill equipped to evaluate academic performance. Faculty must have the widest range of discretion in making judgments as to the academic performance of students and their entitlement to promotion or graduation (435 US 78, 96, n. 6., 98 S. Ct. 948, 958, n. 6).

SUMMARY

The goal of this chapter was to assist faculty in identifying the most prevalent legal issues that arise in nursing education and the potential legal repercussions that could arise from relationships, obligations, and exposure to liability. Educators should consult with their administrators and think about contacting university counsel as soon as they begin to feel uncomfortable in unfamiliar situations. Ethical and social norms have a role in changing laws and regulations. As faculty familiarize themselves with common legal and ethical issues in nursing education, they will become more comfortable addressing these issues. It is important to note that this chapter is a brief overview, and faculty should consult their university legal counsel concerning academic matters with legal implications.

Author's Disclaimer: The case studies in this chapter are not factual. They were developed from the literature, case law, and experience of faculty and administrators. All the names of the characters in the case studies are fictional.

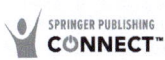

A robust set of instructor resources designed to supplement this text is located at http://connect.springerpub.com/content/book/978-0-8261-8892-2. Qualifying instructors may request access by emailing textbook@springerpub.com.

REFERENCES

Abbott, M. R. B., & Nininger, J. (2021). Academic integrity in nursing education: Policy review *Journal of Professional Nursing, 37*(2), 268–271. https://doi.org/10.1016/j.profnurs.2020.12.006

Alcover, C.-M. (2009). Ombudsing in higher education: A contingent model for mediation in university dispute resolution processes. *Spanish Journal of Psychology, 12*(1), 275–287. https://doi.org/10.1017/S1138741600001682

Alguacil, M., Herranz-Zarzoso, N., Pernías, J. C., & Sabater-Grande, G. (2023). Academic dishonesty and monitoring in online exams: A randomized field experiment. *Journal of Computing in Higher Education*, 1–17. https://doi.org/10.1007/s12528-023-09378-x

American Association of Critical Care Nurses. (2016). *American Association of Critical-Care Nursing standards for establishing and sustaining healthy work environments: A journey to excellence* (2nd ed.). AACN. https://www.aacn.org/WD/HWE/Docs/HWEStandards.pdf

American Association of College of Nursing. (2016). *Advancing healthcare transformation: A new era for academic nursing.* https://www.aacnnursing.org/Portals/0/PDFs/Publications/AACN-New-Era-Report.pdf

American Association of Colleges of Nursing. (2021). *The essentials: Core competencies for professional nursing education.* https://www.aacnnursing.org/Portals/42/AcademicNursing/pdf/Essentials-2021.pdf

American Nurses Association. (2015). *Code of ethics for nurses with interpretive statements.* ANA. https://nursingworld.org/practice-policy/nursing-excellence/ethics/code-of-ethics-for-nurses

Andersson, H., Svensson, A., Frank, C., Rantala, A., Holmberg, M., & Bremer, A. (2022). Ethics education to support ethical competence learning in healthcare: An integrative systematic review. *BMC Medical Ethics, 23*(1), 1–26. https://doi.org/10.1186/s12910-022-00766-z

Anselmi, K. K., Smith Glasgow, M. E., & Gambescia, S. (2014). Using a Student Conduct Committee to foster professionalism among nursing students. *Journal of Professional Nursing, 30*(6), 481–485. https://doi.org/10.1016/j.profnurs.2014.04.002

Board of Curators of the University of Missouri v. Horowitz (435 U.S. 78, 98 S.Ct. 948) (1978).

Chan, D. N. S., Choi, K-C., To, M. H. Y., Ha, S. K. N., & Ling, G. C. C. (2022). Patient privacy protection among university nursing students: A cross-sectional study. *Nursing Ethics, 29*(5), 1280–1292. https://doi.org/10.1177/09697330221085777

Clark, C.M., Gorton, K., & Bentley, A. (2022). Civility: A concept analysis revisited. *Nursing Outlook, 70*(2), 259–270. https://doi.org/10.1016/j.outlook.2021.11.001

Clark, C. M., Landis, T. T., & Barbosa-Leiker, C. (2021). National study on faculty and administrators' perceptions of civility and incivility in nursing education. *Nurse Educator, 46*(5), 276–283. https://doi.org/10.1097/NNE.0000000000000948

De Gagne, J. C., Hall, K., Conklin, J. L., Yamane, S. S., Roth, N. W., Chang, J., & Kim, S. S. (2019). Uncovering cyberincivility among nurses and nursing students on Twitter: A data mining study. *International Journal of Nursing Studies, 89*, 24–31. https://doi.org/10.1016/j.ijnurstu.2018.09.009

De Gagne, J. C., Yamane, S. S., Conklin, J. L. Chang, J., & Kang, H. (2018). Social media use and cybercivility guidelines in U.S. nursing schools: A review of websites. *Journal of Professional Nursing, 34*(1), 35–41. https://doi.org/10.1016/j.profnurs.2017.07.006

Deem, M. J., Vogelstein, E., & Smith Glasgow, M. E. (2020). Integrating ethics across the curricula: Innovations in undergraduate and graduate nursing education. In E. E. Ea & C. M. Alfes (Eds.), *Innovative strategies in teaching nursing: Exemplars of optimal learning outcomes* (pp. 59–67). Springer Publishing Company.

Fontaine, D., Koh, E. H., & Carroll, T. (2012). Promoting a healthy workplace for nursing faculty and staff. *Nursing Clinics of North America, 47*(4), 557–566. https://doi.org/10.1016/j.cnur.2012.07.008

Gasior, M. (2019). *Following policies and procedures and why it's important: Ideas for making sure, your staff knows how to follow procedures.* https://www.powerdms.com/blog/following-policies-and-procedures-why-its-important/

Howard, C. (2013). *The organizational ombudsman.* The American Bar Association

Hudgins, T., Brown, K. D., Layne, D., & Stephens, T. M. (2022). The effect of academic nurse leaders' toxic behaviors. *Journal of Nursing Education, 61*(2), 88–95. https://doi.org/10.3928/01484834-20211213-02

Hunter, R. J., & Shannon, J. H. (2020). A primer on the role of the university's attorney. *Education Quarterly Reviews, 3*(1) 1–9. https://doi.org/10.31014/aior.1993.03.01.113

Kim, S., Jeong, K. S., & Seo, M. H. (2022). Nurses' ethical leadership and related outcome variables: Systematic review and meta-analysis. *Journal of Nursing Management, 30*(7), 2308–2323. https://doi.org/10.1111/jonm.13726

Labrague, L. L., Lorica, J., Nwafor, C. E. van Bogaert, P., & Cummings, G. G. (2020). Development and psychometric testing of the toxic leadership behaviors of nurse managers (ToxBH-NM) scale. *Journal of Nursing Management, 28*(4), 840–850. https://doi.org/10.1111/jonm.13008

Melnyk, B. M., Strait, L. A., Beckett, C., Hsieh, A. P., Messinger, J., & Masciola, R. (2023). The state of mental health, burnout, mattering and perceived wellness culture in doctorally prepared nursing faculty with implications for action. *Worldviews on Evidence-Based Nursing, 20*(2), 142–152. https://doi.org/10.1111/wvn.12632

Moss, A., Rousseau, J., Swartwout, K, Kalensky, M., Gallagher, T., Gorenz, A., & Dickins, K. (2022). Leveraging a successful faculty practice model to recruit and retain early-career nurse faculty. *Nurse Educator, 47*(4), 219–224. https://doi.org/10.1097/NNE.0000000000001177

National Organization of Nurse Practitioner Faculties. (2016). *Benefits of faculty practice partnerships.* https://cdn.ymaws.com/www.nonpf.org/resource/resmgr/statements_&_papers/2016_benefitsoffacultypracti.pdf

Park, H.-K., & Jeong, Y.-W. (2021). Impact of nursing professionalism on perception of patient privacy protection in nursing students: Mediating effect of nursing informatics competency. *Healthcare (Basel), 9*(10), 1364, https://doi.org/10.3390/healthcare9101364

Regents of the University of Michigan v. Ewing (474 U.S. 214, 106 S.Ct. 507) (1985).

Small, S. P., Cashin, G., English, D., & Moran, G. (2024). "It is essentially about treating each other well": Insights from faculty on incivility in nursing education. *Canadian Journal of Nursing Research, 56*(1), 81–94. https://doi.org/10.1177/08445621231204985

Smith Glasgow, M. E., & Colbert, A. M. (2022). Nursing's wicked problems: Partnering with academic leadership to develop solutions. *Nursing Administration Quarterly, 46*(4), 275–282. https://doi.org/10.1097/NAQ.0000000000000545

Smith Glasgow, M. E., Dreher, H. M., Dahnke, M., & Gyllenhammer, J. (2020). *Legal and ethical issues in nursing education: An essential guide.* Springer Publishing Company.

Spitalniak, L. (2022). Ombuds offer colleges conflict resolution in a contentious time. *Higher Ed Dive.* https://www.highereddive.com/news/ombuds-offer-colleges-conflict-resolution-in-a-contentious-time/622153/

Storaker, A., Heggestad, A. K., & Saeteren, B. (2022). Ethical challenges and lack of ethical language in nurse leadership, *Nursing Ethics, 29*(6), 1372–1385. https://doi.org/10.1177/09697330211022415

U.S. Department of Education. (2021). *Family Educational Rights and Privacy Act (FERPA).* https://www2.ed.gov/policy/gen/guid/fpco/ferpa/index.html

Integrating Technology in Education

7

Jennie C. De Gagne

OBJECTIVES

1. Examine the integration of emerging technology tools to support teaching and learning
2. Explore selected instructional technologies and their application to nursing education
3. Assess the infrastructure and classroom alignment required for integrating technology into the teaching-learning process

INTRODUCTION

Integration of technology into education has both transformed learning opportunities and created challenges. Instructional technologies can equip students with essential 21st-century skills and promote critical thinking, creativity, and information literacy. However, in order to leverage these advancements to improve learning outcomes and patient care quality, educators must maintain up-to-date familiarity and proficiency with new technologies as part of their professional development. Nurse educators play a crucial role in adapting technological innovations for use in classrooms, labs, and clinical settings. This chapter (a) examines the role of technology in supporting teaching and learning in nursing education, (b) provides an overview of instructional technologies that are useful in nursing education and their application in a teaching–learning environment, and (c) assesses the infrastructure and classroom alignment required to integrate technology into the teaching-learning process.

BACKGROUND

The role of technology in education has evolved from the initial use of computers and the internet in the 1980s and 1990s to the complex and integrated applications common in the 21st century. The advent of Web 2.0 at the beginning of the 21st century marked a significant shift toward digital communication and networking in education. Social media and online collaboration tools have broadened the scope of nursing education by offering new avenues for interactive learning and professional development; however, adopting and keeping pace with new technologies require thoughtful and informed attention to pedagogical and ethical questions, particularly in ever-evolving fields such as healthcare. Today, the ubiquity of high-powered laptops, tablets, smartphones, and wearable devices has revolutionized teaching and learning methods.

Over the past two decades, the dramatic emergence of advanced technologies such as artificial intelligence (AI), virtual reality (VR), augmented reality (AR), and sophisticated online learning platforms has transformed traditional educational paradigms. The use of AI technologies such as adaptive learning systems, intelligent tutoring systems, and AI-driven analytics has been pivotal in personalizing education, enhancing student engagement, and improving learning outcomes. As we progress through the mid-2020s, the challenge for educators, administrators, and policymakers in nursing education will be to critically assess the impact of advanced technologies on educational quality, student success, and alignment with evolving healthcare practices.

THE INTERNET AND THE WEB

Although the terms *internet* and *the web* are often used interchangeably, they represent different concepts. The internet is a physical network of computers connected by various means (copper wires, fiber optic cables, wireless technologies) to form a global infrastructure of digital communication. On the other hand, the web, or World Wide Web, is a collection of interconnected web pages and applications navigated through hyperlinks and URLs; the web utilizes the internet's infrastructure to facilitate information search and retrieval, thus delivering content including text, audio, video, and other media from the web to users.

Educators who wish to integrate technology into their teaching, especially the use of web conferencing and diverse media content, must understand how this information is transmitted. Transmission speed varies with content type; for example, text transmits faster than multimedia files, which are larger and require more time due to their size. Effective access to media-rich learning content necessitates appropriate internet connections and hardware. The inclusion of internet connection requirements in course syllabi and program descriptions will ensure accessibility for all students, as illustrated in Exhibit 7.1 (which can be adapted for different technologies).

Beyond the internet and web, constantly evolving technologies like virtual simulations, mobile devices, and learner response systems are revolutionizing education.

EXHIBIT 7.1 Sample Syllabi Statement on Internet Connection

General technology requirements for engaging in online or hybrid courses include a reliable broadband internet connection. The most dependable options are fiber optic, cable, and DSL. Although satellite connections, common in rural areas without fiber optic, cable, or DSL access, and wireless cards from mobile internet providers are broadband options, they may be less reliable. These connections can experience intermittent service and slower speeds, potentially disrupting activities such as web conferencing, efficient transfer of course content, and stable connectivity during online assessments in a learning management system.

For tasks that demand high reliability, such as online assessments or web conferencing events like applied demonstrations, using a wireless connection is not advised. Instead, a direct connection to the router using an ethernet cable is recommended to ensure a consistent and robust internet connection.

DSL, digital subscriber line.

Educators must stay informed about emerging instructional technologies in order to adopt the most effective tools for supporting active learning, optimizing time use, enhancing learning outcomes, and preparing students for lifelong learning and careers. Thoughtful strategic planning and evaluation are key to successfully implementing technology in educational settings of all sizes.

TECHNOLOGY TOOLS: PRESENT AND FUTURE

Learning Management Systems

Learning management systems (LMS) are foundational to integrating technology into education; they offer web-based platforms for interactive online learning environments. LMSs enable educators and instructional designers to develop, deliver, and manage online or blended courses that enhance student engagement and learning. Prominent LMSs include proprietary options (e.g., Blackboard, Canvas, Desire2Learn [D2L]) as well as open-source customizable alternatives (e.g., Sakai, Moodle).

Recent advancements in LMS technology have introduced such features as AI integration, including chatbots (also referred to as edubots when used specifically in educational contexts) and adaptive learning technologies, alongside advanced analytics. These enhancements foster personalized learning experiences, provide insights into student performance, and streamline course management. Given the growing emphasis on mobile accessibility, LMSs are increasingly designed for use on smartphones and tablets to meet the needs of mobile learners (Turnbull et al., 2020). Additionally, the rapid growth in online education is spurring continuous development and evolution of LMS platforms that incorporate the latest technological and pedagogical innovations to meet their critical role in digital learning.

Web 1.0 to Web 4.0 in Education

The World Wide Web has evolved from Web 1.0, characterized by static websites that primarily offered reading content, to more interactive and complex phases that have transformed how educational information is delivered and consumed. The one-way flow of information provided by Web 1.0 marked the beginning of online content consumption and emphasized the need for authenticity in digital resources (Singh et al., 2023). The transition to Web 2.0 introduced the "writable web," which fostered user engagement and collaboration through social networking, blogs, wikis, and interactive tools. This phase democratized content creation and enhanced educational practices and learning experiences by integrating applications that support Bloom's digital taxonomy (Akintolu et al., 2022; Singh et al., 2023).

Web 3.0, or the "executable web," has advanced the internet with AI, data analytics, and automation; this current phase emphasizes multimedia-rich content and high-level critical thinking skills in education (Singh et al., 2023). Educators should adapt their teaching methods to include these technologies effectively. The upcoming phase, Web 4.0, or the "trustworthy web," will focus on decentralization, user centricity, and privacy, and will utilize technologies like blockchain to secure online environments. This anticipated phase will enhance digital education with increased security and reliability (Singh et al., 2023). Educators who understand the purposeful progression from Web 1.0 to Web 4.0 will find it easier to navigate the changing digital landscape and leverage new opportunities in digital learning environments.

Cloud Computing in Education

Cloud computing has become increasingly integral to academic institutions, spurred by advancements in hardware, software, and networking. As defined by the National Institute of Standards and Technology (NIST), cloud computing facilitates on-demand access to computing resources like networks, servers, and applications with minimal management effort (Mell & Grance, 2011). This shift toward cloud services enhances institutional flexibility and reduces operating costs, thus offering a significant advantage over traditional IT services (Attaran et al., 2017). Research has illustrated that the rapid adoption of cloud computing in higher education is a key component of contemporary IT strategies (Qasem et al., 2019). Institutions are migrating services like email, file sharing, and student information systems to the cloud, leveraging platforms including Box, Dropbox, Google Drive, and OneDrive.

Despite the advantages of transitioning to cloud computing, there are risks related to management, trust, and control, which must be navigated. Research by Njenga et al. (2019) identified challenges in cloud adoption, especially within developing countries, including infrastructure limitations, data security concerns, and the need to tailor cloud solutions to unique educational contexts. Recommendations for overcoming these obstacles include investing in IT infrastructure, improving data security, and developing scalable, adaptable cloud-based educational models. The current emphasis on cloud computing in education highlights the need for comprehensive strategies that mitigate challenges and capitalize on cloud technology's benefits (Attaran et al., 2017).

Virtual Simulation

The adoption of virtual simulation into health professions education, similar to the transformative adoption of simulators into aviation safety training, is rapidly expanding. However, to effectively integrate virtual simulation into educational curricula, faculty must align its use with learning objectives; faculty collaboration is required to ensure that simulation provides learner enrichment and enhances patient safety without being burdensome. Kononowicz et al. (2019) underscored the shift toward technologically advanced educational methods, including virtual patient simulations, as pivotal in health professions education. Accelerated by the demand for technology-rich simulation environments during the COVID-19 pandemic, this evolution embraces not only virtual patient interactions but also the use of technologies such as electronic health records (EHRs), telemedicine, and wearable sensors (Jeffries et al., 2022).

Simulation environments uniquely combine health IT competencies with practical clinical training. For example, integrating EHR technology with laboratory simulations offers virtual clinical experiences that closely resemble real-world scenarios (Zhang et al., 2019). This fusion enables learners to develop critical thinking skills and make data-driven decisions in a risk-free environment. Consequently, the landscape of simulation in nursing education is rapidly advancing, marked by a trend toward incorporating digital technologies and virtual environments. This progression is vital for enhancing learning experiences and preparing students for success in the rapidly evolving healthcare industry.

Metaverse in Education

The metaverse encompasses immersive technologies such as VR, AR, and extended reality (XR) and is reshaping health professions education. A comprehensive review of related articles from 2013 to 2021 by De Gagne, Randall, et al. (2023) underscored the metaverse's positive effects on nursing student knowledge, confidence, engagement, and performance. In nursing education, the metaverse facilitates simulation of complex medical scenarios (e.g., emergency procedures, patient care, team collaboration exercises), allowing students to practice critical thinking and decision-making skills in realistic settings. Effective integration of the metaverse requires significant infrastructure, faculty training, and consideration of students' comfort with technology (De Gagne, Randall et al., 2023).

The metaverse's support for remote learning expands access to education to a broad student demographic, enables flexible schedules, aligns with digital progression and evolving healthcare expectations, and prepares students for a technologically integrated healthcare future. Its adoption in nursing education requires that educators maintain their ongoing development in digital literacy and address ethical considerations such as data privacy and the psychological impact of immersive technologies. The metaverse signifies a progressive educational approach that can equip nursing students with essential digital and clinical competencies for the healthcare sector's future.

Gaming

Game-based learning (GBL) is an emerging educational approach in health professions education which enables learners to practice and apply knowledge in a safe environment. GBL offers a cost-effective, engaging, and flexible learning solution through serious games and gamification. Beyond promoting technical skills, GBL can be utilized to address essential topics in nursing education, such as health equity, diversity, equity, and inclusion [DEI], according to Copenhaver et al. (2023). GBL uniquely engages students with the concepts of social determinants of health (SDOH) and DEI, thus cultivating empathy, comprehension, and teamwork. This approach is critical for nurturing cultural sensitivity and fostering inclusive healthcare practices (Copenhaver et al., 2023). Furthermore, in a comprehensive review involving 27 randomized controlled trials, Gentry et al. (2019) found GBL to be as (if not more) effective than traditional learning methods and suggested further theory-driven research to solidify findings.

The growing support for serious gaming in education underscores its capacity to engage students and stimulate critical inquiry, thereby enriching the learning experience. Representing a significant paradigm shift in health professions education, GBL offers interactive and immersive learning experiences. As the field evolves, nurse educators and health professionals will need to embrace and integrate these vital technologies into their curricula in order to prepare students for the dynamic and rapidly advancing healthcare environment. For specific examples of universities that are engaging in GBL, refer to Table 7.1.

TABLE 7.1 UNIVERSITY RESEARCH CENTERS EXPLORING GAME-BASED LEARNING

Research Center	Website
American University Game Lab (Washington, DC)	https://www.american.edu/centers/gamecenter
Center for Learning through Games and Simulations (CMU)	https://www.cmich.edu/academics/colleges/liberal-arts-social-sciences/centers-institutes/center-for-learning-through-games-and-simulations
CUNY Games Network	https://commons.gc.cuny.edu/groups/games-teaching-and-learning
Game-Based Education and Advanced Research Studies (GEARS) Lab	https://daytonabeach.erau.edu/about/labs/game-based-education-and-advanced-research
Game Studio at Boise State University	https://www.boisestate.edu/gamestudio/research
Institute for Connected Learning (UCL)	https://www.brunel.ac.uk/research/Groups/Applied-Games-and-Gaming-Research
Interactive Media & Games Division (USC)	https://games.usc.edu
Learning Games Lab (University of North Carolina at Chapel Hill)	https://dlclab.unc.edu/gaming-program
MIT Game Lab	http://gamelab.mit.edu
Serious Games Center at Purdue University	https://education.purdue.edu/research/centers-and-institutes/serious-gaming-center

Clickers and Polling

Audience response systems (ARS), commonly known as "clickers," are gaining momentum in health professions education. Their role in fostering active learning and enhancing student engagement is noteworthy. These systems function as a bridge for two-way communication; they enable immediate feedback on student understanding and cultivate active participation in the learning environment.

Recent technological advancements have transformed ARS from hardware-based clickers to web-based platforms. This evolution allows students to participate using their own mobile devices or laptops, enhancing accessibility and ease of use. Prominent examples of online ARS tools include Poll Everywhere, TurningPoint, Kahoot!, Slido, and Mentimeter; their applications are diverse, extending beyond mere attendance tracking or quiz facilitation to include opinion polls, voting, and group decision-making exercises. The graphical representation of responses, a feature in most e-polling tools, encourages active participation and enables students to visualize diverse viewpoints, thus fostering a dynamic learning atmosphere.

Empirical studies underscore the efficacy of ARS in academic contexts. For instance, Iti and Kadeangadi (2023) revealed that undergraduate medical students using clickers exhibited significantly better academic performance compared to those engaged in traditional group discussions; this finding underscored the ease of use and resultant heightened engagement and participation afforded by ARS. Further, in a study by Anderson et al. (2023) of the impact of higher-order cognitive skill (HOCS) clicker questions on exam performance in a biology course, findings indicated that HOCS clicker questions improved performance in lower-order cognitive skill (LOCS) exam questions but did not significantly affect performance on HOCS exam questions, suggesting that ARS may be particularly effective in consolidating foundational knowledge and preparing students for more complex cognitive tasks.

In nursing education, ARS integration supports active learning and critical thinking, thus addressing the dynamic curricular needs. Despite positive indications of ARS's impact on engagement and outcomes, ongoing research is essential to fully understand its effects on learning and adaptability to learner characteristics. Nurse educators are encouraged to incorporate ARS into their teaching strategies to enhance engagement and support active learning in both traditional and online settings.

Microlearning and Social Media

Microlearning (also called micro- or bite-sized content, micro-courses, or just-enough information) teaches a small learning unit using a step-by-step approach. Microlearning harnesses Web 2.0 technologies such as social media to engage students and promote self-determined learning, also known as heutagogy (De Gagne et al., 2019; Palmon et al., 2021). The ubiquitous Web 2.0 has fueled interest in heutagogy, a learner-centric approach that enables students to access smaller, targeted, and manageable chunks of information available on the web at their convenience (Narayan et al., 2019). A comprehensive scoping review on microlearning in health professions education revealed a diverse array of technology platforms and applications, such as podcasts, short messaging services, microblogging, social networking services, and internet-based applications (De Gagne et al., 2019).

Research highlights microlearning's effectiveness in enhancing knowledge, attitudes, and competencies. Studies by Haghighat et al. (2023) showed significant improvements in trauma care knowledge and learning satisfaction, illustrating microlearning's capacity to engage nursing students at various levels and enhance their learning experiences. Practical examples of its use include integrating digital media and social media channels for interactive learning and case studies. However, challenges such as network connectivity, accessibility, and privacy concerns need to be addressed to ensure equitable access and effective implementation of microlearning strategies.

Despite potential hurdles, the integration of microlearning and social media into health professions education is an evolving trend, and educators should stay abreast of research and best practices to optimize these tools for meaningful educational outcomes (Palmon et al., 2021). The engagement of learners as active participants, coupled with the capabilities of Web 2.0 and mobile technology, hold promise for enriching educational experiences in nursing. A summary of the 17 studies reviewed on microlearning can be accessed at https://mededu.jmir.org/2019/2/e13997.

Mobile Devices in Education

The integration of mobile devices such as smartphones, tablets, iPads, e-book readers, and other emerging technologies into educational settings is transforming the learning landscape. Studies have indicated a positive correlation between technology use and engagement in learning activities (Carstens et al., 2021): The use of mobile devices in education promotes instant access to information, student engagement, and the formation of personal learning networks. Students, faculty, and staff members increasingly arrive on campus equipped with personal mobile devices and expect seamless access to institutional networks and resources. This trend, known as "bring your own device" (BYOD) or the more encompassing "bring your own everything" (BYOE), necessitates that educational institutions provide robust wireless connectivity. The shift toward mobile computing in educational environments aligns with the digital transition of educational publishers, who now offer electronic textbooks, multimedia applications, online videos, and various other digital tools to support faculty and student needs. A successful mobile computing initiative on campus requires institutional support for the necessary infrastructure and pedagogical integration; this includes expanding bandwidth, increasing access points, enhancing network security, and equipping IT staff to manage diverse mobile operating systems. Colleges and universities are reevaluating their IT strategies to address these evolving demands to enhance learning experiences (Livson et al., 2021).

The rapid expansion of BYOD or BYOE complements other trends in higher education, such as virtualization and technology-enriched classrooms. Faculty buy-in and support for these trends are critical to their successful implementation. The "Ithaka S+R US Faculty Survey 2021" (Blankstein, 2022) found that a significant proportion of faculty members characterized themselves as "early adopters" of new education technologies, and many had tried to adopt new technologies after seeing effective use by their colleagues. However, the survey also revealed that faculty remained skeptical about the value of technology in their teaching. Additionally, the survey reported that only a quarter of the faculty had worked with an instructional designer to develop or revise an online course, underscoring the need for greater assistance from instructional designers and more data and feedback on teaching to support nurse educators in effectively integrating technology into their teaching practices.

Learning Analytics

Learning analytics, as defined by the Society for Learning Analytics Research (2024), primarily focuses on collecting, analyzing, and reporting learner data to enhance learning and learning environments. The Horizon Report (Educause, 2020) emphasized the role of learning analytics in interpreting trends from extensive educational datasets to promote a personalized and supportive higher education system. Traditional methods of learning evaluation, such as student evaluations, grades, attrition rates, and faculty input, have been augmented by the digital shift in education; this transition to online platforms has led to an abundance of data, offering new insights into teaching and learning techniques.

Given the challenges to education posed by the COVID-19 pandemic, recent advancements in learning analytics have become crucial for tracking student retention and progression (Jeffries, 2020). The Nursing Universal Retention and Success (NURS) model, as discussed by Bojic et al. (2023), offers a detailed review of learning analytics processes and emphasizes the role of digital assignment materials and the extensive collection of interaction data. Furthermore, research into the motivational profiles of nontraditional practical nurse students indicates that learning analytics can identify varied student motivations, leading to more tailored support (Kleimola et al., 2023).

In nursing education, learning analytics has become a critical tool that transcends traditional evaluation approaches by presenting a data-driven, individualized framework that is especially effective for understanding and aiding the varied motivations of nontraditional nursing students. This shift toward data-informed, dynamic, and inclusive educational practices supported by robust research and evolving educational paradigms will shape the future of nursing education. Economic considerations such as cost impact, return on investment, and the need for lifelong workplace learning will play a significant role in standardizing the use of learning analytics to improve teaching methods and boost student success rates (Pelletier et al., 2023).

Open Educational Resources

Open educational resources (OERs) are instructional materials freely available for public use under open licensing, and thus for faculty use and reuse at no cost, as stated by OER Commons (2024). Originating in the late 20th century, OERs include materials for adoption, adaptation, and distribution within courses. As the costs of higher education rise, universities are increasingly turning to digital textbooks as cost-effective alternatives. OERs reduce the need for expensive textbooks, provide interactive tools for a learner-centered environment, and enhance student engagement (Marín et al., 2022). Librarians play a key role in guiding educators to suitable OERs (Association of College and Research Libraries, 2022).

Recent studies show a growing awareness of OERs among faculty in higher education, indicating a broader acceptance and understanding: Bay View Analytics reported a steady increase in OER awareness, with 72% of faculty acknowledging it in 2023 (Seaman & Seaman, 2023). Research in Technology Enhanced Learning (Marín et al., 2022) also noted varying levels of OER awareness across countries. Table 7.2 provides a list of free digital textbooks and websites exemplifying OERs.

Generative Artificial Intelligence

The integration of generative AI and adaptive learning systems is significantly transforming higher education, including health professions education (De Gagne, 2023b). Advanced technologies such as ChatGPT utilize AI algorithms to

TABLE 7.2 EXAMPLES OF OPEN EDUCATIONAL RESOURCES SITES

Site Name	Website
BCcampus	https://open.bccampus.ca
Canadian Association of Schools of Nursing	https://www.casn.ca/education/5656-2
Community College Consortium for Open Educational Resources	https://www.cccoer.org
MERLOT	https://www.merlot.org
MIT OpenCourseWare (OCW)	https://ocw.mit.edu
OER Commons	https://www.oercommons.org
OpenStax	https://openstax.org
UNESCO OER	https://en.unesco.org/themes/building-knowledge-societies/oer
World Digital Library (WDL)	https://www.loc.gov/collections/world-digital-library/about-this-collection

tailor educational content to the unique needs of individual learners, thus boosting engagement and enhancing overall educational outcomes (Niyozov et al., 2023). The 2023 Educause Horizon Report illuminated key technological and social trends in higher education, particularly emphasizing the increasing demand for flexible learning models aligned with more adaptable educational experiences (Pelletier et al., 2023). AI-enabled LMSs are at the forefront of this transformation, offering personalized learning experiences by adapting content and assessments to individual learner profiles. A prime example is the Artificial Intelligence-enabled Intelligent Assistant (AIIA) framework, which uses AI and Natural Language Processing (NLP) techniques to minimize cognitive load, streamline student assessment, and offer tailored learning support (Sajja et al., 2023).

In nursing education, generative AI and adaptive learning systems are reshaping how students interact with educational content by offering novel and dynamic learning experiences (De Gagne, 2023b). For example, these AI tools are adept at creating realistic simulation scenarios such as patient interviews, thereby enriching interactive and adaptable learning (De Gagne, 2023b). However, some studies have highlighted limitations, particularly in the accuracy of clinical information provided by AI tools like ChatGPT, advising caution in their use for healthcare decision-making (Abujaber et al., 2023; Branum & Schiavenato, 2023). Additionally, concerns have been raised about AI's impact on fundamental nursing values such as empathy and compassion (Abdulai & Hung, 2023). Furthermore, AI integration into nursing education introduces ethical challenges, especially in cyberethics, concerning data privacy, academic integrity, and responsible use of AI-generated content, emphasizing the need for a cautious approach to maintain ethical standards and promote critical thinking (De Gagne, Hwang et al., 2023).

Effective AI integration into nursing education demands a robust infrastructure and strategic alignment in the classroom, provision of the necessary technological resources, comprehensive training, and support for educators (De Gagne, 2023a). Faculty roles are evolving in alignment with the goals of the nursing curriculum to encompass the design and implementation of AI tools. Collaborative efforts among IT professionals, instructional designers, and nurse educators are crucial for crafting a cohesive, technology-enhanced curriculum. Continuous collaboration and research are essential to address challenges and optimize these tools' potential, ensuring future nursing professionals' proficiency in technology use (De Gagne, 2023a).

RETHINKING THE EDUCATION PARADIGM

Technology continues to enhance active learning as it accommodates a variety of learning preferences and facilitates communication, collaboration, and sharing among students. The integration of technology into nursing education should be driven by pedagogical goals to support and facilitate learning, critical thinking, problem-solving, creativity, and innovation rather than by the availability or novelty of a specific technology.

Infrastructure

Investment in infrastructure remains essential for the successful integration of technology into teaching and learning. Schools must support their evolving technological demands. The infrastructure must be secure, available 24/7, able to handle a wide range of applications, and adaptable to new technologies. To accomplish these goals, campuses must develop and implement strategic technology plans that align with the institution's mission and goals. These plans should not be static because new technologies are competing for infrastructure resources on an almost daily basis. The key to success is a commitment from institutional and nursing program leadership to support IT and use technology to improve and maintain institutional performance.

Alignment With Institution and School of Nursing Mission and Goals

Over the past decades, colleges and universities have made substantial investments in technological infrastructure (e.g., course management systems, wireless networks, multimedia classrooms) and a wide array of technology tools to transform teaching and learning. There are many available technologies and various ways of implementing them, so it can be difficult for faculty members, including nurse educators, to keep pace and evaluate whether the use of a technology is affecting learning outcomes.

Evaluation of the success of teaching and learning with technology requires an institutional approach to determine efficiency, effectiveness, sustainability, and quality. A systematic approach may not be appropriate for all technology but is ideal for examining the impact of technologies with broad applicability across the institution. A more individualized approach may be appropriate for specific technologies or in a specialized area of study such as nursing. For technology integration to transform education to its greatest potential, it cannot be used arbitrarily by a few educators only but must be incorporated into the institution's mission and goals. Unless the culture and structure of a school are compatible with and supportive of specific uses of technology, technology integration is not likely to succeed. When technology-enhanced education is part of the mission and goals of an institution, its effect becomes evident in all aspects of the school's programs and fosters an innovative culture that transforms education.

Innovation is often seen as the introduction of new ideas, methods, or devices, yet it also embodies transformations that enhance productivity and quality. Cultivating a culture where this concept is central to the organization's vision and purpose allows institutions to incorporate creative thinking, teaching, and learning beyond conventional methods. By integrating such a mindset into its framework, an institution encourages and supports creativity through practices like coaching, mentoring, hiring, and rewarding faculty and staff.

Constructivism and Technology-Enhanced Learning

The evolution of educational theories, particularly social constructivism, has significantly influenced modern student-centered learning paradigms. Evolved theories advocate for teaching practices that are interactive, problem-based, and enriched with technology to adequately prepare 21st-century learners for a complex, interconnected global society. Constructivism posits that learning is an active process by which learners construct their own understanding and knowledge of the world through having and reflecting on experiences. This concept aligns with ideas on the social and cultural dimensions of learning described by Jerome Bruner in *The Culture of Education* (1996). Current instructional technologies have aligned with constructivist principles to foster environments that challenge students to collaborate effectively and engage actively as self-directed, lifelong learners within and outside formal educational settings.

For nurse educators, key objectives should be (a) leveraging learning theory and best-practice teaching strategies to guide the integration of technology, and (b) aiming for high-quality outcomes. Despite technological advancements that expand educational possibilities, the essence of effective teaching remains constant; it is the methods—now enhanced by technology—which have evolved. Continuous reassessment of curriculum and teaching strategies is vital. For instance, Chickering and Gamson's *Seven Principles for Good Practice in Undergraduate Education* (1987) remains highly relevant in digital classrooms and web-based learning environments, and Chickering and Ehrmann's (1996) insights further underscore how integrating technology can reinforce and extend their principles. Exhibit 7.2 presents these principles as applied in current, technology-enhanced teaching and learning scenarios.

Decision-Making Framework for Technology Selection

The successful use of technology is dependent on the selection and utilization of appropriate tools. Educators who are examining the use of various tools to achieve desired learning outcomes must consider content, format, interface design, and completeness of application. The SECTIONS model is designed to provide

> **EXHIBIT 7.2 Seven Principles for Good Practice in Education Applied to Teaching With Technology**
>
> Encourage contact between student and faculty; utilize various communication platforms (e.g., LMS messaging, video conferencing tools like Zoom, Teams) for continuous and meaningful interactions.
>
> Develop reciprocity and cooperation among students; leverage collaborative digital tools (such as online forums, shared documents, virtual collaboration spaces) for team-based learning and peer interaction.
>
> Use active learning techniques; incorporate advanced simulations, virtual worlds (VWs), interactive demonstrations, and virtual patient interactions for experiential learning.
>
> Give prompt feedback; employ learning management systems (LMS) for immediate formative feedback through quizzes, discussions, and assignments that offer rapid responses and learning enhancement opportunities.
>
> Emphasize time on task; design tasks that encourage preparatory work focused on foundational knowledge, thereby allocating more time for higher-order learning activities like application and creation during class.
>
> Communicate high expectations; facilitate self-directed learning with technology that sets high benchmarks for student engagement in both student–student and faculty–student interactions.
>
> Respect diverse talent and ways of learning; use a variety of teaching technologies to accommodate a range of learning preferences and paces, allowing for repeated content engagement and practice
>
> *Source:* Adapted from Chickering, A. W., & Ehrmann, S. C. (1996). Implementing the seven principles: Technology as lever. *AAHE Bulletin, 49,* 3–6; Chickering, A. W., & Gamson, Z. F. (1987). Seven principles for good practice in undergraduate education. *AAHE Bulletin, 39*(7), 3–6.

educators with technology to integrate into their courses. SECTIONS is an acronym for **s**tudents, **e**ase of use, **c**ost, **t**eaching functions, **i**nteraction, **o**rganizational issues, **n**etworking, and **s**ecurity and privacy. The model allows teachers to answer a series of questions systematically when choosing technologies for their teaching (Bates, 2022). The SECTIONS model can be used to select media for use in campus-based as well as distance education. More information can be found at https://pressbooks.pub/everydayid/chapter/using-sections-to-select-digital-tools.

Technology can provide expanded educational offerings to a broader range of the population, including individuals with less access to higher education or living with disabilities. As there is no single technology that suits all educational environments, experienced educators and skilled developers must plan carefully and choose instructional and delivery media components strategically. It is also critical to match the mechanisms of education technology with appropriate learning environments.

Classroom Redesign

As the educational landscape continually evolves, driven by advancements in technology and progressive learning theories, there is a parallel transformation in classroom design to meet these emerging educational demands. This evolution, which is particularly relevant to nurse educators, has spurred a reevaluation and modernization of teaching approaches, leading to a reimagining and redesigning of physical learning environments.

One notable development has been the creation of active learning classrooms. These spaces are intentionally designed to promote active, student-centered teaching and maximize the room's potential for interactive learning. In such settings, students typically utilize their own computing devices, tapping into the classroom's wireless capabilities for collaborative and interactive learning activities such as small group discussions to brainstorm and develop new ideas under the guidance of educators who play a facilitative and supportive role.

Features of the modern classroom prominently include modular and ergonomic furniture designed to accommodate a range of learning activities and styles. This adaptability allows students to rearrange their learning environment as needed, promoting a sense of independence and deepening their engagement with the learning process. Additionally, technology is a cornerstone in these classrooms, with large LCD screens and other digital tools enhancing group discussions and facilitating interactive, hands-on activities.

In redesigning learning spaces, emphasis has been placed on creating environments that support collaboration, personalization, accessibility, and flexibility. Nurse educators' involvement and enthusiasm are key to the successful implementation and efficacy of these innovative learning spaces.

Flipping the Classroom

The concept of "flipping the classroom" has gained increasing prominence in educational discourse. This approach utilizes technology to move foundational knowledge acquisition outside the classroom, freeing up valuable in-person time for dynamic, practical learning experiences. The model gained particular relevance during the pandemic, spurring the adoption of hybrid teaching approaches (Sampaio & Ramos, 2023). In the flipped classroom model, students independently complete pre-class activities, setting the stage for deeper discussion, application, and synthesis during class time. The classroom becomes a center for collaboration, sharing, and reflection, thus fostering interactive learning. Consequently, the educator transitions from primarily delivering information to facilitating and guiding with an emphasis on critical thinking and problem-solving (Sharom & Kew, 2021).

The ongoing exploration of assistive technologies aims to convert traditional lecture-based learning into active, student-centered engagement (Sampaio & Ramos, 2023). Given the rapid evolution of technologies such as AI, blockchain, the internet of things (IoT), XR, wearables, and biometrics, it is crucial that faculty be prepared not only to teach these concepts but also to facilitate their direct application by students (Sampaio & Ramos, 2023). Successful integration of the flipped classroom model requires both students and educators to adapt to this innovative educational approach.

In health professions education, the flipped classroom has yielded promising outcomes. Research in undergraduate health sciences disciplines has shown related improvements in academic performance, student satisfaction, and self-efficacy which can be attributed to well-structured curricula (Banks & Kay, 2022). However, opinions on the effectiveness of this approach vary, and its impact largely depends on the method and learning context of its implementation. As an educational strategy, the flipped classroom continues to be a focus of research, particularly regarding its effects on academic performance. Despite its challenges, this method offers significant promise for enhancing student engagement and learning outcomes. Nurse educators adopting this strategy should apply effective teaching methods to support learning. Some examples of a flipped classroom model are included in Exhibit 7.3. The success

> **EXHIBIT 7.3 Examples of Flipping the Classroom**
>
> Student-led teaching: Students take on the role of educators by demonstrating their knowledge and assignments through presentations during face-to-face or synchronous online web-conferencing sessions. The faculty member transitions into the role of a facilitator, guiding the learning process.
>
> Team-based learning: This approach ensures that students come to class prepared for learning. It includes the use of individual quizzes with immediate feedback via a learning management system (LMS) assessment. In class, students are placed in teams, retake the quiz as a group, and discuss and collaborate to arrive at correct answers.
>
> Case studies: Cases can be embedded in the academic electronic health record (EHR) and reviewed by students prior to class. During class, students can be placed in teams to navigate the EHR and problem-solve the case.
>
> Educational games: Games such as Jeopardy, Who Wants to be a Millionaire, and Family Feud can be used to review content and foster a collaborative and competitive learning atmosphere. Examples of nursing games can be found at the Merlot website (https://www.merlot.org/merlot/viewMaterial.htm?id=1280129), which hosts over 100 free nursing games used to facilitate learning and make education more interesting.
>
> Chat rooms: These can be used in large classrooms to solicit feedback after mini-lectures or group discussion, allowing all students to have a voice.
>
> Role-playing scenarios: Students can be assigned predetermined roles to perform during class, providing a dynamic and interactive learning experience.
>
> Research and debates: Individual students or teams can be assigned research tasks in preparation for in-class debates on topics such as healthcare, healthcare reform, or patient safety, among others. This strategy encourages critical thinking and active engagement with the subject matter.

of these approaches is influenced by the specific context in which they are applied and how they are implemented. Continuous assessment and adaptation of these strategies are crucial to align them with the evolving learning needs of students.

DEVELOPING FACULTY COMPETENCIES AND MENTORING

Many faculty members in nursing education feel overwhelmed by the rapid advancement of emerging technologies, including LMSs, Web 2.0 technologies, generative AI, and various software applications for classroom and clinical teaching. The essence of faculty development programs lies in their ability to (a) demystify how technological innovations can meet educational outcomes, and (b) propose practical strategies for these achievements. A notable example of such an initiative is the collaboration between the American Association of Colleges of Nursing (AACN) and the Apple education team in 2020, which led to the Digital Innovation Virtual Bootcamp. This initiative aimed to harness cutting-edge technologies to bolster education in classrooms, labs, and clinical settings. Through this program, educators embarked on project implementations at their institutions, partook in dynamic learning techniques, and gained knowledge from the insights of peers and mentors. This model directly catered to the unique demands of nurse educators by combining the knowledge of faculty and instructional designers to showcase pedagogical methods linked with new technologies, thus encouraging continuous collaboration across educational entities.

Technological advancements are set to dramatically revolutionize the healthcare landscape and its associated fields, and it is anticipated that nursing curricula will seamlessly integrate emerging technologies. Richardson et al. (2023) shed light on how nursing schools and accrediting organizations will prioritize innovations. Their research accentuates the role of accrediting bodies in faculty development and outlines obstacles to adopting technologies like AI, blockchain, and the IoT in nursing education. Additionally, by employing the Unified Theory of Acceptance and Use of Technology (UTAUT), their study identified education and training, cost, and complexity as major hurdles to technological assimilation. Richardson and colleagues stated that faculty development programs must take a forward-thinking approach toward incorporating technologies into curricula by ensuring faculty proficiency in their application. They called for a continuous cycle of professional development and support to navigate the dynamic domain of nursing education successfully. Programs like the AACN–Apple Digital Innovation Virtual Bootcamp exemplify the overarching goal of such initiatives: to equip educators with the competencies necessary for the effective use of technology in teaching and mentorship.

Nursing education is poised to evolve—that is, to continue to address identified barriers, harness insights from recent studies, focus on faculty development, and offer education that blends technological innovations with solid pedagogical principles. Faculty development and mentoring programs are critical for achieving an education system that seamlessly integrates emerging technologies, both theoretically and in practice, and equips new generations of nurses with the skills they will need to thrive in technologically advanced healthcare environments.

SUMMARY

This chapter explored the evolving role of technology in nursing education, emphasizing that nurse educators must understand current technological tools and stay informed of emerging technologies. It highlighted the transformation from traditional computer-based learning to diverse interactive tools that have reshaped faculty approaches to teaching. This chapter particularly spotlighted emerging technologies such as the metaverse, generative AI, and gaming for their potential to enhance student learning outcomes. A key focus was on aligning technology with pedagogical best practices to ensure a meaningful integration that supports student learning.

This chapter also (a) described the redesign of learning environments, with emphasis placed on the flipped-classroom model and its role in fostering engaging and effective educational experiences; (b) discussed the need for appropriate infrastructure, resources, and faculty development to ensure successful technology integration into nursing programs; and (c) identified technology as a pivotal element in enhancing both teaching quality and learning experiences in nursing education. As technology continually evolves, its impact on nursing education is anticipated to grow, thus presenting continuous opportunities for innovation and application. Embracing these technological advancements is crucial to effective teaching that prepares future nurses to thrive in a technology-driven healthcare environment.

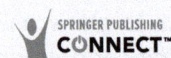 A robust set of instructor resources designed to supplement this text is located at http://connect.springerpub.com/content/book/978-0-8261-8892-2. Qualifying instructors may request access by emailing textbook@springerpub.com.

REFERENCES

Abdulai, A.-F., & Hung, L. (2023). Will ChatGPT undermine ethical values in nursing education, research, and practice? *Nursing Inquiry, 30*, e12556. https://doi.org/10.1111/nin.12556

Abujaber, A. A., Abd-Alrazaq, A., Al-Qudimat, A. R., & Nashwan, A. J. (2023). A Strengths, Weaknesses, Opportunities, and Threats (SWOT) analysis of ChatGPT integration in nursing education: A narrative review. *Cureus, 15*(11), e48643. https://doi.org/10.7759/cureus.48643

Akintolu, M., Dlamini, N., & Letseka, M. (2022). Bloom's taxonomy for the digital age student in a rural African context. *EUREKA: Social & Humanities*, (6), 39–47. http://doi.org/10.21303/2504-5571.2022.002472

Anderson, D. K., Schoenleber, M., & Korshavn, S. (2023). Higher-order clicker questions engage students and prepare them for higher-order thinking activities. *Journal of Microbiology & Biology Education, 24*(1), e00151-22. https://doi.org/10.1128/jmbe.00151-22

Association of College and Research Libraries. (2022). *Welcome to the OER librarian toolkit.* https://acrl.libguides.com/cjcls/oer

Attaran, M., Attaran, S., & Celik, B. G. (2017). Promises and challenges of cloud computing in higher education: A practical guide for implementation. *Journal of Higher Education Theory & Practice, 17*(6), 20–38.

Banks, L., & Kay, R. (2022). Exploring flipped classrooms in undergraduate nursing and health science: A systematic review. *Nurse Education in Practice, 64*, 103417. https://doi.org/10.1016/j.nepr.2022.103417

Bates, A. W. (2022). Choosing and using media in education: The SECTIONS model. In *Teaching in a Digital Age* (3rd ed.). https://pressbooks.bccampus.ca/teachinginadigitalagev3/part/9-pedagogical-differences-between-media

Blankstein, M. (2022). *Research report: Ithaka S+R US Faculty Survey 2021.* https://doi.org/10.18665/sr.316896

Bojic, I., Mammadova, M., Ang, C.-S., Teo, W. L., Diordieva, C., Pienkowska, A., Gašević, D., & Car, J. (2023). Empowering health care education through learning analytics: In-depth scoping review. *Journal of Medical Internet Research, 25*(1), e41671. https://doi.org/10.2196/41671

Branum, C., & Schiavenato, M. (2023). Can ChatGPT accurately answer a picot question? Assessing AI response to a clinical question. *Nurse Educator, 48*(5), 231–233. https://doi.org.10.1097/NNE.0000000000001436

Bruner, J. (1996). *The culture of education.* Harvard University Press.

Carstens, K. J., Mallon, J. M., Bataineh, M., & Al-Bataineh, A. (2021). Effects of technology on student learning. *TOJET: The Turkish Online Journal of Educational Technology, 20*(1), 105–113.

Chickering, A. W., & Ehrmann, S. C. (1996). Implementing the seven principles: Technology as lever. *AAHE Bulletin, 49*(2), 3–6.

Chickering, A. W., & Gamson, Z. F. (1987). Seven principles for good practice in undergraduate education. *AAHE Bulletin, 39*(7), 3–6.

Copenhaver, K., Randall, P. S., & De Gagne, J. C. (2023). Teaching health equity through gaming. *Teaching & Learning in Nursing, 18*(4), 500–502. https://doi.org/10.1016/j.teln.2023.05.014

De Gagne, J. C. (2023a). Renewed urgency: Reimagining roles in nursing and academia amidst rapid AI advancements. *International Journal of Environmental Research and Public Health, 20*(11), 5963. https://doi.org/10.3390/ijerph20115963

De Gagne, J. C. (2023b). The state of artificial intelligence in nursing education: Past, present, and future directions. *International Journal of Environmental Research and Public Health, 20*(6), 4884. https://doi.org/10.3390/ijerph20064884

De Gagne, J. C., Hwang, H., & Jung, D. (2023). Cyberethics in nursing education: Ethical implications of artificial intelligence. *Nursing Ethics*, 9697330231201901. https://doi.org/10.1177/09697330231201901

De Gagne, J. C., Randall, P. S., Rushton, S., Park, H. K., Cho, E., Yamane, S. S., & Jung, D. (2023). The use of metaverse in nursing education: An umbrella review. *Nurse Educator, 48*(3). E73–E78. https://doi.org/10.1097/NNE.0000000000001327

De Gagne, J. C., Park, H., Hall, K., Woodward, A., Yamane, S. S., & Kim, S.-S. (2019). Microlearning in health professions education: Scoping review. *JMIR Medical Education, 5*(2), e13997. https://doi.org/10.2196/13997

Educause. (2020). *2020 horizon report: Teaching and learning edition.* https://library.educause.edu/resources/2020/3/2020-educause-horizon-report-teaching-and-learning-edition

Gentry, S. V., Gauthier, A., Ehrstrom, B. L. E., Wortley, D., Lilienthal, A., Car, L. T., ... & Car, J. (2019). Serious gaming and gamification education in health professions: Systematic review. *Journal of Medical Internet Research, 21*(3), e12994. https://doi.org/10.2196/12994

Haghighat, H., Shiri, M., Esmaeili Abdar, M., Taher Harikandee, S. S., & Tayebi, Z. (2023). The effect of micro-learning on trauma care knowledge and learning satisfaction in nursing students. *BMC Medical Education, 23*(1), 622. https://doi.org/10.1186/s12909-023-04609-2

Iti, J. L., & Kadeangadi, D. M. (2023). Effectiveness of the use of clickers versus group discussion in learning by undergraduate medical students. *Journal of Family & Community Medicine, 30*(3), 219–224. https://doi.org/10.4103/jfcm.jfcm_376_22

Jeffreys, M. R. (2020). Nursing Universal Retention and Success (NURS) model: A holistic, discipline-focused framework. *Journal of College Student Retention: Research, Theory & Practice, 24*(3), 650–675. https://doi.org/10.1177/1521025120939254

Jeffries, P. R., Bushardt, R. L., DuBose-Morris, R., Hood, C., Kardong-Edgren, S., Pintz, C., Posey, L., & Sikka, N. (2022). The role of technology in health professions education during the COVID-19 pandemic. *Academic Medicine, 97*(3), S104–S109. https://doi.org/10.1097/ACM.0000000000004523

Kleimola, R., López-Pernas, S., Väisänen, S., Saqr, M., Sointu, E., & Hirsto, L. (2023). Learning analytics to explore the motivational profiles of non-traditional practical nurse students: A mixed-methods approach. *Empirical Research in Vocational Education and Training, 15*(1), 11. https://doi.org/10.1186/s40461-023-00150-0

Kononowicz, A. A., Woodham, L. A., Edelbring, S., Stathakarou, N., Davies, D., Saxena, N., Car, L. T., Carlstedt-Duke, J., Car, J., & Zary, N. (2019). Virtual patient simulations in health professions education: Systematic review and meta-analysis by the digital health education collaboration. *Journal of Medical Internet Research, 21*(7), e14676. https://doi.org/10.2196/14676

Livson, M., Ulanova, K. L., Pertsev, V. V., Dudynov, S. V., & Novikov, A. V. (2021). The Influence of BYOD on Results of Students' Learning. *Propósitos y Representaciones, 9*(SPE3), e1265. https://doi.org/10.20511/pyr2021.v9nSPE3.1265

Marín, V. I., Zawacki-Richter, O., Aydin, C. H., Bedenlier, S., Bond, M., Bozkurt, A., Conrad, D., Jung, I., Kondakci, Y., Prinsloo, P., Roberts, J., Veletsianos, G., Xiao, J., & Zhang, J. (2022). Faculty perceptions, awareness and use of open educational resources for teaching and learning in higher education: A cross-comparative analysis. *Research and Practice in Technology Enhanced Learning, 17*(1), 11. https://doi.org/10.1186/s41039-022-00185-z

Mell, P., & Grance, T. (2011). *The NIST definition of cloud computing* (Special Publication 800-145). The National Institute of Standards and Technology, United States Department of Commerce.

Narayan, V., Herrington, J., & Cochrane, T. (2019). Design principles for heutagogical learning: Implementing student-determined learning with mobile and social media tools. *Australasian Journal of Educational Technology, 35*, 86–101. https://doi.org/10.14742/ajet.3941

Niyozov, N., Saburov, S., Ganiyev, S., & Olimov, S. (2023). AI-powered learning: Revolutionizing technical higher education institutions through advanced power supply fundamentals. *E3S Web of Conferences, 461*, 01092. https://doi.org/10.1051/e3sconf/202346101092

Njenga, K., Garg, L., Bhardwaj, A. K., Prakash, V., & Bawa, S. (2019). The cloud computing adoption in higher learning institutions in Kenya: Hindering factors and recommendations for the way forward. *Telematics and Informatics, 38*, 225-246. https://doi.org/10.1016/j.tele.2018.10.007

Open Educational Resources Commons. (2024). *Getting started with OER.* https://www.oercommons.org

Palmon, I., Brown, C. S., Highet, A., Kulick, A. A., Barrett, M. E., Cassidy, D. E., Herman, A. E., Gomez-Rexrode, A. E., O'Reggio, R., Sonnenday, C., Waits, S. A., & Wakam, G. K. (2021). Microlearning and social Media: A novel approach to video-based learning and surgical education. *Journal of Graduate Medical Education, 13*(3), 323. https://doi.org/10.4300/JGME-D-20-01562.1

Pelletier, K., Robert, J., Muscanell, N., McCormack, M., Reeves, J., Arbino, N., & Grajek, S. (2023). *2023 EDUCAUSE Horizon Report, Teaching and Learning Edition* https://library.educause.edu/-/media/files/library/2023/4/2023hrteachinglearning.pdf?la=en&hash=195420BF5A2F09991379CBE68858EF10D7088AF5.

Qasem, Y. A. M., Abdullah, R., Jusoh, Y. Y., Atan, R., & Asadi, S. (2019). Cloud computing adoption in higher education institutions: A systematic review. *IEEE Access, 7*, 63722–63744. https://doi.org/10.1109/ACCESS.2019.2916234

Richardson, E. L., Gordon, J., Ginnetti, R., Cochran, R., Conklin, S., Oetjen, R., & Oetjen, D. (2023). Are Nursing faculty future-ready? The effects of emerging technologies on nursing education. *Journal of Nursing Education, 62*(12), 689–700. https://doi.org/10.3928/01484834-20231006-04

Sajja, R., Sermet, Y., Cikmaz, M., Cwiertny, D., & Demir, I. (2023). *Artificial intelligence-enabled intelligent assistant for personalized and adaptive learning in higher education* (arXiv:2309.10892). arXiv. https://doi.org/10.48550/arXiv.2309.10892

Sampaio, L. A., & Ramos, M. H. T. (2023). Transforming teaching in health: Exploring the advantages of the flipped classroom active methodology. *Research, Society & Development, 12*(7), e14512742637. https://doi.org/10.33448/rsd-v12i7.42637

Seaman, J. E., & Seaman, J. (2023). *Digitally established: Educational resources in U.S. higher education, 2023*. https://www.bayviewanalytics.com/reports/digitallyestablished-2023.pdf

Sharom, K., & Kew, S. N. (2021). A conceptual framework on technology integration in english writing flipped classroom. *IOP Conference Series: Materials Science & Engineering, 1051*(1), 012010. https://doi.org/10.1088/1757-899X/1051/1/012010

Singh, J., Singh, A. K., & Singla, M. (2023). Recent trends in e-learning using Web 4.0. In D. Goyal, A. Kumar, V. Piuri, & M. Paprzycki (Eds.), *Proceedings of the Third International Conference on Information Management and Machine Intelligence* (pp. 167–173). Springer Nature. https://doi.org/10.1007/978-981-19-2065-3_20

Society for Learning Analytics Research. (2024). *What is learning analytics?* https://www.solaresearch.org/about/what-is-learning-analytics

Turnbull, D., Chugh, R., & Luck, J. (2020). Learning management systems, an overview. In A. Tatnall (Ed.), *Encyclopedia of Education and Information Technologies* (pp. 1052–1058). Springer International Publishing. https://doi.org/10.1007/978-3-030-10576-1_248

Zhang, H., Mörelius, E., Goh, S. H. L., & Wang, W. (2019). Effectiveness of Video-assisted debriefing in simulation-based health professions education: A systematic review of quantitative evidence. *Nurse Educator, 44*(3), E1–E6. https://doi.org/10.1097/NNE.0000000000000562

Teaching in Online Learning Environments

Jennie C. De Gagne

8

OBJECTIVES

1. Describe the roles and responsibilities of educators as facilitators in the online learning environment
2. Examine instructional technologies and resources that can help nurse educators select and incorporate new strategies into their online teaching
3. Evaluate the process of reconceptualizing for designing and evaluating online courses and modules

INTRODUCTION

Teaching and learning in the online environment signify a profound transformation from the centuries-old tradition of classroom-based education. The advent of the web, originally designed to facilitate communication and information sharing, has seamlessly transitioned into a pivotal educational platform. Online education leverages this digital medium to overcome the geographical and scheduling barriers inherent in traditional education, thus offering invaluable opportunities for learners constrained by distance or personal commitments.

The COVID-19 pandemic underscored the indispensable role of online learning as a means of continuing education amid global crises. As healthcare systems faced unprecedented challenges, the need for competent nursing professionals reached new heights. Higher education institutions, particularly nursing schools, swiftly expanded their digital offerings, incorporating both hybrid and fully online courses and programs to cater to emergent needs and student preferences. The postpandemic landscape has seen a persistent shift toward hybrid learning models, reflecting a broader acceptance and integration of digital education modalities across the board.

This chapter explores the nuanced distinctions between online and traditional classroom teaching and emphasizes the dynamic roles and responsibilities that educators assume as facilitators in the digital domain. It delves into the complexities of course content, teaching strategies, and the important task of designing and refining online learning environments. Additionally, the discussion encompasses the interaction dynamics within online courses, the strategic application of educational technologies, and methodologies for assessing online program effectiveness. Special attention is dedicated to the critical need for accessibility and usability, and guidance is provided on how to make online education accessible, responsive, and inclusive for all learners.

DEFINITIONS

Instructors venturing into online teaching may encounter a variety of terms that have broadened to elucidate the evolving landscape of education: *Distance learning*, traditionally characterized by the physical separation between instructor and student, has broadened to include not just correspondence courses but also remote and online learning modalities (Atkinson, 2023); its definition has evolved to reflect a shift from traditional mail-based correspondence courses to the dynamic incorporation of multimedia and e-learning strategies that enrich knowledge transmission. *E-learning*, which initially focused on digital content delivery, now integrates diverse media and digital resources to offer interactive educational experiences; this approach has been enhanced by predictive analytics and machine learning, marking a shift toward personalized and adaptive learning experiences (Akhmedova et al., 2023).

Online learning, or *web-based learning*, utilizes the internet to streamline educational processes; the pandemic notably accelerated its adoption, establishing online learning as a standard in educational settings (Oliver Del Olmo, 2021). *Hybrid* or *blended learning* merges online and face-to-face elements, employing texts, multimedia, hyperlinks, and virtual case studies to cater to different learning preferences and needs. This blend not only supports practical skill development but also offers theoretical learning flexibility, fostering engagement and knowledge application in varied settings.

Interaction in online learning environments manifests in three forms: instructor–student, student–student, and student–content. Interaction can occur *synchronously*, with real-time engagement, or *asynchronously*, with participation occurring according to individual schedules. Asynchronous interactions enable message exchanges on dedicated platforms, which facilitate convenient peer and content engagement. Conversely, synchronous interactions demand real-time participation, anchoring the learning experience in immediacy.

The emergence of remote, virtual, and hybrid learning terminologies, propelled by the COVID-19 pandemic, highlights the adaptability and resilience within education (Raghunathan et al., 2022). These modalities ensure continuity in learning despite disruptions, and equip nursing students for healthcare challenges. The pandemic era has undeniably spurred educational innovation by encouraging the integration of effective distance education strategies to meet evolving needs.

ADVANTAGES AND DISADVANTAGES OF ONLINE LEARNING

Online learning utilizes the internet to expand access to educational resources significantly. This mode of learning allows students to interact with course materials and engage in educational activities at any time and place, provided they have internet access. Emphasizing a student-centered approach, online learning offers rich, dynamic interactions and a flexible learning environment. However, it necessitates a level of computer literacy among students and depends on the compatibility of hardware and software. Additionally, online learning systems may encounter technical issues that can disrupt their operation. The diverse implications of this learning modality are summarized in Table 8.1, which outlines the primary advantages and challenges associated with online education.

TABLE 8.1 ADVANTAGES AND DISADVANTAGES OF ONLINE LEARNING

Advantages	Disadvantages
▪ *Accessibility*: Learning materials and resources are accessible around the clock, enabling students to access them 24/7 from any location with an internet connection. ▪ *Flexibility*: The online learning environment allows students to learn at their own pace, accommodating their personal and professional commitments. ▪ *Reduced Time and Space Barriers*: Online learning eliminates the need for physical presence in a classroom, saving time and potentially reducing educational costs. ▪ *Diverse Learning Experiences*: The use of multimedia and interactive tools in online learning can enhance the educational experience by catering to different learning preferences. ▪ *Enhanced Digital Literacy*: Navigating online learning platforms can improve students' digital skills to prepare them for the current and future workforce.	▪ *Technical Skills Requirement*: Students must possess not only fundamental computer skills but also the ability to navigate various online learning platforms, troubleshoot common technical issues, and effectively utilize collaborative tools and resources. ▪ *Self-Motivation and Discipline*: Success in online learning demands high levels of motivation and self-discipline from students. ▪ *Limited In-Person Interaction*: Online learning may offer fewer opportunities for face-to-face interactions with peers and instructors, which can impact the learning experience. ▪ *Technical Issues*: A dependence on technology means that system failures can limit access to learning materials and disrupt educational processes. ▪ *Access and Compatibility*: Not all students have reliable internet or compatible technology, which creates barriers to equitable online learning access.

PREVALENCE OF ONLINE COURSES

The landscape of online courses and degree programs has continued to evolve, with significant transformation and expansion reflecting a steady increase in enrollments annually. Recent data from the National Center for Education Statistics (2023) provide an updated perspective on the trends in distance education enrollment, particularly in the context of the shifts induced by the COVID-19 pandemic. In fall 2021, about 9.4 million undergraduate students, or 61% of the undergraduate cohort, registered for at least one distance education course, a substantial shift from 36% in 2019 to 75% in 2020. Notably, 4.4 million undergraduates, which is 28% of this population, pursued their studies entirely online in 2021, showcasing fluctuations from 15% in 2019 to 44% in 2020.

A pronounced preference for enrolling in institutions within their own state was observed among students opting for exclusively online courses, with 74% choosing in-state institutions and 23% selecting out-of-state options. The engagement in distance education varied significantly across different types of institutions, underscoring diverse patterns of adoption among public, private nonprofit, and private for-profit entities. On the postbaccalaureate level, approximately 1.8 million students engaged in at least one online course in fall 2021, with 1.3 million of these students opting for exclusively online formats; these numbers indicate a sustained integration and acceptance of online learning and distance education in the higher education ecosystem and signal a dynamic evolution in educational paradigms, with online learning emerging as an essential strategy for institutions, notwithstanding the challenges that necessitate greater acceptance and integration. The trajectory suggests an ongoing shift toward educational offerings that are more flexible, accessible, and tailored to diverse learning needs and preferences.

The emergence of massive open online courses (MOOCs) has introduced complexities to traditional education models. Since their inception in 2008, and their proliferation from Stanford University in 2011, MOOCs have been instrumental in enhancing the efficiency and productivity of higher education institutions, despite ongoing debates about their impact on educational practices, as highlighted by Nath et al. (2014) and further explored by Liu et al. (2023). MOOC platforms such as Coursera® (http://www.coursera.org), edX (https://www.edx.org), Khan Academy (https://www.khanacademy.org), and Udemy (https://www.udemy.com) have democratized access to education, reaching over 220 million learners globally (Shah, 2021).

The discourse on online course enrollment sizes underscores the nuanced impact they have had on various aspects of education, including pedagogical strategies, institutional finances, and faculty workload (Taft et al., 2019). Research suggests that a differentiated approach to class size based on intended learning outcomes should be considered, with larger classes for foundational learning and smaller groups for advanced intellectual engagement (Taft et al., 2019). As the prevalence of online courses and MOOCs continues to rise, their multifaceted effects on student outcomes and institutional efficiency, as well as how these effects are influenced by course design, institutional support, and student characteristics, will remain areas of active investigation.

SUCCESSFUL ONLINE COURSES

Online courses can facilitate learning as they offer flexibility, accessibility, and a wide range of educational opportunities that extend beyond traditional geographical limitations. Their effectiveness is grounded in best practices and foundational principles that were inspired by the seminal work of Chickering and Ehrmann (1996) and are essential for successful online courses, such as engaging student–faculty interaction, fostering mutual student support, employing active learning techniques, providing timely feedback, emphasizing effective time management, communicating high expectations, and accommodating diverse learning preferences. The principles for good online teaching practice are summarized in Exhibit 8.1.

1. *Good practice encourages contact between students and faculty.* Teachers can contact each student with a text or an e-mailed video greeting to extend a warm welcome before the course begins. As facilitators, teachers conference with students via media chat or Zoom and through asynchronous communication on a discussion

board. A question-and-answer forum allows students to interact with faculty and fellow students.

2. *Good practice develops reciprocity and cooperation among students.* Students interact with one another via postings on the discussion board. Upon entering the course, students are directed to a forum where they introduce themselves and are assigned to small group rooms where they complete assignments in discussion groups and have asynchronous or synchronous discussions with their teacher and peers.

3. *Good practice uses active learning techniques.* Teachers use active teaching strategies to keep students actively involved in their learning, help them develop ideas, and show them how to link theory and practice. Online strategies include discussions, debates, concept maps, case studies, and group work using collaborative learning tools such as wikis.

4. *Good practice gives prompt feedback.* Timely, meaningful, and detailed feedback is an important element of effective online teaching. Feedback provides students with specific information about their progress and success in the course. The teacher develops a schedule for feedback, communicates it to the students, and follows it. Rubrics can be used to provide clear and standardized feedback. Quizzes or educational games can help students identify how well they are mastering the content and learning objectives.

5. *Good practice emphasizes time on task.* The time required to complete coursework assigned in an online class should be the same as in a traditional class: an estimated minimum of 3 hours per week for a 14-week course, or 6 hours per week for a 7-week course (i.e., 42 hours per credit). In a 3-credit course, for example, students should spend a minimum of 9 hours weekly on coursework. Sharing this rule with students should help them to plan and organize their coursework load.

6. *Good practice communicates high expectations.* At the beginning of the course, teachers should provide students with a list of rules and policies for online learning. This information is usually included in the course syllabus. For courses with face-to-face and online sections, and for which the syllabus cannot be changed, the teacher should create a manual for the online section of the course that includes its policies. For example, the manual might include (a) a definition and description of the items on menus or tools, (b) netiquette, (c) the day of the week on which the modules start, and (d) expectations for the student and teacher. Expectations for participation and posts should be clearly delineated, and students should be held accountable for following the policies; if policies are not followed, the student(s) should receive feedback detailing expected changes in behavior.

7. *Good practice respects diverse talents and ways of learning.* Teachers can include design strategies to engage all students in the course by (a) using broad and open-ended questions to encourage critical thinking and open feedback; (b) basing evaluations on a variety of assignment formats, such as papers, videos, or presentations; and (c) designing group assignments with multiple components so that students can choose to complete components suited to their individual learning preferences.

> **EXHIBIT 8.1 Principles of Good Practice in Online Teaching**
>
> Good practice encourages contact between students and teachers.
> Good practice develops reciprocity and cooperation among students.
> Good practice uses active learning techniques.
> Good practice gives prompt feedback.
> Good practice emphasizes time on task.
> Good practice communicates high expectations.
> Good practice respects diverse talents and ways of learning.

Source: Chickering, A. W., & Ehrmann, S. C. (1996). *Implementing the seven principles: Technology as lever* (pp. 1–7). American Association for Higher Education Bulletin. https://sphweb.bumc.bu.edu/otlt/teachinglibrary/technology/seven_principles.pdf

SUCCESSFUL ONLINE STUDENTS

A variety of online assessment tools are available to help students determine whether online learning matches their schedule, learning preferences, self-motivation, and technological skills. Websites such as the Penn State Behrend eLearning Assessment (https://behrend-elearn.psu.edu/weblearning/questionnaire/ORQ.HTM) and North Carolina Central University's Online Readiness Questionnaire (https://nccuonline.nccu.edu/student-resources/am-i-ready-to-take-online-courses) offer insights on how to evaluate whether online education fits individual needs. Additionally, platforms such as YouTube provide resources to guide students in selecting online courses that align with their learning preferences and circumstances.

Personal circumstances significantly influence the decision to pursue online learning. Many students juggle full-time employment and family responsibilities, so they require a learning schedule that accommodates these demands. Success in online education necessitates daily dedication to coursework and offline study, timely completion of assignments, and effective use of academic resources. Collaborative learning and emotional support play crucial roles in mitigating the potential isolation associated with online education. Respectful communication, sensitivity to peers' feelings, and a commitment to a supportive learning community are vital for cultivating a positive and inclusive online learning environment.

In the post-COVID-19 era, the demand for online education has increased, leading to a greater focus on the characteristics and preferences of adult learners for online, hybrid, or in-person programs. Research by Gardner et al. (2022) highlighted that course-taking preferences among adult learners are influenced by age, marital status, and motivation for attending college. Such findings can help to support adult learner degree completion through online program enrollment.

The Illinois Online Network (ION, 2022b) specifies essential strategies for student success in online learning environments, as detailed in Exhibit 8.2.

SUCCESSFUL ONLINE FACILITATORS

In online education, the educator transcends traditional teaching paradigms to embrace the role of facilitator of learning. This significant shift necessitates (a) an adaptation in interaction styles to better support and enhance student learning,

> **EXHIBIT 8.2 Strategies for Students' Success When Learning Online**
>
> Adaptability: Willingness to share life, work, and educational experiences as part of the learning process.
>
> Communication Proficiency: Comfort expressing oneself in writing, given the virtual classroom's reliance on written communication.
>
> Self-Motivation and Discipline: Understanding the responsibility that accompanies the freedom and flexibility of the online environment.
>
> Proactive Engagement: Communicating difficulties promptly, whether related to technology or course content.
>
> Time Management: Committing 4 to 15 hours weekly per course; acknowledging the extensive time and commitment required.
>
> Goal Alignment: Meeting or exceeding the program's minimum requirements; recognizing the convenience, not the ease, of online education.
>
> Critical Engagement: Openness to critical thinking and decision-making as core components of the learning process.
>
> Reflective Participation: Contributing meaningfully to discussions after thoughtful consideration of responses.
>
> Community Involvement: Regular participation in virtual classroom activities to foster a collaborative learning environment.
>
> Technology Utilization: Proficiency in using the required technology effectively.
>
> *Source:* Illinois Online Network. (2022b). *What makes a successful online student?* https://www.uis.edu/ion/resources/tutorials/pedagogy/successful-online-student

(b) a comprehensive understanding of online pedagogy, and (c) a talent for organizing instructional resources that cater to diverse learning needs. Facilitators act primarily as guides to the wealth of resources available, bringing rich experience paired with academic credentials into the virtual classroom. Their online presence radiates openness, concern, flexibility, and authenticity, and sets a welcoming and supportive tone for the learning environment.

Successful online facilitators are known for their competent, clearly written communication; their instructions and feedback are easily understandable and actionable. They are committed to ensuring that the rigor and value of online-facilitated learning equals that of traditional educational models. These educators possess the skills to steer students toward critical thinking to enhance their learning outcomes, and encourage students to integrate theoretical knowledge with practical, real-world scenarios, thereby preparing them for the complexities of the professional world.

The ION (2022a) delineates key strategies for amplifying facilitator effectiveness in online learning environments, as detailed in Exhibit 8.3.

Effective Facilitation of Online Forum

Facilitating discussion can be an art: decisions about where to add input, what input to add, and how to direct the discussion can be approached in various ways. Some approaches work better than others, and facilitators may need to refine their practices over time. Good facilitation posts should identify a relevant idea or question from a participant, add ideas or perspectives to help "flesh out" the topic, and examine it more critically. Online teachers should actively interact with their students

> **EXHIBIT 8.3 Strategies for Facilitator Effectiveness in Online Learning Environments**
>
> Leverage Diverse Experiences: Integrate life, work, and educational experiences into teaching to enrich learning.
>
> Enable Application of Theory: Facilitate the easy translation of theoretical concepts into practical applications to ensure that students can apply what they learn.
>
> Supply Practical Tools: Provide resources that empower students to apply theoretical concepts in practical scenarios.
>
> Foster Continuous Improvement: Encourage students to seek improvement and provide them with opportunities to do so.
>
> Accommodate Needs: Tailor learning experiences to accommodate students' unique needs and preferences.
>
> Engage in Active Feedback: Solicit and attentively listen to student feedback and apply it to enhance the learning experience.
>
> Prioritize Student Success: Keep students informed of their progress and actively contribute to their success.
>
> Offer Constructive Feedback: Provide timely and insightful feedback on assignments, discussions, and quizzes.
>
> Adapt Teaching Methods: Embrace methods suitable for online learning; minimize traditional lecturing and tests of memorization in favor of interactive, application-based learning and case analysis.
>
> Cultivate Respectful Interaction: Maintain a respectful and polite online presence; ensure constructive interactions and support students' needs and desires.
>
> *Source:* Illinois Online Network. (2022a). *Pedagogy and learning: What makes a successful online facilitator?* https://www.uis.edu/ion/resources/tutorials/pedagogy/successful-facilitator

in discussions and consistently guide them toward learning objectives. Teachers can facilitate discussion by highlighting and building upon ideas from the week's topics and learning objectives, and they can encourage students to consider readings more critically, delve into unexplored topics, or consult sources that they may have overlooked. Follow-up questions at the end of a facilitation post entice critical thinking and are helpful for stimulating additional discussion. The following A-B-C approach is a tool for facilitating effective online discussions:

- **A**cknowledge the student's input,
- **B**uild on that input by adding relevant thoughts and integrating the text and/or alternate perspectives, and
- **C**onclude the message with a pointed follow-up question to move the discussion forward.

When facilitating online discussions, the teacher should use a warm tone yet maintain a professional approach, thus "leading by example." By reflecting a careful and positive attitude in their writing, teachers not only set a tone for students but also improve their own practice.

Student interactions on the discussion forum create a record of participation and engagement. Although learning outcomes for the course dictate whether online discussions are graded, students need timely and constructive evaluation of their work. If students' online discussion posts are graded, the teacher should offer constructive critiques and suggestions for improvement. Using a predesigned rubric allows the teacher to clarify how students' work will be assessed and graded. The use of a rubric is especially useful to teaching assistants who help with large online courses. Examples of online discussion rubrics can be found at https://topr.online.ucf.edu/discussion-rubrics.

Cybercivility and Cyberethics in Online Education

Online learning environments demand the same level of civility expected in traditional classrooms; all involved share the responsibility of fostering a positive atmosphere. Despite concerted efforts to address cyberincivility (i.e., disrespectful or disruptive behavior in digital spaces), rude and troublesome behaviors present an ongoing problem that can negatively impact personal, professional, and academic well-being (De Gagne et al., 2016; De Gagne, Cho et al., 2023). This problem extends to e-mails, social media, online forums, and videoconferencing platforms like Zoom, which emerged as a significant channel for classroom interaction during the COVID-19 pandemic. The need to address cyberincivility should be considered critical and constant.

Research indicates that faculty behavior during videoconferencing significantly impacts students' emotional health, with negative emotions linked to perceived incivility and unfair treatment (Alt et al., 2022). Because negative experiences and perceived insecurity can reduce participation or lead to course withdrawal, it is essential that the teacher create a safe space for expressing concerns and collaboratively finding solutions. Solutions proposed by students are often more readily accepted and successful. Educators must remain sensitive to students' emotional needs and cultivate a supportive online environment.

Effective online instruction extends beyond content delivery to communication that builds trust within the classroom. The teacher's voice can be a crucial tool for engaging students, alleviating feelings of isolation, and promoting a culture of cybercivility (Cribb, 2023). Addressing uncivil behavior with prompt, private communication is essential. Such interactions should acknowledge student frustrations while emphasizing the importance of adhering to community norms.

Cultivating cybercivility is a complex process that demands a focus on emotional well-being, instructional strategies, technological skills, and the development of a supportive online environment. All participants in the learning environment, including teachers, must be dedicated to maintaining a respectful and productive space. At the core of these efforts lies cyberethics, which outlines guidelines for ethical online behavior (De Gagne, Cho et al., 2023; De Gagne, Hwang et al., 2023).

Cyberethics encompasses a broad array of considerations, including privacy, security, intellectual property rights, and online decorum. As online interactions grow, a thorough understanding of cyberethics is increasingly vital for guiding individual conduct and institutional policies. Faculty must craft curricula that incorporate ethical considerations into online learning and embrace best practices for digital citizenship (De Gagne, Cho et al., 2023; De Gagne, Hwang et al., 2023). A seamless integration of cybercivility and cyberethics can improve the quality of online education as well as prepare students to handle the complexities of digital interactions with integrity and respect.

ONLINE PEDAGOGY

Online pedagogy is rooted in constructivism and social learning theories, thus it approaches learning as a dynamic, interactive process. Constructivism suggests that learners actively construct knowledge by engaging in cycles of action and reflection, effectively building on prior experience to develop an understanding of its connection with real-world situations. This learning approach is characterized by its active nature: It prompts learners to immerse themselves in hands-on activities facilitated by technological advancements. Furthermore, it emphasizes interaction and utilizes tools such as discussion boards and videoconferencing to stimulate dialogue and collaboration among participants.

Within the digital landscape, these pedagogical underpinnings have been pivotal in crafting effective educational experiences that are deeply meaningful because they are tailored to the individual learner's context. Technology's role in this educational approach enhances the active components of learning to enable a more vibrant engagement with the material and concepts at hand. Simultaneously, the interactive dimension is expanded through digital communication tools, which serve to cultivate the sense of belonging and collective exploration essential for social learning.

Figure 8.1 delineates the steps and processes of a pedagogical framework for establishing an online learning environment in which theoretical insights and technological advancements converge to facilitate comprehensive learning journeys. This model highlights the deliberate and thoughtful integration of pedagogical strategies and digital tools to deliver an educational experience that is both enriching

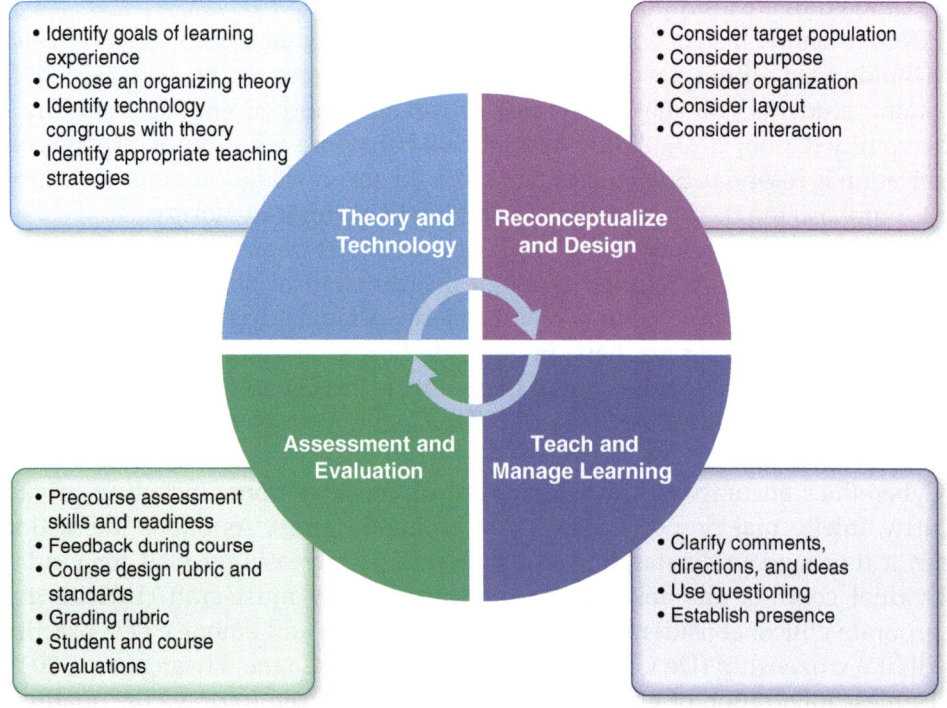

Figure 8.1 Stages and process of creating an online learning environment.

and universally accessible, irrespective of geographical constraints. By adopting this approach, online pedagogy aspires to replicate the intricacy and interactivity found in traditional classroom settings while leveraging the unique capabilities of digital technologies to broaden educational horizons.

TECHNOLOGY REPORTS

Two pivotal reports that have significantly contributed to our understanding of technology's role in education offer a comprehensive overview of the trends and strategies reshaping the educational landscape: The annual Campus Computing Survey, an integral part of the ongoing Campus Computing Project™, delves into the integration of information technology within American higher education, illuminating the digital infrastructure, tools, and policies that are reshaping campuses nationwide (www.campuscomputing.net). This survey provides a detailed analysis of how colleges and universities are adopting and adapting to technological advancements and highlights the progress and challenges of implementing effective digital solutions.

The *EDUCAUSE Horizon Report*® annually identifies emerging technologies poised to impact teaching and learning. The 2023 edition highlights six key areas: AI-enabled applications, generative AI, blended learning modalities, hyflex courses, microcredentials, and fostering student belonging (Educause, 2023). These areas reflect the current swift adoption of online and hybrid learning models and highlight the evolving demands on educators to engage students effectively through online pedagogy. For instance, the rapid integration of AI and blended learning modalities reflects a shift toward more personalized, flexible learning environments that cater to diverse student needs and preferences. Hyflex courses and microcredentials, on the other hand, reflect a growing emphasis on offering students multiple pathways to learning and certification, thereby enhancing accessibility and inclusivity in higher education.

The insights from the *EDUCAUSE Horizon Report* align with the technological trends and challenges identified in the Campus Computing Survey; collectively, they emphasize (a) the importance of fostering student belonging and creating supportive, engaging online communities that promote student retention and success; and (b) the critical need for strategic faculty development to equip educators with the skills and knowledge required to leverage technologies effectively and ensure that students not only remain engaged but also thrive in online and hybrid learning environments.

Technology in Online Learning

The evolution of online learning has been significantly influenced by technologies that enrich educational experiences. Ensuring accessibility for all students, including those with disabilities, remains a paramount goal. The Universal Design for Learning (UDL) framework, grounded in interdisciplinary research, aims to create inclusive and effective online learning environments. UDL addresses key challenges such as technical skill gaps, limited assistive technology, and insufficient digital accessibility (Fakhru et al., 2022).

Learning Management Systems (LMSs) such as Canvas and Moodle have been instrumental in streamlining online education by providing essential services such as interactive platforms, content distribution, and progress monitoring. The COVID-19 pandemic expedited the integration and refinement of these systems and underscored their value in the digital education landscape (Badaru & Adu, 2022). Furthermore, the incorporation into virtual classrooms of active learning strategies (ranging from polls and discussions to simulations and project-based learning) is gaining momentum, facilitated by digital tools to enhance student engagement, promote collaboration, and enrich the learning experience (Martynyuk & Orlovska, 2023). Despite technological and pedagogical advancements, challenges pertaining to digital accessibility, student engagement, and rapid technological shifts persist. Addressing these challenges through strategies such as adopting the UDL framework, integrating active learning techniques, and regularly evaluating LMS platforms is essential for the continuous improvement of online learning environments.

Accessibility and Usability in Online Nursing Education

In nursing education, the expanding role of technology underscores the need to make online learning platforms accessible and user-friendly for all students. Ensuring accessibility to an inclusive learning environment is an ethical duty and a practical necessity for nurse educators. The UDL framework provides guidelines for making online materials engaging and accessible to students with diverse abilities.

The UDL framework, which is grounded in the latest research from neuroscience, computer science, and digital accessibility, advocates for flexible and adaptable learning experiences tailored to meet diverse needs. It emphasizes three core principles crucial for the creation of inclusive online learning spaces: (a) provision of multiple means of representation, (b) action and expression, and (c) engagement (CAST, 2018). These principles advocate for a delivery of educational content in various formats (e.g., text, video, audio, images) to accommodate different learning styles and preferences. Furthermore, they support offering students diverse ways to demonstrate their knowledge and interact with the material in order to enhance their motivation and participation.

Implementing the UDL framework involves a multifaceted approach. Nurse educators are guided to offer content in various formats (e.g., videos with captions, audio, simulations) in order to make materials widely accessible. Flexible assessments (e.g., essays, presentations) allow students to express knowledge using methods that cater to their individual strengths. The course design should prioritize easy navigation and consistency, ensuring straightforward access to resources in the LMS. Moreover, the teacher must select technologies that are compatible with assistive devices so that all students can engage fully with the content in a supportive and diverse learning community (CAST, 2018).

Developed by the World Wide Web Consortium (W3C) in 2008, the Web Content Accessibility Guidelines (WCAG) constitute the international standard for digital content accessibility. These guidelines are indispensable for nurse educators as they offer a detailed framework for creating accessible online materials that are perceivable, operable, understandable, and robust for users with disabilities, thus ensuring that the online learning environment is inclusive and equitable.

Beyond accessibility, the usability of online learning platforms is important for nurturing a positive and effective educational experience; intuitive design principles should be employed that render LMS and digital tools straightforward and easy to navigate. Offering comprehensive technical support and training for essential online tools can significantly enhance the learning experience. Moreover, regular feedback and evaluation mechanisms are crucial for continually assessing and improving the accessibility and usability of online courses. Engaging students, particularly those with disabilities, in this feedback process enables the identification and rectification of potential barriers, thereby ensuring that online nursing education remains dynamic, responsive, and inclusive.

HOW TO CREATE ONLINE LEARNING ENVIRONMENTS

Transforming a traditional classroom course into an effective online learning experience entails more than simply digitizing existing materials; this process, known as reconceptualization, requires educators to adapt and redesign the course content to address the unique advantages and challenges of online education.

Reconceptualization

Reconceptualizing a course involves a comprehensive review and adaptation to align the content with institutional goals, leverage cutting-edge technology, and target the expertise and needs of both faculty and students. This critical process leads to informed decisions about the course structure, including the methods of presenting content and organization of modules or units.

A significant benefit of online learning is its capacity to reach a wide audience, making educational programs accessible to students far beyond the physical boundaries of a campus. This aspect is especially valuable for programs with a statewide or national scope. Additionally, online platforms offer the advantage of long-term access to course materials. Such accessibility is useful for programs offered multiple times throughout the year, as it allows students to revisit resources as needed, thereby accommodating diverse learning preferences and schedules.

Unlike traditional course settings that can accommodate large numbers of students, online courses often have smaller enrollment, fostering a more personalized, interactive learning experience that enables individualized attention. Institutions should first consider whether online education aligns with their mission and vision, then confirm the availability of essential resources such as digital learning platforms, technical and instructional support, digitally literate faculty, and effective marketing strategies for online programs. Transitioning to online education necessitates a thorough evaluation of the available technology, including hardware and software, to maintain and facilitate access to online courses. Investment in technology infrastructure must be justified by demonstrating its potential to enhance educational outcomes.

Preparing faculty for online instruction is equally critical. Development programs should encompass online pedagogy, course management, student assessment, and the ethical aspects of online education. Employing interactive digital tools and multimedia resources in training can empower faculty to deliver engaging and impactful online learning experiences. Moreover, fostering a collaborative community among online educators encourages the exchange of best practices and innovative teaching strategies.

Student readiness for online learning must be assessed to ensure that course enrollees possess or can acquire the necessary technological tools and skills. Introducing students to online learning through orientations and providing ongoing technical support, particularly at the course outset, is fundamental. Academic success in online education can be supported by enhancing students' access to academic resources, including online tutoring and library services. A seamless reconceptualization ensures that the resulting online course not only aligns with the instructor's capabilities but also addresses students' learning requirements comprehensively.

How to Design Online Courses and Modules

Strategic development of an online course that achieves its objectives and outcomes entails identifying the target population, establishing the purpose and objectives, organizing the course content, ensuring easy navigation, creating an appealing page layout, and choosing suitable interaction methods.

The target population refers to the learners. Educators should evaluate students' existing knowledge and learning preferences and consider their varied characteristics, such as age, interests, computer literacy, socioeconomic status, and motivation, before adopting diverse strategies for module design. Educators must select appropriate technologies to meet the broad spectrum of student needs.

The design should reflect the course's purpose and objectives. The structure of a didactic learning environment differs from that of a seminar course. A skills workshop might necessitate a distinct arrangement for laboratory experiences compared to a traditional classroom setting. Similarly, clinical components may require a different organizational approach than conventional lab experiments.

A well-organized course is pivotal for facilitating seamless transitions between sections. Students should be able to efficiently locate essential materials with no more than three mouse clicks; such navigational ease is crucial for maintaining student engagement and reducing frustration. Moreover, maintaining a consistent structure across modules can significantly enhance the speed and ease of information retrieval in subsequent sections. Design consistency not only aids navigation but also helps students develop a sense of familiarity with the course layout, making their learning experience more intuitive and user-friendly.

The design of the page layout should prioritize clarity, readability, and consideration of the target population's needs. Font size, header styles, and color schemes can enhance readability and aesthetic appeal. The CRAP (**C**ontrast, **R**epetition, **A**lignment, **P**roximity) principles are valuable guidelines for creating visually engaging layouts (Williams, 2014). More information about the use of the CRAP principles in online learning can be found at https://lewisu.edu/writingcenter/pdf/crap-resource-revised-pub.pdf.

Interactions in online courses can be asynchronous or synchronous to fulfill varied educational needs. Asynchronous platforms such as discussion boards, blogs, and wikis support the exchange of ideas and feedback between individuals or groups in both open and closed formats. Conversely, synchronous tools, such as videoconferencing, enable real-time interactions for office hours, student conferences, and seminars but require careful scheduling and clear agendas to optimize engagement and learning outcomes.

Quality First

Any nursing program, school of nursing, or institution that incorporates online pedagogy must maintain standards of quality equivalent to those for traditional educational approaches. To this end, a variety of comprehensive evaluation frameworks have been developed which employ diverse terminologies such as benchmarks, pillars, indicators, dimensions, best practices, and paradigms to outline criteria for quality assessment. Frameworks such as the Online Learning Consortium (OLC) Scorecard and Quality Matters (QM) are notable for assessing online programs against quality indicators; these frameworks are grounded in best practices for teaching and learning, and incorporate principles of sound instructional design and insights derived from educational research. Moreover, they provide tools for evaluating, developing, and enhancing student learning environments, and advocating for a model of continuous improvement.

The Online Learning Consortium Quality Scorecard

The OLC's Open SUNY Course Quality Review (OSCQR) scorecard is a prime example of a tool designed for the meticulous review and enhancement of online course quality with a focus on instructional design and accessibility (OLC, 2024). The OSCQR scorecard for online programs delineates 50 indicators across six critical categories:

1. Course Overview and Information: Establishes the foundation of the course and outlines objectives, expectations, and resources.
2. Course Technology and Tools: Assesses the integration and accessibility of technological resources used to facilitate learning.
3. Design and Layout: Evaluates the course's visual and structural organization to ensure a coherent and engaging learning experience.
4. Content and Activities: Reviews the relevance, quality, and interactivity of course materials and learning activities.
5. Interaction: Measures the effectiveness of communication channels among students, and between students and instructors.
6. Assessment and Feedback: Analyzes the alignment of assessments with learning objectives and the timeliness and constructiveness of feedback.

A key advantage of the OLC scorecard is its open-license nature and the flexibility it offers for customization to align with specific institutional needs. The OSCQR rubric provides institutions with a powerful tool to pinpoint areas for enhancement and facilitate a targeted approach to elevating the quality of their online offerings (OLC, 2024).

Quality Matters Rubric

QM is a faculty-centered, peer-reviewed process designed to assess and certify the quality of online and blended courses (MarylandOnline, 2024). QM offers various membership levels that provide access to a suite of resources, including course review tools, professional development opportunities, and an expansive community dedicated to online teaching and learning. All resources are designed to elevate the educational experience in accordance with the QM rubric's eight general standards:

1. Course Overview and Introduction: Sets the stage for the course by offering clear directions for getting started and navigating the course components.
2. Learning Objectives (Competencies): Articulates clear, measurable learning objectives or competencies that guide the learner's experience.
3. Assessment and Measurement: Ensures assessments are aligned with learning objectives and provide a clear measure of student achievement.
4. Instructional Materials: Evaluates the relevance and quality of instructional materials for supporting the course's educational goals.
5. Learning Activities and Learner Interaction: Focuses on engaging learning activities and meaningful interaction to foster active learning.
6. Course Technology: Assesses whether the technology used enhances learning outcomes and supports the course's instructional needs.
7. Learner Support: Addresses the availability and accessibility of support services essential for student success.
8. Accessibility and Usability: Ensures that the course is designed to be accessible to all students, including those with disabilities.

Schools engaging with the QM organization benefit from a comprehensive framework that emphasizes quality assurance and student-centered learning. Educators and institutions can apply the QM rubric to enhance their online and blended courses, thus committing to an ongoing process of improvement and innovation in teaching.

HOW TO TEACH AND MANAGE ONLINE LEARNING ENVIRONMENTS

In the evolving landscape of online education, faculty members play a pivotal role as facilitators who guide students toward achieving their learning objectives with precision and empathy. A preparatory stage is crucial for students to acclimate to the course's demands and structure, so teachers should provide an accessible syllabus that details clear expectations well before the course commences. To further student engagement, teachers can introduce the course a few days prior to its official start through an innovative approach such as a scavenger hunt, which not only acquaints students with the course layout but also injects an element of enjoyment and discovery into the learning process. For instance, directing students to use the course roster to determine the number of their peers who are enrolled would encourage familiarity with the platform's features.

Orientation to the course management system is indispensable, particularly for newcomers to the online nursing program; it serves as a vital reference point, equipping students with the necessary tools and confidence to navigate the digital learning environment successfully. Equally important is the establishment of cybercivility and cyberethics guidelines to ensure a respectful and conducive online learning atmosphere.

Throughout the course, the instructor's roles are multifaceted and dynamic. Foremost among these is the timely correction of errors, a task that underscores the importance of the instructor's vigilance and proactive engagement. For example, a misinterpretation by the first student to comment on a discussion post could lead others astray; therefore, the instructor's prompt intervention to correct misunderstandings and ensure the integrity of course discussions is essential. This active involvement conveys to students that their contributions are valued and scrutinized for accuracy, which helps to foster a culture of precision and accountability.

Another critical function is the clarification of student contributions in relation to the course's objectives and outcomes. By paraphrasing a student's post (e.g., "I think you are saying that . . .") and summarizing its key points, the instructor can bridge any gaps in understanding, relate insights to practical scenarios, and enrich the learning experience with real-world relevance. Furthermore, innovative questioning techniques such as the "sandwich" method, which layers positive feedback with a probing question, stimulate deeper cognitive engagement and critical analysis among students; this approach not only validates the student's initial input but also challenges them to consider broader implications and perspectives.

The concept of instructor *presence* is integral to cultivating a vibrant and interactive online learning community. It is the tangible manifestation of the instructor's active participation and investment in the course. Strategies to enhance presence include engaging with discussion boards, making timely announcements, incorporating humor, and dynamically adjusting course content to reflect ongoing progress. Such actions signal to students that the instructor is not just a figurehead but an active, responsive participant in their learning journey. Moreover, personalizing the learning experience through storytelling, or sharing relevant anecdotes or examples, can help the instructor add depth to the course content and foster a connection that transcends the virtual barrier. Creating a repository of stories related to course modules not only enhances the instructor's online persona but also allows students to learn from a rich, contextual backdrop to which they can relate.

ASSESSMENT AND EVALUATION

Evaluating online learning requires approaches distinct from those used in traditional classroom settings. This necessity stems from several unique aspects of online education, including the need for students to self-assess readiness, the importance of ongoing feedback, and the prerequisite for courses to be fully developed and functional before they are accessed by students.

Students should be assessed before the course begins, during the learning experience, and at the end of the learning experience; the course should be evaluated before it goes live, during the learning experience, and at the end of the learning experience. Pre-course student assessments might include surveys on computer literacy and readiness, while ongoing evaluations could involve journals, quizzes, and discussion contributions. Summative assessments at the end of modules or the course could take the form of exams, presentations, or papers.

The use of grading rubrics is highly recommended to clarify expectations for assignments; there are options for creating custom rubrics or adopting those available in public galleries such as RCampus™ (2024). These tools facilitate transparent and consistent grading practices. Further discussion and examples of rubrics for assessment in nursing courses is provided in Chapter 15.

Course evaluation is critical at multiple stages: prior to launch to ensure functionality; continuously throughout for real-time adjustments; and after completion for overall effectiveness. Techniques such as the "pulse check" provide informal, formative feedback that allows instructors to gauge and respond to student needs. Summative evaluations, including surveys of students and faculty, offer insights into satisfaction and areas for improvement.

Evaluating the effectiveness of online learning and quality of education delivered involves collaboration with course leadership and program teams. The Kirkpatrick four levels of evaluation offer a comprehensive framework for examining online programs and outcomes. Starting with learners' reactions, this framework assesses emotional and intellectual responses, highlighting satisfaction and engagement; it then evaluates the depth of learning, focusing on acquired knowledge, skills, and attitudes, and the learners' readiness to apply these in practice (Kirkpatrick Partners, 2024). Next, the model analyzes behavior changes, observing how learners apply their knowledge in real-world settings, which serves as a practical measure of the course's impact on their professional actions. Finally, it assesses tangible results, such as improvements in patient safety or care quality, which illustrate the direct benefits of the learning on healthcare. Drawing on years of evidence that support educational program evaluation methods, the Kirkpatrick model offers online educators a diverse array of formative approaches to assess outcomes across the teaching–learning continuum (Kirkpatrick Partners, 2024).

SUMMARY

Online education in nursing has expanded rapidly, propelled by the push toward hybrid and fully online programs which took place during the COVID-19 pandemic. This chapter explored the evolving role of educators as facilitators, the integration of instructional technologies, and the critical aspects of designing and assessing online courses. It delved into the dynamics of online interaction, the strategic use of educational technologies, and the methods for evaluating the effectiveness of online programs. Although online learning offers the benefits of accessibility and flexibility, it requires technical proficiency, self-motivation, and readiness to tackle potential technical challenges. The growth in online course enrollment signals a shift toward more adaptable, accessible education and underscores the importance of active learning, student–faculty interaction, and continuous feedback for success. This chapter emphasized the need for quality in online learning environments and suggested that, as technology advances, so too will the methods and quality of online nursing education.

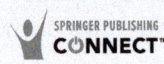

A robust set of instructor resources designed to supplement this text is located at http://connect.springerpub.com/content/book/978-0-8261-8892-2. Qualifying instructors may request access by emailing textbook@springerpub.com.

REFERENCES

Akhmedova, M. G., Ibragimov, G. I., Kryukova, N. I., Galchenko, N. A., Lutskovskaia, L. Y., Sizova, Z. M., & Minkin, M. R. (2023). Uncovering patterns and trends in online teaching and learning for STEM education. *Contemporary Educational Technology, 15*(3), ep444. https://doi.org/10.30935/cedtech/13363

Alt, D., Itzkovich, Y., & Naamati-Schneider, L. (2022). Students' emotional well-being, and perceived faculty incivility and just behavior before and during COVID-19. *Frontiers in Psychology, 13*, 849489. https://doi.org/10.3389/fpsyg.2022.849489

Atkinson, S. P. (2023). Definitions of the terms open, distance, and flexible in the context of formal and non-formal learning. *Journal of Open, Flexible and Distance Learning, 26*(2), 18–28. https://doi.org/10.61468/jofdl.v26i2.521

Badaru, K. A., & Adu, E. O. (2022). Platformisation of education: An analysis of South African universities' learning management systems. *Research in Social Sciences & Technology, 7*(2), 66–86. https://doi.org/10.46303/ressat.2022.10

CAST. (2018). *Universal design for learning guidelines version 2.2.* https://udlguidelines.cast.org

Chickering, A. W., & Ehrmann, S. C. (1996). *Implementing the seven principles: Technology as lever.* (pp. 1–7). American Association for Higher Eeducayion Bulletin. https://sphweb.bumc.bu.edu/otlt/teachinglibrary/technology/seven_principles.pdf

Cribb, M. (2023). The power of the voice in facilitating and maintaining online presence in the era of Zoom and Teams. *Teaching English as a Second or Foreign Language, 27*(2), 1–14. https://doi.org/10.55593/ej.27106int

De Gagne, J. C., Choi, M., Ledbetter, L., Kang, H., & Clark, C. M. (2016). An integrative review of cybercivility in health professions education. *Nurse Educator, 41*(5), 239–245. https://doi.org/10.1097/NNE.0000000000000264

De Gagne, J. C., Cho, E., Randall, P. S, Hwang, H., Wang, E., Yoo, L., Yamane, S., Ledbetter, L. S., & Jung, D. (2023). Exploration of cyberethics in health professions education: A scoping review. *International Journal of Environmental Research & Public Health, 20*(22), 7048. https://doi.org/10.3390/ijerph20227048

De Gagne, J. C., Hwang, H., & Jung, D. (2024). Cyberethics in nursing education: Ethical implications of artificial intelligence. *Nursing Ethics, 31*(6), 1021–1030. https://doi.org/10.1177/09697330231201901

Educause. (2023). *2023 Horizon report: Teaching and learning edition.* https://library.educause.edu/resources/2023/5/2023-educause-horizon-report-teaching-and-learning-edition

Fakhru, A.-N., Khalily, H., Khadr, K., Dirgham, R., & Ayyash, R. (2022). Online learning challenges for students with disabilities: Digital accessibility and universal design for learning solutions. *Hebron University Research Journal, 17*(2), 241–286. https://doi.org/10.60138/17220229

Gardner, A. C., Maietta, H. N., Gardner, P. D., & Perkins, N. (2022). Online postsecondary adult learners: An analysis of adult learner characteristics and online course taking preferences. *American Journal of Distance Education, 36*(3), 176–192. https://doi.org/10.1080/08923647.2021.1928434

Illinois Online Network. (2022a). *Pedagogy and learning: What makes a successful online facilitator?* https://www.uis.edu/ion/resources/tutorials/pedagogy/successful-facilitator

Illinois Online Network. (2022b). *What makes a successful online student?* https://www.uis.edu/ion/resources/tutorials/pedagogy/successful-online-student

Kirkpatrick Partners. (2024). *The New World Kirkpatrick Model.* https://www.kirkpatrickpartners.com/Our-Philosophy/The-New-World-Kirkpatrick-Model

Martynyuk, O., & Orlovska, O. (2023). Introducing active language learning techniques into a virtual classroom: Reflection on the American practices. *Comparative Professional Pedagogy, 13*(1), 44–52. https://doi.org/10.31891/2308-4081/2023-13(1)-6

MarylandOnline. (2024). *Quality matters program.* https://www.qualitymatters.org

Liu, Z., Xiong, H., & Sun, Y. (2023). Will online MOOCs improve the efficiency of Chinese higher education institutions? An empirical study based on DEA. *Sustainability, 15*(7), 5970. https://doi.org/ 10.3390/su15075970

Nath, A., Karmakar, A., & Karmakar, T. (2014). MOOCs impact in higher education institution: A pilot study In Indian context. *International Journal of Engineering Research & Applications, 4*(7), 156–163.

National Center for Education Statistics. (2023). *Undergraduate enrollment. Condition of education*. U.S. Department of Education, Institute of Education Sciences. https://nces.ed.gov/programs/coe/indicator/cha

Oliver Del Olmo, S. (2021). COVID-19 and the autonomous university of Barcelona: Current trends on language teaching and learning strategies. In R. Nebojša, A. Anastasia, F. Maria, & S. Josef (Eds.), The world univ*ersities' response to COVID-19: R*emote online language teaching (pp. 321–336). Research-publishing.net. https://doi.org/10.14705/rpnet.2021.52.1281

Online Learning Consortium. (2024). *OLC OSCQR course design review*. https://onlinelearningconsortium.org/consult/oscqr-course-design-review

Raghunathan, S., Darshan Singh, A., & Sharma, B. (2022). Study of resilience in Learning environments during the Covid-19 Pandemic. *Frontiers in Education, 6*. https://doi.org/10.3389/feduc.2021.677625

Rcampus. (2024). *Rubric gallery*. http://www.rcampus.com/rubricshellc.cfm

Shah, D. (2021). *By the numbers: MOOCs in 2021*. https://www.classcentral.com/report/mooc-stats-2021

Taft, S. H., Kesten, K., & El-Banna, M. M. (2019). One size does not fit all: Toward an evidence-based framework for determining online course enrollment sizes in higher education. *Online Learning, 23*(3). https://doi.org/10.24059/olj.v23i3.1534

Williams, R. (2014). *The non-designer's design book* (4th ed.). Peachpit Press.

World Wide Web Consortium. (2008). *Web Content Accessibility Guidelines (WCAG) 2.0*. https://www.w3.org/TR/2008/REC-WCAG20-20081211

Incorporating Simulation in Nursing Education: Overview, Essentials, and the Evidence

9

Kristina T. Dreifuerst, Pamela R. Jeffries, Katie A. Haerling, and Michelle Aebersold

OBJECTIVES

1. Describe types of simulations in nursing and strategies of implementing different types of simulations into the nursing curriculum
2. Critique various debriefing approaches and their use in nursing education
3. Describe evaluation processes to use when developing and implementing simulations
4. Review developments in simulation practices, research, and credentialing

INTRODUCTION

Simulations provide opportunities for learners to apply and demonstrate nursing knowledge, skills, and attitudes in an on-campus, safe, and controlled environment before going into the traditional off-campus clinical setting. However, in the current environment of complex clinical environments, increased patient acuity, and limited clinical placements, simulations also serve a broader role as a supplement to, or replacement for, traditional clinical experiences. Moreover, the simulation environment can be used for teaching and assessing competence in prelicensure and graduate nurses, playing an increasingly important role in both formative and summative evaluation.

This chapter provides an overview of types of clinical simulations in nursing. The importance of creating realism in the simulations is also discussed. In addition, design and implementation of simulations within a nursing curriculum, and debriefing and evaluation processes to use when developing and implementing clinical simulations, are presented. Finally, the evidence regarding the use of clinical simulations, beyond asking whether the pedagogy actually works and how to make it work best, are highlighted.

TRADITIONAL SIMULATION

Different modalities of simulations provide varying degrees of fidelity, or the ability of the simulation environment to replicate the actual clinical environment (Loke et al., 2020). This fidelity, or realism, allows the learner to engage within the simulation's physical, psychological, and environmental elements (Lioce et al., 2020). Likewise, different simulation modalities have different costs and offer varied benefits (Haerling & Miller, 2024). Educators should select the appropriate type of simulation to meet the required competencies.

Manikin-Based Simulation

Manikin-based simulation has been used for hundreds of years, including both the bronze acupuncture teaching statues from the Song Dynasty in China as well as "Mrs. Chase," the classic nursing manikin used for task training since 1922 (Herrmann, 2008; Owen, 2012). Manikins vary in the amount and degree of technology built into the device and the level of fidelity they offer. Simulation fidelity is defined as the extent to which a simulated experience is real or believable to the participants (Lioce et al., 2020). Fidelity can be thought of as two dimensional: engineering fidelity, or how authentic the simulation looks and feels, and psychological fidelity, or how realistic the behaviors and actions required mimic what is anticipated or expected (Loke et al., 2020).

All simulations need learner objectives (International Nursing Association of Clinical Simulation and Learning [INACSL] Standards Committee, 2021e). Some learning objectives and competencies to be developed require simple resources, such as performing an intramuscular injection on an orange, while other learning objectives require higher levels of fidelity to create a realistic experience for the learners, such as a decompensating patient in the operating room. Fidelity is important to consider when developing simulations for learners because it reflects the level of engagement that will be expected of participants as they are involved in the experience (MacLean et al., 2019).

Manikins that are life-sized, have realistic anatomical structures, and contain technology that dynamically mimics changes in human physiology, are called high-fidelity human patient simulators (HPSs), whereas other full-sized manikins that may only partially, or not as realistically, mimic physiological changes are called medium- fidelity HPSs. Low- fidelity HPSs are task trainers that are static and typically represent one function of the human body, such as an arm model used to practice venipuncture. These are particularly useful for novice students learning basic skills and general principles of patient care (Loke et al., 2020; MacLean et al., 2019).

High-fidelity HPSs are best used when learners are expected to successfully care for a patient with multiple physiological assessments contained within the simulation scenario. These manikins allow for changes of physiological parameters within the simulation, either by programming ahead of the simulation or by changing the parameters in real time within the simulation. This allows faculty to evaluate the learner's ability to rapidly respond to changes in the patient's condition or demonstrate the physiological effects of any nursing interventions. Multiple physiological parameters, including pupil dilation/constriction, respiratory and cardiac signs (breath and heart sounds, pulses, blood pressure, pulse oxygenation), and abdominal signs (bowel sounds) may be programmed depending on the type of high-fidelity HPS used in the scenario. High- fidelity HPSs also allow learners to practice and refine psychomotor skills, such as basic and advanced life support contextually to mimic total patient care. When the simulation scenario requires only a limited number of physiological changes or simple to complex task training, using a medium- or low- fidelity HPS may be more appropriate. The simulation design should reflect the type of simulator used (INACSL Standards Committee, 2021i).

Moulage is another option to enhance fidelity that nurse educators can consider. Moulage incorporates the use of makeup, clothing, and wigs to enhance the patient appearance to fit the story. Wax, latex, artificial fluids, and simulation enhancers can be used to simulate injury, disease, aging, and make other physical enhancements to the manikin (Stokes-Parish et al., 2019). Adding moulage to the simulator increases the realism for the learner and can make the simulation experience more authentic for holistic learning.

Fidelity in simulation is intended to immerse the learner in a realistic experience that represents a clinical setting or client care situation. Attention to having realistic equipment and creating a representative physical environment impacts the believability of the simulation experience for many learners and may impact clinical learning. Low-, medium-, and high-fidelity simulations can all be valuable learning environments when they are incorporated into the curriculum with associated learning objectives for nursing students (INACSL Standards Committee, 2021i).

Standardized Patients

A standardized patient (SP) is a person who engages in specialized training to portray a patient with a specific condition. With this training, SPs are able to portray their role consistently within every simulated clinical scenario; however, the context in which SPs are working determines the amount of consistency and accuracy required of multiple people playing the same role or the single individual repeating the role for different learners. For example, when the simulation is used for high stakes assessment, SPs may need to act in a standardized manner so each learner can be evaluated consistently (Doyle et al., 2024). During these simulations, the SP will be trained not to go off script, embellish the response, or provide additional information that was not asked by the learner. To do this, the SP rehearses the role with the simulation faculty or facilitator to ensure that each learner experiences the same patient portrayal. In formative educational settings, standardization may not be critical to the simulation design. In these cases, trained SPs have the autonomy to respond within the scenario with more flexibility in response to the learner (Lewis et al., 2017). It is important to note also that sometimes an individual or another learner with little or no training is enlisted to role-play a part in a simulation. In this case, this individual is not an SP, and there is no assurance that the role will be played in the same manner for each simulation.

SPs may be further subdivided according to the objective of the simulation and the role that they play. Within the simulation, they can portray patients, but also may function as the teacher, evaluator, or both. For example, SPs may be used to teach and evaluate physical examination skills such as a head-to-toe assessment. Some SPs obtain further education and training to evaluate the learner for either formative or summative evaluation including high-stakes simulation. Objective structured clinical examinations (OSCEs) are a series of skill-based stations where learners demonstrate skills or care for a variety of patients according to a predetermined time-limited schedule for each station. SPs are often used to portray these patients and may participate in the evaluation of the learner as well.

Incorporating SPs within a simulation program requires planning and sufficient funds to hire and train them. They can be trained actors, college students in other programs, or community members. The Association for Standardized Patient Educators (ASPE) is an excellent resource and can be accessed at www.aspeducators.org. Additional human and fiscal resources may be required to coordinate the SP program within the school; however, most programs that use SPs report that the experience is valuable and worth the funding if it is intentionally designed, embedded intentionally into the curriculum with specific objectives, and includes consistent outcome evaluation (Rutherford-Hemming et al., 2019).

EXTENDED REALITY SIMULATIONS

The use of technology-mediated simulations is becoming an integral part of nursing education. The term extended reality (XR) is an umbrella term used to group these new modalities. XR includes technology-mediated experiences enabled with a wide spectrum of hardware and software applications. XR is immersive and interactive (XRSI, n.d.). There are three XR technologies that are increasing in use: augmented reality (AR), immersive virtual reality (IVR), and mixed reality (MR). AR is a digital overlay of content in the real world using a tablet or smartphone. IVR is a fully immersive experience viewed through a head-mounted display (HMD) in which the learner does not see the real world, only the digital world. MR, viewed through an HMD, blends the real world with digital content in a way that both environments can interact with each other (X Reality Safety Intelligence [XRSI], n.d.). Screen-based simulation or desktop VR is not considered a part of XR, but is an interactive experience where learners interact with the environment displayed on a computer using a keyboard and mouse or touchpad (Shorey & Ng, 2021). All of these technology-mediated experiences have a role to play in nursing education but, to be most effective, should be aligned with learning outcomes or competencies.

The use of XR in healthcare education has been studied, and early results are promising. A systematic review by Foronda and colleagues (2020) examined virtual simulation in nursing education and its impact on learning outcomes. The modalities used in the selected studies included screen-based simulations, virtual worlds, and virtual environments. Overall, the majority of learners showed improved outcomes, suggesting these types of technologies support learning in nursing education. A recent comparison of IVR to traditional simulation evaluated studies that directly compared the two modalities (Foronda et al., 2024). Of the 15 studies included, eight showed no difference, four indicated traditional/in-person simulation had better outcomes, and three reported IVR had better outcomes. The results of this review highlight the fact that learning outcomes may be related to matching the intended outcomes of the simulation to the technology or method chosen.

The use of IVR simulation is becoming more available as companies developing this type of learning have matured and can offer robust and varied scenarios in the IVR space. HMDs, which are now commercially available, do not require being attached to a computer and are affordable. Current HMDs can deliver high quality graphics and do not cause as much cyber or motion sickness as did earlier models. The important consideration when implementing IVR simulations is to adhere to Healthcare Simulation Standards of Best Practice™ (HSSOBP; Standards Committee, 2021c, 2021d) and to adjust in the debriefing phase to account for the fact that the facilitator often does not see what the learner is doing, and each learner has a slightly different experience.

Some principles to keep in mind when using IVR simulations include:

- Providing an orientation to the equipment.
- Allowing learners to practice in the virtual environment to learn how it works.
- Debriefing the learners in a way that allows them to describe their own experience.
- Limiting the amount of time in the HMD to about 20 to 30 minutes initially.
- Providing an alternative for the few learners who do not tolerate the HMD.

IVR is an emerging technology that can be aligned to learning outcomes such as communicating with patients, team communication skills, priority setting, and managing multiple patients (Salcedo et al., 2022). It does not have the haptic ability to teach hands-on skills at this time. However, the use of MR can be used for more skill-based learning simulations. MR can combine an HMD with actual simulation manikins or task trainers. The HMDs used in MR have the ability to show the learner the physical environment with an overlay of digital content. For example, learners inserting an intravenous catheter using an MR HMD can see an overlay of the arm vasculature as they perform that procedure. Another use of MR is to provide a digital avatar that overlays on a simulation manikin and provides a more interactive experience. Currently there are few commercial applications available for this type of learning, and the HMDs used are more expensive, limiting this technology. However, as this area of simulation matures, it is likely more options will be available. Table 9.1 provides some examples of uses for XR technologies.

TABLE 9.1 SELECT XR MODALITIES

XR Modality	Equipment Used	Use
Desktop Virtual Reality (screen-based)	Computer, tablet, mouse, touchpad	Engage students in simulation experiences where they can examine and interview patients, plan care for care needs, or explore a community.
Augmented Reality	Phone, tablet	Project human anatomy to gain a 360-degree view. Use with QR codes on a manikin to display images such as wounds or skin rashes.
Mixed Reality	Headset for mixed reality: Microsoft HoloLens 2®, Apple Vision Pro™	Combine with manikins to practice procedures with digital overlays. Project digital patients or anatomy and interact at a high level of engagement and realism.

(continued)

TABLE 9.1 SELECT XR MODALITIES (continued)

XR Modality	Equipment Used	Use
Immersive Virtual Reality	Standalone headsets for IVR: Meta Quest 2 or 3™, PICO Neo3™	Provide care to patients in an immersive environment that can recreate a hospital or clinic environment. Allows for interaction with patients, family members, and other healthcare team members. Blocks out the real environment so the student is completely immersed in the virtual environment with a 360-degree view.

XR, extended reality.

Source: Aebersold, M., Lee, D., & Nelson, J. (2022). Using augmented and immersive virtual reality in nursing education. In P. R. Jeffries (Ed.). *Clinical simulations in nursing education: Advanced concepts, trends, and opportunities* (2nd ed., pp.177–194). National League for Nursing/Wolters Kluwer.

XR technologies continue to move forward as a viable learning modality for simulation-based activities in nursing education. They have several advantages over other methods because of the technology. They can provide individual learning experiences where the learner can independently care for patients and make decisions. They provide rich data analytics that are user specific to assist learners in self-reflection and improving their own skills.

INTEGRATION OF SIMULATION INTO THE CURRICULUM

Simulations offer a rich opportunity to improve student learning and achieve desired outcomes throughout a nursing curriculum. Simulations can be used in a variety of ways by faculty to meet different learning objectives, ranging from knowledge acquisition to application of a theoretical concept, demonstration of skills contextually within a complete clinical situation, professional role development, and development and evaluation of learner competency (Cole, 2023; Coyne et al., 2021; Keddington & Moore, 2019; Moore & Hawkins-Walsh, 2020).

One common use of simulation is to create a clinical experience for learners that they may not experience otherwise. This experience may supplement or replace clinical hours or a clinical day for any type of patient care within a nursing curriculum. While nurse educators often think about simulation mimicking the acute or intensive care environments, simulation can also be used to replicate long-term, hospice, outpatient, home, and community care. For example, a simulation can mimic a school nursing environment, a community center, and a clinic just as easily as a hospital room. Creativity, intentional design, SMART (**S**pecific, **M**easurable, **A**chievable, **R**elevant, and **T**ime-Bound) objectives, and thoughtful curricular integration are key to optimal application of simulation (INACSL Standards Committee, 2021i).

Simulation also allows all learners in a program to experience patient care situations deemed critical for professional practice, which cannot be guaranteed in a clinical setting. These can be referred to as low-frequency, high- impact experiences.

For example, it might be considered critical for all program graduates to know how to assess and care for a diabetic patient with significant hypoglycemia. While all learners could be assigned a diabetic patient in a traditional off-campus clinical setting, there is no guarantee that they would all provide care for a patient with hypoglycemia. Yet this experience can be granted consistently to every learner using simulation. Simulations also can create clinical experiences that are rare in clinical practice but potentially life -threatening and require prompt recognition and intervention. Clinical simulations can be developed to provide learners with a practice setting or a type of experience that is difficult to offer because of a variety of factors such as limited clinical sites, lack of qualified faculty in a specialty area, or geographic remoteness. For example, it may be difficult to place all of the nursing students into a labor and delivery environment, and there may be limited inpatient pediatric units. In those cases, simulation can be used to meet the learning objectives including care for mothers during childbirth and children of all ages.

Likewise, simulations are intended to replicate true clinical practice. While historically the scenarios were designed with a critical event or change in patient status, such as a rapidly deteriorating patient, simulations mimicking true practice offers an opportunity for learners to also experience patient care without a crisis. These simulations might include a focus on unchanged patient assessment, noticing trends, patient education, care of multiple patients, delegation, or different types of communication. These simulations, referred to as high- frequency–low-impact are important for preparing nursing graduates for transition to practice. All simulations should be leveled throughout the curriculum, building and varying in complexity, intention, and ambiguity. When selecting or writing simulations, faculty should create experiences that help students develop and demonstrate competencies for professional practice.

Simulation can also be incorporated into traditional didactic courses in addition to its use in clinical courses. This use assists learners in linking the content between theory and practice. For example, class content could present the facts about a myocardial infarction and standard care of these patients. Following this classroom presentation, learners could participate in a simulation that allows them to apply those facts to assessment and care for a simulated patient with a myocardial infarction. Using another approach, the content could be presented via the simulation, with learners given materials to prepare for the experience with the goal that knowledge would be attained through the simulation.

A mechanism of introducing increasingly complex simulations into a curriculum is to use an unfolding case. In an unfolding case, learners are introduced to a particular patient repeatedly at different points in the care continuum within a simulation, throughout a course, or throughout the curriculum. The patient scenario becomes more complex and requires different assessment skills or interventions on the part of the nurse. For example, in a psychiatric mental health class, learners could be introduced to a patient with depression. Later in the semester the students may "meet" the same patient, but this time the patient is suicidal. The learners interact with the same patient again at a later date in a different course, such as community health, when they are making a home health visit. During the home visit, learners can observe the patient interacting with their family and home environment.

Another way to add complexity to a simulation is to repeat the same case but use a modified or an unfolding version (Johnson et al., 2020). This could occur after debriefing one aspect of a simulation, when the learners switch roles and repeat or continue the scenario in a slightly different way. For example, the first scenario might have the postpartum patient with normal vaginal discharge after delivery. When the simulation is repeated, the patient develops signs and symptoms of a postpartum hemorrhage, and the nurse needs to identify the difference as well as the appropriate nursing actions. Each of these simulations offers different opportunities for teaching and learning.

Simulation can play an important role in developing professional roles and behaviors in nursing students. In addition to learning to think and act like a nurse, students need to learn how to work with other healthcare professions. Interprofessional (IP) and interdisciplinary simulations develop improved team communication and foster high-quality and safe patient care (Hodgkins et al., 2020; INACSL Standards Committee, 2021h). IP simulations can represent basic to complex interactions in patient care. For example, beginning learners might be involved in a simulation where a patient has an abnormal laboratory value. The nurse would be responsible for identifying the problem, contacting the physician, and receiving and acting on new medical orders. The physician would be responsible for evaluating the data presented by the nurse, making a diagnosis, and providing appropriate medical orders. With more advanced learners, an IP simulation might reflect a difference of opinion as to best care or an ethical dilemma related to possible care and treatment options. Other team members that should be incorporated include physical therapists, respiratory therapists, nutritionists, social workers, and pharmacists, among others.

In IP simulations, learners typically portray roles within their own profession. They learn about other professions by observing others portray their role in the simulation and through the discussion in debriefing (INACSL Standards Committee, 2021h). A variety of simulation experiences may be used to help learners understand the roles and responsibilities of other healthcare providers and to create empathy for the experiences of other professions. In IP simulations the debriefing often includes interdisciplinary aspects as well as a disciplinary focus (Hodgkins et al., 2020).

Simulation also can be used as a method to evaluate learner knowledge, abilities, and competency (INACSL Standards Committee, 2021d; Keddington & Moore, 2019). In introductory courses, learners might have to identify normal or abnormal heart or breath sounds; in more advanced courses they might be required to demonstrate competency, for example, by recognizing deterioration of a patient's status and taking appropriate action. Faculty need to reach a philosophical consensus and interrater reliability when using simulation as an evaluation tool (Tiffany et al., 2021). Is the desired outcome to bring all learners to a certain level of ability or competency prior to allowing them to progress in the curriculum? This would typically indicate that learners would have multiple opportunities to attempt the simulation, with assistance to improve as needed. Or is the intent of the graded simulation to prevent progression of students unable to demonstrate a certain level of ability or competency? These simulations, used for competency evaluation, are known as high-stakes simulations and might mean learners would have only one opportunity to pass the simulation. Another similar situation is when a grade is associated with the simulation. For all graded and high-stakes simulations, a grading rubric is needed (INACSL Standards Committee, 2021d). Faculty should reach a curricular consensus as to how to evaluate a simulation

> **EXHIBIT 9.1 Checklist for Implementation of a Simulation**
>
> Create or select the simulation scenario and objectives.
> Determine your resources:
> - number of manikins or SPs available,
> - number of simulation rooms available, and
> - number of faculty available to assist in running the simulation.
>
> Determine the time needed to run the scenario and debriefing.
> Determine the time needed to allow all learners to participate in the simulation:
> - number of learner groups and
> - include time to rotate groups.
>
> Determine the date(s) and time(s) the simulation will run.

and establish interrater reliability using the instrument prior to implementation (Tiffany et al., 2021).

IMPLEMENTATION OF SIMULATIONS

Once simulation experiences have been mapped to the curriculum and the best methodology of presenting them has been identified by faculty, implementation can begin (Exhibit 9.1). To create an effective learning experience, faculty should carefully plan all aspects relevant to running the simulation (INACSL Standards Committee, 2021g). Using simulation as a teaching strategy cannot be done successfully as a spur-of-the-moment decision.

The first step in simulation design is the creation or selection of the simulation scenario (INACSL Standards Committee, 2021i). This might be done with several content experts writing and reviewing a draft of the simulation after consulting the literature to ensure that current guidelines for evidence-based practice are met. A template is helpful to provide a standardized structure for the simulation and to guarantee that key aspects are not overlooked; resources for faculty are available at the National League for Nursing's (NLN) Simulation Innovation Research Center (SIRC; sirc.nln.org). Specific learning objectives and learner outcomes should be identified and should reflect what learners can actually accomplish in the allotted time given their skills and abilities (INACSL Standards Committee, 2021e). A detailed description related to staging the scene should include factors such as how the manikin or patient will "look," what equipment needs to be in the room, what supplies the learner will need to perform in the simulation, what props will add realism, what information needs to be in the patient's medical record, and how the patient will respond (verbally, physiologically) to interventions made by the nurse. All of these details must be considered, planned, and directly written into the simulation scenario (INACSL Standards Committee, 2021i).

An alternative to writing simulations is using premade or purchased scenarios. These have the advantage that the content has, in most circumstances, having been reviewed by experts and determined to accurately reflect current standards of practice. Pre-made or purchased simulations may be adjusted to meet local differences in care practices or to level the simulation to meet the learner's abilities at a given point in the curriculum. For faculty just learning to use simulation, this simplifies the process of incorporating simulation into the curriculum.

The remainder of planning and implementing simulations into a course involves practical issues of facilitating a simulation (INACSL Standards Committee, 2021g). A primary consideration is how much time will be needed for the prebriefing, simulation, and debriefing. Prebriefing should be designed as a component of the simulation. Prebriefing incorporates both prep work for learners as well as a briefing to set the stage for the experience (INACSL Standards Committee, 2021f). Often, prebriefing is 15 to 30 minutes, scenarios run 10 to 30 minutes, and debriefing takes at least two or three times the length of the scenario or longer, but these are generalizations. Many factors go into the timing decisions of simulation planning, including the complexity of the simulation, the level and roles of the learners, and the outcomes of the experience. It also is important to consider the total number of learners participating in simulation and the amount of time available (INACSL Standards Committee, 2021e).

Here is an example: A basic simulation of 10 minutes also has 20 minutes of prebriefing and 30 minutes of debriefing time. It will therefore take 60 minutes for each group of learners to complete the simulation. If you have 50 learners, and you want them to participate in the simulation in groups of five, and each group needs 60 minutes for the simulation and debriefing, it will take more than 10 hours to run the simulation if you only have one manikin or SP to use at a time and the environment needs to be reset for each new group.

Next consider how much time you have available. Are you using class time (e.g., a 50-minute time period)? This amount of time is not sufficient to run the simulation. At least 60 minutes is needed for one group, plus the additional time that is needed to rotate learners and reset the room for the next group. For this reason, many programs utilize several manikins or SPs concurrently.

In addition to time, there are other resources that should be considered. The number of simulation rooms and manikins or SPs that can be used at a single time is only one important variable. Additional rooms for debriefing are also critical as the simulation space can be used for one or two additional groups while the first group is debriefing. Therefore, it is also important to consider how many faculty members and simulation staff are familiar with the pedagogy and technology and can be available to assist with facilitating the simulation and leading the debriefing to ensure that simulation resources are allocated appropriately. Faculty need to plan thoroughly for a simulation experience and consider all aspects needed to run the simulation and debriefing smoothly. Attention to detail is important and using a simulation template can be helpful. Sufficient time should be allotted to design, plan, and implement simulations into the curriculum. When the simulation experience runs smoothly, faculty and staff are less stressed, and learners receive a more positive learning experience.

DEBRIEFING

Debriefing is an important component of learning in simulation. Typically, debriefing immediately follows a simulation as an opportunity for the nursing students and teachers to review the experience, discuss, and learn from what did or did not happen (Dreifuerst, 2009; INACSL Standards Committee, 2021b; Onello & Forneris, 2018; Rivière et al., 2019)

During debriefing, teachers can guide learners to discuss, analyze, and synthesize their thoughts and feelings about the experience. It is also a time to carefully review the thinking, actions, and clinical decisions that occurred during the simulation (Bradley et al., 2020; Dreifuerst, 2015; Kolbe et al., 2023) and discuss options and alternatives to improve the nursing care or patient outcomes. Because of the sensitive nature of the discussion, holding the debriefing in a comfortable private area, away from the actual simulated patient environment, is an important consideration (Turner et al., 2024). There are many ways to debrief; however, it is common for faculty and learners to first review what occurred and then focus the discussion on feedback including what went right, what went wrong, and what should be done differently, then move to reflection focused on the thinking and actions including assimilation, accommodation, and anticipation (Lee et al., 2020; Seibert, 2023).

Debriefing is a constructivist, reflective teaching strategy (Johnson, 2020). It commonly involves an interactive discussion between the learners who were directly involved in the simulation scenario, the learners who observed the simulation, and the debriefer (Johnson, 2019). These lively discussions should use the learning objectives or outcomes as a guide. Debriefing using this format becomes a type of formative feedback, which is intended to change thinking and behaviors when the learner encounters similar issues later in clinical practice (INACSL Standards Committee, 2021b).

The debriefer typically guides the debriefing experience by acting as a mentor, coach, or clinical teacher depending on the situation, learners, and simulation outcomes. The debriefer's role in the debriefing process can vary because it is dependent on the skill level of the participants, how much guidance is needed to keep the discussion flowing, and the outcome of the simulation. Debriefers generally are more active when the learners are novices and new to simulation and when there has been an emotional experience by one or more of them. Likewise, the debriefer can guide the discussion to provide additional support when negative outcomes or poor learner performances have occurred. As the learners gain experience and knowledge, they assume a more active role in the discussion and the debriefer can become more of a guide and less of a facilitator (Kolbe et al., 2023).

Guiding the discussion can involve the use of many communication strategies by the debriefer. These include incorporation of open-ended questions, active listening, Socratic questioning, restating, rephrasing, and leading questions. These techniques may require training and practice by the debriefer prior to the actual simulation experience (INACSL Standards Committee, 2021b; Seibert, 2023). Continuing education opportunities to learn evidence-based debriefing practices and strategies are available from a variety of venues, including formal education sessions and informal peer coaching. These are also opportunities to learn new ways and methods that can be used to debrief learners in simulation. The importance of faculty development and training in debriefing to ensure consistent outcomes cannot be overlooked (Bradley, 2019; INACSL Standards Committee, 2021c; Jeffries et al., 2015).

Debriefing Methods

There are many debriefing methods that are used in healthcare simulations. While many of these methods share similar practices, each has unique attributes that support different learners and environments (Lee et al., 2020). Reflection and feedback are essential components of debriefing regardless of the method used (Walsh & Sethares, 2022). Recalling the events of the simulation is important to understand the behaviors, decision-making, and patient outcomes in the simulation. Reflecting also solidifies learning from the experience, particularly when attention is paid to reflecting-in-action, reflecting-on-action, and reflecting-beyond-action (Dreifuerst, 2009; Schön, 1983).

Different debriefing methods can be used to guide the reflective process (Exhibit 9.2). Some of the more common debriefing methods include Plus Delta, Debriefing for Meaningful Learning© (DML), Debriefing with Good Judgment, Gather-Analyze-Summarize (GAS), and Promoting Excellence and Reflective Learning in Simulation (PEARLS).

Variations of the Plus-Delta debriefing method are popular in interdisciplinary healthcare simulations. This method emphasizes providing feedback including what went well (plus) and what could be done better or differently (delta, which is the Greek symbol for change), by soliciting reflective responses from the learners involved in the simulation (Fanning & Gaba, 2007). This method is not difficult and is easily adapted to many different types of simulations and learners.

EXHIBIT 9.2 Debriefing Methods

Plus -Delta
- What went right?
- What would you change?

Debriefing for Meaningful Learning (DML)
- Recall
- Unpack and uncover thinking and actions
- Reflection-in-action
- Reflection-on-action
- Reflection-beyond-action

Debriefing with Good Judgment
- Statement of advocacy or assertion
- Request for clarification or inquiry

Gather-Analyze-Summarize (GAS)
- Pull together pertinent information
- Discuss details of what went well and what did not
- Review all aspects of the experience in the context of the debriefing discussion

Promoting Excellence and Reflective Learning in Simulation (PEARLS)
- Reaction phase
- Description phase
- Analysis phase
- Learner self-assessment
- Feedback and teaching
- Summary phase

DML is a structured method that emphasizes uncovering the relationship between thinking and actions to foster reflection-in-action, reflection-on-action, and reflection-beyond-action; clinical reasoning; and thinking like a nurse (Dreifuerst et al., 2021; Huang et al., 2023; Loomis et al., 2022; Schön, 1983). A premise of this method is that the debriefer is a clinician or a clinical teacher with knowledge about the patient population. Following recollection of the experience, the debriefer guides the reflective process of uncovering the learner's thinking that underpinned their actions and decisions during the simulation and how that thinking informed assimilation, accommodation, and anticipation (Dreifuerst, 2015). DML debriefing is best assessed using the Debriefing for Meaningful Learning Evaluation Scale (DMLES) (Bradley, 2019). The DMLES assesses observable behaviors anchored in the DML debriefing. The items in the DMLES are closely aligned with the process of DML and assess each of the behaviors that should be present when using this method for debriefing and how well the behaviors were done.

In the Debriefing with Good Judgment method, the debriefer uses advocacy–inquiry to focus on a particular component of the simulation because the learner involved in the experience has done something unexpected or unanticipated (Rudolph et al., 2007). The discussion begins with a statement of advocacy or assertion about what was observed from the teacher's perspective, followed by a question or request for clarification about their thinking and actions from the learners in a nonthreatening way (Rudolph et al., 2007). This leads to a discussion that also includes feedback.

The GAS method uses a three-step debriefing process (American Heart Association, 2010). Teachers guide the learners to integrate or gather all of the pertinent information about the simulation experience, including what occurred, the decisions that were made, and outcomes. Next, the learners and facilitator analyze the information that has been gathered using the objectives for the simulation as well as what went right and what did not. Finally, everything that has been discussed is summarized to reinforce learning.

PEARLS represents a method of debriefing that advocates educators' intentional use of a variety of debriefing strategies to individualize the discussion to meet particular learner needs and unique learning environments. When debriefing using PEARLS, the debriefer can choose from different strategies to ensure the discussion includes reactions, descriptions, and analysis (Cheng et al., 2016; Høegh-Larsen et al., 2022).

Regardless of the method used, debriefing that includes reflection and revisiting of the events and actions to understand behaviors, decision-making, and the impact on patient outcomes is an essential part of simulation learning. Additionally, debriefing should consider the objectives of the experience, yet debriefers need to be careful to debrief the actual experience and not what was hoped would happen. Therefore, including an intentional method of recalling the events of the simulation is an important initial step of debriefing. Assessing the quality of debriefing is also important. Another tool that can be used to assess all debriefing methods is the Debriefing Assessment for Simulation in Healthcare© (DASH), which is available in three versions (https://harvardmedsim.org/debriefing-assessment-for-simulation-in-healthcare-dash/). Finally, learners should be actively involved in the debriefing discussion regardless of their role as participant or observer in the simulation, and everyone should have an opportunity to clarify anything that was uncertain during the simulation and debriefing (Johnson, 2019). It cannot be overstated that faculty who use simulation should have training and assessment in debriefing to be able to facilitate this important component of student learning (Bradley et al., 2023; Cheng et al., 2017; INACSL Standards Committee, 2021b; Woda et al., 2022).

SIMULATION THEORY

Simulation presents many opportunities for evaluation. It is commonly used for evaluating the learning or performance of the simulation participant, but there are other aspects of simulation that also can be evaluated. One way to examine the various opportunities for evaluation within simulation is by looking at the National League for Nursing's (NLN) Jeffries Simulation theory (Jeffries, 2022). There are seven concepts in the theory: *Context, Background, Design, Facilitator, Educational Strategies, Participant,* and *Outcomes,* and each represents an opportunity for evaluation (Figure 9.1). The concepts in the NLN Jeffries Simulation Theory are described briefly with opportunities for evaluation within each concept.

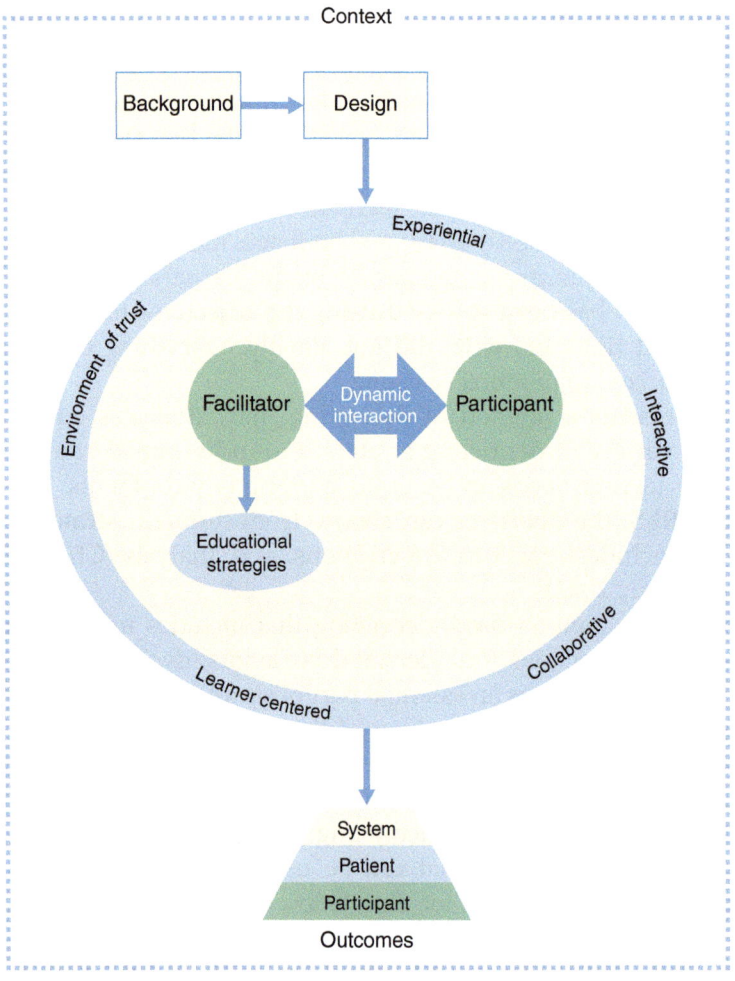

Figure 9.1 Diagram of the National League for Nursing's Jeffries Simulation Theory©.
Source: Jeffries, P. R. (Ed.). (2022). *The NLN Jeffries Simulation Theory.* Wolters Kluwer/National League for Nursing. Reprinted by permission, 2024.

SIMULATION EVALUATION

The HSSOBP: Outcomes and Objectives (INACSL Standards Committee, 2021e), and Evaluation of Learning and Performance (INACSL Standards Committee, 2021d) provide excellent starting points for thinking about simulation evaluation.

All aspects of a simulation or simulation program can be assessed. Based on the assessment data, evaluations including decisions and modifications can be made. Each of the simulation standards and the criteria they outline provide benchmarks for assessment and evaluation. For example, the standards provide guidance on deciding the type and timing of assessment and evaluation of learners using simulation in addition to guidance on the use of tools and instruments (INACSL Standards Committee, 2021d). Criteria for formative and summative assessment of learners using simulation can also be incorporated into competency-based education models and frameworks (Keddington & Moore, 2019). To that end, understanding how outcomes and objectives are incorporated into simulation is important (INACSL Standards Committee, 2021e) in addition to identifying the target of the evaluation.

Kirkpatrick and Kirkpatrick (2019) describe four levels that are helpful for categorizing or identifying the target of an evaluation. These levels, as they apply to simulation participant evaluation, include (a) Level 1: *Participants' reactions* to the simulation activity, (b) Level 2: *Participants' learning* from the simulation activity, (c) Level 3: Changes in *participants' behavior* as a result of the simulation activity, and (d) Level 4: Longer-term *results* or *outcomes* that take place because of the simulation activity. The category of learning (Level 2) may be further divided using the three domains of learning: cognitive, affective, and psychomotor. While many simulation evaluations seek to cover multiple levels and learning domains, using Kirkpatrick's language helps to describe the foci of the particular evaluation strategy.

Evaluations become increasingly more difficult, but potentially more meaningful, as they progress from Level 1 (reaction) to Level 4 (results). For example, it is much easier to ask participants to rate their level of satisfaction with a simulation activity (Level 1: reaction) or assess participant knowledge before and after a simulation activity (Level 2: learning [cognitive]) than it is to determine whether a simulation activity impacts how participants performed in the clinical environment (Level 3: behavior) or changes in patient outcomes (Level 4: results). However, the effort to produce such evaluations is commensurate with their potential impact. Yet, the information provided by Levels 3 and 4 evaluations has much greater impact than the information provided by the lower levels of evaluation (Levels 1 and 2).

Planning the Simulation Evaluation

One of the first steps in planning an effective simulation participant evaluation is to identify the purpose and focus of the evaluation. This includes determining the stakes of the evaluation: formative, summative, or high stakes (INACSL Standards Committee, 2021d). Answering the following questions can also help frame the purpose and focus of the evaluation: Which level from Kirkpatrick and Kirkpatrick's (2019) levels of evaluation should be the focus (reaction, learning, behavior, or results)? Is there a specific learning objective, technical skill, or ability such as clinical judgment that needs to be assessed? Who will be the focus of the evaluation, individuals or groups?

Once the purpose and focus of the evaluation have been determined, the next step is to design an effective simulation-based evaluation. If the evaluation is going to include an observation-based assessment such as a checklist or rubric completed by a rater while they watch the simulation, it is essential to ensure the simulation experience includes the opportunity for simulation participants to observably demonstrate their achievement of the learning objective, technical skill, or cognitive, affective, or psychomotor abilities being measured. If the rater cannot see the participant demonstrating the behavior, the rater cannot score it. The simulation should be appropriately timed depending upon the stakes of the evaluation. For example, a formative evaluation may take place in the middle of a course whereas a summative or high-stakes evaluation will likely take place at the end of a course or program of learning.

Selecting or developing an appropriate evaluation instrument is the next key step in the evaluation process. The type of evaluation instrument will vary depending upon the objective of the evaluation or competency to be assessed (INACSL Standards Committee, 2021d). For example, a simple procedural checklist may be appropriate for a specific technical skill. The use of an existing simulation evaluation instrument is highly recommended, as the development of a new simulation evaluation instrument requires extensive investment of time and resources.

If the objective of the evaluation is to measure clinical judgment ability, the simulation scenario must include opportunities for the participant to demonstrate clinical judgment and an instrument such as the Lasater Clinical Judgment Rubric (LCJR) may be applicable (Lasater, 2007; Lasater & Nielsen, 2024). The LCJR is an 11-item rubric based on Tanner's (2006) Model of Clinical Judgment. Each of the four aspects of clinical judgment— Noticing, Interpreting Responding, and Reflecting— are rated using multiple items and a scale ranging from beginning through accomplished. The LCJR has demonstrated high reliability and validity.

Another well-accepted instrument for simulation participant evaluation, which has established high reliability and validity (Manz et al., 2022), is the Creighton Competency Evaluation Instrument (C-CEI(R); https://www.creighton.edu/nursing/academics/competency-evaluation-instrument). There are 23 items on the CCEI, reflecting competencies in Assessment, Communication, Clinical Judgment, and Patient Safety. Scoring options for each competency include (a) demonstrates, (b) does not demonstrate, and (c) not applicable, which can be used to assess learners in a variety of clinical contexts.

Carefully selecting and training raters to complete the evaluation instrument that will be used with the simulation will help ensure valid and reliable results (INACSL Standards Committee, 2021c). This may be as simple as identifying a qualified individual who will complete all the evaluations in one session, or as complex as selecting and training a group of raters and assessing important criteria such as interrater reliability. With these decisions made, the next steps include collecting, interpreting, and reporting evaluation data. Additional guidelines on assessment and evaluation that are relevant to simulation evaluation are provided in Chapters 15 to 17.

While many of the characteristics of clinical evaluation are relevant to using simulation for learner assessment, simulation also offers evaluation opportunities that may not exist in traditional clinical environments. These include the ability to (a) create and standardize scenarios to isolate and elicit specific participant skills and behaviors, (b) allow multiple participants to engage in a given scenario or an individual participant to engage in a given scenario multiple times, and (c) allow a participant to make errors without endangering a patient. Simulation also holds enormous promise for learner evaluation beyond the clinical environment. These evaluations may be implemented as an alternative or adjunct to classroom assessment, including the current multiple-choice examinations used for academic progression and licensure, or may be employed for formative and summative assessment of competency. Thoughtful planning and focus on higher levels of evaluation that reflect knowledge, skills, and attitudes attained through the use of simulation are important to the ongoing development of simulation pedagogy.

DEVELOPMENTS IN SIMULATION RESEARCH, REGULATION, AND CREDENTIALING

Credentialing, and Regulation

The use of simulation-based education continues to grow, and leaders in healthcare education consistently cite simulation as a top research priority. Consequently, the body of literature examining best practices for simulation-based education is expanding rapidly. With well over 200 papers related to simulation published annually, it continues to be the largest area of pedagogical research in healthcare education.

While a decade old now, the National Council of State Boards of Nursing's landmark national simulation study exploring the amount of traditional clinical time that could be substituted with high-quality clinical simulation (Hayden et al., 2014) remains the gold standard informing academic and regulatory decisions about simulation use in nursing education. This national, multisite, longitudinal study included three groups of participants ($n = 666$) across 10 different schools of nursing (five baccalaureate and five associate degree programs) in the United States. One group, serving as the control, had less than 10% of clinical time replaced with clinical simulations, another group had 25% of clinical time replaced with simulations, and a third group had up to 50% of clinical time replaced with simulation across seven different courses. The clinical practice time was replaced with controlled, immersive clinical simulations in four semesters of a generic baccalaureate and an associate degree nursing program (Hayden et al., 2014).

Findings from this seminal study included: (a) Up to 50% of traditional clinical hours may be replaced with high-quality simulation in all core courses across the prelicensure nursing curriculum. (b) This 50% replacement with simulation can be effectively used in various program types, in different geographic areas, and in urban and rural settings with good educational outcomes. (c) NCLEX-RN® pass rates were unaffected by the substitution of simulation throughout the curriculum; therefore, all groups were equally prepared for entry into practice as a new graduate RNs. (d) Policy decisions about the use and amount of simulation in nursing should depend on the use of best practices in simulation (Hayden et al., 2014). As a result, guidelines for state boards of nursing regulators and leaders in schools of nursing have been developed with variance across states and programs (Bradley et al., 2019).

Developments in Simulation Regulation

Since publication of the National Council of State Boards of Nursing Simulation Study (NSS), there have been significant developments in the regulation of simulation in nursing education. Smiley and Martin (2023) compared nursing regulation of simulation in 61 jurisdictions between the years 2014 and 2022. The number of jurisdictions with explicit, simulation-specific regulations for prelicensure RN education programs nearly doubled between 2014 and 2022, going from 21 in the year 2014 to 41 in the year 2022. Nursing regulatory bodies appear to be following the evidence from the NSS. This is reflected by the number of jurisdictions allowing up to 50% of clinical time to be replaced with simulation which rose from 1 in the year 2014 to 23 in the year 2022. Regulation of licensed vocational nurse (LVN) and licensed practical nurse (LPN) education programs is following a similar trajectory (Smiley & Martin, 2023). Additional changes in regulation include how to count or give credit for time spent in simulation toward required clinical time and how to ensure the quality of simulation. To that end, there is emerging evidence and interest about counting each hour spent in simulation as 2 hours of required clinical time (1:2 ratio; Curl et al. 2016; Haerling et al., 2023; Sullivan et al., 2019). Regulatory bodies are currently considering how this might impact future regulation, education, and outcomes as the use of simulation continues to rise.

Developments in Simulation Credentialing

Credentialing in simulation is offered to individuals by the Society for Simulation in Healthcare (SSH), an international organization dedicated to healthcare simulation (https://www.ssih.org/credentialing/certification). These credentials define and recognize achievement of best practices in simulation pedagogy and operations. Simulation centers can also pursue accreditation through the SSH (https://www.ssih.org/credentialing/accreditation) to demonstrate evidence of dedicated resources (personnel and equipment) whose mission is specifically targeted toward improving patient safety and outcomes through assessment, research, advocacy, and education using simulation. Additionally, INACSL offers a Healthcare Simulation Standards Endorsement™ program. This endorsement recognizes simulation programs that demonstrate excellence consistently using the core four HSSOBP (INACSL Standards Committee, 2021a, 2021b, 2021f, 2021g), which serve as the Cornerstone of Best Practice in Simulation (https://www.inacsl.org/cornerstones-of-best-practice).

SUMMARY

Simulations provide opportunities for learners to apply and demonstrate nursing knowledge, skills, and attitudes in an on-campus, safe, and controlled environment before going into the traditional off-campus clinical setting. However, in the current complex clinical environments, increased patient acuity, and limited clinical placements, simulations serve a broader role as a supplement to, or replacement for, traditional clinical experiences. Moreover, the simulation environment can be used for teaching and assessing competence in prelicensure and graduate-level nurses, playing an increasingly important role in both formative and summative evaluation.

This chapter provided an overview of types of simulations in nursing. In addition, the design and implementation of simulations within a nursing curriculum, models of debriefing, and evaluation processes to use when developing and implementing clinical simulations were presented. Finally, the chapter presented developments in simulation research, credentialing, and regulation. The rapid infusion of innovative technology associated with high-fidelity manikins, sophistication of gaming, the impact of the use of SPs, the proliferation of screen-based simulation, and the rapid adoption of AR, VR, and immersive VR all contribute to the rise in simulation, use in nursing education today. As the discipline moves toward a competency-based education model, there will be a continued need for research into best practices for simulation use and its impact on healthcare in the future.

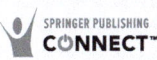 A robust set of instructor resources designed to supplement this text is located at http://connect.springerpub.com/content/book/978-0-8261-8892-2. Qualifying instructors may request access by emailing textbook@springerpub.com.

REFERENCES

Aebersold, M., Lee, D., & Nelson, J. (2022). Using augmented and immersive virtual reality in nursing education. In P. R. Jeffries (Ed.). *Clinical simulations in nursing education: Advanced concepts, trends, and opportunities* (2nd ed., pp. 177–194). National League for Nursing/Wolters Kluwer.

American Heart Association. (2010). GAS Model of Debriefing *debriefing*. http://members.nata.org/education/f/ATEC2015/GAS-Model-of-Debriefing.pdf

Bradley, C. S. (2019). Impact of training on use of debriefing for meaningful learning. *Clinical Simulation in Nursing, 32*(C), 13–19. https://doi.org/10.1016/j.ecns.2019.04.003

Bradley, C. S., Johnson, B. K., & Dreifuerst, K. T. (2020). Debriefing: A place for enthusiastic teaching and learning at a distance. *Clinical Simulation in Nursing, 49*, 16–18. https://doi.org/10.1016/j.ecns.2020.04.001

Bradley, C. S., Johnson, B. K., Dreifuerst, K. T., White, P., Conde, S. K., Meakim, C. H., Curry-Lourenco, K., & Childress, R. M. (2019). Regulation of simulation use in United States prelicensure nursing programs. *Clinical Simulation in Nursing, 33*, 17–25. https://doi.org/10.1016/j.ecns.2019.04.004

Bradley, C. S., Johnson, B. K., Woda, A., Hansen, J., Loomis, A., & Dreifuerst, K. T. (2023). The impact of single-dose Debriefing for Meaningful Learning training on debriefer quality, time, and outcomes: Early evidence to inform debriefing training and frequency. *Nursing Education Perspectives, 44*(6), E33–E38. https://doi.org/10.1097/01.Nep.0000000000001163

Cheng, A., Grant, V., Huffman, J., Burgess, G., Szyld, D., Robinson, T., & Eppich, W. (2017). Coaching the debriefer: Peer coaching to improve debriefing quality in simulation programs. *Simulation in Healthcare, 12*(5), 319–325. https://doi.org/10.1097/sih.0000000000000232

Cheng, A., Grant, V., Robinson, T., Catena, H., Lachapelle, K., Kim, J., Adler, M., & Eppich, W. (2016). The promoting excellence and reflective learning in simulation (PEARLS) approach to health care debriefing: A faculty development guide. *Clinical Simulation in Nursing, 12*(10), 419–428. https://doi.org/10.1016/j.ecns.2016.05.002

Cole, H. S. (2023). Competency-based evaluations in undergraduate nursing simulation: A state of the literature. *Clinical Simulation in Nursing, 76*, 1–16. https://doi.org/10.1016/j.ecns.2022.12.004

Coyne, E., Calleja, P., Forster, E., & Lin, F. (2021). A review of virtual-simulation for assessing healthcare students' clinical competency. *Nurse Education Today, 96*, 104623. https://doi.org/10.1016/j.nedt.2020.104623

Curl, E., Smith, S., Chisholm, L., McGee, L., & Das, K. (2016). Effectiveness of integrated simulation and clinical experiences compared to traditional clinical experiences for nursing students. *Nursing Education Perspectives, 37* (2), 72–77.

Doyle, A. J., Sullivan, C., O'Toole, M., Tjin, A., Simiceva, A., Collins, N., Murphy, P., Anderson, M. J., Mulhall, C., Condron, C., Nestel, D., MacAulay, R., McNaughton, N., Coffey, F., & Eppich, W. (2024). Training simulated participants for role portrayal and feedback practices in communication skills training: A BEME scoping review: BEME Guide No. 86. *Medical Teacher, 46*(2), 162–178. https://doi.org/10.1080/0142159X.2023.2241621

Dreifuerst, K. T. (2009). The essentials of debriefing in simulation learning: A concept analysis. *Nursing Education Perspectives, 30*(2), 109–114.

Dreifuerst, K. T. (2015). Getting started with debriefing for meaningful learning. *Clinical Simulation in Nursing, 11*(5), 268–275. https://doi.org/10.1016/j.ecns.2015.01.005

Dreifuerst, K. T., Bradley, C. S., & Johnson, B. K. (2021). Using Debriefing for Meaningful Learning with screen-based simulation. *Nurse Educator, 46*(4), 239–244. https://doi.org/10.1097/nne.0000000000000930

Fanning, R. M., & Gaba, D. M. (2007). The role of debriefing in simulation-based learning. *Simulation in Healthcare, 2*(2), 115–125. https://doi.org/10.1097/SIH.0b013e3180315539

Foronda, C. L., Fernandez-Burgos, M., Nadeau, C., Kelley, C. N., & Henry, M. N. (2020). Virtual simulation in nursing education: A systematic review spanning 1996 to 2018. *Simulation in Healthcare, 15*(1), 46–54. https://doi.org/10.1097/sih.0000000000000411

Foronda, C. L., Gonzalez, L., Meese, M. M., Slamon, N., Baluyot, M., Lee, J., & Aebersold, M. (2024). A comparison of virtual reality to traditional simulation in health professions education: A systematic review. *Simulation in Healthcare, 19*(1S), S90–S97. https://doi.org/10.1097/sih.0000000000000745

Haerling, K., Kmail, Z., & Buckingham, A. (2023). Contributing to evidence-based regulatory decisions: A comparison of traditional clinical experience, mannequin-based simulation, and screen-based virtual simulation. *Journal of Nursing Regulation, 13*(4), 33–43. https://doi.org/10.1016/S2155-8256(23)00029-7

Haerling, K., & Miller, C. (2024). A cost-utility analysis comparing traditional clinical, mannequin-based simulation, and virtual simulation activities. *Journal of Nursing Education, 63*(2), 79–85. https://doi.org/10.3928/01484834-20231205-04

Hayden, J., Smiley, R., Alexander, M. A., Kardong-Edgren, S., & Jeffries, P. J. (2014). The NCSBN national simulation study: A longitudinal, randomized, controlled study replacing clinical hours with simulation in prelicensure nursing education. *Journal of Nursing Regulation, 5*(Suppl. 2), S3–S40. https://doi.org/10.1016/S2155-8256(15)30062-4

Herrmann, E. K. (2008). Remembering Mrs. Chase. Before there were smart hospitals and Sim-Men, there was "Mrs. Chase." *Imprint, 55*(2), 52.

Hodgkins, S. R., Marian, K. M., Shrader, S., Averett, E., Crowl, A., Kalender-Rich, J. L., & Johnston, K. (2020). A case of anaphylaxis: IPE simulation as a tool to enhance communication and collaboration. *Journal of Interprofessional Education & Practice, 18*, 100303. https://doi.org/10.1016/j.xjep.2019.100303

Høegh-Larsen, A. M., Ravik, M., Reierson, I. Å., Husebø, S. I. E., & Gonzalez, M. T. (2022). Pearls debriefing compared to standard debriefing effects on nursing students' professional competence and clinical judgment: A quasi-experimental study. *Clinical Simulation in Nursing, 74*. 38–48. https://doi.org/10.1016/j.ecns.2022.09.003

Huang, C.-Y., Lee, C.-H., Lin, P.-H., Lu, W.-J., Lin, R.-J., Hung, C.-Y., Li, P.-C., & Chung, C.-H. (2023). Effectiveness of Debriefing for Meaningful Learning (DML) combined with empathy map on prelicensure nursing students' competency: A quasi-experimental study. *Clinical Simulation in Nursing, 81*, 101427. https://doi.org/10.1016/j.ecns.2023.101427

International Nursing Association of Clinical Simulation and Learning Standards Committee, Bowler, F., Klein, M., & Wilford, A. (2021a). Healthcare simulation standards of best practice™ Professional integrity. *Clinical Simulation in Nursing, 58*, 45–48. https://doi.org/10.1016/j.ecns.2021.08.014

International Nursing Association of Clinical Simulation and Learning Standards Committee, Decker, S., Alinier, G., Crawford, S. B., Gordon, R. M., Jenkins, D., & Wilson, C. (2021b). Healthcare simulation standards of best practice™ the debriefing process. *Clinical Simulation in Nursing, 58*, 27–32. https://doi.org/10.1016/j.ecns.2021.08.011

International Nursing Association of Clinical Simulation and Learning Standards Committee, Hallmark, B., Brown, M., Peterson, D. T., Fey, M., Decker, S., Wells-Beede, E., Britt, T., Hardie, L., Shum, C., Arantes, H. P., Charnetski, M., & Morse, C. (2021c). Healthcare simulation standards of best practice™ Professional development. *Clinical Simulation in Nursing, 58*, 5–8. https://doi.org/10.1016/j.ecns.2021.08.007

International Nursing Association of Clinical Simulation and Learning Standards Committee, McMahon, E., Jimenez, F. A., Lawrence, K., & Victor, J. (2021d). Healthcare simulation standards of best practice™ Evaluation of learning and performance. *Clinical Simulation in Nursing, 58*, 54–56. https://doi.org/10.1016/j.ecns.2021.08.016

International Nursing Association of Clinical Simulation and Learning Standards Committee, Miller, C., Deckers, C., Jones, M., Wells-Beede, E., & McGee, E. (2021e). Healthcare simulation standards of best practice™ Outcomes and objectives. *Clinical Simulation in Nursing, 58*, 40–44. https://doi.org/10.1016/j.ecns.2021.08.013

International Nursing Association of Clinical Simulation and Learning Standards Committee, McDermot, D. S., Ludlow, J., Horseley, E., & Meakim, C. (2021f). Healthcare simulation standards of best practice™ prebriefing: Preparation and briefing. *Clinical Simulation in Nursing, 58*, 9–13. https://doi.org/10.1016/j.ecns.2021.08.008

International Nursing Association of Clinical Simulation and Learning Standards Committee, Persico, L., Belle, A., DiGregorio, H., Wilson-Keates, B., & Shelton, C. (2021g). Healthcare simulation standards of best practice™ Facilitation. *Clinical Simulation in Nursing, 58*, 22–26. https://doi.org/10.1016/j.ecns.2021.08.010

International Nursing Association of Clinical Simulation and Learning Standards Committee, Rossler, K., Molloy, M. A., Pastva, A. M., Brown, M., & Xavier, N. (2021h). Healthcare simulation standards of best practice™ simulation-enhanced interprofessional education. *Clinical Simulation in Nursing, 58*, 49–53. https://doi.org/10.1016/j.ecns.2021.08.015

International Nursing Association of Clinical Simulation and Learning Standards Committee, Watts, P. I., McDermott, D. S., Alinier, G., Charnetski, M., Ludlow, J., Horsley, E., Meakim, C., & Nawathe, P. A. (2021i). Healthcare simulation standards of best practice™ Simulation design. *Clinical Simulation in Nursing, 58*, 14–21. https://doi.org/10.1016/j.ecns.2021.08.009

Jeffries, P. R. (Ed.). (2022). *The NLN Jeffries Simulation Theory.* Wolters Kluwer/National League for Nursing.

Jeffries, P. R., Dreifuerst, K. T., & Kardong-Edgren, S. (2015). Faculty development when initiating simulation programs: Lessons learned from the NCSBN simulation study. *Journal of Nursing Regulation, 5*(4), 17–23. https://doi.org/10.1016/S2155-8256(15)30037-5

Johnson, B. K. (2019). Simulation observers learn the same as participants: The evidence. *Clinical Simulation in Nursing, 33*(4), 26–34. https://doi.org/10.1016/j.ecns.2019.04.006

Johnson B. K. (2020). Observational experiential learning: Theoretical support for observer roles in health care simulation. *Journal of Nursing Education, 59*(1), 7–14. https://doi.org/10.3928/01484834-20191223-03

Johnson, C. E., Kimble, L. P., Gunby, S. S., & Davis, A. H. (2020). Using deliberate practice and simulation for psychomotor skill competency acquisition and retention: A mixed-methods study. *Nurse Educator, 45*(3), 150–154. https://doi.org/10.1097/nne.0000000000000713

Keddington, A. S., & Moore, J. (2019). Simulation as a method of competency assessment among health care providers: A systematic review. *Nursing education perspectives, 40*(2), 91–94. https://doi.org/10.1097/01.Nep.0000000000000433

Kirkpatrick, J., & Kirkpatrick, W. (2019). *An introduction to the new world Kirkpatrick model.* Kirkpatrick Partners.

Kolbe, M., Grande, B., Lehmann-Willenbrock, N., & Seelandt, J. C. (2023). Helping healthcare teams to debrief effectively: Associations of debriefers' actions and participants' reflections during team debriefings. *BMJ Quality & Safety, 32*(3), 160–172. https://doi.org/10.1136/bmjqs-2021-014393

Lasater, K. (2007). Clinical judgment development: Using simulation to create an assessment rubric. *Journal of Nursing Education, 46*(11), 496–503. https://doi.org/10.3928/01484834-20071101-04

Lasater, K., & Nielsen, A. (2024). The Lasater Clinical Judgment Rubric: 17 Years Later. *Journal of Nursing Education, 63*(3), 149–155. https://doi.org/10.3928/01484834-20240108-05

Lee, J., Lee, H., Kim, S., Choi, M., Ko, I. S., Bae, J., & Kim, S. H. (2020). Debriefing methods and learning outcomes in simulation nursing education: A systematic review and meta-analysis. *Nurse Education Today, 87*, 104345. https://doi.org/10.1016/j.nedt.2020.104345

Lewis, K. L., Bohnert, C. A., Gammon, W. L., Hölzer, H., Lyman, L., Smith, C., Thompson, T. M., Wallace, A., & Gliva-Mcconvey, G., (2017). The Association of Standardized Patient Educators (ASPE) Standards of Best Practice (SOBP). *Advances in Simulation, 2*(1). https://doi.org/10.1186/s41077-017-0043-4

Lioce, L., Downing, D., Chang, T. P., Robertson, J. M., Anderson, M., Diaz, D. A., Spain, A. E., & the Terminology and Concepts Working Group. (2020). *Healthcare simulation dictionary–Second edition* (AHRQ Publication No. 20-0019). Agency for Healthcare Research and Quality. https://doi.org/10.23970/simulationv2

Loke, J. C. F., Lee, B. K., Loh, S., & Noor, A. M. (2020). High fidelity full sized human patient simulation manikins: Effects on decision making skills of nursing students. *Journal of Nursing Education and Practice, 4*(7), 31–40. https://doi.org/10.5430/jnep.v4n7p31

Loomis, A., Dreifuerst, K. T., & Bradley, C. S. (2022). Acquiring, applying and retaining knowledge through Debriefing for Meaningful Learning. *Clinical Simulation in Nursing, 68*, 28–33. https://doi.org/10.1016/j.ecns.2022.04.002

MacLean, S., Geddes, F., Kelly, M., & Della, P. (2019). Realism and presence in simulation: Nursing student perceptions and learning outcomes. *Journal of Nursing Education, 58*(6), 330–338. https://doi.org/10.3928/01484834-20190521-03

Manz, J. A., Tracy, M., Hercinger, M., Todd, M., Iverson, L., & Hawkins, K. (2022). Assessing competency: An integrative review of the Creighton Simulation Evaluation Instrument (C-SEI) and Creighton Competency Evaluation Instrument (C-CEI). *Clinical Simulation in Nursing, 66*, 66–75. https://doi.org/10.1016/j.ecns.2022.02.003

Moore, J., & Hawkins-Walsh, E. (2020). Evaluating nurse practitioner student competencies: Application of entrustable professional activities. *Journal of Nursing Education, 59*(12), 714–720. https://doi.org/10.3928/01484834-20201118-11

Onello, R., & Forneris, S. G. (2018). Clinical conversations. In S. G. Forneris & M. K. Fey (Eds), *Critical conversations: The NLN guide for teaching thinking* (pp. 49–58). Wolters Kluwer.

Owen, H. (2012). Early use of simulation in medical education. *Simulation in Healthcare, 7*(2), 102–116. https://doi.org/10.1097/SIH.0b013e3182415a91

Rivière, E., Jaffrelot, M., Jouquan, J., & Chiniara, G. (2019). Debriefing for the transfer of learning. *Academic Medicine, 94*(6), 796–803. https://doi.org/10.1097/acm.0000000000002612

Rudolph, J. W., Simon, R., Rivard, P., Dufresne, R. L., & Raemer, D. B. (2007). Debriefing with good judgment: Combining rigorous feedback with genuine inquiry. *Anesthesiology Clinics, 25*(2), 361–376. https://doi.org/10.1016/j.anclin.2007.03.007

Rutherford-Hemming, T., Alfes, C. M., & Breymier, T. L. (2019). A systematic review of the use of standardized patients as a simulation modality in nursing education. *Nursing Education Perspectives, 40*(2), 84–90. https://doi.org/10.1097/01.NEP.0000000000000401

Salcedo, D., Regan, J., Aebersold, M., Lee, D., Darr, A., Davis, K., & Berrocal, Y. (2022). Frequently used conceptual frameworks and design principles for extended reality in health professions education. *Medical Science Educator, 32*(6), 1587–1595. https://doi.org/10.1007/s40670-022-01620-y

Schön, D. A. (1983). *The reflective practitioner: How professionals think in action.* Basic Books.

Shorey, S., & Ng, E. D. (2021). The use of virtual reality simulation among nursing students and registered nurses: A systematic review. *Nurse Education Today, 98*, 104662. https://doi.org/10.1016/j.nedt.2020.104662

Seibert, S. A. (2023). Scaffolding questions to foster higher order thinking. *Teaching and Learning in Nursing, 18*(1), 185–187. https://doi.org/10.1016/j.teln.2022.09.008

Smiley, R., & Martin, B. (2023). Simulation in nursing education: Advancements in regulation, 2014–2022. *Journal of Nursing Regulation, 14*(2), 5–9. https://doi.org/10.1016/S2155-8256(23)00086-8

Stokes-Parish, J., Duvivier, R., & Jolly, B. (2019). Expert opinions on the authenticity of moulage in simulation: A Delphi study. *Advances in Simulation, 4*(1), 16. https://doi.org/10.1097/01.NEP.0000000000000095

Sullivan, N., Swoboda, S. M., Breymier, T., Lucas, L., Sarasnick, J., Rutherford-Hemming, T., Budhathoki, C., & Kardong-Edgren, S. (2019). Emerging evidence toward a 2:1 clinical to simulation ratio: A study comparing the traditional clinical and simulation settings. *Clinical Simulation in Nursing, 30*(3), 34–41. https://doi.org/10.1016/j.ecns.2019.03.003

Tanner C. A. (2006). Thinking like a nurse: A research-based model of clinical judgment in nursing. *The Journal of Nursing Education, 45*(6), 204–211. https://doi.org/10.3928/01484834-20060601-04

Tiffany, J. M., Hoglund, B. A., Holland, A. E., Schug, V., Blazovich, L., & Bambini, D. (2021). Promoting fair evaluation of learning during clinical simulation: Knowing yourself, your team, and your tool. *Clinical Simulation in Nursing.* https://doi.org/10.1016/j.ecns.2021.05.009

Turner, S., Rabbani, R., & Harder, N. (2024). Location! location! location! comparing simulation debriefing spaces. *Clinical Simulation in Nursing, 87*, 101504. https://doi.org/10.1016/j.ecns.2023.101504

Walsh, J. A., & Sethares, K. A. (2022). The use of guided reflection in simulation-based education with prelicensure nursing students: An integrative review. *Journal of Nursing Education, 61*(2), 73–79. https://doi.org/10.3928/01484834-20211213-01

Woda, A., Hansen, J., Dreifuerst, K. T., Johnson, B. K., Loomis, A., Cox, N., & Bradley, C. S. (2022). Debriefing for Meaningful Learning: Implementing a train-the-trainer program for debriefers. *The Journal of Continuing Education in Nursing, 53*(7), 321–327. https://doi.org/10.3928/00220124-20220603-08

X Reality Safety Intelligence. (n.d.). *The XRSI taxonomy of XR*. Retrieved March 1, 2024, from https://xrsi.org/definitions

Teaching in a Clinical and Interprofessional Education Setting

III

Clinical Teaching in Nursing

10

Lisa K. Woodley and Leslie M. Sharpe

OBJECTIVES

1. Describe the importance of effective teaching in learning laboratories and clinical settings
2. Examine principles of effective clinical teaching
3. Describe models of clinical teaching and their application in nursing education
4. Discuss the process of clinical teaching
5. Analyze challenges associated with clinical teaching in nursing, along with strategies to mitigate them
6. Explain special considerations for working with advanced practice registered nursing students

INTRODUCTION

The clinical teacher plays a pivotal role in shaping the learning experience for nursing students in the clinical setting. Given this critical function, it is imperative that clinical teachers demonstrate effective teaching behaviors and adhere to best practices in nursing education, inspiring their students in the process. This chapter elucidates why learning laboratories and clinical settings are integral components of nursing education. It addresses the principles of clinical teaching and explores various models thereof, including telehealth experiences, community-based learning projects, experiential learning opportunities, global clinical experiences, and remote preceptorships. The clinical teaching process is thoroughly described, covering aspects such as assessing learners' needs and outcomes, planning clinical activities, organizing faculty and students, conducting site visits, and effectively leveraging feedback. Challenges inherent in clinical teaching are acknowledged, with strategies proposed to mitigate these issues. Specific attention is paid to considerations when working with advanced practice registered nurses (APRNs) as graduate students.

IMPORTANCE OF EFFECTIVE TEACHING IN LEARNING LABORATORIES AND CLINICAL SETTINGS

Learning laboratories and clinical experiences remain cornerstones of nursing education. They afford learners hands-on experience in real-world healthcare environments, where students apply theoretical knowledge gained in the classroom to practical situations. These settings play a crucial role in the socialization of nursing students into the profession as students learn professional norms, values, and ethical standards by interacting with patients, families, healthcare teams, and educators (Oermann, 2022). In these learning spaces, students develop a deep understanding of nursing concepts, psychomotor skills, communication, teamwork, and leadership abilities necessary for professional practice.

Learning Laboratories

Learning laboratories, also known as resource centers or skills laboratories, provide safe environments for students to develop psychomotor skills and become acquainted with the professional role of the nurse (Durham & Baker, 2022). Learning laboratories are sometimes referred to as on-campus clinical experiences, highlighting similarities with clinical practice settings, since they promote foundational knowledge, skills, and attitudes essential for nursing practice. Educators in learning laboratories help students understand that psychomotor skills are one aspect of nursing practice, but critical thinking, judgment, and sound decision-making are also emphasized (Durham & Baker, 2022). Through guided practice and supervision focused on patient safety and quality care, students are facilitated in achieving learning competencies (Perez-Perdomo & Zabalegui, 2024).

Much like the clinical experience, a successful learning laboratory should be integrated throughout the curriculum, offering students regular opportunities for deliberate practice. Skills acquisition occurs in a psychologically safe environment, where the focus is on learning without fear of negative consequences. Collaboration is key, with students and educators sharing responsibility for learner competencies. Learning laboratory educators provide opportunities for repeated practice and feedback ensures skill retention (Durham & Baker, 2022). Many learning laboratories incorporate simulations using computerized manikins and virtual reality (VR) tools, which enhance learning and application to realistic patient care scenarios. Simulations and VR are discussed in more detail in Chapter 9.

Clinical Experiences

Clinical experiences provide a bridge between classroom learning, learning laboratories, and professional nursing practice, equipping students with knowledge, skills, and attitudes needed to provide safe and competent care (Arkan et al., 2018; Gcawu & van Rooyen, 2022). By actively engaging in patient care under the guidance of experienced clinical educators and preceptors, students develop essential clinical competencies, critical thinking abilities, and decision-making skills. Clinical experiences immerse students in diverse patient populations, healthcare settings, and interdisciplinary teamwork, expanding their perspectives and preparing them to deliver holistic, patient-centered care. Students cultivate professionalism, empathy, and resilience, shaping them into confident and compassionate nurses prepared for the challenges of current healthcare environments (Al-Daken et al., 2024).

Given that the clinical environment is an essential component of nursing education and resources and sites are limited, clinical teachers must maximize learning opportunities. To do this, they must exhibit highly effective clinical teaching behaviors. Without skilled clinical teachers, students may develop poor habits and feel disconnected from theory. Effective clinical educators bridge theory–practice gaps, instill meaning in learning, and boost student confidence (Al-Daken et al., 2024; Arkan et al., 2018). They foster problem-solving, decision-making, reflective skills, creative thinking, and skill development for students (Munangatire et al., 2023). As such, clinical teachers are fundamental in students' clinical experiences, influencing learning outcomes regardless of available experiences.

PRINCIPLES OF EFFECTIVE CLINICAL TEACHING

Key principles underpin effective clinical teaching in nursing. First, educators must establish a supportive learning environment where students can actively and safely apply their knowledge through patient care engagement and critical reflection. Clinical teachers need to ensure integration of current research and best practices into their own actions and decision-making processes as well as those of their students. They must guide students in fostering critical thinking and clinical reasoning, helping them to analyse patient situations and make sound judgments based on evidence. Clinical teachers cultivate professionalism and ethical practice, instilling in students the professional values, ethical standards, and accountability necessary for responsible nursing practice (McNeill et al., 2023; Oermann, 2022).

Establishing a supportive learning environment is vital in the clinical environment. This entails creating an atmosphere where students feel not only comfortable, but actively participate in their own learning journey. Students should feel safe to ask questions, voice concerns, and engage in discussions without fear of judgment. Moreover, educators should foster an atmosphere where students feel supported and making mistakes is viewed as a part of the learning process rather than a failure (Juan et al., 2023). Clinical teachers should reassure students that the role of the clinical teacher is not just to evaluate, but rather to educate, mentor, and help students learn (Hamaideh et al., 2024; Stubin, 2021). Keeping clinical feedback instructional and not overly personal or critical can increase student motivation to learn (Oermann et al., 2022). By cultivating a supportive learning environment, educators can facilitate greater student engagement, foster confidence, and promote deeper learning experiences that prepare students for the challenges of professional nursing practice.

Research suggests that effective clinical teachers exhibit a variety of behaviors to foster student learning. Knox and Mogan's (1985) seminal study reported that effective clinical teaching behaviors fall within the categories of (a) nursing competence, (b) teaching ability, (c) interpersonal relations, (d) personality traits, and (e) evaluation skills. Nursing competence involves having up-to-date knowledge and effectively communicating it to students to promote clinical judgment. Teaching abilities include helping students organize care and being well-prepared and organized. Interpersonal relations are demonstrated through mutual respect, active listening, and supportive yet challenging interactions. Personal characteristics include approachability, enthusiasm, humility, and a sense of humor. Evaluation skills reflect fair and constructive feedback aimed at facilitating learning (Knox & Mogan, 1985).

Adopting evidence-based teaching practices in the clinical environment is key to both teacher and student success. Research has shown that thoughtfully orienting students to the clinical setting, planning for each clinical day, engaging in ongoing student assessment, possessing emotional intelligence, and role-modeling professional practice are essential (Abdelkader et al., 2021; Gcawu & van Rooyen, 2022;

Mosca, 2019). Collaboration between clinical and classroom faculty is also vital to the academic success of students and a consistent, positive learning environment (Al-Daken et al., 2024).

As adult consumers of education, nursing students hold expectations of clinical learning. Munangatire et al. (2023) note that when student expectations and their actual experiences do not align, learning is hampered. Thus, clinical faculty must ensure that they assess student expectations while helping them apply theory to practice and develop reflection skills (Munangatire et al., 2023). However, underrepresented minority students experience a unique intersectionality of roles and challenges in the clinical setting, which includes the scarcity of role models in nursing from similar backgrounds and feelings of not belonging (Woodley & Lewallen, 2020). Therefore, clinical teachers must prioritize creating a supportive environment where *all* students feel valued. By being dedicated to student success and showing genuine interest in each student, clinical teachers foster positive faculty–student relationships and model key nursing values of caring, compassion, and empathy (Woodley & Lewallen, 2020).

MODELS OF CLINICAL TEACHING

Traditional models of clinical teaching in prelicensure nursing programs involve one clinical teacher with a small group of around six to 10 students. These experiences typically take place within inpatient settings, but can also incorporate long-term care environments, outpatient areas, and community-based settings. The shortage of clinical teachers and clinical sites provides the impetus for exploring alternate, novel models of clinical instruction.

Innovative models of clinical teaching in non traditional settings offer diverse and immersive opportunities for student learning and skill development. Simulations in the learning laboratory, discussed further in Chapter 9, use equipment and realistic scenarios to replicate clinical situations in a controlled, safe environment. These experiences promote practice of clinical skills and decision-making under realistic conditions and integrate skills related to diversity, equity, and inclusion (Daya et al., 2023; Durham & Baker, 2022). Integrating simulations at all education levels improves clinical reasoning skills and patient care quality (Perez-Perdomo & Zabalegui, 2024). VR and augmented reality (AR) technologies are immersive, where students practice clinical skills and decision-making virtually in settings that closely resemble real-world healthcare (Pardue et al., 2023).

Telehealth clinical experiences foster student engagement with patient consultations, telemonitoring, and telemedicine visits. For example, students may participate in virtual clinic sessions where they interact with patients via video-conferencing technology, conduct assessments, and collaborate with healthcare providers to develop care plans (Dzioba et al., 2022). This virtual interaction not only builds telecommunication skills, but also prepares students for the increasing digitalization of healthcare services.

Community-based learning projects immerse students in population health initiatives, such as health screenings, health education programs, and community outreach events. Students may work with public health departments, community clinics, and non profit organizations to address healthcare disparities and promote health education in underserved communities (Brennan et al., 2024). These experiences enrich students' understanding of social determinants of health and the importance of community engagement in public health.

Experiential learning projects involve students in research, quality improvement initiatives, and case studies, providing hands-on experience in healthcare innovation and problem-solving. Students may participate in research projects exploring healthcare disparities, quality improvement projects aimed at enhancing patient safety, or case studies analyzing complex patient cases and treatment options. Through these projects, students can apply theoretical knowledge in real-world settings.

Global health clinical experiences offer students the opportunity to participate in international clinical rotations, medical missions, and cultural immersion programs. For example, students may travel to low-resource environments to provide healthcare services to underserved populations, participate in health education initiatives, and learn about global health challenges and solutions. These experiences broaden student understanding of global health issues and healthcare systems while promoting cultural humility. Reflective journaling during this type of experience can be especially powerful in fostering the development of student cultural competencies (Massarelli, 2023).

Preceptorship models with undergraduate students can take place in a wide variety of settings and can serve as a complement to a traditional clinical experience or as a stand-alone opportunity. For instance, students in a traditional inpatient pediatric setting can spend a portion of their clinical time in other practice areas. Examples can include a 1-day preceptorship experience in a pediatric critical care setting, a primary care clinic, or a perioperative setting. These experiences expose students to different aspects of the patient care trajectory, a wide variety of nursing roles, and a glimpse into potential career interest areas. Rosli et al. (2022) note that preceptored clinical models play an important role in nursing students' professional socialization, fostering responsibility, confidence, skill acquisition and facilitating student transition to practice.

Remote preceptorships connect students with experienced practitioners in rural or underserved areas, engaging them in direct patient care under supervision or via telecommunication technology. These models of clinical teaching enhance student independence and prepare them for the complexities of health disparities and patient-centered care (Chicca & Shellenbarger, 2021). Additionally, they offer a unique opportunity for students to learn adaptability, and resourcefulness in diverse healthcare environments, further enriching their clinical competencies and cultural sensitivity.

PROCESS OF CLINICAL TEACHING

Clinical teaching includes identifying learning outcomes, assessment of learner needs, planning clinical activities, guiding students, and providing feedback (Oermann et al., 2022). Clinical evaluation is discussed in Chapter 17.

Learning Outcomes

Intended learning outcomes for students relate to three domains of learning: cognitive, psychomotor, and affective learning. Cognitive learning reflects students' growing knowledge level, ability to engage in clinical reasoning and problem-solving, development of higher-level thinking skills, and capacity to relate their knowledge to the care that they are providing (Oermann et al., 2022). Faculty can foster cognitive learning outcomes through engaging in patient-centered discussions, prompting students to consider multiple perspectives, posing rigorous yet supportive questions teaching students how to *think* rather than memorize, and offering frequent, specific feedback on knowledge application (Juan et al., 2023).

Psychomotor learning reflects students' skill acquisition, including the ability to perform skills in a safe, effective, and accurate manner (Oermann et al., 2022). Psychomotor learning outcomes are fostered by clinical teacher role modeling and hands-on practice. Through group simulations and practice sessions, students enhance their organization, priority setting, and time-management skills, complemented by role modeling and resource sharing.

Affective learning involves the development of professional attitudes, beliefs, and values that are an integral part of nursing practice (Oermann et al., 2022). Faculty provide clear expectations and directions, role-model professional behaviors, and leverage their interpersonal skills to develop and challenge students within the affective domain of learning (Hamaideh et al., 2024; Stubin, 2021). This nurturing of the affective domain is crucial for fostering empathetic, ethical, and responsive nursing professionals who are well-prepared to meet the emotional and psychological needs of their patients.

Apart from the planned learning outcomes, students may also experience unintended learning outcomes during clinical experiences. These outcomes can be positive, like sparking interest in a specialty area, or negative, such as loss of confidence or disengagement. These outcomes heavily depend on the clinical teacher's interactions with students in the clinical setting (Stubin, 2021).

Learner Needs Assessments

Creating an effective learning experience in the clinical setting begins with assessing individual learner characteristics and learning needs. Nurse educators work with students from various backgrounds, cultures, ethnicities, genders, ages, work experiences, and education levels. For example, clinical faculty in prelicensure programs may teach associate-degree students transitioning from licensed practical nurse (LPN) or medic roles, traditional baccalaureate students, and accelerated second-degree nursing students. Similarly, educators in APRN programs will teach students with diverse work, life, and professional practice experience. Nurse educators need to explore how each student learns best, identify learning gaps, and provide guidance accordingly.

Planning Clinical Activities

Creating an Effective Learning Environment

Planning student activities in the clinical setting begins with creating a safe and enjoyable learning environment. As clinical teachers orient themselves to the clinical environment and patient population, they develop collaborative relationships with staff, establish a partnership before the course even begins, and establish clear expectations. It is important to recognize that teachers and students are guests in the healthcare setting and interactions with staff should reflect this.

Clinical Orientation

A well-planned student orientation is one in which the clinical teacher establishes a positive, well-organized learning environment. For instance, if the teacher arrives late, lacks prepared materials, and fails to engage students, they may appear disorganized and uncaring. This can make students uncertain about expectations or hesitant to ask questions. Before or during orientation, the teacher should share resources such as clinical expectations, the clinical schedule, an outline of a typical day in the setting, descriptions of assignments, documentation examples, site- and specialty-dependent resources, and the clinical evaluation tool.

Clinical orientation provides an opportunity for teachers to get to know students individually and establish the climate of the group. Clinical teachers should clearly communicate the expectation that students will learn from and support each other to prevent competition and group polarization. In settings where teachers are off-site, orientation discussions should emphasize the importance of communication, outlining when and how students should contact faculty and what to expect during site visits. Table 10.1 provides some key questions to ask students during orientation.

TABLE 10.1 SAMPLE QUESTIONS WITH RATIONALES FOR USE IN CLINICAL ORIENTATION

What are students excited and nervous about as they begin this clinical experience?	- Encourages students to share personal perceptions and promotes affective learning. - Establishes the clinical group and setting as a safe learning environment. - Highlights the significance of student engagement and transparency in the teacher–student relationship.
What are the students' expectations of the clinical teacher or preceptor?	- Facilitates open discussion about student expectations. - Enhances group cohesiveness. - Clarifies potential misconceptions. - Establishes a partnership learning climate with shared responsibility between students and teacher.

What are the clinical teacher's or preceptor's expectations of students in the clinical setting?	- Presents the educator's expectations after student expectations are addressed.
	- Saves valuable time during the clinical experience.
	- Topics to cover include:
	  • Clinical preparation
	  • Supervision requirements
	  • Learning activities
	  • Non patient care activities
	  • Prohibited skills and behaviors
	  • Practicum activity progression

(continued)

TABLE 10.1 SAMPLE QUESTIONS WITH RATIONALES FOR USE IN CLINICAL ORIENTATION (continued)

What are the ways in which individual students in the clinical setting learn best?	▪ Communicates care for individual students. ▪ Respects students as unique, adult learners. ▪ Encourages students to reflect on their learning styles or preferences. ▪ Promotes accountability for their own learning.
Are individual students visual, auditory, and/or kinesthetic learners?	▪ Guides clinical teachers in tailoring teaching methods to individual student learning styles or preferences.
What is at least one personal goal that each student has in terms of this clinical experience?	▪ Helps students guide their own learning, promoting personal and professional growth. Asking students about their personal goals helps them become personally invested in their learning.

EXHIBIT 10.1 Sample Clinical Guidelines to Share with Students in Orientation

Clinical teacher contact information

Clinical site contact numbers

Clinical site information (short description of the clinical setting where students are practicing, including phone number, typical patient population, types of common patient and family problems, common interventions, typical staffing, etc.)

Procedure for absence or lateness

Clinical practice preparation (process, student and teacher roles, clinical worksheets, pre-conferences, etc.)

Expected student behaviors (important actions if unsure about care, treatments, or have questions; need for communication and sharing pertinent information about patient with educator, preceptor, staff; dress code and why important; new orders and process; documentation; etc.)

Written assignments and submission information

Given the volume of information shared during orientation, providing a printed or electronic copy of key faculty expectations is helpful, as students may not remember all verbal details. Exhibit 10.1 includes sample guidelines to share with students during clinical orientation. Morandini (2022) recommends using screencasting technology to create a video for clinical preparation, offering visual and verbal guidance on patient care flow, guidelines, and role expectations. This approach supports students' learning by boosting their confidence and preparedness.

Orientation to the clinical setting should include discussion of the clinical agency's electronic medical record (EMR) and documentation system. If students are not able to document care in the EMR, the clinical teacher or preceptor should review the school's documentation process for that clinical experience. Many nursing programs teach students to document care in academic EMR applications.

Selecting Clinical Assignments

Clinical teachers align patient assignments and clinical activities with intended learning competencies and achievement of clinical objectives. While students often focus on specific psychomotor skill practice, clinical teachers ensure a more comprehensive approach to learning including consideration of patient diagnoses, backgrounds, and health histories. Opportunities for interdisciplinary communication, patient advocacy, ethical discussions, and family-centered care are invaluable. Tracking student experiences in a simple spreadsheet helps ensure varied learning experiences. Selection of patient assignments can be faculty led, student directed depending on learner experience, or take a shared approach (Mella, 2021). Soliciting student input into patient assignment fosters collaboration, respect, and mutual trust.

Clinical teachers should explore alternative patient assignment approaches beyond the traditional one-student-to-one-patient option. In an inpatient setting, students can work in pairs to care for a more complex patient, or care for a group of more stable patients. Students can engage in learning leadership or management skills through shadowing charge nurses or acting in a mock charge nurse role with their peers. In outpatient settings, students can work in small groups to assess and screen communities and engage in service learning. Peer teaching and mentoring programs can pair students with more advanced peers or healthcare professionals to promote collaboration and knowledge exchange.

The use of specific and individualized forms where clinical teachers post patient assignments in a clinical setting prevents miscommunication and promotes coordinated care across the healthcare team. These forms should include teacher contact information, student schedules, and designated activities for the day while clarifying that staff nurses remain the primary patient caregivers. Clinical teachers must be mindful of patient privacy laws and avoid sharing identifying details on assignment forms. An example patient assignment form for hospital or long-term care settings is available in Exhibit 10.2 and can be adapted for other models of clinical teaching.

In some locations within the United States, boards of nursing outline specific skills that students may not perform under any circumstances. Clinical nurse educators should be aware of this information to avoid putting the student, patient, family, staff members, or themselves at risk. Learning objectives should become more complex as students progress through a given clinical course and throughout the nursing program. Patient assignments and other clinical learning activities

---

EXHIBIT 10.2 Sample Nursing Student Assignment Sheet for a Prelicensure Program

School of Nursing

Course Number and Name

Clinical Teacher, Credentials

Email Address and Contact Phone Number

Dates of Care:

Clinical Activities: Nursing students are responsible for the following activities: Basic care of the assigned patient including hygiene, assisting with patient nutrition, vital signs, intake and output, and assessments. The assigned staff nurse remains the primary caregiver for the patient.

Clinical Hours:

should reflect this increasing complexity and this information should be communicated clearly to students and staff.

Organization for Faculty and Students

Organization is crucial for a smooth clinical experience, especially given the multiple responsibilities clinical teachers and preceptors have to students, patients, and healthcare teams. Being well-prepared for the clinical experience, selecting appropriate learning activities, and providing clear directions are essential strategies. Providing guidance on how students can access support, such as through a pager system or texting, enhances communication and organization. The better organized and prepared clinical teachers are, the more effective they will be as educators. Teachers can also provide students with tools to help them organize their patient care. Some clinical teachers provide students with course-specific tools, such as what information they need to know about their patients prior to engaging in their care. Other tools can also be used, such as time sequence plans to provide structure for the day's organization.

Clinical Conferences

Clinical conferences are vital for learning, problem-solving, and gaining insights into patient care. When structured well, they reinforce the clinical setting as a safe learning environment, enabling students to reflect on their experiences and enhance clinical judgment (Kelly et al., 2019). Clinical educators should establish a collaborative team dynamic, fostering an atmosphere where students can freely ask questions, challenge ideas, and engage in respectful debate. Encouraging high-level questioning during group conferences stimulates student engagement and teamwork. If students struggle with higher-level questions, clinical teachers can rephrase and transition to lower-level questions to boost confidence. Clinical conferences may occur in person during or at the end of the clinical day, depending on the clinical experience model, or on a different day in a face-to-face or virtual format.

Preconference

Preconferences, a type of clinical conference held before patient care, serve multiple purposes. They allow clinical teachers to assess students' knowledge and understanding of patients, foster critical thinking, and encourage group discussion. Teachers ask questions to develop students' thinking skills and apply theory to practice, while also facilitating discussions on nursing priorities, anticipated outcomes, and potential scenarios. Focused discussions on students' assigned patients facilitate comparisons of individuals, their support systems, and situations, aiding in understanding patients' experiences at different illness stages. Students can also assess the impact of family, culture, or health trajectories. During preconference, clinical teachers may assign student buddies for the day, where students learn about each other's patient(s), provide support, report to each other for breaks, and gain additional patient exposure. Preconferences can offer students the chance to briefly present their assigned patients to the group, helping them practice conciseness and develop verbal handoff skills. Finally, clinical teachers can use preconference time to check on their students' well-being, address practical issues, and plan for the day.

Postconference

Postconferences offer a variety of learning opportunities. While they commonly occur at the end of the clinical day, timing should be chosen thoughtfully to maximize learning. Factors like student fatigue and avoiding distractions from patient care should be considered. Online postconferences conducted asynchronously after the clinical practicum may allow students more time for reflection but may be difficult to schedule (Hannans, 2019).

Postconferences provide students with the opportunity to debrief, addressing challenging experiences or unanswered questions (Kelly et al., 2019; Oermann et al., 2022). Strategies like role-playing, active listening, peer feedback, and group discussions offer support and stimulate learning. Clinical teachers can guide reflection with questions such as, "What would you do differently and why?" or "How will today's learnings influence your future clinical practice?" Kelly et al. (2019) recommend that clinical nurse educators follow similar debriefing standards as those used in simulations, where critical feedback is shared while safeguarding the feelings of learners.

Postconferences offer many opportunities for student learning. Students can share clinical perspectives, teach each other, build confidence, and foster teamwork. Assignments may involve presenting patients and comparing care with published evidence, while peers ask the student presenter questions. These activities foster problem-solving and oral communication skills that nurses need to successfully engage in healthcare team discussions. Table 10.2 outlines a variety of additional creative strategies for use in clinical postconferences (Hensel et al., 2020; Kelly et al., 2019; Oermann, 2022).

Written Clinical Assignments

Written clinical assignments can cater to a variety of learning objectives in clinical practice. Cognitive learning can be fostered through concise written assignments with guided questions aligned with clinical objectives, where students are asked to appraise patient safety, develop a plan for developmental needs, or plan a patient teaching session. To promote affective learning outcomes, students may be asked to write journal reflections on their patient interactions, including what went well, what did not, changes for future practice, and impactful events during the experience (Massarelli, 2023). Besides facilitating exploration of clinical situations, these assignments also hone writing skills and the capacity to articulate ideas clearly and succinctly (Oermann, 2022).

Clinical Site Visits for Prelicensure Students

In the final semester of many prelicensure nursing programs, students engage in precepted experiences with registered nurses. Clinical site visits are crucial for monitoring student progress, providing feedback, and ensuring competency development. Close collaboration among the clinical teacher, preceptor, and student is essential for meeting course objectives and fostering skill application to patient care. Consistency in site visits, including timing, frequency, and interactions, is vital for effective evaluation and feedback. During site visits, faculty and preceptors can provide feedback and formative evaluations to support student learning and development. Yun et al. (2022) note the need for preceptor education, support, and two-way feedback to improve quality of patient care and lessen the transition shock for new graduates.

Before or during the initial site visit, the clinical teacher should establish communication preferences among the educator, preceptor, and student. They should also review course outcomes, competencies, expectations, and evaluation tools. When feasible, subsequent visits aim to observe preceptor–student interactions. Site visits allow students to discuss patient care experiences, engage in higher-level questioning to promote critical thinking, and identify areas for improvement and personal

TABLE 10.2 STRATEGIES TO ENHANCE STUDENT LEARNING DURING CLINICAL POSTCONFERENCES

Strategy	Explanation and Rationale
Pass the Problem	<ul><li>Students present a clinical situation or problem they encountered.</li><li>Another student analyzes the presented situation.</li><li>A third student critiques the analysis provided.</li><li>This strategy, when conducted supportively and openly, fosters critical thinking and highlights the significance of multiple solutions to clinical problems.</li></ul>
One-Minute Care Plan	<ul><li>Students draw an algorithm related to their patient's care.</li><li>They identify nursing priorities and track their progress throughout the day.</li><li>Students then share their ideas with their peers.</li><li>This activity encourages creativity among students.</li></ul>
Online Tools for Reflections	<ul><li>Utilize platforms like futureme.org™ (www.futureme.org) where students can write reflections as letters to themselves.</li><li>Letters are scheduled for delivery via email at a future date.</li><li>This exercise enables students to reflect on their clinical experiences, fears, or aspirations.</li><li>Upon rereading the letter at a later date, students can observe their professional growth by comparing their initial thoughts to their current perspectives.</li></ul>
Clinical Cases	<ul><li>Present opening case scenarios to students, followed by additional patient information as they respond.</li><li>Cases foster group teamwork and boost students' self-confidence.</li><li>Walking students through a clinical judgment model within a case allows them to recognize and analyze patient cues, prioritize hypotheses, generate solutions, take action, and evaluate outcomes.</li><li>Cases provide a safe environment for students to learn clinical judgment skills and receive feedback.</li></ul>
Nursing Rounds	<ul><li>During nursing rounds, students present their patients and the care they have provided to peers, clinical teachers, staff nurses, and/or other healthcare professionals.</li><li>Nursing rounds facilitate learning to confidently and concisely present information about patients, advocate for them, collaborate with the healthcare team, ask questions, and consider various approaches to care.</li></ul>

(continued)

TABLE 10.2 STRATEGIES TO ENHANCE STUDENT LEARNING DURING CLINICAL POSTCONFERENCES (continued)

Strategy	Explanation and Rationale
Student Presentations	- Encourage students to share key points about their patients from previous experiences, highlighting one aspect of nursing care that intrigued them. - Students retrieve a nursing article related to evidence-based practice concerning the highlighted aspect of nursing care and compare it with their observed or engaged care. - Foster critical thinking by having other students pose questions to the presenter or allow the presenter to ask questions of the group. - Enhances students' cognitive skills and self-confidence during communication.
Lab Blitzes	- Utilize occasional clinical conferences for group discussions on key patient data, like poorly understood laboratory results. - Employ creative strategies during laboratory blitzes, such as reviewing EMR records confidentially in a private group space to apply content. - Task students with analyzing the results, determining potential diagnoses, and identifying nursing priorities based on the laboratory data.
Ten Key Questions to Ask Yourself About Your Patient	- Encourage students to ask each other about varying aspects of their patients, such as priorities, medications, lab results, diagnostics, and other examples. - Fosters a deeper understanding of various aspects of patient care and implications through guided inquiry and discussion.

goals. Confidential meetings among faculty, students, or and/or preceptors can also be arranged during site visits as needed.

Feedback in the Clinical Setting

Prompt, specific, and regular feedback, both verbal and written, is critical to the learning process and allows students to correct mistakes before they become patterns. This approach ensures fair summative evaluations, reduces student anxiety, and fosters a mentoring environment. Effective feedback incorporates specificity, transparency, honesty, and encouragement. Rather than simply pointing out shortcomings, teachers should provide balanced feedback that acknowledges strengths and areas for improvement. Feedback should remain instructional rather than punitive, since teacher observations can be a significant stressor for nursing students. Feedback should be delivered sensitively, avoiding public settings or situations that may cause the student to feel criticized, such as in front of patients, peers, or staff (Toqan et al., 2023; Yildirim & Terzioglu, 2022).

TABLE 10.3 EXAMPLE OF iSoBAR FORMAT FOR GIVING FEEDBACK

After observing a beginning student perform a bed bath, a clinical educator might provide this feedback:

Identify	"As your clinical instructor, I'd like to take a moment to review your care of Mr. X."
Situation	"As we discussed, providing personal hygiene for a patient is a deeply personal and an important role for the nurse."
Observations	"I noticed that you were respectful of Mr. X and asked him if this was a good time for his bath. I also saw that you took great care in ensuring his comfort and privacy while you cleaned him."
Background	"As we discussed in orientation, you need to complete a bed bath on a variety of patients during this practicum so that you can gain confidence and competence in carrying out this skill."
Agreed Plan	"Next week, let's plan on you caring for a patient who will be able to help less with their care, so that you can continue building on these skills."
Read-Back	Confirm with the student their understanding of the plan.

iSoBAR, identify, situation, observations, background, agreed plan, read-back.

Russell (2019) proposes providing feedback throughout the learning process using the iSoBAR framework. The iSoBAR acronym stands for **i**dentify (introducing your role in providing student feedback), **s**ituation (why you are giving feedback), **o**bservations (giving examples from the student's clinical practice), **b**ackground (how the feedback relates to clinical learning objectives or planned learning), **a**greed plan (for continued learning), and **r**ead-back (confirming that the student has understood the feedback and plan; Russell, 2019). Table 10.3 provides an iSoBAR feedback example.

In clinical experiences where the teacher is not on site, additional support and feedback are crucial from both the teacher and the preceptor. The preceptor, working directly with the student, should offer immediate feedback during observations and during a debriefing session at the end of the day. This session should encompass overall performance feedback, achieved goals, and future objectives. Trust and open communication among the student, preceptor, and clinical teacher are requisite for providing effective feedback.

OVERCOMING COMMON CHALLENGES IN CLINICAL TEACHING

Clinical teachers have a responsibility not only to their students, but also to patients, families, communities, and the nursing profession to prepare skilled graduates ready for today's healthcare arena. Unfortunately, many clinical teachers lack formal preparation for their teaching role. Teachers may possess clinical competence and hold a graduate degree related to APRN but lack experience or formal training in *how* to teach or thrive in an academic setting. Furthermore, an overall shortage of nurse faculty, which is a major contributing factor to the current global nursing shortage, means that the recruitment and retention of effective full-time clinical faculty with current clinical expertise is difficult (Margolis et al., 2024; McPherson, 2019). As a result, nursing programs are turning to many part-time and adjunct faculty to teach students in clinical and learning laboratory settings. Unless these clinical faculty are well mentored and supported, they may leave their new role, perpetuating the faculty shortage (McPherson, 2019).

Challenges can arise for clinical teachers in nursing. For example, generational differences among educators and students requires adaptability. Clinical teachers may find themselves teaching multiple generations of students simultaneously, such as Millennial students craving highly stimulating learning environments and opportunities to multitask, digitally native Generation Z students known for quick decision-making, and baby boomers pursuing nursing as a second or third career (Hampton et al., 2020; Lewis-Pierre, 2019; Licas & Torres, 2024; Williams, 2019). Nurse educators must appraise and integrate generational characteristics, learner backgrounds, values, work styles, and technological proficiencies while using innovative and creative approaches for effective student engagement.

Stress can pose a significant challenge in the clinical environment for both students and clinical teachers. Student stress is associated with fear of making a mistake, unrealistic performance expectations, and personal challenges (Hamaideh et al., 2024; Toqan et al., 2023). Non native speakers of the school's language, especially international students, face added stress in clinical placements due to language and cultural differences (Lim et al., 2023). High stress levels impede students' capacity to concentrate, make sound clinical decisions, and interact effectively with patients and healthcare teams (Hamaideh et al., 2024) Unchecked, this stress may lead to burnout, decreased motivation, decreased quality of life, lower academic performance, uncertainty about professional identity, and compromised mental health among students (Araújo et al., 2023; Hamaideh et al., 2024).

Identifying and addressing student stress allows clinical teachers to offer suitable support, resources, and interventions that foster resilience and promote positive learning outcomes. Clinical teachers can alleviate stress among non native student speakers by fostering a nurturing environment, using a strength-based approach, facilitating transcultural socialization opportunities, and demonstrating acceptance of students' cultural and language backgrounds (Lim et al., 2023). Given that clinical teachers' own actions and behaviors can also affect student stress levels, educators should be mindful of these interactions and how their communication impacts students. Clinical teachers who foster a supportive, respectful, and interpersonal environment reduce student stress and enhance student success (Stubin, 2021). Toqan et al. (2023) emphasize that clinical settings should be viewed as opportunities for learning more than a stage for evaluating theoretical knowledge.

Student stress is linked to emotional intelligence (Yildirim & Terzioglu, 2022). Clinical faculty help nursing students manage their emotions by fostering in-person and online spaces where students candidly discuss challenging situations with peers and faculty (Yildirim & Terzioglu, 2022). Nursing staff incivility can trigger heightened student emotions (Foreman, 2023). Clinical teachers should help vulnerable student groups navigate such behaviors by using methods like debriefing, role-playing, timely feedback, and post-conference discussions (Foreman, 2023).

Clinical teachers also face stressors in the clinical setting. Table 10.4 outlines some of these stressors, along with suggestions to mitigate them (Gcawu & van

TABLE 10.4 FACULTY STRESSORS IN THE CLINICAL SETTING AND ACTIONS FOR MITIGATION

Faculty Stressors in the Clinical Setting	Actions for Mitigation
Managing Large Clinical Groups	▪ Plan clinical sessions in advance. ▪ Break down the groups into smaller, manageable subgroups considering the students' levels of experience and any specific learning needs. ▪ Clearly communicate expectations to students regarding their roles, responsibilities, and behavior during clinical sessions. ▪ Utilize peer teaching and collaborative learning among students. ▪ Delegate tasks to experienced students or clinical assistants. ▪ Organize student activities and rotations to maximize efficiency.
Time Constraints in Short Clinical Rotations	▪ Prioritize learning objectives and focus on essential skills. ▪ Streamline documentation processes to save time. ▪ Use simulation labs or virtual clinical experiences to supplement short rotations. ▪ Provide pre clinical preparation to optimize time spent in clinical settings.
Balancing Student Learning With Patient Safety	▪ Emphasize the importance of patient safety in all clinical activities. ▪ Set clear expectations for student behavior and responsibilities. ▪ Supervise closely and intervene when necessary to ensure patient safety. ▪ Provide opportunities for reflection and debriefing after clinical experiences.
Being Viewed as Visitors in Their Clinical Teaching Setting	▪ Build rapport with clinical staff through effective communication and collaboration. ▪ Demonstrate expertise and professionalism in clinical teaching. ▪ Offer to assist with clinical duties when appropriate to integrate into the clinical environment. ▪ Advocate for the value of nursing education and its role in improving patient care.
Lacking Formal Teaching Preparation	▪ Seek professional development opportunities in teaching and instructional design. ▪ Collaborate with experienced educators or mentors for guidance and support. ▪ Utilize resources such as textbooks, online courses, and workshops focused on teaching in clinical settings.

(continued)

TABLE 10.4 FACULTY STRESSORS IN THE CLINICAL SETTING AND ACTIONS FOR MITIGATION (continued)

Faculty Stressors in the Clinical Setting	Actions for Mitigation
Teaching Outside Primary Area of Clinical Expertise	▪ Update knowledge and skills through continuing education and self-study. ▪ Collaborate with colleagues or experts in the specific area for guidance. ▪ Focus on fundamental nursing principles and critical thinking skills applicable across specialties.
Having Students Being Used as Nursing Staff Rather Than Focusing on Their Learning Needs	▪ Advocate for clear delineation between student learning activities and nursing staff responsibilities. ▪ Communicate with clinical staff and administrators about the importance of protecting students' learning time. ▪ Provide guidance and support to students in navigating their roles in clinical settings.
Witnessing Student and Staff Conflict	▪ Address conflicts promptly and objectively. ▪ Facilitate open communication and active listening among all parties involved. ▪ Provide conflict resolution training or resources for students and staff. ▪ Foster a supportive and respectful learning environment.
Working With Poorly Prepared and Failing Students	▪ Offer additional support and resources for struggling students, such as tutoring or remediation programs. ▪ Provide constructive feedback and guidance for improvement. ▪ Collaborate with academic advisors or support services to address underlying issues affecting student performance.
Fulfilling Lengthy Organizational Compliance Requirements	▪ Develop efficient systems for documentation and compliance tracking. ▪ Delegate tasks related to compliance when possible. ▪ Advocate for streamlined processes or resources to support compliance efforts. ▪ Prioritize tasks based on urgency and impact on patient care and student learning.
Receiving Less Than Desirable Compensation and Teaching Contracts	▪ Advocate for fair compensation and benefits through professional organizations or unions. ▪ Negotiate for improved terms in teaching contracts, such as workload, schedule, and compensation. ▪ Consider the overall satisfaction and rewards derived from teaching as motivation during challenging times.

Rooyen, 2022; Margolis et al., 2024; McPherson, 2019; Oermann et al., 2022; Ryan & McAllister, 2020; Yang & Chao, 2018).

The COVID-19 pandemic heightened stress levels of students and faculty alike in the clinical setting, requiring clinical teachers to be flexible and adapt creative teaching methodologies in response to suspension of training in-person (Al-Rawajfah et al., 2022; McKay et al., 2022). Students faced heightened anxiety and stress related to remote learning, lockdown measures, and anticipation of entering the nursing workforce during the pandemic, requiring clinical teachers to provide psychological support (Al-Rawajfah et al., 2022). The stress during this period also impacted clinical faculty, many of whom were simultaneously working at the bedside, leading to significant pressure from their dual roles. Adaptability and flexibility from both students and faculty were essential for a smooth transition to remote learning. Faculty used innovative teaching methods, such as virtual and computer-based simulations with, in some cases, faculty-created storyboards or unfolding cases to provide context for learning (Hensel et al., 2020; Roberts & Mazurak, 2022). Technology leveraged for virtual clinical content focused on helping students achieve learning outcomes (Roberts & Mazurak, 2022). Despite the stress, faculty found joy in positive teaching experiences and student learning during the pandemic, fostering deeper connections with students (Al-Rawajfah et al., 2022; McKay et al., 2022).

ADVANCED PRACTICE REGISTERED NURSE CLINICAL TEACHING CONSIDERATIONS

While the planning of the clinical experiences for the APRN has similarities to the prelicensure student, there are some distinct considerations. The experience with the clinical preceptor is a fundamental component of the educational experience for the APRN student (American Association of Colleges of Nursing [AACN], 2021a). The clinical experience provides the opportunity for APRN students to translate the knowledge learned in the classroom to their experience providing direct patient care (Gigli et al., 2022; Pleshkan, 2024). Working one-on-one with a preceptor in the clinical setting, APRN students begin transitioning from their role as an RN to the APRN role where they gain practical experience with advanced physical assessment, clinical reasoning, and developing a plan of care, allowing them to develop competence in cognitive, psychomotor, and affective learning (AACN, 2021b). In the clinical setting, APRN students learn to function within the clinical team, gaining self-confidence, developing a professional identity, as well as a sense of professional belonging (AACN, 2021b).

APRNs are highly sought after in the U.S. job market, with an expected growth rate of 38% between 2022 and 2032 (United States Bureau of Labor Statistics, 2023), thus requiring schools to be prepared for an influx of students. In the United States, APRN students are currently required to complete a minimum 500 practice hours (AACN, 2023). However, the American National Task Force's (NTF) 2022 Standards for Quality Nurse Practitioner Education has proposed increasing the direct clinical practice hours required for students to 750 hours (NTF, 2022). Unfortunately, a shortage of qualified preceptors is a primary limiting factor for schools of nursing increasing admissions of APRN students (Pleshkan, 2024). APRN preceptors cite many barriers to precepting students including time constraints in a busy clinical setting (Pleshkan, 2024), space limitations, limited access to EMRs, reduction in productivity, and lack of monetary compensation (Gigli et al., 2022; Hawkins, 2019; Pleshkan, 2024; Renda et al., 2022). Gigli et al. (2022) found that almost a third of nurse practitioners (NPs) surveyed reported that the employers did not allow them to precept. Furthermore, some NPs reported a lack of desire to precept, with over a third stating they had never been asked to do so (Gigli et al., 2022). On the other hand, additional barriers include exhaustion from continuous precepting and feeling overwhelmed by the sheer number of precepting requests (Miura et al., 2020).

Students, placement coordinators, and program directors face significant obstacles in securing clinical sites for APRN students. Larger hospital systems often pose greater challenges than smaller, privately owned practices due to existing contractual agreements (Hawkins, 2019). U.S. Medicare and Medicaid reimbursement structures prioritize medical resident placements over APRN students. Competition for sites is further intensified by other health professions students (medical students, physician assistant [PA] students), especially since preceptors are typically compensated for medical and PA students. Finally, non preceptor gatekeepers (practice managers) and complex administrative requirements within large systems increase the burden of securing placements (Hawkins, 2019).

To facilitate program expansion and accommodate more APRN students, barriers to finding appropriate preceptors must be addressed. Aside from the obvious financial compensation from schools, many preceptors desire incentives, such as access to university library privileges, presentation of current information about new medications and current clinical guidelines from students, and preceptor hour verification to count toward recertification hours (Miura et al., 2020; Renda et al., 2022). Additionally, many preceptors request formal preceptor education. Support from systems or practices includes increasing preceptor workload flexibility to spend more teaching time with students and facilitating student access and training within EMRs (Pleshkan, 2024). All incentives require an intentional multipronged approach to address the needs of more clinical sites and preceptors.

The National Organization of Nurse Practitioner Faculties (NONPF) and the American Association of Nurse Practitioners (AANP) joined forces to develop expectations around the clinical experience for the APRN (Pitts et al., 2019). They developed a checklist to guide preceptors and faculty to assist in providing a strong clinical experience to support the didactic portion of the program. The checklist includes recommendations for establishing the clinical rotation, orientation needs, clinical experience, communication, and evaluation.

In considering the course expectations and learning outcomes specific to the course, thoughtful and careful attention is required when selecting a site and preceptor. This requires that those making site and preceptor selections also have knowledge and understanding of student needs. For example, a beginning student or a student that requires a higher level of support may benefit from a site with a lower volume of patients (Pitts et al., 2019). Further, rotating students through diverse sites allows the students to experience a wide variety of populations (urban versus vs. rural, underserved and uninsured vs. adequately insured). Before the students arrive at the site, the school should provide the preceptor with the course syllabus, objectives, weekly schedule of topics, and preceptor expectations. Additionally, the preceptor should clearly communicate availability (start date and available days of the week) and expectations for professional attire. Finally, to enhance efficiency and develop competence in documentation and autonomous clinical decision-making, the preceptor and site director should arrange orientation to the EMR before the clinical rotation commences (Pleshkan, 2024).

Orientation to the site and the healthcare team will enhance success at the site. During orientation, the preceptor is encouraged to provide the student with a brief introduction about themselves and an introduction to the clinical team, site, and policies. It is also helpful to provide information about patient demographics, including most common diagnoses (Pitts et al., 2019; Pleshkan, 2024). Clinical teachers should guide APRN students in identifying learning needs so that the student and preceptor can create SMART (specific, measurable, achievable, relevant, time-based) learning goals for the rotation (Pitts et al., 2019; Theard et al., 2021). The preceptor and student can then negotiate progression from observation to increased independence with patient visits (Pitts et al., 2019).

Many factors coalesce to enhance the safety and connection in the learning environment. The preceptor can start each clinical experience by reviewing the patient schedule and recommending an appropriate caseload for the day (Pitts et al., 2019). Approachability of the preceptor is an important factor to foster a safe learning experience (Pitts et al., 2019; Pleshkan, 2024). Additionally, using a framework of growth mindset fosters a clinical experience that allows a student the opportunity to grow and thrive (Theard et al., 2021). In addition to creating learning goals for the student, expectations for progression should be clear and the preceptor and clinical teacher should clearly communicate how they will follow up with the learner. Seeking and providing active feedback on how to better support the student's needs and acknowledging their growth and effort can also foster a healthy and positive learning environment (Theard et al., 2021).

Numerous reliable strategies exist for the preceptor to build the skills, competencies, and confidence of the student learner. For the beginning student, modeling and observation may be effective. In this situation, the preceptor models clinical skills and professional behaviors while the student observes how a preceptor approaches patients and starts the conversation. As the student progresses, the preceptor can assess the ability of the student to obtain a patient history, report pertinent physical exam findings, generate differential diagnoses, choose diagnostic tests, and determine a plan of care with the use of case presentations. Direct questioning may be useful to assess and enhance clinical reasoning skills (Mallinson, 2021). The preceptor may also encourage the student to think aloud to reflect and verbalize rationales for making clinical decisions. Coaching is also helpful when the preceptor guides a student through a procedure.

Clinical faculty-graded case analyses improve the APRN student's ability to analyze a case according to current evidence-based guidelines and articulate the evidence base for practice decisions. This requires a collaborative effort between the student, clinical faculty, and preceptor. Clinical faculty can have students use reflective journaling to supplement the clinical experience as a useful tool for developing and reinforcing critical thinking skills. McNeill et al. (2023) recommend reflective journaling for students to describe how selected competencies can be met.

Lazarus (2016) offers several practical strategies to maximize teaching in a busy advanced-practice clinical setting. One strategy, the one-minute preceptor (OMP) approach, is preceptor-guided and focuses on developing a differential diagnosis and management plan. The preceptor asks the student for the most probable differential diagnosis with supporting evidence. Then, the preceptor shares concise, tailored teaching points based on the case, reinforcing areas of success and providing constructive feedback (Gatewood & De Gagne, 2019; Lazarus, 2016). In a systematic review of the OMP, Gatewood and De Gagne (2019) found this method to be effective, acceptable to both students and preceptors, and helpful for increasing assessment and feedback on clinical reasoning.

The five-minute preceptor (FMP) is a variation of the OMP. While this method takes slightly more time than the OMP, it provides additional teaching depth. The FMP extends the OMP approach by allowing the student to start an interaction with a case summary. Next, the steps of the traditional OMP are completed and then the preceptor concludes with some brief teaching while addressing any student errors (Lazarus, 2016). This approach offers more *cognitive preceptorship* when the preceptor explains the rationale for the medical decision-making process (Pleshkan, 2024).

The SNAPPS technique (**s**ummarize the case, **n**arrow and **a**nalyze the differential, **p**robe the preceptor [ask clarification questions], **p**lan management, and **s**elect a case-related issue for **s**elf-directed learning) is a learner-centered approach that facilitates discussion between the APRN student and preceptor (Lazarus, 2016). This technique requires both preceptor and student understanding of the method, with the student assuming more responsibility for leading the teaching encounter. Thus, it may be better suited for highly motivated or advanced learners.

Other preceptor responsibilities when working with APRN students include creating the final steps of a clinical checklist (Pitts et al., 2019). Preceptors must have strong communication skills to guide and encourage student learning. They also need to be able to communicate feedback with clinical faculty on student performance and learning progression. Finally, preceptors must verify student clinical hours and be available for virtual or face-to-face visits with clinical faculty.

APRN clinical experiences involve evaluation of student competencies (Pitts et al., 2019). While clinical evaluation is covered in more depth in Chapter 17, evaluation of APRN student competencies is briefly addressed here. Clinical site visits for precepted experiences are essential for monitoring student experiences, providing feedback, and evaluating progress (NTF, 2022). These visits necessitate a close relationship among the clinical teacher, preceptor, and student to ensure fulfilment of course objectives and the development of essential student competencies. The preceptor is responsible for observing and completing the formal preceptor evaluation of student clinical performance. Clinical faculty can utilize virtual visits or face-to-face visits to meet the NTF requirements. The benefits of face-to-face clinical visits include the opportunity for clinical teachers to evaluate the site and to directly observe student interactions with patients and the preceptor (Bice & Parker, 2019). The downsides to face-to-face visits, especially when student clinical sites may be in rural or underserved areas, are the burden in terms of faculty time and institutional resources related to travel costs (Bice & Parker, 2019; Harris et al., 2020). As for virtual site visits, they may have the benefits of being less stressful and more convenient. If preceptors identify student concerns during a virtual site visit, a face-to-face visit is warranted. Overall, APRN programs may find benefit in utilizing a combination of virtual and onsite clinical supervision visits.

SUMMARY

Clinical teaching and learning laboratories are cornerstones of skill development and professional identity formation in nursing education. Clinical teachers must optimize learning opportunities due to resource limitations, drawing on key principles such as creating a supportive learning environment, integrating research, fostering critical thinking, and promoting professionalism. Effective teaching practices are required for both traditional and innovative models of clinical instruction and to address the diverse challenges faced by nursing students, particularly underrepresented populations. Unique considerations also exist in clinical teaching for APRN students. Clinical faculty should focus on overcoming barriers to placement, careful site and preceptor selection, orientation strategies, and ongoing support mechanisms to enhance APRN student success in clinical practice.

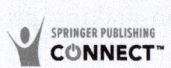

A robust set of instructor resources designed to supplement this text is located at http://connect.springerpub.com/content/book/978-0-8261-8892-2. Qualifying instructors may request access by emailing textbook@springerpub.com.

REFERENCES

Abdelkader, A. M., El-Aty, N. S. A., & Abdelrahman, S. M. (2021). The relationship between self-confidence in learning and clinical educator's characteristics by nursing students. *International Journal of Nursing Education, 13*(2), 1–10. http://doi.org/10.37506/ijone.v13i2.14614

Al-Daken, L., Lazarus E. R., Al Sabei, S. D., Alharrasi, M., & Al Qadire, M. (2024). Perception of nursing students about effective clinical teaching environments: A multi-country study. *SAGE Open Nursing, (10),* 1–10. http://doi.org/10.1177/23779608241233146

Al-Rawajfah, O. M., Al Hadid, L., Madhavanprabhakaran, G. K., Francis, F., & Khalaf, A. (2022). Predictors of effective clinical teaching—nursing educators' perspective. *BMC Nursing, 21*(55), 1–9. https://doi.org/10.1186/s12912-022-00836-y

American Association of Colleges of Nursing. (2021a). *APRN clinical preceptor resource guide.* https://www.aacnnursing.org/Education-Resources/APRN-Education/APRN-Clinical-Preceptor-Resources-Guide

American Association of Colleges of Nursing. (2021b). *The essentials: Core competencies for professional nursing education.* https://www.aacnnursing.org/Portals/0/PDFs/Publications/Essentials-2021.pdf

American Association of Colleges of Nursing. (2023). *The essentials: Core competencies for professional nursing education: Frequently asked questions.* https://www.aacnnursing.org/Portals/0/PDFs/Essentials/Essentials-Revised-Frequently-Asked-Questions.pdf

Araújo, A. A. C., de Godoy, S., Maia, N. M. F. E. S., de Oliveira, R. M., Vedana, K. G. G., de Sousa, A. F. L., Wong, T. K. S., & Mendes, I. (2023). Positive and negative aspects of psychological stress in clinical education in nursing: A scoping review. *Nurse Education Today, 126,* 105821. https://doi.org/10.1016/j.nedt.2023.105821

Arkan, B., Ordin, Y., & Yilmaz, D. (2018). Undergraduate nursing students' experience related to their clinical learning environment and factors affecting their clinical learning process. *Nurse Education Practice, 29,* 127–132. https://doi.org/10.1016/j.nepr.2017.12.005

Bice, A. A., & Parker, D. L. (2019). Piloting virtual clinical site visits in a family nurse practitioner program. *Journal of Nursing Education, 58*(3), 160–164. https://doi.org/10.3928/01484834-20190221-06

Brennan, K., Woodley, L., & Winstead, C. (2024). Bridging the gap: Innovating undergraduate public health nursing education through a service-learning health fair project. *Public Health Nursing, 41*(4), 825–828. https://doi.org/10.1111/phn.13324

Chicca, J., & Shellenbarger, T. (2021). Preparing, maintaining, and evaluating remote preceptorships: Considerations for nurse educators. *Teaching and Learning in Nursing, 16*, 396–400. https://doi.org/10.1016/j.teln.2021.04.006

Daya, S., Illangasekare, T., Tahir, P., Bochatay, N., Essakow, J., Ju, M., & van Schaik, S. (2023). Using simulation to teach learners in health care behavioral skills related to diversity, equity, and inclusion: A scoping review. *Simulation in Healthcare, 18*(3), 312–320. https://doi.org/10.1097/SIH.0000000000000690

Durham, C., & Baker, C. (2022). Learning laboratories as a foundation for nursing excellence. In M. H. Oermann, J. C. De Gange, & B. C. Phillips (Eds.), *Teaching in nursing and the role of the educator* (3rd ed., pp. 183–207). Springer Publishing Company.

Dzioba, C., LaManna, J., Perry, C. K., Toerber-Clark, J., Boehning, A., O'Rourke, J., & Rutledge, C. (2022). Telehealth competencies: Leveled for continuous advanced practice nurse development. *Nurse Educator, 47*(5), 293–297. https://doi.org/10.1097/NNE.0000000000001196

Foreman, R. (2023). Cognitive rehearsal: Teaching nursing students to address incivility in the clinical setting. *Nurse Educator, 49*(2), E107–E108. https://doi.og/10.1097/NNE.0000000000001494

Gatewood, E., & De Gagne, J. C. (2019). The one-minute preceptor model: A systematic review. *Journal of the American Association of Nurse Practitioners, 31*(1), 46–57. https://doi.org/10.1097/JXX.0000000000000099

Gcawu, S. N., & van Rooyen, D. (2022). Clinical teaching practices of nurse educators: An integrative literature review. *Health SA Gesondheid, 27*, 1728. https://doi.org/10.4102/hsag.v27i0.1728

Gigli, K. H., & Gonzalez, J. D. (2022). Meeting the need for nurse practitioner clinicals: A survey of practitioners. *Journal of the American Association of Nurse Practitioners, 34*(8), 991–1001. https://doi.org/10.1097/JXX.0000000000000749

Hamaideh, S., Abuhammad, S., Abu Khait, B., Al-Modallal, H., Hamdan-Mansour, A., Masa'deh, R., & Alrjoub, S. (2024). Levels and predictors of empathy, self-awareness, and perceived stress among nursing students: A cross sectional study. *BMC Nursing, 23*(131). https://doi.org/10.1186/s12912-024-01774-7

Hampton, D., Welsh, D., & Wiggins, A. (2020). Learning preferences and engagement level of generation Z nursing students. *Nurse Educator, 45*(3), 160–164. https://doi.org/10.1097/NNE.0000000000000710

Hannans, J. (2019). Online clinical post conference: Strategies for meaningful discussion using VoiceThread. *Nurse Educator, 44*(1), 29–33. https://doi.org/10.1097/NNE.0000000000000529

Harris, M., Rhoads, S. J., Rooker, J. S., Kelly, M. A., Lefler, L., Lubin, S., Martel, I. L., & Beverly, C. J. (2020). Using virtual site visits in the clinical evaluation of nurse practitioner students: Student and faculty perspectives. *Nurse Educator, 45*(1), 17–20. https://doi.org/10.1097/NNE.0000000000000693

Hawkins, M. D. (2019). Barriers to preceptor placement for nurse practitioner students. *Journal of Christian Nursing: A Quarterly Publication of Nurses Christian Fellowship, 36*(1), 48–53. https://doi.org/10.1097/CNJ.0000000000000519

Hensel, D., Cifrino, S., & Conover, K. (2020). A cohesive plan for virtual clinical education to teach clinical judgment using unfolding cases. *Nurse Educator, 45*(6), 289–290. https://doi.org/10.1097/NNE.0000000000000920

Juan, S., Esseiva, Z., Mccrae, J., & Nielsen, R. (2023). Anxiety provoking behaviors of nursing clinical instructors and effects on undergraduate nursing students' wellbeing: A mixed methods design. *Nurse Education in Practice, 66*, 103517. https://doi.org/10.1016/j.nepr.2022.103517

Kelly, S. H., Henry, R., & Williams, S. (2019). Using debriefing methods in the postclinical conference. *American Journal of Nursing, 119*(9), 56–60. https://doi.org/10.1097/01.NAJ.0000580280.87149.12

Knox, J., & Mogan, J. (1985). Important clinical teacher behaviors as perceived by university nursing faculty, students, and graduates. *Journal of Advanced Nursing, 10*(1), 25–30. https://doi.org/10.1111/j.1365-2648.1985.tb00488.x

Lazarus, J. (2016). Precepting 101: Teaching strategies and tips for success for preceptors. *Journal of Midwifery & Women's Health, 61*(1), 11–21. https://doi.org/10.1111/jmwh.12520

Lewis-Pierre, L. (2019). Preparing for the next generation of educators and nurses: Implications for recruitment and educational innovations. *The ABNF Journal, 30*(2), 35–36.

Licas, P., & Torres, G. (2024). Feedback preferences of generation Z nursing students: A conjoint analysis. *Teaching and Learning in Nursing, 19*(2), e449–454. https://doi.org/10.1016/j.teln.2024.01.012

Lim, E., Kalembo, F., Bosco, A., Ngune, I., Adebayo, B., & Brown, J. (2023). "It's not their fault": Clinical facilitators' experiences supporting English as second language students. *Collegian, 30*(1), 9–16. https://doi.org/10.1016/j.colegn.2022.05.006

Mallinson, T. (2021). An exploratory study into the teaching of clinical examination skills in advanced practice. *British Journal of Nursing, 30*(12), 712–720. https://doi.org/10.12968/bjon.2021.30.12.712

Margolis, M., Clancy, C., Hayes, R., Sullivan-Marx, E., Wetrich, J., & Broome, M. (2024). How academia can help to grow—and sustain—a robust nursing workforce. *Nursing Outlook, 72*(1), 102017. https://doi.org/10.1016/j.outlook.2023.102017

Massarelli, J. (2023). Enhancing nursing students' cultural competency: Reflective journaling while traveling abroad. *Nursing Education Perspectives, 44*(1), 52–53. https://doi.org/10.1097/01.NEP.0000000000001061

McKay, M., Pariseault, C., Whitehouse, C., Smith, T., & Ross, J. (2022). The experience of baccalaureate clinical nursing faculty transitioning to emergency remote clinical teaching during the COVID-19 pandemic: Lessons for the future. *Nurse Education Today, 111*, 1–7. https://doi.org/10.1016/j.nedt.2022.105309

McNeill, C., Walker, T. & Stephens, U. (2023). Reflective journaling: Assessing competencies for advanced practice nursing students. *Nurse Educator, 48*(4), 203. https://doi.org/10.1097/NNE.0000000000001369

McPherson, S. (2019). Part-time clinical nursing faculty needs: An integrated review. *Journal of Nursing Education, 58*(4), 201–206. https://doi.org/10.3928/01484834-20190321-03

Mella, A. (2021). An integrative literature review on selecting patient assignments for undergraduate nursing students in the clinical setting. *Nurse Education Today, 107*, https://doi.org/10.1016/j.nedt.2021.105103

Miura, M., Daub, K., & Hensley, P. (2020). The one-minute preceptor model for nurse practitioners: A pilot study of a preceptor training program. *Journal of the American Association of Nurse Practitioners, 32*(12), 809–816. https://doi.org/10.1097/JXX.0000000000000300

Morandini, S. (2022). Clinical preparation strategy. *Nurse Educator, 48*(1), E20. https://doi.org/10.1097/NNE.0000000000001273

Mosca, C. (2019). The relationship between emotional intelligence and clinical teaching effectiveness. *Teaching and Learning in Nursing, 14*, 97–102. https://doi.org/10.1016/j.teln.2018.12.009

Munangatire, T., Tomas, N., & Asino, H. M. M. (2023). Nursing students' experiences and expectations of clinical learning: A qualitative study. *Nurse Education Today, 124*, 105758. https://doi.org/10.1016/j.nedt.2023.105758

National Task Force. (2022). *Standards for quality nurse practitioner education: A report of the national task force on quality nurse practitioner education* (6th ed.). https://www.nonpf.org/page/NTFStandards

Oermann, M. H., Shellenbarger, T., & Gaberson, K. B. (2022). *Clinical teaching strategies in nursing* (7th ed.). Springer Publishing Company.

Pardue, K. T., Holt, K., Dunbar, D-M., & Baugh, N. (2023). Exploring the development of nursing clinical judgment among students using virtual reality simulation. *Nurse Educator, 48*(2), 71–75. https://doi.org/10.1097/NNE.0000000000001318

Perez-Perdomo, A., & Zabalegui, A. (2024). Teaching strategies for developing clinical reasoning skills in nursing students: A systematic review of randomized controlled trials. *Healthcare, 12*(1), 90. https://doi.org/10.3390/healthcare12010090

Pitts, C., Padden, D., Knestrick, J., & Bigley, M. B. (2019). A checklist for faculty and preceptor to enhance the nurse practitioner student clinical experience. *Journal of the American Association of Nurse Practitioners, 31*(10), 591–597. https://doi.org/10.1097/JXX.0000000000000310

Pleshkan, V. (2024). A systematic review: Clinical education and preceptorship during nurse practitioner role transition. *Journal of Professional Nursing: Official Journal of the American Association of Colleges of Nursing, 50*, 16–34. https://doi.org/10.1016/j.profnurs.2023.10.005

Renda, S., Fingerhood, M., Kverno, K., Slater, T., Gleason, K., & Goodwin, M. (2022). What motivates our practice colleagues to precept the next generation? *Journal for Nurse Practitioners, 18*, 76–80. https://doi.org/10.1016/j.nurpra.2021.09.008

Roberts, M., & Mazurak, J. (2022). Virtual clinical experiences in nursing education: Applying a technology-enhanced storyboard technique to facilitate contextual learning in remote environments. *Nursing Education Perspectives, 43*(4), 260–261. https://doi.org/10.1097/01.NEP.0000000000000883

Rosli, N., Choo, T., & Idris, D. (2022). Impact of preceptorship models for undergraduate nursing students and its implementation: Systematic review. *International Journal of Nursing Education, 14*(1), 111–118. https://doi.org/10.37506/ijone.v14i1.17764

Russell, K. (2019). The art of clinical supervision: Strategies to assist with the delivery of student feedback. *Australian Journal of Advanced Nursing, 36*(3), 6–13.

Ryan, C. L., & McAllister, M. M. (2020). Professional development in clinical teaching: An action research study. *Nurse Education Today, 85*, 104306. https://doi.org/10.1016/j.nedt.2019.104306

Stubin, C. A. (2021). Keeping nursing student stress in check: Strategies from clinical nursing faculty. *Journal of Nursing Practice Applications & Reviews of Research, 11*(1), 1–8. https://doi.org/10.13178/jnparr.2021.11.01.1007

Theard, M. A., Marr, M. C., & Harrison, R. (2021). The growth mindset for changing medical education culture. *EClinicalMedicine, 37*, 100972. https://doi.org/10.1016/j.eclinm.2021.100972

Toqan, D., Ayed, A., Malak, M. Z., Hammad, B. M., ALBashtawy, M., Hayek, M., & Thultheen, I. (2023). Sources of stress and coping behaviors among nursing students throughout their first clinical training. *SAGE Open Nursing, 9*, 1–7. https://doi.org/10.1177/23779608231207274

U.S. Bureau of Labor Statistics. (2023). *Occupational outlook handbook: Nurse anesthetist, nurse midwives, and nurse practitioners*. https://www.bls.gov/ooh/healthcare/nurse-anesthetists-nurse-midwives-and-nurse-practitioners.htm

Williams, C. A. (2019). Nurse educators meet your new students: Generation Z. *Nurse Educator, 44*(2), 59–60. https://doi.org/10.1097/NNE.0000000000000637

Woodley, L. K., & Lewallen, L. P. (2020). Acculturating into nursing for Hispanic / Latinx baccalaureate nursing students: A secondary data analysis. *Nursing Education Perspectives, 41*(4), 235–240. https://doi.org/10.1097/01.NEP.0000000000000627

Yang, C., & Chao, S-Y. (2018). Clinical nursing instructors' perceived challenges in clinical teaching. *Japan Journal of Nursing Science, 15*(1), 50–55. https://doi.org/10.1111/jjns.12167

Yildirim, H. S., & Terzioglu, F. (2022). Nursing students' perceived stress: Interaction with emotional intelligence and self-leadership. *Perspectives in Psychiatric Care, 58*(4), 1381–1387. https://doi.org/10.1111/ppc.12940

Yun, B., Su, Q., Ye, X., Wu, Y., Chen, L., Zuo, Y, Liu, J., & Han, L. (2022). The relationships between clinical teaching behavior and transition shock in newly graduated nurses. *Nursing Open, 10*, 2107–2117. https://doi.org/10.1002/nop2.1458

Weaving Interprofessional Education Into Nursing Curricula

11

Karen T. Pardue, Shelley Cohen Konrad, and Dawn-Marie Dunbar

OBJECTIVES

1. Describe foundational frameworks for interprofessional education (IPE)
2. Identify core competencies for IPE
3. Examine the content and processes for integrating IPE into nursing curricula
4. Describe in-person and online teaching strategies for IPE in the classroom, simulation, and clinical learning environments

INTRODUCTION

There is growing evidence to support interprofessional education (IPE) as an essential pedagogy to improve team-based collaborative practice. Collaborative care delivery has been shown to favorably impact patient/population health outcomes such as reduced length of hospital stay, reduction in medical errors, enhanced patient education, and greater patient and provider satisfaction (Cadet et al., 2023). Over the last decade, many universities have integrated IPE competencies into curricular and cocurricular learning. Most health professions' accrediting bodies, including all three in nursing, advance standards that mandate incorporation of collaborative team-based competencies as part of the program of study (Interprofessional Education Collaborative [IPEC], 2023). According to the 2022 American Interprofessional Health Collaborative (AIHC) survey, IPE learning experiences have made "… substantive inroads into required curricula" (IPEC, 2023, p. 8) as evidenced by reports of growing student participation in interprofessional (IP) activities coupled with required programmatic expectations and longitudinal IP exposure (IPEC, 2023).

The IPE initiative can be traced back more than two decades when the Institute of Medicine (IOM) identified alarming rates of medical errors and patient safety concerns stemming from ineffective provider communication and poor collaboration (IOM, 2000). The IOM called on educators to respond by reforming health profession curricula to include IP and collaborative, team-based competencies as a requisite component of academic preparation (Greiner & Knebel, 2003).

Numerous national and international reports, including the World Health Organization (WHO, 2010), Robert Wood Johnson Foundation's *Future of Nursing*

(2011), the American Association of Colleges of Nursing's (AACN) *Essentials* (2021), and IPEC's Core Competencies for Interprofessional Collaborative Practice: Version 3 (IPEC, 2023) offer the nursing profession a blueprint for active engagement and leadership in IP care delivery. The need for duality of focus on both disciplinary and IP preparation understandably presents a daunting challenge for faculty, as the configuration of most nursing and health profession programs still reflects siloed curricula. Such curricular designs produce nursing and health profession graduates who have little to no knowledge of what their respective colleagues do and are insufficient in teaching ways to effectively work as a team.

Building collaborative competencies in nursing education is crucial, preparing future clinicians to work in IP teams and ensuring effective person-centered care while mitigating provider burnout. This chapter explores the content, pedagogical theories, and processes for weaving IPE and collaborative learning into nursing curricula. Foundational frameworks are provided, along with examination of in-person and virtual didactic, simulation, and clinical experiences that promote collaborative practice capabilities across the continuum of care.

FOUNDATIONAL FRAMEWORKS

Defining Interprofessional Education

IPE is defined as events where multiple professions engage in learning together, sharing knowledge and insights in order to enhance teamwork and improve the quality of healthcare delivery (Centre for the Advancement of Interprofessional Education [CAIPE], 2024). Collaborative practice is similarly defined as opportunities whereby practitioners learn together through working together (CAIPE, 2024). WHO augments these definitions, contending that IPE occurs when students "… representing two or more professions learn about, from, and with each other to enable effective collaboration and improve health outcomes for the patients and populations they serve" (2010, p. 13). These definitions are well accepted and are frequently referenced in the IPE literature.

Interprofessional Collaboration

The word *collaboration* is derived from the Latin word *collaborare*, meaning "to labor, to work with and together" (LatDict, 2016, para 1). Collaboration requires interaction between participants, characterized by reciprocal giving and receiving of information and a mutual working relationship centered on trust, respect, and psychological safety (the belief that one can express their perspectives without fear of negative repercussions; Lackie et al., 2023). Practitioners should be proficient in applying collaboration skills in any team settings they are part of.

IPEC's *Interprofessional Core Competencies for Collaborative Practice* (IPEC, 2011, 2016, 2023) have been globally influential and provide an indispensable educational resource to prepare learners for IP practice. First published in 2011 and then revised in 2016 and 2023, the competency guidelines advance critical constructs of team-based, patient-centered, safe, and equitable practice. The framework proposes that the *way* healthcare is delivered is as important to patient outcomes as is the *type* of care that is provided. It supports the creation of intentional learning experiences between health disciplines to prepare a future collaborative workforce.

Core Competencies for Interprofessional Practice

In 2009, six national health profession associations, which included nursing, established a collaborative to examine the nature and development of IPE. In 2016, IPEC expanded its membership to 22 national education and health organizations. The first expert panel report was published in 2011, asserting that the goal of IP collaborative practice is the provision of safe, high-quality, patient and family-centered care. The report identified four broad competency domains as characterizing IP collaborative practice:

- Values and Ethics for IP Practice,
- Roles and Responsibilities for Collaborative Practice,
- IP Communication Practices, and
- IP Teamwork and Team-Based Practice.

These four competency domains were reaffirmed in 2023 and remain as foundationally relevant today as when originally published. The 2023 IPEC *Core Competencies* emphasize guiding assumptions applying person-centeredness, cultural responsivity, equity, and accessibility to IP learning and practice. Competency tenets recognize the variable, ever-changing nature of IP clinical settings and the diversity of institutions. Competencies encompass skills such as effective communication, active listening, mutual respect, shared decision-making, conflict resolution, and understanding of various disciplinary roles. The framework integrates concepts from the Triple Aim (Berwick et al., 2008) with additional content from the Quadruple Aim (Bodenheimer & Sinsky, 2014) and the Quintuple Aim (Nundy et al., 2022), as well as the tenets of social justice and health equity. In combination, the 2023 IPEC report promotes high-level competency attainment so that different professions and institutions can adapt the competencies for local use (IPEC, 2023).

The updated version contains a total of 33 subcompetency statements which have been broadened to achieve wide applicability across diverse settings and populations. Table 11.1 presents a sample of the updated core competency domains with sample subcompetency statements.

In addition to participating as a care team member, nurses commonly assume care coordination roles in inpatient, ambulatory, or community-based settings. The Canadian Interprofessional Health Collaborative (CIHC) identifies *collaborative leadership* as critical to best practice. Collaborative leadership is grounded in relational strength, whereby the healthcare team determines the member most equipped for leadership given the needs of the situation (CIHC, 2010). Facilitation is at the heart of collaborative leadership, as are the tenets of value and respect for every team member.

Collaborative leadership is a final important IP competency for inclusion in nursing education. Collaborative leaders employ well-developed listening and communication skills to ensure all team members know what is expected of them in their execution of patient care. They are responsible for establishing a culture of psychological safety in which all participants feel comfortable and confident providing input (Lackie et al., 2023).

TABLE 11.1 FOUR INTERPROFESSIONAL CORE COMPETENCY 2023 DOMAINS WITH SAMPLE SUBCOMPETENCY STATEMENTS

IPEC Competency Domain and Definition	Sample Subcompetency Statement
Values and Ethics (VE) Work with team members to maintain a climate of shared values, ethical conduct, and mutual respect (p. 16).	VE2: Advocate for social justice and health equity of persons and populations across the lifespan (p. 16). VE5: Value the expertise of health professionals and its impact on team functions and health outcomes (p. 16).
Roles and Responsibilities (RR) Use the knowledge of one's own role and team members' expertise to address individual and population health outcomes (p. 17).	RR2: Collaborate with others within and outside of the health system to improve health outcomes (p. 17). RR5: Practice cultural humility in interprofessional teamwork (p. 17).
Communication (C) Communicate in a responsive, responsible, respectful, and compassionate manner with team members (p. 18).	C3: Communicate clearly with authenticity and cultural humility, avoiding discipline-specific terminology (p. 18). C5: Practice active listening that encourages ideas and opinions of other team members (p. 18).
Teams and Teamwork (TT) Apply values and principles of the science of teamwork to adapt one's own role in a variety of team settings (p. 19).	TT3: Practice team-reasoning, problem-solving, and decision-making (p. 19). TT4: Use shared leadership practices to support team effectiveness (p. 19).

Source: Interprofessional Education Collaborative. (2023). *IPEC core competencies for interprofessional collaborative practice: Version 3.* Interprofessional Education Collaborative.

THEORETICAL FRAMEWORKS TO SUPPORT INTERPROFESSIONAL EDUCATION

IPE differs from disciplinary education in that the primary focus is on participation and interaction among diverse learners, as opposed to teachers imparting specific content. As such, IPE is grounded in social engagement, thus numerous theories are useful for nurse educators when designing and implementing shared learning experiences.

Theories for Designing IPE Learning Experiences

No single theory is universally accepted for IPE; rather, most endeavors reflect a blend of education and social engagement theories to achieve collaborative learning outcomes (Hean et al., 2018). Principles of adult learning provide a solid underpinning for IPE (Hean et al., 2018). Knowles (1984) advanced the concept of andragogy and the belief that engaged adult learners are motivated and assume responsibility for their educational experiences. Adults seek relevant educational opportunities, making connections between new learning and their current and past life experiences (Knowles, 1984).

Kolb's theory of experiential learning (1984) is a foundational framework often employed for successful integration of IPE. Kolb proposes learning occurs when students move through four discrete phases which are defined as: (a) concrete experience (new material is presented); (b) reflective observation (observing, considering, and mentally reviewing the new material); (c) abstract conceptualization (analysis and generation of questions about the material); and (d) active experimentation (application or testing of new learning to the real-world situation).

Social engagement models support classic education theory in the development of IPE. Contact hypothesis, initially proposed by Hewstone and Brown (1986), contends that attitudinal change is fostered when participants have the opportunity to actively learn together. Learning with others establishes new relationships and results in the questioning of negative stereotypes, myths, and assumptions as new associations are formed. Moreover, Haruta and Yamamoto (2020) report medical and health profession students cultivated new connections when united in an IP clinical-shadowing experience. When utilizing contact hypothesis in IPE design, it is important that learners be of comparable stages of development, hold equal status in the experience, and be bound together via common educational or patient-care goals (Haruta & Yamamoto, 2020).

The Communities of Practice Framework (CoP) reflects constructivist theory and the active role learners play in building new knowledge and capabilities together (Wenger-Trayner & Wenger-Trayner, 2015). This orientation advances collaborative problem-solving to address "real-world" issues, during which participants engage in peer-to-peer learning, active questioning, and robust discussion (Wenger-Trayner & Wenger-Trayner, 2015). This framework has been expanded to include interactions in the online environment and is commonly referred to as communities of inquiry (Evans & Perry, 2023). Constructivist approaches support future IP practice, developing students' communication, teamwork, and problem-solving skills.

Relational learning theory builds upon other theories that emphasize the merits of interpersonal connection, communication, and establishment of psychologically safe learning venues (Lackie et al., 2023). Relational pedagogy focuses on *how* content is taught rather than the content itself. With IPE, instructors are encouraged to model cross-disciplinary connections and integrate the relevance of partnerships with others when teaching in their specific profession.

Curricula based in relational principles embed opportunities for students to discover and capitalize on the distinctive skills and expertise of others while working together. IPE curricular integration can be accomplished by, for example, commenting on the role of another discipline when teaching about chronic illness, or including articles authored by professionals from other disciplines in course syllabi. These simple acts of inclusivity foster students' curiosity about professional roles and generate a pathway for IP socialization.

Relational pedagogy further promotes critical thinking and cultural responsivity, a focus that aligns well with IPEC's (2023) expanded emphasis on population health, equity, and social justice. IP case scenarios can be designed with social determinants of health, social justice, and health disparities in mind; students can also explore how access to care, transportation, literacy, and stigma may affect outcomes for the patient, provider, and healthcare team.

Model for Conceptualizing Process of Interprofessional Student Learning

In combination, the aforementioned theories provide a foundation for shaping and implementing collaborative learning. Cahn and colleagues (2018) encourage programs to explicitly weave the IPEC competencies throughout the curricula, thereby formalizing and scaffolding learning that is developmentally appropriate for students. The University of British Columbia's (UBC) model for IPE is an enduring one and serves as a faculty guide in developing IPE across the curriculum (Charles et al., 2010).

The initial stage in the UBC model is *exposure*. Exposure learning is introductory and provides a foundation for success in future IP collaborations (Charles et al., 2010). Exposure learning is appropriate for novice prelicensure learners and involves bringing students together from diverse professions to begin to learn about collaborative practice. Sample topics reflective of the exposure stage of IPE might include:

- What is IP practice?
- Why does IP collaborative practice matter?
- What are the roles and responsibilities of various health profession disciplines?
- What are the myths and/or stereotypes associated with different health professions?
- What are critical elements inherent in high-functioning teams?
- What are communication tools and techniques that promote optimal team functioning?

Exposure to IP is especially successful when presenting a common topic to diverse learners, thus promoting cross-disciplinary discussion. For example, students can be brought together to learn about the exigencies of childhood asthma and divided into small IP groups to discuss what each profession has learned and how they might address the diagnosis in practice. This exposure method is adaptable to both in-person and online instructional formats.

Immersion represents the second stage in the UBC model, involving more advanced learners with beginning clinical practice experience (Charles et al., 2010). The immersion stage challenges students to work with each other, using their emerging professional knowledge and skills to determine how disciplinary roles and collaborative teamwork contribute to high-quality patient/family care delivery (Charles et al., 2010). Examples of immersion learning include:

- IP teams of students analyzing a complex or unfolding case study,
- IP disciplines participating in a shared in-person or virtual simulation,
- IP teams of students learning telehealth and telecollaboration skills,
- Diverse health profession disciplines examining a standardized patient (patient actor),

- IP disciplines coordinating a clinical plan of care with a patient, and
- IP students participating in a service-learning project in a community or clinical setting.

Mastery is the final stage of learning conceptualized in the UBC model (Charles et al., 2010). The mastery phase represents advanced practice and is generally limited to postlicensure learners in graduate or doctoral education, or practicing clinicians engaged in continuing education. Mastery is realized through substantial clinical practice and involves high-level critical thinking as well as deep self-reflection on one's own IP experiences and practices (Charles et al., 2010).

CURRICULAR CONSIDERATIONS

Nurse educators often take the lead in championing IP learning, and meaningful curricular integration requires significant planning with disciplines outside of nursing. The following are a select number of pedagogical considerations essential for successful IPE design and implementation.

Learning Outcomes

A first step in successful curriculum design involves the identification of desired learning outcomes from collaborative experiences (Hean et al., 2018; Pardue, 2015). Nurse educators need to explicitly determine the desired knowledge, skills, behaviors, and/or attitudinal changes students will demonstrate at the conclusion of IPE. These capabilities should align with the four IPEC competency domains (IPEC, 2023), and for that reason, it is recommended that the sub-competencies, as explicated in the 2023 IPEC competency report, be used as a blueprint (Pardue, 2015). Extensive coordination among faculty planners is required to ensure collective affirmation of agreed upon outcomes. The sample competencies previously presented in Table 11.1 provide examples of outcomes-based IPE learning.

Consistent with any curriculum planning, IP knowledge, skills, and behaviors should be formally introduced at an appropriate time for learning (exposure stage), and subsequently reinforced later on in the curriculum through experiential opportunities (immersion stage). Cahn et al. (2018) advocates for nurse educators to create a systematic IPE plan, thereby formally mapping the anticipated timing and activities for IP competency development.

LEARNER CONSIDERATIONS

A second early consideration in IP learning is identifying potential programs and participants for collaborative education. This process can be challenging, as health profession education is disciplinarily nuanced, thereby reflecting diverse timepoints for student IPE readiness. Thibault (2011) referred to this mutual time for IPE readiness as curricular "sweet spots," requiring faculty to become well-acquainted with their partnering program(s) to ascertain parallel time frames for student preparation. This design also renders "asymmetrical" education encounters (Thibault, 2011), bringing together learners from dissimilar academic years and even different degree levels (e.g., prelicensure nursing and doctoral physical therapy) for IPE. This requires intentional coordination between nursing faculty and other disciplines in planning and delivering effective IPE for all students.

Class size, disciplinary distribution, and timing are other important learner considerations (El-Awaisi et al., 2021). Class size addresses the actual number of participants for collaborative education, considering questions such as how large are the disciplines being assembled, and is there space to accommodate shared learning. In planning for IPE, it is not necessary to include all professions in every event; such design becomes unwieldy and does not mirror actual clinical practice. To promote active student engagement, groups are generally divided into smaller subgroups or teams. Successful group dynamics appear to be best supported by limiting subgroup size to no more than 10 participants (El-Awaisi et al., 2021).

Disciplinary distribution presents a second consideration, as an equal mix of disciplines serves to foster equality of voice and equitable interaction. Ensuring a balanced composition of students supports team functioning and negates the opportunity for dominance by any one profession (Konrad et al., 2017). Longitudinal opportunities for collaborative learning are viewed as best practice as learners become familiar with other professions and engage with them while advancing through developmental levels (Khalili & Price, 2022). Repeated interactions among learners supports IP identity formation and provides authentic learning to achieve the goals of IPE.

Timing for IPE is another feature requiring attention by nurse faculty and their IP colleagues. There is robust debate in the IPE community as to the best time to introduce collaborative learning. On the one hand, novice learners typically have limited clinical experience, rendering concepts of team functioning and conflict resolution as abstract and lacking context (Lanning et al., 2021). Alternatively, the early introduction of IPE can reduce disciplinary stereotyping and promote healthy dialogue and collaboration among all professions (El-Awaisi et al., 2021). Early learners describe numerous benefits from introductory IPE exposure, including increased awareness of roles and responsibilities, enhanced communication skills, and the benefits of teamwork and IP problem-solving (Lanning et al., 2021). Early introduction parallels the UBC model of exposure, laying a foundation for future collaborative learning once students gain more knowledge about their own profession (Charles et al., 2010).

In 2020, the COVID-19 pandemic required learners to fully transition from in-person classrooms to virtual learning platforms. While the sudden closures of onsite education created chaos forcing students and faculty to quickly adapt to online methodologies, it also opened new opportunities for IPE. According to researchers, levels of IPE and collaborative learning increased significantly during the pandemic in both educational and clinical settings (Evans & Perry, 2023; Langlois et al., 2020). Virtual learning sidestepped logistical barriers such as space and timing and offered novel approaches to simulation, case-based instruction, and participation across campuses and institutions previously thought to be insurmountable. Langlois and colleagues (2020) refer to this wholesale migration to online as the "silver lining," enhancing IPE and revolutionizing education and healthcare practice (p. 587).

FACULTY ROLE

The constructivist theories that underpin IPE inform the faculty role and associated approaches to instruction. Most faculty are comfortable and familiar with traditional lectures and the role faculty play imparting information to students. However, successful IPE relies on student interaction and the role of faculty in active facilitation, modeling, and debriefing. This technique of facilitation requires faculty to

> **EXHIBIT 11.1 Tips and Techniques for Successful IPE Facilitation**
>
> Are there common, agreed-upon learning objectives?
> Are two or more professions involved?
> Are the sessions interactive?
> Are contributions of different members encouraged?
> Has psychological safety been established?
> Are learners, not teachers, doing most of the talking?
> Are IP communication strategies employed?
> Is there time planned for a focused debrief based on IP competencies?
> Are faculty trained in IP facilitation?

IPE, interprofessional education.

invite, guide, and encourage collaborative exchange, rendering a psychologically safe environment to explore similarities, differences, and potential conflict (Evans & Perry, 2023). Skillful facilitators pay close attention to team formation and group dynamics to anticipate and intervene as issues arise. IP facilitation is a complex and demanding role and it is recommended that faculty be afforded additional training and support (Evans & Perry, 2023). Exhibit 11.1 offers select tips and techniques that support successful IPE facilitation.

In addition to facilitation, faculty can model collaboration through cross-professional interaction during IPE instruction. The rationale for intentional faculty interaction is based on the observation that students regard IPE seriously when they see their own instructors actively engaged in communication, teamwork, and problem-solving—the very behaviors targeted through IP learning (El-Awaisi et al., 2021; Lanning et al., 2021). Conversely, when faculty are disengaged with IPE, their students assume a similar posture and may render the experience as "soft" and "unimportant." Faculty role modeling is a critical consideration in planning and implementing IPE.

The technique of debriefing is another important constructivist consideration with IP learning. Debriefing involves revisiting important conversations, examining changed assumptions, and exploring new insights gleaned from a given educational experience. IPE commonly culminates in a formal debriefing session which may be conducted by instructors or by more advanced students. Oftentimes, advanced students are well-equipped to debrief an IPE experience, providing powerful role modeling for learners. Additionally, students may debrief with standardized patients following IP simulation and receive direct feedback on their demonstration of IPEC competencies, cultural responsiveness, and patient-/person-centeredness. Throughout the debriefing process, faculty should maintain a focus on IP competencies and behaviors versus discipline-specific clinical content.

DIDACTIC LEARNING

Didactic learning is a common instructional format for introducing nursing students to IPE and reflects UBC exposure-level learning. A didactic approach supports a uniform educational experience for all participants and can be delivered in numerous ways. For example, some institutions require that all incoming students take part in an IPE session as part of their overall orientation. A mandatory session acknowledges the critical importance of IPE, explicitly recognizing that collaborative competencies are essential to best practice and not, as previously mentioned, "soft" knowledge and skills. IPE sessions introduce core IP competencies and promote future IPE cocurricular activities, providing students with opportunities to apply their developing knowledge and skills. In some cases, students are invited to participate in a brief IPE activity to get to know each other and to illustrate how IPE is applied in practice.

Early learners are eager to gain knowledge of their own discipline; thus, integration of IPE must explicitly connect the dots between nursing education and collaborative competencies. Educators may present answers to such questions as: Why is it important for nurses to know the skill set of an occupational therapist? What specialized skills are necessary for teamwork and how can nurses advance patient care when working on a team? How do nurses and their patients benefit from a collaborative, psychologically safe environment? In the classroom, faculty may use modules, videos, and interactive strategies to expose students to basic tenets of IPE competencies. Numerous low- or no-cost IPE resources exist to assist faculty, a number of which are depicted in Table 11.2. Interactive instructional methods offer students a glimpse into the processes of team-based care in day-to-day practice.

TABLE 11.2 RESOURCES FOR DEVELOPING INTERPROFESSIONAL LEARNING

Resource/URL	Description
Guide to Effective Interprofessional Education Experiences in Nursing Education https://www.nln.org/docs/default-source/uploadedfiles/default-document-library/ipe-toolkit-krk-012716.pdf?sfvrsn=7b00d30d_0	A free guide for designing and implementing effective interprofessional education (IPE) and collaborative practice experiences in nursing. Website includes sample lesson plans for didactic, simulation, and clinical education; a guide to creating an institutional culture of collaboration; and program- evaluation strategies to assess IPE impact and evidence-based teaching practices.
National Center for Interprofessional Practice and Education (NCIPE) https://nexusipe.org/informing/about-national-center. Video Library: https://nexusipe.org/search/site/videos Catalog of IP Research Instruments: https://nexusipe.org/advancing/assessment-evaluation-start.	NCIPE offers a range of resources to support interprofessional education, practice, and research. Their video library covers contemporary topics and training for classrooms and faculty development, and their catalogue of IP research instruments is extensive.

(continued)

TABLE 11.2 RESOURCES FOR DEVELOPING INTERPROFESSIONAL LEARNING *(continued)*

Resource/URL	Description
American Interprofessional Health Collaborative (AIHC) https://aihc-us.org/	AIHC is an organization for students, health professionals, educators, researchers, administrators, and community members engaged in interprofessional education and collaborative practice. The organization aims to improve health outcomes and health equity in partnership with NCIPE.
Institute for Health Improvement (IHI) Open School https://www.ihi.org/education/ihi-open-school	The IHI Open School is an interprofessional online educational community that offers students, trainees, professionals, health systems, and institutions of higher learning the skills and support network to become leaders in healthcare.
Interprofessional.Global https://interprofessional.global/	Interprofessional.Global is an international group that facilitates exchange between worldwide interprofessional education and collaborative practice (IPECP) networks. The agency offers workshops, updated information, and brings like-minded people and organizations together to share new ideas to improve global healthcare.

Inviting cross-professional guest speakers is another approach providing early exposure to various disciplines nursing students will work alongside in future practice. In collaboration with the guest speaker, teachers are charged with prompting peer discussion that highlights similarities and differences in roles, explores communication and teamwork know-how, and imparts respect for the various roles professional and support staff play.

Case-based learning (CBL) and collaborative group projects are instructional activities which shed light on the advantages of IP collaboration. The aim of team-centered CBL is for students to learn from each other and become aware of the distinctive and shared disciplinary roles in patient care. Successful CBL scenarios involve clinical situations uniformly familiar to students, thereby requiring faculty awareness of the timing of curricular concepts across the participating professions. Cross-disciplinary group projects unite students in examining a common health or social concern, such as bullying or environmental hazards. Both assignments (CBL or group project) require students to work with counterparts from another profession or, at the very least, study how another discipline might address the problem at hand. Student posters or oral presentations serve as summative products, as students demonstrate their IP process, describe cross-disciplinary learning, and invite input from other participants to extend teachable moments.

As noted earlier, virtual platforms are now commonly being used for IPE. Students from multiple professions can take part in synchronous online learning where they are introduced to new content and skills common across disciplines. A key feature of online IPE instruction is facilitation that encourages interactive student participation, presents content gleaned from multiple viewpoints, and asks questions to spark IP exchange (Evans & Perry, 2023).

Asynchronous learning offers student opportunities to interact on their own when schedules and curricular constraints are obstacles to face-to-face exchange. Faculty can coordinate shared assignments whereby students are required to contact classmates for information about their professions or solicit a multidisciplinary opinion about a case scenario. Discussion boards can also support student engagement and contribution from various professions and perspectives.

Facilitation and faculty modeling are pivotal to successful IPE didactic instruction, especially during the exposure phase. New learners may struggle with the relevance of IPE and may already consider themselves proficient communicators and team players. Ironically, engagement in IP team-based activities reveals to these students how very difficult collaborative teamwork can be and why explicit IPE instruction is necessary. Introducing students to the concept of productive struggle early on (Mylopoulos et al., 2018) reduces anxiety about the difficulties they may encounter in the IP learning or practice environment. Struggling through collaborative care plan development or a joint patient interview provides students opportunity to learn from each other and problem-solve as a team. Productive struggle resolution does not necessarily mean learners come up with the "right" answer but rather, that they have communicated effectively and capitalized on each other's distinctive expertise to best serve their patient.

In 2014, the Josiah Macy Jr. Foundation (2014) called on educators to integrate patients and families as partners in health profession education. Stories of patients *from* patients are perhaps the most transformative learning experiences for students. Patient stories told in nonclinical, real-life terms remind students that anyone could face a life-altering health situation at any time. Inviting patients and family members to share their care experience narratives has the added benefit of explicating how collaboration is successful or unsuccessful. Table 11.3 offers sample teaching and learning strategies appropriate for IPE didactic instruction.

SIMULATION LEARNING

The simulation laboratory provides an unparalleled experiential learning environment for cultivating and assessing IP capabilities. Clinical simulation was initially piloted in the 1950s and emerged as an indispensable instructional modality during the COVID-19 pandemic (Langlois et al., 2020). Consistent with prior definitions, IP simulation (IPE-SIM) occurs when faculty, facilitators, and students from two or more disciplines participate together in a shared simulation experience to realize mutually identified goals or learning outcomes (Decker et al., 2015, p. 294).

IPE-SIM reflects an immersive, performance-based strategy (Charles et al., 2010), focused on the skills of teamwork, communication, and problem-solving.

TABLE 11.3 SAMPLE ACTIVE LEARNING STRATEGIES FOR DIDACTIC INTERPROFESSIONAL EDUCATION IPEC COMPETENCY WITH SAMPLE ACTIVE LEARNING STRATEGY

Values/Ethics for IP Practice	Roles and Responsibilities for IP Practice
<ul><li>Assemble students into small IP groups with access to the internet.</li><li>Direct students to a pre selected case study at the AHRQ Patient Safety Network (PSNet). PSNet is home to hundreds of Web Morbidity & Mortality (WebM&M) real-life case studies. https://psnet.ahrq.gov/webmm-case-studies.</li><li>Choose a case study reflecting the various disciplines and levels of the IP learners.</li><li>Prompt students to analyze the case from an interprofessional perspective, examining how IP teamwork, communication, and knowledge of roles/responsibilities might impact the outcome.</li></ul>	<ul><li>Assemble students into small IP groups with access to the internet.</li><li>Assign students to complete a web quest in researching similarities and differences in roles and responsibilities of various health professions (e.g., roles/responsibilities for occupational therapy, physical therapy, speech and language therapy, leisure therapy). Once completed, have students create a visual or graphic to capture their findings.</li></ul>
IP Communication	**IP Teamwork and Team-based Practice**
<ul><li>Assemble students into small IP groups and provide TeamSTEPPS 3.0 communication resources. Materials are free at the AHRQ website: https://www.ahrq.gov/teamstepps-program/index.html<ul><li>Instruct students to become familiar with communication tools such as SBAR, CUS, Teach-back.</li><li>Have students review the Team STEPPS 3.0 patient video: Tara.</li><li>Debrief with students and have them list the supportive and nonsupportive communication techniques conveyed in the video. Explore verbal, nonverbal, and technical communication strategies that promote patient safety and quality care. Have students consider, "Is patient engagement a provider skill or a provider trait?" or "Can engagement approaches be learned?"</li></ul></li></ul>	<ul><li>Assemble students into small IP groups. Assign students to work together completing a teamwork activity found on the web (e.g., paper chain challenge, Lego® tower challenge, marshmallow/ spaghetti challenge). Debrief the experience by analyzing the process:<ul><li>How did your group work as a unit?</li><li>What was the process like?</li><li>Did a leader emerge? If so, how did this happen?</li><li>Who assumed what role in completing the activity?</li><li>What did the team do when different ideas were offered?</li><li>Any observations about communication?</li><li>Who negotiated? How were problems solved?</li><li>What would you do differently next time?</li><li>For the winning team:</li><li>What was your process like?</li><li>How does this compare with the other teams?</li></ul></li></ul>

AHRQ, Agency for Healthcare Resources and Quality; CUS, concerned, uncomfortable, safety (issue); IP, interprofessional; SBAR, situation, background, assessment, recommendation (or request).

The simulation lab provides students with opportunities to enact behaviors characteristic of collaborative health professions practice (Astbury et al., 2021). Attention to the *process* of care and working together as a team differentiates IPE-SIM from discipline-specific simulation, thus requiring joint faculty collaboration and the co-development of multidisciplinary scenarios to achieve IP learning outcomes.

A team-based approach to simulation development, which involves faculty using their own clinical experiences as a guide, renders scenario cocreation that is both authentic and relevant for the involved disciplines. Scenario learning objectives should be guided by the IPEC competencies and subcompetencies (2023) and jointly agreed upon by the planning team. IPE-SIM should provide learners with the opportunity to elicit knowledge, demonstrate behaviors, and convey attitudes reflective of collaborative practice. An IP scenario does not have to be complex to be effective, but it must reflect real-life patient and provider encounters.

One common IPE-SIM pitfall occurs when too many disciplines are involved at the same time, or different professions are linked in a manner that does not reflect the realities of clinical practice. In such situations, students quickly disengage, as provider relationships are forced, unnatural, and artificial. The development team should be aware of social hierarchy and stereotypes (e.g., all surgeons are headstrong, all nurses are female), which could influence the learning outcomes and learner future performance (El-Awaisi et al., 2021). The planning team needs to consider authentic clinical situations and the professions most likely to collaborate, as well as the points in the care delivery continuum where these collaborations naturally occur.

An example IPE-SIM cocreated by an IP faculty workgroup addresses the collaborative care of a young woman with life-altering injuries from a motor vehicle accident. Chronic pain, loss of mobility, self-care deficits, previously unidentified dental issues, financial concerns, and questions about childbearing options characterize the issues set forth in this multisession IPE-SIM. Consistent with the IPEC 2023 revisions, case implications were expanded to include critical social determinants and health equity issues impacting this woman and her family. This unfolding case was designed so that student IP teams could assess and prioritize needs and propose an integrated care plan for the simulated patient and her partner as care progressed across the continuum from acute hospitalization to rehabilitation to home.

Students from nursing, osteopathic medicine, physician assistant, dental hygiene, dental medicine, social work, pharmacy, and occupational and physical therapy all provided meaningful contributions at various points across the care continuum. The IP exchange and multisession sequence allowed students to become acquainted with one another and their varied expertise. This served to enhance student understanding of the rigors and benefits of collaboration and fostered an appreciation for what it takes to become an effective person-centered team in real-world practice. Participating IPE-SIM students described gaining confidence in their own professional identity and an enhanced ability to communicate and work effectively on a team (Konrad et al., 2017). Students further reported that recognizing the knowledge overlap between professions increased the team's capacity to provide safe and efficient care.

The organizational framework of IPE-SIM reflects the same best practice process found in any discipline-specific simulation experience, including a prebrief, simulation, and debrief. IP debriefing can be challenging for even the most experienced simulation facilitators, yet the temptation to digress into discipline-specific clinical content is bypassed when clear IPE learning objectives guide the debriefing. Chapter 9 provides an excellent overview and helpful guidance for the design and implementation of simulation.

While there are numerous valid methods for debriefing (see Chapter 9), a number of best practices guide effective IP debriefing. First and foremost, it is critically important to foster a psychologically safe and respectful environment (Lackie et al., 2023), as such climate encourages candid communication and reflection among diverse disciplinary participants who are likely unfamiliar with each other. Lackie and colleagues (2023) instruct strategies by which IP faculty can model psychological safety through demonstrating curiosity, approachability, and respect. Facilitators should be alert for any cognitive frames relating to differences, biases, and/or clinical hierarchies, as psychologically safe environments engender conversation which may uncover such attitudes. If this occurs, IP faculty should be prepared to lead participants in additional discussion, exploring strategies to address issues and advance collaboration. Successful IP debriefing is also supported when IP faculty predetermine a consistent set of postsimulation questions. Aligning the debriefing questions with the IPE competencies ensures that discussions are relevant and contribute to the cultivation of essential IP skills. Finally, the recognition that the debriefing process involves diverse learners with varying levels of experience serves to ensure each participant can meaningfully engage in and benefit from the simulation. One indicator of success is when students articulate how IPE-SIM will change or influence their future practice because of the experience and opportunity for reflection.

There are numerous challenges that commonly arise in the design and delivery of IPE-SIM, and anticipating obstacles is an important step in the planning process. As discussed with didactic programming, logistical impediments include finding a common time for IPE-SIM in light of differing calendars and schedules. Institutions may be reticent to provide sufficient faculty release time for shared IPE-SIM development or, similarly, dedicate adequate faculty coverage during the execution of an IPE-SIM (Astbury et al., 2021). Financial support may also be problematic in determining how and which program resources will be used to fund IPE-SIM. Additionally, faculty may express discomfort in working with learners of differing educational levels and varied clinical experiences (Astbury et al., 2021).

Addressing these challenges requires flexibility, creativity, and "out of the box" thinking. Early collaboration with administration can clarify the importance of IPE-SIM, which may render protected time and financial investments at an institutional level. Providing administration with an overview as to how simulation meets learning outcomes for different disciplines highlights the advantages of common infrastructure and financial investment. Additionally, careful consideration should be given to the level of fidelity needed for the IPE-SIM experience. Faculty need to weigh the benefits of using high- or low-fidelity manikins, standardized patients, or multiplayer virtual reality (VR) simulation platforms. Importantly, fidelity should enhance rather than distract from the learning experience.

Various IP communication strategies serve as effective tools for addressing disciplinary scheduling. Learners do not necessarily need to be in the same physical space during simulation, as they can successfully share information through texts, phone calls, discussion boards, or synchronous platforms such as Zoom (Evans & Perry, 2023). As an example, while participating in an on-campus high-fidelity simulation, baccalaureate nursing students sought consultation from off-site pharmacy students using previously provided cell phone contacts. In addition, Zoom has been successfully employed to mimic telehealth encounters engaging IP students from diverse locations. These exemplars provide an opportunity for students to collaborate in real time by caring for simulated patients while maintaining different program-specific schedules. Thoughtful IP faculty planning can successfully mitigate structural issues with IPE.

The integration of advanced technologies, such as VR, offers a forward-thinking approach to address the traditional costly barriers of space, equipment, and specialized faculty to guide high-fidelity simulation (Shin et al., 2019). Virtual simulation (VS) and VR have emerged as scalable alternatives, providing immersive and interactive learning environments that allow for spatial presence beyond the capabilities of conventional methods (Foronda et al., 2020). VR, in particular, has shown promise in nursing and physician collaborative training, promoting students' psychomotor performance, cognitive knowledge, and IP capabilities related to communication, teamwork, leadership, and self-confidence (Foronda et al., 2020; Shin et al., 2019). The ongoing evolution of these technologies and their integration into IPE-SIM reflect an exciting trend toward improving both the efficiency and effectiveness of healthcare education while preparing learners for interdisciplinary practice.

CLINICAL LEARNING

IP clinical learning is experiential in nature, providing an opportunity for students to apply concepts and theories learned in the classroom to the care of actual patients, families, and communities. This represents an immersion level of learning (Charles et al., 2010), as students are engaged not only in providing disciplinary-focused care but also in delivering care as a member of a health team. A recent shift in IP clinical learning emphasizes the need for academic and clinical partners to unify IPE learning for both students and clinical providers (Brandt et al., 2023). The aim of this intentional connection is to identify what patients and local health systems need and then link IP opportunities to create a practice responsive workforce. As such, IP clinical education involves students and current health professionals working and learning together to achieve desired targeted outcomes and provide equitable clinical care for the communities they serve (Brandt et al., 2023).

It is well acknowledged that IP clinical learning experiences will be variable, as not every student will have the same opportunity with clinical IPE. Select clinical settings and care foci should reflect a culture and inherent disposition supportive of teamwork and collaboration. Rich IP clinical learning experiences are common for nursing students engaged in geriatrics, hospice, rehabilitation, long-term care, substance use treatment, and rural health rotations.

IP clinical learning may be realized through numerous approaches. Job shadowing is one potential activity, allowing students to observe other professions in action and leading them to consider such questions as: How does the practice of the observed discipline compare with nursing practice? What roles overlap? Are IP competencies being applied and if not, why not? Further, observing in vivo demonstration of others' skills encourages students to reflect on how and when working together serves to achieve best practice. Such experiences also illustrate referral processes, explicating how and why nursing recommends the expertise of another discipline. Faculty prompts further guide student reflection, debriefing, and critical observation. Following job shadowing, students might orally present their experiences related to communication, roles, and teamwork as part of a clinical postconference. Alternatively, students may journal on their shadowing experience, providing time for reflection on disciplinary approaches, dialogue observed, and application for future practice.

Patient rounding presents another experience for IP clinical learning. This setting-dependent practice provides an opportunity for students to engage and problem-solve with patients and other health disciplines involved in care delivery. The patient rounding experience may assume numerous forms: observational in noting team participant interactions or direct if providing care to the featured patient(s). Rounding also provides nursing students the chance to observe leadership skills and identify differences in approaches or styles in leading care teams. These observations constitute useful topics for clinical postconference, supporting analysis of the impact of leadership approaches on clinical care delivery and patient outcomes.

Some clinical settings (e.g., hospice, long-term care) commonly conduct case conferences to assess how care is being provided and to establish future clinical goals. Ideally, case conferences are patient centered, thereby including perspectives not only from providers but also the patient, family members, or caregivers. Participation in or observation of case conferences affords nursing students additional experience in examining how communication, teamwork, and collaboration impact the process and outcomes of clinical care. The opportunity to debrief these observations with cross-professional classmates adds considerable value to the case conference learning experience.

Intentionally designed IP service learning offers nursing students hands-on opportunities to interface with individuals while working collaboratively with multidisciplinary classmates. Recognized as a means for enhancing student awareness of social issues and the needs of communities, service learning is increasingly being used as a learning tool to help students develop interprofessional teamwork skills (Dunn & Konrad, 2019). As with simulation, collaborative service learning is cocreated by a faculty team to ensure IP learning objectives are met within the context of addressing a real need in the community. An exemplar of IP service learning is a biannual vital sign screening that occurs in an older adult communal residence. IP student teams offer a roster of screenings and work together with older adult residents and staff to provide updated health information which can then be shared with their health providers. A debrief follows during which students share what they learned with and from each other and about the needs of older adults who may or may not be receiving routine care. Other natural venues which support IP service learning include school systems, childcare centers, and correctional facilities. These settings support the application of core IP competencies and promote improved outcomes for those receiving services (Dunn & Konrad, 2019).

Through interaction with IP colleagues, nursing faculty may discover other professional disciplines during clinical rotations occurring in conjunction with their clinical group. This presents potential for shared pre- or postconferences, as well as an opportunity for collaborative care planning. If the rotation involves community health, it might be possible to arrange joint IP home visiting experiences. Faculty collaboration and creativity are essential in discovering and advancing IP clinical learning for nursing students.

EVALUATION OF INTERPROFESSIONAL EDUCATION

Evaluation of IPE outcomes begins with a clear identification of the desired IP knowledge, skills, and attitudes. Early IPE endeavors involve exposure or introduction of foundational concepts; thus, student learning can be determined through direct assessment such as examinations, student writing/reflections, or focus groups. Faculty collaboration during IPE exposure experiences should determine what artifacts will be used as evidence of student learning. Foundational outcomes commonly address participant knowledge about communication, roles, and responsibilities, and the process of collaboration, as well as determination of changes in attitudes or perceptions about teamwork. Although there is value in validating that students have cognitively grasped collaborative practice principles, what matters more is whether students demonstrate IP capabilities when providing actual patient care. As a result, an IPE evaluation plan generally assumes a longitudinal, multistep design.

Immersion learning supports student performance of collaborative behaviors and is accomplished through simulation or observation in the clinical setting. It is important to clearly identify the action or behavior to be evaluated, with IP competency statements subsequently integrated into simulation performance rubrics or as items on clinical evaluation tools. This process invites students and supervising faculty to narratively describe situations and associated actions or behaviors that evidence collaborative practice capabilities. Valid and reliable IP tools are available at the National Center for Interprofessional Practice and Education website (https://nexusipe.org/). Each instrument featured at the National Center is accompanied by a description explaining use, target audience, intended outcome/competency, and authorship. The National Center is an invaluable resource for nurse educators in the IPE evaluation process.

Rapid cycle evaluation is an expedient method to assess the efficacy of IP learning methods and programs (Zakocs et al., 2015). Information obtained through rapid cycle evaluation is used to revise and improve learning activities and to confirm to students that their input is thoughtfully considered and integrated with future programming. Continuous student feedback informs faculty about which methods are well received by students and whether they are meeting proposed learning outcomes.

Finally, questions addressing IP learning may be incorporated into departmental/college alumni satisfaction surveys. Students may not realize the value of collaborative practice lessons until they are well engaged in postlicensure day-to-day practice. Obtaining graduate feedback regarding their IPE learning informs curricular efficacy and supports future refinements and improvements.

SUMMARY

This chapter provides pedagogical guidance in the design, implementation, and evaluation of IPE in nursing education. Opportunities for broad curricular integration, including didactic, simulation, and clinical learning, were explored. Numerous exemplars and resources were provided to support faculty newly embarking on IP teaching and learning. It is essential for nursing education to adopt and integrate IPE, thereby cultivating nursing graduates who are knowledgeable about disciplinary roles and responsibilities and competent in communication, teamwork, and collaborative leadership. Learning together for future practice supports national calls for health professions education reform and produces practice-ready nurses prepared for today's collaborative, team-based workforce.

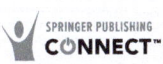 A robust set of instructor resources designed to supplement this text is located at http://connect.springerpub.com/content/book/978-0-8261-8892-2. Qualifying instructors may request access by emailing textbook@springerpub.com.

REFERENCES

American Association of Colleges of Nursing. (2021). *The essentials: Core competencies for professional nursing education.* https://www.aacnnursing.org/Portals/42/Academic Nursing/pdf/Essentials-2021.pdf

Astbury, J., Ferguson, J., Silverthorne, J., Willis, S., & Schafheutle, E. (2021). High fidelity simulation-based education in pre-registration healthcare programmes: A systematic review of reviews to inform collaborative and interprofessional best practice. *Journal of Interprofessional Care, 35*(4), 622–632. https://doi.org.10.1080/13561820.2020.1762551

Berwick, D., Nolan, T., & Whittington, J. (2008). The triple aim: Care, health, and cost. *Health Affairs, 27*(3), 759–769. https://doi.org/10.1377/hlthaff.27.3.759

Bodenheimer, T., & Sinsky, C. (2014). From triple aim to quadruple aim: Care of the patient requires care of the provider. *Annuals of Family Medicine, 12*(6), 573–576. https://doi.org/10.1370/afm.1713

Brandt, B. F., Dieter, C., & Arenson, C. (2023). From the Nexus vision to the NexusIPE™ learning model. *Journal of Interprofessional Care, 37*(supp.1), S15–S27. https://doi.org/10.1080/13561820.2023.2202223

Cadet, T., Cusimano, J., McKearney, S., Honaker, J., O'Neal, C., Taheri, R., Uhley, V., Zhang, Y., Dreker, M., & Cohn, J. (2023). Describing the evidence linking interprofessional education interventions to improving the delivery of safe and effective patient care: A scoping review. *Journal of Interprofessional Care, 38*(3), 476–485. https://doi.org/10.1080/13561820.2023.2283119

Cahn, P. S., Tuck, I., Knab, M. S., Doherty, R. F., Portney, L. G., & Johnson, A. F. (2018). Competent in any context: An integrated model of interprofessional education. *Journal of Interprofessional Care, 32*(6), 782–785. https://doi.org/10.1080/13561820.2018.1500454

Canadian Interprofessional Health Collaborative. (2010). *A national interprofessional competency framework: Quick reference guide.* https://phabc.org/wp-content/uploads/2015/07/CIHC-National-Interprofessional-Competency-Framework.pdf

Centre for the Advancement of Interprofessional Education. (2024). *About CAIPE.* https://www.caipe.org/about

Charles, G., Bainbridge, L., & Gilbert, J. (2010). The University of British Columbia model of interprofessional education. *Journal of Interprofessional Care, 24*(1), 9–18. https://doi.org/10.3109/13561820903294549

Committee on the Robert Wood Johnson Foundation Initiative on the Future of Nursing at the Institute of Medicine. (2011). *The future of nursing: Leading change, advancing health.* https://nap.nationalacademies.org/catalog/12956/the-future-of-nursing-leading-change-advancing-health

Decker, S. I., Anderson, M., Boese, T., Epps, C., McCarthy, J., Motola, I., & Scolaro, K. (2015). Standards of best practice: Simulation standard VIII: Simulation-enhanced interprofessional education (SIM-IPE). *Clinical Simulation in Nursing, 11*(6), 293–297. https://doi.org/10.1016/j.ecns.2015.03.010

Dunn, K., & Konrad, S. C. (2019). Stronger when combined: Lessons from an interprofessional, jail-based service-learning project. *Partnerships: A Journal of Service-Learning and Civic Engagement, 10*(1), 117–128.

El-Awaisi, A., Sheikh Ali, S., Abu Nada, A., Rainkie, D., & Awaisu, A. (2021). Insights fromhealthcare academics on facilitating interprofessional education activities. *Journal of Interprofessional Care, 35*(5), 760–770. https://doi.org/10.1080./13561820.2020.1811212

Evans, S., & Perry, E. (2023). An exploration of perceptions of online asynchronous and synchronous interprofessional education facilitation strategies. *Journal of Interprofessional Care, 37*(6), 1010–1017. https://doi.org/10.1080/13561820.2023.2213718

Foronda, C. L., Fernandez-Burgos, M., Nadeau, C., Kelley, C. N., & Henry, M.N. (2020). Virtual simulation in nursing education: A systematic review spanning 1996 to 2018. *Simulation in Healthcare, 15*(1), 46–54. https://doi.org/10.1097/SIH.0000000000000411

Greiner, A. C., & Knebel, E. (2003). *Health professions education: A bridge to quality*. National Academies Press.

Haruta, J., & Yamamoto, Y. (2020). Realist approach to evaluating an interprofessional education program for medical students in clinical practice at a community hospital. *Medical Teacher, 42*(1), 101–110. https://doi.org/10.1080/0142159X.2019.1665633

Hean, S., Green, C., Anderson, E., Morris, D., John, C., Pitt, R., & O'Halloran, C. (2018). The contribution of theory to the design, delivery, and evaluation of interprofessional curricula: BEME Guide No. 49. *Medical Teacher, 40*(6), 542–558. https://doi.org/10.1080/0142159X.2018.1432851

Hewstone, M., & Brown, R. (1986). Contact is not enough: An intergroup perspective on the "contact hypothesis." In M. Hewstone & R. Brown (Eds.), *Contact and conflict in intergroup encounters* (pp. 1–44). Blackwell.

Konrad, S. C., Cavanaugh, J., Hall, K., Rodriguez, K., & Pardue, K. T. (2017). A five-session interprofessional team immersion program for health professions students. *Journal of Interprofessional Education & Practice, 6*, 49–54. https://doi.org/10.1016/j.xjep.2016.12.007

Institute of Medicine. (2000). Kohn, L. T., Corrigan, J. M., & Donaldson, M. S. (Eds.). *To err is human: Building a safer health system*. National Academies Press. https://doi.org/10.17226/9728

Interprofessional Education Collaborative. (2011). *Core competencies for interprofessional collaborative practice: Report of an expert panel*. https://ipec.memberclicks.net/assets/2011-Original.pdf

Interprofessional Education Collaborative. (2016). *Core competencies for interprofessional collaborative practice: 2016 update*. https://ipec.memberclicks.net/assets/2016-Update.pdf

Interprofessional Education Collaborative. (2023). *Core competencies for interprofessional collaborative practice: Version 3*. https://www.ipecollaborative.org/assets/core-competencies/IPEC_Core_Competencies_Version_3_2023.pdf

Josiah Macy Jr. Foundation. (2014). *Partnering with patients in education and health care transformation*. https://macyfoundation.org/news-and-commentary/partnering-with-patients-in-education-and-health-care-transformation

Khalili, H., & Price, S. L. (2022). From uniprofessionality to interprofessionality: Dual vs dueling identities in healthcare. *Journal of Interprofessional Care, 36*(3), 473–478. https://doi.org/10.1080/13561820.2021.1928029

Knowles, M. (1984). *The adult learner: A neglected species* (3rd ed.). Gulf Publishing.

Kolb, D. (1984). *Experiential learning: Experiences as the source of learning and development*. Prentice Hall.

Lackie, K., Hayward, K., Ayn, C., Stilwell, P., Lane, J., Andrews, C., Dutton, T., Ferkol, D., Harris, J., Houk, S., Pendergast, N., Persaud, D., Thillaye, J., Mills, J., Grant, S., & Munroe, A. (2023). Creating psychological safety in interprofessional simulation for health profession learners: A scoping review of the barriers and enablers. *Journal of Interprofessional Care, 37*(2), 187–202. https://doi.org/10.1080/13561820.2022.2052269

LatDict. (2016). *Collaborare*. https://latin-dictionary.net/search/latin/collaborare

Langlois, S., Xyrichis, A., Daulton, B. J., Gilbert, J., Lackie, K., Lising, D., MacMillan, K., Najjar, G., Pfeifle, A. L., & Khalili, H. (2020). The COVID-19 crisis silver lining: Interprofessional education to guide future innovation. *Journal of Interprofessional Care, 34*(5), 587–592. https://doi.org/10.1080/13561820.2020.1800606

Lanning, S., Pardue, K., Eliot, K., Goumas, A., Kettenbach, G., Mills, B., Lockeman, K., Breitbach, A., & Gunaldo, T. P. (2021). Early-learners' expectations of and experience with IPE: A multi-institutional qualitative study. *Nurse Education Today, 107*, 105142. https://doi.org/10.1016/j.nedt.2021.105142

Mylopoulos, M., Steenhof, N., Kaushal, A., & Woods, N. N. (2018). Twelve tips for designing curricula that support the development of adaptive expertise. *Medical Teacher, 40*(8), 850–854. https://doi.org/10.1080/0142159X.2018.1484082

Nundy, S., Cooper, L. A., & Mate, K. S. (2022). The quintuple aim for health care improvement: A new imperative to advance health equity. *Journal of the American Medical Association, 327*(6), 521–522. https://doi.org/10.1001/jama.2021.25181

Pardue, K. T. (2015). A framework for the design, implementation, and evaluation of interprofessional education. *Nurse Educator, 40*(1), 10–15. https://doi.org/10.1097/NNE.0000000000000093

Shin, H., Rim, D., Kim, H., Park, S., & Shon, S. (2019). Educational characteristics of virtual simulation in nursing: An integrative review. *Clinical Simulation in Nursing, 37*, 18–28. https://doi.org/10.1016/j.ecns.2019.08.002

Thibault, G. E. (2011). Interprofessional education: An essential strategy to accomplish the future of nursing goals. *Journal of Nursing Education, 50*(6), 313–317. https://doi.org/10.3928/01484834-20110519-03

Wenger-Trayner, E., & Wenger-Trayner, B. (2015). *Introduction to communities of practice*. http://wenger-trayner.com/introduction-to-communities-of-practice

World Health Organization. (2010). *A framework for action on interprofessional education & collaborative practice*. https://www.who.int/publications/i/item/framework-for-action-on-interprofessional-education-collaborative-practice

Zakocs, R., Hill, J., Brown, P., Wheaton, J., & Friere, K. E. (2015). The data-to-action framework: A rapid program improvement process. *Health Education & Behavior, 42*(4), 471–479. https://doi.org/10.1177/1090198115595010

Academic–Practice Partnerships

12

Elizabeth Gatewood

OBJECTIVES

1. Describe historical and current trends in academic–practice partnerships
2. Identify the steps required to establish a sustainable academic–practice partnership using one framework
3. Articulate the values and opportunities for effective models of faculty practices

INTRODUCTION

Academic–practice partnerships are pivotal in preparing nurses to excel in increasingly complex health systems. Such collaborations, between nursing educational programs and clinical settings, are crafted to bridge the gap between academic preparation and practical realities of nursing work. Defined as intentional relationships characterized by mutual goals, respect, and shared knowledge, these partnerships aim to enhance the educational experiences of nursing students, thereby improving patient care quality and safety (American Association of Colleges of Nursing [AACN], 2023).

This chapter provides effective strategies for forming and maintaining meaningful academic–practice partnerships. It explores the roles and responsibilities inherent in collaborations between nursing schools and clinical environments, presenting various models of clinical training within these partnerships. Additionally, the chapter discusses the significance of these partnerships and the vital roles that nurse educators play in fostering sustainable, effective collaborations that propel contemporary models of clinical nursing education forward.

EVOLUTION OF ACADEMIC–PRACTICE PARTNERSHIPS

Historically, academic–practice partnerships were established for a wide range of purposes relevant to advancing religious missions, delivery of patient care, research, government programs, and hospital initiatives. Educational institutions and clinical entities began developing alliances and partnerships with the aim to further research, develop pathways to address healthcare provider shortages, and provide educational opportunities for learners. The continuing nursing shortage, access to healthcare, and the need for continuous quality care and improved patient safety reflect ongoing shared interests among academic and healthcare service organizations. As a result, academic programs, service agencies, and regulatory or policy–making bodies continue to align and leverage resources to meet the challenges of educating the healthcare workforce and building safer delivery systems (AACN, 2016; AACN/American

Organization of Nurse Executives [AACN/AONE], 2023). These organizations and partnerships recommit to improving patient experience and health outcomes through academic–practice partnerships. Academic-practice partnerships must be mutually beneficial to further the goal of healthcare equity and access.

The 2016 AACN report, *Advancing Healthcare Transformation*, also known as the Manatt Report, highlighted opportunities for the future of academic nursing and the nursing profession (AACN, 2016). While this report focuses on nursing and academic health centers (AHCs), much can be applied to the development of academic–practice partnerships outside of the AHC setting. For academic–practice partnerships, the implications of this report are calling for nursing to be a full partner in the practice setting, engaging faculty in practice with the partner, and in the development of nurses at all levels, including creating nurse-led care models.

In 2018, the AACN and AONE joined forces to address models of care and to strengthen practice and academic alignment (American Organization for Nursing Leadership [AONL], 2018). The new strategic advisory group seeks to advance the earlier work of the AACN and AONE. The committee has two strategic priorities focusing on leveraging practice and academic leaders. The first priority calls for the development and implementation of a nursing leader campaign to influence leaders in practice and academia about the need for partnerships that address workforce shortages using new models for learning and care (AONL, 2018). The second priority focuses on collaboration between academic and practice leaders in the identification of opportunities and challenges when creating effective partnerships (AONL, 2018). The AACN and AONE continue to work to identify exemplar academic–clinical practices, ascertain challenges, and provide support to contribute to the impact and success of these partnerships (AACN/AONE, 2023)

CURRENT STATUS OF ACADEMIC–PRACTICE PARTNERSHIPS

Academic–practice partnerships overcome challenges faced by academic institutions and clinical practices. On the academic side, schools of nursing are challenged to meet the educational training of nursing programs due to a shortage of clinical opportunities and faculty. The AACN (2016) and others (Padilla & Kreider, 2020; Petges et al., 2020; Roach & Hooke, 2019) highlight the value and significance of partnerships in improving the quality and effectiveness of nursing education and have called for support and collaboration among stakeholders. Collaboration is necessary to maximize the use of limited resources and build capacity to educate more nurses. Clinical practices and institutions are struggling with a shortage of providers and experts in quality improvement and implementation science. Practices, therefore, benefit from partnerships by developing a pathway for future nurses, ensuring up-to-date patient care, developing access to expert nurses for support on quality improvement projects, and increasing patient access through faculty practices. The ultimate purpose of formal academic–practice relationships is to advance nursing practice and to improve the health of the public (AACN, 2012). In 2015, the AACN and AONE reviewed and modified the guidelines to address the changing environment of academic–practice partnerships (AACN, 2018).

Partnerships are evolving in significance, purpose, structure, and expected outcomes. Examples of academic–practice partnerships focus on educating nurses, sharing resources, and undertaking projects on nursing student clinical education, evidence-based practice initiatives, interprofessional education (IPE), and professional development or academic progression programs. In academic–practice partnerships, both members of the partnership benefit. Within the partnership model, students, practice-setting nurses, and academic programs benefit. Engagement of faculty not only in practice, but as valuable members of the practice organization, can lead to examination of current trends, issues, and problems experienced within the practice environment from a new perspective.

ESTABLISHING MEANINGFUL PARTNERSHIPS

The AACN–AONE Task Force recognized the significance of academic–practice partnerships in empowering nurses to drive change and advance health. While these relationships are broadly defined, key guiding principles were identified and endorsed by both the AACN and AONE (AACN, 2012). These eight guiding principles provide a useful framework for nurse leaders in both academic and practice settings to understand the development of meaningful relationships (Exhibit 12.1).

The ability to establish and sustain effective partnerships is based on shared mission, values, and trust. Relationships are built through effective, clear communication and commitment to addressing conflicts collaboratively. Opportunities for moving from contractual affiliations to meaningful partnerships exist from carefully planning initial discussions to evaluating outcomes. However, the efforts involved in developing and sustaining strong collaborative relationships are complex and time-consuming, and often influenced by personal commitments or individual representation within the organization.

An interactive toolkit was developed by the AACN–AONE in 2012 and revised in 2015 to guide nursing leaders in the development, growth, and evaluation of

---

EXHIBIT 12.1 AACN–AONE Guiding Principles for Academic–Practice Partnerships

Collaborative relationships between academia and practice are established and sustained

Mutual respect and trust are the cornerstones of the practice–academia relationship

Knowledge is shared among partners

A commitment is shared by partners to maximize the potential of each registered nurse (RN) to reach the highest level within their individual scope of practice

A commitment is shared by partners to work together to determine an evidence-based transition program for students and new graduates that is both sustainable and cost-effective

A commitment is shared by partners to develop, implement, and evaluate organizational processes and structures that support and recognize academic or educational achievements

A commitment is shared by partners to support opportunities for nurses to lead and develop collaborative models that redesign practice environments to improve health outcomes

A commitment is shared by partners to establish infrastructures to collect and analyze data on the current and future needs of the RN workforce

---

AACN, American Association of Colleges of Nursing; AONE, American Organization of Nurse Executives.
Source: American Association of Colleges of Nursing and American Organization of Nurse Executives Task Force on Academic–Practice Partnerships. (2012). Guiding principles for academic-practice partnerships. https://www.aacnnursing.org/our-initiatives/education-practice/academic-practice-partnerships/the-guiding-principles-for-academic-practice-partnerships.

academic–practice partnerships. The toolkit is available at https://www.aacnnursing.org/our-initiatives/education-practice/academic-practice-partnerships/implementation-tool-kit. The toolkit includes specific questions for developing and sustaining partnerships, exemplars of strong academic–practice partnerships, and other resources. The successful implementation of an academic–practice partnership to increase educational capacity requires supportive relationships, goodness of fit, flexibility, and communication (Teel et al., 2011). These themes are described in Table 12.1.

In a systematic review of the evidence, Nabavi et al. (2012) identified four stages related to the formation and implementation of academic and service partnerships. The stages, outlined in Table 12.2, are applicable to a variety of partnerships and create a framework for identifying structures, processes, procedures, and outcomes.

TABLE 12.1 FOUR THEMES CONTRIBUTING TO SUCCESSFUL IMPLEMENTATION OF ACADEMIC–PRACTICE PARTNERSHIP

Theme	Application Strategy

Supportive relationships	Students, faculty, and preceptors (clinical staff) form a core triad:
	■ Elements of supportive relationships:
	  • Pairing of student and preceptor
	  • Orientation of preceptors by faculty
	  • Faculty role as advocate between student and preceptor
	■ Continuity of clinical rotations in a single clinical agency

Goodness of fit	Planning for and assessing the innovation for an appropriate "fit." This includes: ■ An organizational culture that values and supports innovation ■ Recognition of vital roles of faculty and preceptors including various forms of financial support ■ Assessment and identification of potential participants (students, preceptors, faculty) and program components for the best "fit"
Flexibility	The partnership stakeholders recognize: ■ Organizational culture, structure, rules, and needs that will influence partnership ■ Willingness to change ■ Value of feedback from students, faculty, preceptors to adapt and change
Communication	Multiple modes of communication foster effective use of resources and information to meet the needs of students, faculty, and clinical partners in the partnerships (printed literature; interviews of students, faculty, and preceptors; websites and portals; e-mail and telephone communication; regularly scheduled face-to-face meetings with all stakeholders)

Source: Adapted from Teel, C. S., MacIntyre, R. C., Murray, T. A., & Rock, Z. (2011). Common themes in clinical education partnerships. *Journal of Nursing Education, 50*(7), 365–372. https://doi.org/10.3928/01484834-20110429-01

TABLE 12.2 FOUR STAGES OF FORMATION AND IMPLEMENTATION OF ACADEMIC–SERVICE PARTNERSHIPS

Four Stages	Examples
Mutual potential benefits Discovery of interests or issues which could be served by resources of a partnership	- Nursing workforce shortage - Insufficient number of clinical placements to support increasing enrollments - Insufficient number of qualified/clinically competent faculty - Development of evidence-based practice, including translation of nursing research into practice
Moving from competitor to collaborator Planning and development of a cooperative structural framework that includes identification and coalition of stakeholders	- Senior leadership from each partner (academic, service, legislative, regulatory agencies) or other stakeholders identify mutual interests and set mission, goals, plans, timelines, and deadlines: - Executive/management committee or advisory council
Shared decision or policy making Structure that facilitates interaction between partners	- Task force or working groups formed to promote interaction in a partnership. Focus and activities are to implement mission of partnership and develop methods, including supervision or oversight, identification of roles and responsibilities, framework for decision-making, and training needs across organizations in partnership - Development of job descriptions - Affiliation agreement and contract auditing - Regulatory education and compliance monitoring - Preceptor development - Continuing education/staff development
Joint practice—Process of cooperation between the academic and service organizations to meet mutual goals	- New structures and procedures in a partnership bring change to roles and responsibilities for employees in each organization and for students (e.g., faculty appointments, models of precepting/supervising students, use of service learning, IPE)

Mutually beneficial outcomes
Three realms of benefits to an effective academic–service partnership:
  1. Service/practice
  2. Education
  3. Profession
	- Career progression path for clinical nurses into education
	- Clinical nurse job satisfaction
	- Increase in number of clinical faculty
	- Increased educational capacity
	- Supportive learning environments
	- Improved employment and recruitment opportunities

IPE, interprofessional education.
Source: Adapted from Nabavi, F. H., Vanaki, Z., & Mohammadi, E. (2012). Systematic review: Process of forming academic service partnership to reform clinical education. *Western Journal of Nursing Research, 34*(1), 118–141. https://doi.org/10.1177/0193945910394380

STRUCTURAL FOUNDATIONS OF ACADEMIC–PRACTICE PARTNERSHIPS

Capacity Management

Nursing programs are increasingly under pressure to admit and educate more students, given the demand to ease the nursing shortage and meet the healthcare needs of an aging population. Applications to baccalaureate and graduate nursing programs in the United Sates have been steadily increasing since 2000 (AACN, 2023). Despite a slight dip in 2022 (1.4% decrease in enrollment), 78,200 qualified applications were denied due to insufficient faculty, clinical sites, clinical preceptors, and budget constraints (AACN, 2023). Similarly, 23% of qualified applicants to associate degree nursing programs in 2021 were turned away (National League for Nursing, 2023).

Although there are limited fiscal capital and human resources, nursing leaders recognize the expertise across education and practice that is needed to address complex challenges in improving patient safety, quality care, and cost-effective outcomes. When determining the capacity relevant to preparing nurses, nursing administrators consider the organization's mission and values and the impact on patient care delivery, patient outcomes, and nursing staff resources. For example, hiring policies related to educational preparation required for nursing positions and accreditation, such as Magnet™, have begun to provide the framework for the type of academic degree programs the agency will host. Many decisions to host students in the service agency also consider the time; number of resources needed, including personnel, equipment, and space; costs associated with those resources; and the overall number of placement requests from nursing programs. Examples of service agency variables in determining clinical capacity are depicted in Table 12.3.

TABLE 12.3 EXAMPLES OF SERVICE AGENCY VARIABLES IN DETERMINING CLINICAL CAPACITY

Operational Systems	Clinical Services
<ul><li>Determination and monitoring of affiliation agreements/contracts and associated policies that determine roles and responsibilities of the partnership</li><li>Providing The Joint Commission standards required for orientation of nonemployees, which includes students, related to basic life safety and agency operations/resources</li><li>Electronic medical record access and medication dispensing systems for student use, which includes training, surveillance of proper use, and troubleshooting resources</li></ul>	<ul><li>Hours of agency operation</li><li>Types of patient services offered and location of services</li><li>Opening or closing and expansion of patient care units or services</li><li>Changing staffing, skill mix, patient acuity, and census levels that reflect productivity metrics and patient outcome indicators</li><li>Existing and anticipated competency-based education, training, and orientation needs of experienced and newly hired staff</li><li>Supply levels of personal protective equipment</li><li>Safety for nonemployees in the environment</li></ul>

Service agencies may also examine clinical placement requests in terms of their experience and familiarity with the academic curriculum, model of student supervision used for clinical education, and previous experiences with student performance. Agencies carefully consider requests for preceptorships in terms of the availability of staff with appropriate credentials and educational background, availability and costs associated with preceptor development courses, and preceptor incentives. The workload distribution and impact on productivity when clinical staff assume a heavy responsibility for clinical education during a preceptorship are important factors in determining capacity. Assessment and identification of healthy clinical work environments are other critical considerations.

Nurse educators from both academic and practice settings should consider the systems, frameworks, and practices that support nurses in developing competence to deliver safe and quality patient care across settings and the continuum of care. This is the first step in determining if the clinical unit is appropriate and ready to develop clinical learning experiences and student placements. Nursing programs continue to establish partnerships with ambulatory care, primary care clinics, outpatient care settings, and community-based sites (refugee centers, day treatment centers, respite care centers, and walk-in care centers) to augment student learning experiences.

Academic and practice partnerships may use centralized computer or web-based programs to standardize student placement processes. Additional purposes and functions of these programs are to monitor student placement numbers at clinical sites and on units, identify sites and units not being used but with the potential for development to support clinical learning and course objectives, and improve information sharing between nursing programs and service agencies for decision-making about current and future needs for clinical placements. Using data derived from placement platforms, including efficacy and quality measurement, to drive innovations in clinical education is an opportunity for further research. Financial models for the sustainability of centralized clinical placement platforms are also evolving, with costs shared between academic and service partners or covered through student use fees.

Clinical Affiliation Agreements

The clinical practice environment for students is defined through written agreements jointly designed to benefit academic and practice partners with ongoing evaluation and continuous improvement (AACN, 2021). The clinical affiliation agreement is a tool used by a healthcare agency and an academic program to provide clinical learning experiences for students. Exhibit 12.2 lists areas often included in a clinical affiliation agreement.

Clinical affiliation agreements typically have multiple clauses that serve to protect the healthcare agency and academic program. It is common for the affiliation agreement to be reviewed by legal counsel, risk management, human resources, and agency and nursing program administration to ensure that all interests are represented. The healthcare agency and academic program have mandates to structure the affiliation agreement. However, the intent of the partnership is to provide a supportive learning environment and associated clinical experiences for students. The leadership structure of each organization determines the signature authority to establish an affiliation agreement.

> **EXHIBIT 12.2 Content Areas of a Clinical Affiliation Agreement**
>
> Shared purpose of healthcare agency and nursing program
> Term period of agreement and renewal
> Scope of clinical placement
> Responsibilities of the healthcare agency
> Responsibilities of the academic program
> Joint responsibilities
> Employment status
> Payment status
> Insurance and other provisions

Although the affiliation agreement provides the framework for clinical learning experiences, it is essential to recognize that the collaboration between academic program faculty and representatives from the healthcare agency is critical to selecting appropriate learning environments and experiences to facilitate the achievement of specific learning outcomes. The collaborative effort extends to determining the type of student supervision required in the clinical environment or model of clinical instruction used.

Associated internal policies within the healthcare agency may also support affiliation agreements and student placements. Policies describe the circumstances under which students may have clinical experiences as part of an academic program. Accountability of agency personnel and students is identified in these policies, which include the steps in the process for clinical placement of students, orientation of students to the agency, and methods for determining and evaluating clinical placements in the agency. Recordkeeping of placements and audits of compliance with aspects of the affiliation agreement are also components of an agency's policy. Course faculty, students, and nurses interfacing with the students need to be aware of the policies related to the presence of students in the practice setting. Revisiting the policies with appropriate individuals each term can create a clear framework of expectations, responsibilities, and rules related to clinical experiences.

ALLIANCE FOR CLINICAL EDUCATION

The Alliance for Clinical Education (ACE) is an example of an academic–practice partnership that represents more than 70 nursing schools, healthcare organizations, and professional and regulatory entities in the Denver, Colorado, metropolitan area and surrounding region. ACE aims to promote collaboration between practice and education in preparing a nursing workforce for the future. The ACE group meets quarterly as a forum to share ideas and information and to make recommendations surrounding best practices, community standards, and regulatory compliance to provide the optimum clinical student learning experiences (ACE, 2015).

This alliance between education and healthcare organizations not only addresses clinical nursing education issues as a primary focus but also serves as a forum to connect and inform members of initiatives and changes affecting nursing workforce development occurring within individual organizations, the State of Colorado Board of Nursing, the Colorado Area Health Education Councils, the Colorado Center for

Nursing Excellence, and the Colorado Nurses' Association. The ACE bylaws, scope of work, meeting minutes, and documents are open-source materials and can be found at https://www.coloradonursingcenter.org/alliance-for-clinical-education.

MODELS OF CLINICAL EDUCATION

Quality clinical experiences are intended to give students time and opportunity to synthesize professional values, roles, and cognitive and psychomotor skills into emerging practice competencies. Support of practice outcome competencies along the education continuum, including transition into professional practice, should be a shared priority for academic and service partnerships. With a changing landscape of healthcare delivery models and reimbursement, academic and service entities are adding process improvement, research and quality improvement methodologies, and outcomes evaluation into examining the success of their partnerships in preparing the future healthcare workforce (Roach & Hooke, 2019). The boundaries of teaching and learning environments in which partnerships function continue to be challenged by paradigm shifts and innovations. For example, Petges et al. (2020) present their participatory action research (PAR) model as one that engages participants actively to address the gaps identified by the academic and clinical practice partner. Their model used eight steps to explore and create new student learning opportunities within nine clinical delivery systems.

Traditionally, the nursing education model in the United States consists of an academic faculty member or clinical nurse educator providing direct supervision of several students in the application of knowledge and skills acquired in the classroom, laboratory, or simulation setting to assigned patients. The model includes scheduling students in a patient care setting for set days per week and scheduling and rotating students in different healthcare agencies to meet different population competencies. Students are required to complete preclinical preparation work and other learning activities such as reflection. A recent integrative review found that the clinical nurse educator engages in planning for the experience, facilitation of learning, evaluation of students' skills, modeling, work-based assessment, and clinical teaching in the simulation lab (Gcawu & van Rooyen, 2022). Alternatives to traditional models of clinical education have been developed. Six types of clinical education models within academic–practice partnerships that reflect collaboration and innovation are described.

Interprofessional Education

The need for IPE and core competencies for interprofessional (IP) collaborative practice were discussed earlier in Chapter 11. Developing well-functioning teams is a priority because of the complexity of care delivery and the need for care coordination among the many providers a single patient may encounter. IP collaboration focuses on activities that promote integrated models of education and practice among students in health professions, including the value of each discipline as a full partner in delivering and determining quality and safe patient care. Students learn the professional role and scope of practice of their profession and, through IPE, develop an awareness of other health professional roles and the convergence of those roles to achieve the common goal of optimal patient outcomes.

IPE may occur in the classroom, through simulation, activities in the clinical setting, or a combination of these throughout health professions programs. Teaching strategies and learning opportunities to reframe relationships and use collaboration, negotiation, and communication skills are foundational in developing IP partnerships as a standard in professional practice. During the implementation of IPE initiatives or associated activities, the clinical teacher may be able to renegotiate traditional roles and responsibilities among staff and establish new ways of working that promote IP competencies.

Peer Teaching and Learning

Peer teaching and learning is a collaborative and cooperative teaching strategy where students are active and equal partners in the learning process. It can allow students to practice skills that they will utilize in their future profession and can foster a more personalized learning experience (Pålsson et al., 2021). In practice, peer teaching and learning may involve multiple students taking shared responsibility for an assigned patient, collaborating in care, and providing emotional support and feedback through discussions and assisting with physical skills and tasks.

Empirical research highlights the benefits of this method, particularly in small group settings which are conducive to interaction and support. These settings enable the provision of immediate, formative feedback, enhancing the learning experience (Knight & Brame, 2018). Additionally, students have reported greater satisfaction and an increase in self-confidence as direct outcomes of peer teaching (Usman & Jamil, 2019). Further investigation into peer learning dynamics revealed that unintended collaborative interactions often spur growth across various competencies, underscoring the role of peer interactions in educational advancement (Pålsson et al., 2021).

Peer teaching and learning may also enhance student access to, and involvement in, planned learning activities, potentially easing the demand on faculty resources. However, effective peer learning requires appropriate faculty supervision (Coffman et al., 2020; Usman & Jamil, 2019). Important considerations in implementing this educational approach include identifying the specific content and skills that are suitable for peer-assisted learning, determining the level of involvement and collaboration required from faculty or healthcare agency staff, and addressing any incompatibilities among students. By carefully navigating these factors, institutions can maximize the benefits of peer teaching and learning, fostering an educational environment that not only supports academic achievement but also prepares students for professional responsibilities in healthcare settings.

Service Learning

Service learning (SL) is a strategy that combines community service with instruction and reflection to enhance learning, promote civic responsibility, and strengthen communities (Hefferman, 2001). In this model, students engage in activities that are mutually identified by academic and community partners to benefit the community while connecting these experiences to their academic learning (Marcilla-Toribio et al., 2022). These partnerships may involve individual academic–clinical collaborations or be part of broader agreements with health systems, such as operating a mobile health clinic within a larger health network.

The process of reflection is a key component of SL, setting it apart from mere volunteerism. This may include journaling or participating in structured debriefing sessions (Bennett et al., 2016). SL has been linked to increased student knowledge in areas such as social activism, healthcare equity (Lee & Kelley-Petersen, 2018), cultural diversity (Bartleet et al., 2019), and the development of leadership skills (Foli et al., 2014).

An integrative review by Marcilla-Toribio et al. (2022) highlighted the positive impact of SL on outcomes like teamwork and communication skills. Students reported increased empathy, a deeper questioning of their own prejudices, and a stronger commitment to their professions. Further, a qualitative systemic review and meta-synthesis found that students often found SL challenging but rewarding, noting an increase in confidence, clinical skills, leadership abilities, cultural awareness, and personal and professional growth (Zhu et al., 2022). SL models are versatile and can be applied to a wide range of community needs, including health screening programs, flu vaccination clinics, wellness initiatives for underserved populations or elderly individuals, food delivery services, friendly visitor programs, participation in health policy legislative sessions, and faith-based outreach efforts.

Clinical Scholar Model

The clinical scholar model (CSM) originated in 1984 as a joint initiative between the University of Colorado School of Nursing—Auschutz Medical Campus, and the University of Colorado Hospital. The model has expanded in the past three decades. The service agencies include acute care hospitals, county public health, and mental health and rehabilitation facilities. The financial modeling of the CSM varies among service agencies and correlates with overall student progression, placement needs, and curriculum objectives. Clinical scholars are expert nurses in service agencies who plan and coordinate students' clinical experiences, teach students, and contribute to evaluating their clinical competencies. Additionally, these nurses participate in training offered by their agency, the academic partner, or an external agency to introduce them to the concepts related to creating successful student learning experiences within the practice arena.

Qualifications and attributes of the clinical scholar include:

- Expert nurse who exemplifies professionalism and relationship-centered care in practice and conveys a passion for teaching and learning, particularly in the clinical setting
- An employee of the healthcare agency, with time dedicated to planning, coordinating, teaching, and evaluating student clinical experiences
- Master's prepared in nursing
- Minimum of 5 years' experience in a nursing specialty practice and 2 years of employment within the healthcare agency
- Recruited within the healthcare agency based on experience in practice and as a preceptor
- Jointly interviewed and hired by the college of nursing and the healthcare agency

Clinical scholars are invaluable to clinical education, coordinating placements and learning experiences, providing consistent instruction and supervision, and contributing to the evaluation of students' clinical competencies. They facilitate streamlined communication and act as liaisons to staff, helping integrate students smoothly into the clinical setting. Their involvement promotes consistency in educational experiences, enhances the relevance of clinical learning, and facilitates necessary curricular modifications. Tasked with treating every student interaction with respect and care, clinical scholars focus on collaboration, education, and evaluation to create an environment conducive to both learning and professional growth. These contributions not only bolster educational quality but also foster a collaborative atmosphere that supports student development.

Dedicated Education Units

The dedicated education unit (DEU) model, originated in the late 1990s at Flinders University of South Australia School of Nursing, exemplifies an effective academic–service partnership (Edgecombe et al., 1999). This model creates a triadic relationship among students, clinical nursing staff, and faculty members, designed to optimize the learning environment through collaborative efforts among clinical nurses, agency management, and academic faculty (Moscato et al., 2013). The key features of the DEU model are:

1. The clinical unit is an optimal teaching/learning environment.
2. The primary goal is student achievement of learning outcomes.
3. The DEU is used solely by one nursing program.
4. The commitment to attain an optimal practice environment for students and staff is shared through collaborative work efforts and communication.
5. Staff nurses, who indicate a desire to teach, are prepared for the clinical teaching role, and nursing faculty members from the academic program support the staff nurse in the instructor role.
6. Students are paired with the staff nurse, who is a clinical teacher (Moscato et al., 2013).

The essence of the DEU model is the pivotal educational role played by staff nurses in facilitating students' acquisition of knowledge and skills (Moscato et al., 2013). Successful partnerships within DEUs are characterized by collaboration, respect, trust, goodwill, and equal participation (Marcellus et al., 2021). This model has proven effective in enhancing critical thinking skills among nursing students and is highly favored by students for the support it provides (Hooper et al., 2020). Furthermore, the DEU model supports the teaching and learning of quality improvement and safety competencies, reduces student anxiety, and builds trust and confidence in students (Rusch et al., 2018). DEUs are not limited to traditional acute care or medical–surgical units but are also implemented in varied patient care settings such as long-term care, maternal–newborn units, and intensive care units.

DEUs enhance the capacity of clinical agencies, allowing for increased student enrollments and accommodation of more students in practice settings compared to traditional preceptor models (Marcellus et al., 2021). Research indicates high satisfaction among both students and staff with the clinical teaching and learning experiences within DEUs (Rusch et al., 2018). In a mixed-methods study, Hooper et al. (2020) found that students and preceptors believed the DEU model better facilitated student learning. Additional benefits of DEUs include increased satisfaction among staff nurses, who feel valued for their clinical expertise, and fostering of teamwork to create a supportive learning environment. This model also encourages nurses to pursue further education (Fusner & Melnyk, 2019). Moreover, DEU agency partners have reported reduced orientation times for new graduate nurses who have undergone DEU clinical experiences, emphasizing the staff's appreciation for the students they have educated (Sharpnack et al., 2014; Smyer et al., 2015).

Faculty Practice Model

The faculty practice model empowers faculty members to engage in clinical settings, taking responsibility for patient outcomes. This model emerged in response to the disconnect between didactic faculty teaching in research and practice and patient care. Integrating practice with education proves beneficial for both academic institutions and practice sites. The AACN and the National Organization of Nurse Practitioner Faculties (NONPF) support this model, underscoring the importance of faculty maintaining up-to-date clinical knowledge and skills (AACN, 2021). A defining feature of faculty practice is that faculty members remain actively involved in all academic facets, including teaching, scholarship, and service, distinguishing faculty practice from roles such as preceptor or clinical instructor.

Benefits of the faculty practice model include enhanced educational and patient outcomes, opportunities for scholarly collaboration, and pathways for nurturing future faculty (Gonzales et al., 2023a, 2023b). Specifically, within education, faculty practice improves learner assessment (Gonzales et al., 2023a). Challenges include achieving promotion or tenure, limited space and clinical hours, and demanding productivity metrics (Gonzales et al., 2023a, 2023b). Faculty, students, and administrators view faculty practice as positively impacting education (Gonzales et al., 2023a).

The faculty practice agreement can be established within an affiliation agreement between academic and practice institutes or as a standalone contract. Common barriers such as financial constraints necessitate having a dedicated individual or office to manage faculty practice contracts. Key contract considerations should include competitive hourly rates, renegotiation terms, productivity expectations, precepting responsibilities, and provisions for sick leave (Gonzales & Stoltman, 2020). Agreements can be structured as fee for service, where the practice setting compensates the institution for the faculty's time, which in turn pays the faculty. Alternatively, agreements might involve dual appointments in both the academic and practice settings. Monitoring the outcomes of these agreements is crucial to ensure satisfaction for both academic and clinical partners. Once established, these contracts allow faculty to focus on educating students, providing care, engaging with nurses, and conducting scholarly work.

Within the faculty practice model, various configurations exist. Some models involve a single practice setting where multiple faculty members work on different days or hours. This arrangement familiarizes staff and patients with the educational environment and facilitates faculty coverage of ongoing responsibilities, easing patient handoffs. However, it may lead to clinics or rotations that do not integrate well with larger health practice settings. This stand-alone practice can be organized through a joint appointment agreement or operated by an academic institution. Another model permits faculty members to practice for a set number of hours within a stand-alone unit. Here, faculty bring students on-site on their working days, allowing students to observe faculty interactions with the IP team. While this model enriches the learning experience, it may complicate ongoing clinical responsibilities when the faculty member is absent. This setup is typically arranged through a fee-for-service model.

Students benefit from learning in both practice and classroom settings under faculty guidance, gaining insights into current practices and linking didactic learning with practical application. Nurses in practice settings have opportunities to influence nursing education in response to the growing complexity of patient care. They can collaborate with students and faculty on quality improvement projects to enhance patient health outcomes. Faculty members also use their practical experiences to inform and update academic curricula.

The practice leadership network within the AACN recently released a tool kit providing a framework for faculty practice, available for download here: https://www.aacnnursing.org/faculty-tool-kits. Additionally, NONPF has updated its tool kit for faculty practice in 2023, accessible to members at: https://www.nonpf.org/news/631972/Faculty-Practice-Tool-Kit-2nd-Edition-2023.htm.

ROLES OF PARTICIPANTS IN PARTNERSHIPS

In any partnership, the value of the mission must be demonstrated and supported first and most fundamentally by the chief nurse officer and nursing school dean or director. The challenge is to establish working relationships through awareness of mutual goals, develop trust and effective communication, and engage to ensure that affiliations move to meaningful partnerships. After the partnership is established, the value of the partnership should be continuously embraced and cultivated by nurse leaders, faculty, and staff responsible for the planning, implementation, and evaluation. Nursing faculty and agency staff activities influence the relationship and contribute to meeting needs and achieving goals. Roles and responsibilities at each level are important determinants of the effectiveness of the partnership.

A vast range of opportunities for effective partnerships and collaboration await faculty from the academic program and nurses at the staff or unit leader level at the clinical agency. Mutual respect, valuing, and investment are demonstrated through presence, engagement, and effective faculty and unit staff communication. Nurse educators and clinical faculty impact the quality of the partnership through planning and preparation for the student learning experiences with unit managers and staff. Students who demonstrate readiness and professionalism contribute to developing a meaningful and valued role for the team and delivering quality and safe care. The appropriate level of student engagement, including expectations for patient assessment, nursing interventions, documentation, and supervision, should be clarified to the team members. Team member roles and responsibilities should be explained to the student.

Staff nurses who are prepared for the students' presence and learning needs and are recognized for their expertise feel valued for their contributions to clinical education. The faculty can support the nurse educators through the development of clinical teaching skills. The relationship of faculty and clinical teachers with the nursing staff and nurse leaders at the patient care unit or service level is critical to an effective partnership. Additional evidence of the partnership may include volunteer faculty appointments, preceptor training, student scholarships, participation in unit-based or nursing education committees relevant to quality and safety, and competency development.

SUSTAINING PARTNERSHIPS

The principles outlined in the AACN/AONE documents provide an excellent framework for academic and practice partners to use in the creation of their agreement. Multiple resources are available at www.aacnnursing.org/Academic-Practice-Partnerships. Essential principles for developing and sustaining a trusting and respectful partnership include a shared mission, vision, and goals. The partnership must build on shared strengths and assets while balancing power between the partners. Norms for communication, processes, roles, and policies need to be carefully delineated and followed. The establishment of routine communication that provides feedback in a timely manner allows for quality improvement changes to occur. Additionally, outcome measures that are mutually agreed on are critical to the evaluation of the partnership. The AACN–AONE task force developed outcome metrics, available for download here: https://www.aacnnursing.org/our-initiatives/education-practice/academic-practice-partnerships/partnership-expectation-and-outcome-matrix. The partnership is collaborative and supports everyone's success while sharing responsibility. Partnerships take time to develop and need planned feedback loops to be successful.

FUTURE OF ACADEMIC–PRACTICE PARTNERSHIPS

One of the long-term goals of academic and practice partnerships is to transform clinical education, patient outcomes, and clinical care. This includes partnering with nursing faculty and researchers across both environments. To transform clinical education and address the real-world complexities of healthcare encountered by students, teaching and practice innovations should be coupled with teamwork and collaboration among health professionals in academic and service organizations. Students' experiences of these innovative training models within academic–practice partnerships are positive, with improved clinical learning (Pedregosa et al., 2020). As doctor of nursing practice (DNP) programs continue to grow with a focus on implementation science, there is a burgeoning opportunity to further develop and expand academic–practice partnerships. These collaborations have already demonstrated their effectiveness in supporting quality improvement and enhancing patient outcomes (Phillips et al., 2019). The landscape for creating new and innovative academic–practice partnerships is expanding, promising significant impact on healthcare education and delivery.

SUMMARY

Academic–practice partnerships are continually catalyzing innovations in clinical education, drawing from rich experiences, contextual knowledge, and empirical data. These partnerships serve as potent agents of change within nursing education, fostering engagement among students, faculty, clinical staff, and nursing administrators to develop evidence-based educational models. Essential to the formation of these partnerships are guiding principles rooted in shared missions and values. Once established, these collaborations support a variety of clinical education models that yield mutual benefits to both academic institutions and practice settings. Notable models include IPE, peer teaching and learning, the CSM, SL, DEU, and the faculty practice model. The collaborative design of these partnerships is crucial for selecting the most suitable model and securing successful outcomes, which ultimately enhance patient health outcomes. These partnerships are poised to further evolve, offering new opportunities to assess their effects on the transition to professional practice, nurse retention, patient outcomes, and broader organizational impacts.

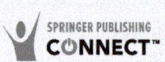

A robust set of instructor resources designed to supplement this text is located at http://connect.springerpub.com/content/book/978-0-8261-8892-2. Qualifying instructors may request access by emailing textbook@springerpub.com.

REFERENCES

Alliance for Clinical Education. (2015). *By-laws*. http://www.coloradonursingcenter.org/documents/ace/bylaws_042015.pdf

American Association of Colleges of Nursing. (2012). *The guiding principles for academic-practice partnerships*. https://www.aacnnursing.org/our-initiatives/education-practice/academic-practice-partnerships/the-guiding-principles-for-academic-practice-partnerships

American Association of Colleges of Nursing. (2016). *Advancing healthcare transformation: A new era for academic nursing*. https://www.aacnnursing.org/portals/42/publications/aacn-new-era-report.pdf

American Association of Colleges of Nursing. (2018). *AACN and AONE join forces to address nursing workforce issues*. https://www.aonl.org/aacn-and-aone-join-forces-advance-new-models-care-and-address-nursing-workforce-issues

American Association of Colleges of Nursing. (2021). *The essentials: Core competencies for professional nursing education*. https://www.aacnnursing.org/Portals/0/PDFs/Publications/Essentials-2021.pdf

American Association of Colleges of Nursing. (2023). *New data show enrollment declines in schools of nursing, raising concerns about the nation's nursing workforce*. https://www.aacnnursing.org/news-data/all-news/new-data-show-enrollment-declines-in-schools-of-nursing-raising-concerns-about-the-nations-nursing-workforce

American Association of Colleges of Nursing and American Organization of Nurse Executives Task Force on Academic–Practice Partnerships. (2023). *Academic-practice afternoon of dialogue summary report*. https://www.aacnnursing.org/Portals/0/PDFs/Reports/AONL-AACN-Afternoon-of-Dialogue-Summary-March-2023.pdf

American Organization for Nursing Leadership. (2018). *AACN and AONE join forces to address nursing workforce issues*. https://www.aonl.org/aacn-and-aone-join-forces-advance-new-models-care-and-address-nursing-workforce-issues

Bartleet, B.-L., Bennett, D., Power, A., & Sunderland, N. (2019). Service learning with first peoples: A framework to support respectful and reciprocal learning. *Intercultural Education*, 30(1), 15–30. https://doi.org/10.1080/14675986.2018.1528526

Bennett, D., Sunderland, N., Bartleet, B.-L., & Power, A. (2016). Implementing and sustaining higher education service-learning initiatives. *Journal of Experiential Education*, 39(2), 145–163. https://doi.org/10.1177/1053825916629987

Coffman, J. M., McConkey, M. J., & Cole, J. (2020). Effectiveness of video-assisted, self-directed, and peer-guided learning in the acquisition of surgical skills by veterinary students. *Veterinary Surgery*, 49(3), 582–589. https://doi.org/10.1111/vsu.13368

Edgecombe, K., Wotton, K., Gonda, J., & Mason, P. (1999). Dedicated education units: 1 A new concept for clinical teaching and learning. *Contemporary Nurse, 8*(4), 166–171. https://doi.org/10.5172/conu.1999.8.4.166

Foli, K. J., Braswell, M., Kirkpatrick, J., & Lim, E. (2014). Development of leadership behaviors in undergraduate nursing students: A service-learning approach. *Nursing Education Perspectives, 35*(2), 76–82. https://doi.org/10.5480/11-578.1

Fusner, S., & Melnyk, B. M. (2019). Dedicated education units: A unique evaluation. *Journal of Doctoral Nursing Practice, 12*(1), 102–110. https://doi.org/10.1891/2380-9418.12.1.102

Gcawu, S. N., & van Rooyen, D. R. (2022). Clinical teaching practices of nurse educators: An integrative literature review. *Health SA Gesondheid (Online), 27*, 1–9. http://doi.org/10.4102/hsag.v27i0.1728

Gonzales, K., Holmes, L., Klein, A., Hanish, A., & Struwe, L. (2023a). Faculty practice as an educational strategy: Student, faculty, and administrator perspectives. *Nurse Educator, 48*(4), 214–219. https://doi.org/10.1097/nne.0000000000001367

Gonzales, K., Holmes, L., Klein, A., Struwe, L., & Hanish, A. (2023b). Academic nursing and faculty practice. *Nurse Educator, 48*(2), E53–E58. https://doi.org/10.1097/nne.0000000000001305

Gonzales, K., & Stoltman, A. (2020). Optimization of faculty practice. *Journal of Professional Nursing, 36*(1), 56–61. https://doi.org/10.1016/j.profnurs.2019.06.013

Hefferman, K. (2001). Service-learning in higher education. *Journal of Contemporary Water Research and Education, 199*(1), 1–8.

Hooper, R. A., AlMekkawi, M., Williams, G., Thompson, B., & Zeeman, M. (2020). Nursing Students' perceptions of the dedicated education unit model in 2 UAE hospitals. *Dubai Medical Journal, 3*(2), 61–69. https://doi.org/10.1159/000508714

Knight, J. K., & Brame, C. J. (2018). Peer instruction. *CBE - Life Sciences Education, 17*(2), 1–4. https://doi.org/10.1187/cbe.18-02-0025

Lee, K. A., & Kelley-Petersen, D. J. (2018). Service learning in human development: Promoting social justice perspectives in counseling. *Professional Counselor, 8*(2), 146–158. https://doi.org/10.15241/kal.8.2.146

Marcellus, L., Jantzen, D., Humble, R., Sawchuck, D., & Gordon, C. (2021). Characteristics and processes of the dedicated education unit practice education model for undergraduate nursing students: A scoping review. *JBI Evidence Synthesis, 19*(11), 2993–3039. https://doi.org/10.11124/JBIES-20-00462

Marcilla-Toribio, I., Moratalla-Cebrián, M. L., Bartolomé-Guitierrez, R., Cebada-Sánchez, S., Galán-Moya, E. M., & Martínez-Andrés, M. (2022). Impact of Service-Learning educational interventions on nursing students: An integrative review. *Nurse Education Today, 116*, 105417. https://doi.org/10.1016/j.nedt.2022.105417

Moscato, S. R., Nishioka, V. M., & Coe, M. T. (2013). Dedicated education unit: Implementing an innovation in replication sites. *Journal of Nursing Education, 52*(5), 259–267. https://doi.org/10.3928/01484834-20130328-01

Nabavi, F. H., Vanaki, Z., & Mohammadi, E. (2012). Systematic review: Process of forming academic service partnership to reform clinical education. *Western Journal of Nursing Research, 34*(1), 118–141. https://doi.org/10.1177/0193945910394380

National League for Nursing. (2023). *NLN releases new survey results of nursing schools & programs showing persistent challenges to addressing the nursing shortage.* https://www.nln.org/detail-pages/news/2023/09/25/nln-releases-new-survey-results-of-nursing-schools-programs-showing-persistent-challenges-to-addressing-the-nursing-shortage

Padilla, B. I., & Kreider, K. E. (2020). Communities of practice: An innovative approach to building academic–practice partnerships. *Journal for Nurse Practitioners, 16*(4), 308–311. https://doi.org/10.1016/j.nurpra.2020.01.017

Pålsson, Y., Mårtensson, G., Swenne, C. L., Mogensen, E., & Engström, M. (2021). First-year nursing students' collaboration using peer learning during clinical practice education: An observational study. *Nurse Education in Practice, 50*, 102946. https://doi.org/10.1016/j.nepr.2020.102946

Pedregosa, S., Fabrellas, N., Risco, E., Pereira, M., Dmoch-Gajzlerska, E., Şenuzun, F., Martin, S., & Zabalegui, A. (2020). Effective academic-practice partnership models in nursing students' clinical placement: A systematic literature review. *Nurse Education Today, 95*, 104582. https://doi.org/10.1016/j.nedt.2020.104582

Petges, N., Sabio, C., & Hickey, K. (2020). An academic and clinical practice partnership model: Collaboration toward baccalaureate preparation of RNs. *Journal of Nursing Education, 59*(4), 203–209. https://doi.org/10.3928/01484834-20200323-05

Phillips, J. M., Phillips, C. R., Kauffman, K. R., Gainey, M., & Schnur, P. L. (2019). Academic–practice partnerships: A win-win. *Journal of Continuing Education in Nursing, 50*(6), 282–288. https://doi.org/10.3928/00220124-20190516-09

Roach, A., & Hooke, S. (2019). An Academic-Practice Partnership: Fostering collaboration and improving care across settings. *Nurse Educator, 44*(2), 98–101. https://doi.org/10.1097/NNE.0000000000000557

Rusch, L. M., McCafferty, K., Schoening, A. M., Hercinger, M., & Manz, J. (2018). Impact of the dedicated education unit teaching model on the perceived competencies and professional attributes of nursing students. *Nurse Education in Practice, 33*, 90–93. https://doi.org/10.1016/j.nepr.2018.09.002

Sharpnack, P. A., Koppelman, C., & Fellows, B. (2014). Using a dedication education unit clinical education model with second-degree accelerated nursing program students. *Journal of Nursing Education, 53*(12), 685–691. https://doi.org/10.3928/01484834-20141120-01

Smyer, T., Gatlin, T., Tan, R., Tejada, M., & Feng, D. (2015). Academic outcome measure of a dedicated education unit over time. Help or hinder? *Nurse Educator, 40*(6), 294–297. https://doi.org/10.1097/NNE.0000000000000176

Teel, C. S., MacIntyre, R. C., Murray, T. A., & Rock, Z. (2011). Common themes in clinical education partnerships. *Journal of Nursing Education, 50*(7), 365–372. https://doi.org/10.3928/01484834-20110429-01

Usman, R., & Jamil, B. (2019). Perceptions of undergraduate medical students about peer assisted learning. *Professional Medical Journal, 26*(8), 1283–1288. https://doi.org/10.29309/TPMJ/2019.26.08.3870

Zhu, Z., Xing, W., Liang, Y., Hong, L., & Hu, Y. (2022). Nursing students' experiences with service learning: A qualitative systematic review and meta-synthesis. *Nurse Education Today, 108*, 105206. https://doi.org/10.1016/j.nedt.2021.105206

Curriculum Development IV

Competency-Based Education in Nursing

13

Gerry Altmiller

OBJECTIVES

1. Compare competency-based education (CBE) principles with traditional teaching and learning structures
2. Use the American Association of Colleges of Nursing (AACN) *Essentials* as a framework for designing CBE and assessment
3. Demonstrate strategies for creating a curricular infrastructure to support CBE
4. Review learning activities and strategies for implementing competency-focused teaching and competency-based assessment

INTRODUCTION

Traditionally, nurse educators have developed curricula focused on the acquisition of knowledge and skills, believing that with knowledge, learners would have the basis to be practice ready. Research suggests, however, that this approach has left graduate nurses unprepared for the demands of current clinical practice. Kavanagh and Szweda (2017) studied 5000 nurses who had recently passed the National Council Licensure Exam (NCLEX®) and found that only 23% could recognize a patient problem and take it to resolution. Subsequent studies indicated that this statistic worsened after the COVID-19 pandemic (Kavanagh & Sharpnack, 2021), clearly demonstrating that knowledge alone does not equate to competency and creating a call to action for nurse educators to adopt a different approach for preparing future nurses for practice.

Additional impetus for change has been the increasing complexity of nursing work, ongoing employer dissatisfaction with the abilities of new-to-practice nurses, and the release of the American Association of Colleges of Nursing (AACN) *The Essentials: Core Competencies for Professional Nurse Education* (henceforth, *Essentials*; AACN, 2021). Along with reframing the focus of nursing education to align with quality and safety competencies, the *Essentials* call for nurse educators to adopt competency-based pedagogy across the curriculum. The National League for Nursing (NLN) also recognizes the significance of CBE as a modality for better preparing the nursing workforce, publishing the Vision Statement: *Integrating Competency-Based Education in the Nursing Curriculum* (NLN, 2023). Although the new emphasis on CBE and assessment may be a challenge for faculty, CBE has set the stage for an exciting and creative period of innovation in nursing education.

This chapter prepares educators for developing and implementing CBE in their nursing program. CBE as a learning model is described and compared to traditional teaching and learning structures. The AACN *Essentials* are used as a framework for designing CBE and assessment. CBE follows a backward design, which is explained in this chapter. Backward design also can be used to build the infrastructure that supports the adoption of CBE across the curriculum. Other content includes entrustable professional activities, how to develop program and course outcomes stated as competencies, curriculum mapping for CBE, and learning activities and strategies for implementing competency-focused teaching and competency-based assessment. Many examples are provided throughout this chapter.

COMPETENCY-BASED EDUCATION AS A LEARNING MODEL

A definition of CBE, adapted from Frank et al. (2010), is an outcomes-based approach to the design, implementation, assessment, and evaluation of nursing education programs using an organizing framework of competencies. Competencies are observable abilities of students that can be measured (Oermann, 2022). With CBE, the focus shifts from the content or the structure and process for how content is presented to the outputs of the instruction: Of key importance is what the individual can do because of what has been learned. In this way, it is a pedagogy that is learner-centered, focusing on the individual's ability to perform within one's professional context. Implementing CBE requires a restructuring of how nursing education is developed, delivered, and evaluated (Table 13.1).

TABLE 13.1 COMPARISON OF TRADITIONAL NURSING EDUCATION AND COMPETENCY-BASED EDUCATION

Construct	Traditional Approach	Competency-Based Approach
Structure	Didactic concentration	Personalized plan with supports
Instruction	Teacher centered: Lecture delivery	Student centered: Application activities
Assessment/Evaluation	Summative evaluation May have one opportunity to meet requirement Emphasis on knowledge	Frequent formative assessments with feedback Emphasis on performance outcomes
Grading	Norm referenced; comparison to others in class May be norm referenced (comparison to others in class) or criterion referenced (related to criteria, independent of other learners)	Criterion referenced
Progression	Based on meeting minimum standard of course	Based on safe performance for professional context

Copyright Gerry Altmiller, 2024. Reprinted by permission, 2024.

Covert et al. (2019) identified five characteristics of competencies: (1) They are focused on outcomes; (2) they reflect what has been learned; (3) they are expressed in observable, measurable behavior; (4) they become the standard for judging competency independent of any other person's performance; and (5) they inform learners and other interested parties about what is expected of the learner. Competency is developed on a continuum over time. Wittmann-Price and Gittings (2021) offer some concrete steps based on Miller's pyramid of competence (1990) to describe how learners demonstrate the development of competency in nursing (Figure 13.1). Correctly answering low-level, multiple-choice questions on a test demonstrates the learner "knows" facts. This is an important first step because knowledge is a constituent of competency (Rotthoff et al., 2021). When learners use those facts to work through case studies, solve problems presented in vignettes, or perform diagnostic reasoning, they are demonstrating that they "know how" to use those facts as part of clinical reasoning. In standardized simulation, as learners make decisions based on assessment findings and provide appropriate care, they "show how" the facts they know and the clinical reasoning they are developing can be applied in standardized controlled situations. However, the true measure of competency in nursing education comes from observations of performance where the learner "does" the work in a professional context, whether that be in providing direct care or in completing work that indirectly relates to patient care and nursing work.

Competency is a set of expectations that, when put into action collectively, demonstrate what learners can do with what they know. Nursing education has historically embraced the cognitive domain, frequently measured by Bloom's taxonomy (1956), the psychomotor domain measured in the skills laboratory or in the clinical setting, and the affective domain, often evaluated based on interactions between

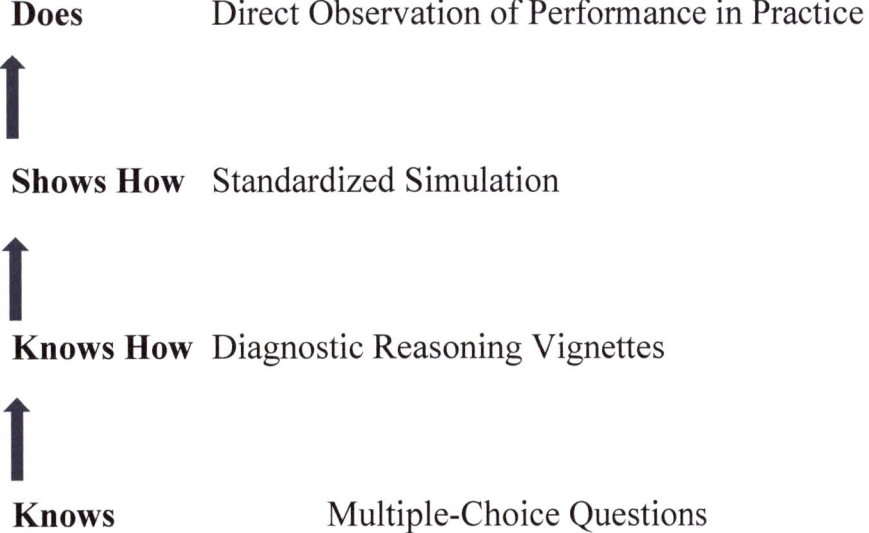

Figure 13.1 Development of competence.

Source: Miller, G. E. (1990). The assessment of clinical skills/competence/performance. *Academic Medicine, 65*(9), S63–67. https://doi.org/10.1097/00001888-199009000-00045; Wittmann-Price, R. A., & Gittings, K. K. (2021). *Fast facts about CBE in nursing.* Springer Publishing Company.

Copyright Gerry Altmiller, 2024. Reprinted by permission, 2024.

students and faculty. Moving toward CBE, the learning domains are a composite of knowledge, skills, and attitudes, and are evaluated together as a whole to determine the competency of the individual.

Consider the graduate student in a nurse anesthetist program. An expected competency is to safely intubate patients. Competency requires that the student have nursing knowledge of anatomy and physiology as well as skills to insert an endotracheal tube. Additionally, the student needs clinical reasoning abilities to determine if the patient requires sedation, effective communication skills as these events frequently occur under duress, and a professional demeanor as the team leader during the intubation. With CBE, the assessment of the student would be based on the entire intervention, because to assess any of these requirements individually does not assess competency. Competency in this example is the combined demonstration of knowledge, skills, and attitudes that allow for safe intubation.

CBE follows a backward design (Figure 13.2). The first step is that the desired results of the course are determined by the educator based on the curriculum plan. These desired results should be reflected in the student learning outcomes for the course and stated as competency statements. Simply put, educators consider what they want the learner to be able to do. Next, the educator determines the evidence needed to validate that learning has occurred and creates assessments to capture that validation. The assessments might be papers, projects, clinical performance evaluations, simulations, or any other observable and measurable demonstration of abilities. The final step is then to plan learning experiences and instruction to align with the course outcomes and support the learner in successfully completing the assessments to demonstrate competency.

Competency is developed on a continuum where the learner acquires and refines clinical judgment skills in increasingly more complex situations. New learning builds on previous learning. Clearly defined progression indicators determined by faculty at different points serve as the signal that competency is achieved, and the learner can progress in the program. Figure 13.3 demonstrates how the expectation of competency for safe medication administration evolves as the learner progresses through the program and develops the clinical judgment needed to manage increasingly complex situations related to medication administration. At the beginning of the program, the expectation may be that the learner would be able to correctly retrieve medications from the dispenser using the medication administration record (MAR). Because every assessment should have a judgment opportunity, at this early stage, the judgment may be that the medication order requires splitting a tablet or doubling tablets for the correct dose.

As the learner moves through the program, the complexity increases. Near the midpoint for the learner enrolled in a first medical-surgical nursing course, the expectation might be to retrieve medications associated with cardiac disease and diabetes from the MAR. During this phase of learning and assessment, the learner must consider the patient's blood pressure and blood glucose level prior to administration, using clinical judgment to determine if it is safe for the patient to receive the medications. The greatest complexity occurs toward the end of the program

Student Learning/Course Outcomes ⟹ Assessments ⟹ Learning Activities

Figure 13.2 Backward design for competency-based education.

Fundamentals Course	
Use MAR to obtains medications from PYXIS™	*Judgment*: Need to divide a tablet in half to get the correct dose
Medical-Surgical 1 Course	
Use MAR to obtain cardiac and diabetic medications from PYXIS™	*Judgment*: Need to consider BP and blood glucose level
Medical-Surgical 2 Course	
Use MAR to obtain cardiac, diabetic, and antibiotic medications from PYXIS™	*Judgment*: Need to consider BP and blood glucose level; patient due for hemodialysis treatment; and patent has a respiratory infection

Figure 13.3 Competency development with increasingly complex situations course outcome: Administers medication safely.
BP, blood pressure; MAR, medication administration record; PYXIS™, BD Pyxis™ medication station.
Copyright Gerry Altmiller, 2024. Reprinted by permission, 2024.

where the learner must consider additional factors such as a pending hemodialysis treatment or acute illness when making decisions regarding medication administration to demonstrate sound clinical reasoning and safe nursing judgment.

In true CBE, learners progress through the program at their own pace, which can create challenges for educators working within the current structure of higher education. Nursing education is moving toward a modified competency-based model that requires students to assume responsibility for seeking out experiences and be accountable for their learning. While there is a plan for each course with a start and end date, struggling students would be provided with additional resources and opportunities. Large class sizes may make this personalization of student learning more difficult to implement.

ASSESSMENT OF COMPETENCY

Competency is assessed using tools that measure the observable behaviors that successful performers demonstrate while working in any given job. The difficulty for nurse educators is that no one objective, reliable tool for measuring competency exists because competency is context driven. Learners may demonstrate competency in one area of nursing practice and not in another and, therefore, opportunities to apply what is learned in multiple contexts are required. Multiple measures in varying contexts by different assessors provide a wider range of data for making judgments about the learner's performance (Oermann, 2022).

Competency-based assessments are criterion referenced, meaning the evaluation of performance is independent of others and based solely on the individual's ability to demonstrate achievement of designated outcomes. Performance assessment in nursing education frequently involves a norm-referenced approach, for example, in an examination where educators make decisions to discard poor performing items or curve grades based on overall class performance. Faculty will continue to use quizzes and examinations as evaluation strategies because knowledge is a constituent of competency (Rotthoff et al., 2021). Examination questions, however, do not measure competency; if they are well written, they may be measures of clinical judgment. Therefore, while quizzes and examinations will continue to be important assessments, they cannot serve as a demonstration of competency.

Formative and summative assessments are essential in CBE, but not all assessments require grading. Frequent formative assessments serve to track student progress and provide an opportunity for performance gaps to be identified and addressed through feedback designed to enhance learning. Summative assessments serve to evaluate student abilities against predetermined standards or progression indicators at a specified point. Types of assessments may include tests and quizzes to measure requisite knowledge, case studies, simulations, papers, presentations, projects, portfolios, objective structured clinical examinations (OSCE), and direct observations of performance.

Rubrics have long been used in academic and clinical settings to define performance expectations, increase objectivity in grading, standardize the evaluation method, and provide transparency. Rubrics include the criteria or performance behaviors to be assessed and a scoring system for rating if the learner met them. Many rubrics also include quality descriptors to further explain the criterion to be rated. Rubrics should describe specific observations identified as "anchors" that clarify the academic standard for competency. Anchors target judgment based on the underlying subject matter. It is important that rubric items are clear enough that subjectivity is decreased between observers and that items are developed for the abilities acquired by the learner so far. Having more than one observer scoring the performance increases reliability. With limited numbers of faculty, educators may consider having students serve as observers and use rubrics to score each other's performance as this will help them to develop competency in engaging in peer evaluation, a subcompetency of AACN *Essential's* Domain 9.

Competency-based clinical evaluations that state increasing performance expectations as learners move through the program can serve as evidence of the learner's growth on the competency continuum. Clinical evaluations cannot be one-size-fits-all in nursing education as it is important that evaluation instruments demonstrate the evolving complexity and growth expectation of learners' clinical performance (Altmiller, 2019). Clinical evaluations based on the Quality and Safety Education for Nurses (QSEN) competencies can be easily adapted for use with the AACN *Essentials* as both are in alignment with the core competencies originally developed by the Institute of Medicine (now the National Academy of Medicine) competencies (2003), which remain current in practice and are required for all healthcare professionals to this day.

Entrustable professional activities (EPAs) have been used in medical education since their introduction in 2005 (ten Cate, 2013), but are new as a framework for organizing, implementing, and assessing competency in nursing education. EPAs translate competencies into practice and are focused on essential professional activities identified as units of professional practice that an individual should be able to perform in a clinical context. Grounded in the concept of trust, decisions regarding competency are based on assessments of the perceived amount of supervision an individual requires to function in a safe and effective manner.

EPAs are observable activities comprised of multiple tasks that detail the real-world knowledge, skills, and attitudes that learners must perform competently to be deemed trustworthy to practice unsupervised (Corrigan et al., 2022). Because it is not possible to assess everything a care provider is expected to demonstrate, EPAs serve as carefully determined, deliberate samples of essential knowledge, skills, and attitudes that are representative of core professional requirements (Humphrey-Murto et al., 2017). Examples are conducting a physical and history on a patient or documenting a clinical encounter in the patient record (Association of American Medical Colleges [AAMC], 2014). Assessment strategies for EPAs include direct observation, simulation, and OSCE. Development and use of EPAs for nursing education are expected to expand in coming years.

DEVELOPING THE INFRASTRUCTURE FOR COMPETENCY-BASED EDUCATION

Backward design can also be used to build the infrastructure that supports the adoption of CBE across the curriculum. Educators can follow a three-step process to bring curriculum into alignment with national standards and CBE. The first step is to develop end-of-program outcomes that align with the chosen standards for each degree program and certificate program. The second step is to map the curriculum for what already exists in the program that is competency based. This allows educators to see where competency-based activities and assessments exist and where more are needed. The third step is to develop course outcomes as competency statements, including outcomes that can address the gaps identified through the mapping. Once the infrastructure is in place, faculty can continue the ongoing work to adapt teaching and assessment processes to be competency based.

Program Outcomes Aligned With Standards as Competency Statements

Developing end-of-program outcomes stated as competencies and aligned with accepted national standards is the first step in building the infrastructure needed to support CBE. The program outcomes provide an endpoint for achievement and become the guide to curriculum planning. The criteria for program outcomes may be the 10 AACN *Essentials* domains (AACN, 2021), the QSEN competencies (QSEN Institute, 2022), or some other criteria that align with the school's accrediting body. While the domains and competencies may overlap in many situations, for those aligning with the AACN *Essentials*, developing one program outcome for each of the 10 domains establishes the focus of the outcome and captures the language and nuance of each domain. This creates clarity for faculty and students.

Developing program outcomes can be difficult for faculty. Table 13.2 demonstrates an intuitive process whereby faculty use a worksheet (Appendix B) to create a new/revised outcome by combining language from the *Essential* domain descriptor with language from the school's current end-of-program outcome. Faculty should consider the mission and vision of the institution to ensure these are represented in the revised outcomes. In schools with graduate programs, faculty should develop the bachelor of science in nursing (BSN) program outcomes first. Once the BSN outcomes have been created, a column can be added to develop master of science (MSN) program outcomes. Lastly, a column for doctor of nursing (DNP) outcomes can be developed. Developing end-of-program outcomes this way engages all faculty in the work of determining the outcomes for the entirety of the school's programs while allowing them to view the outcomes on a single form to ensure that each degree is more complex in competency expectation.

When using the *Essentials* as the standard, BSN students are required to achieve Level 1 competencies. Examples of competency for BSN students may be to apply, provide, implement, use, and demonstrate these domains. Graduate students are required to achieve Level 2 competencies. Program outcomes for MSN students should demonstrate greater leadership capacity. Examples of competency may be that they interpret, translate, direct, coordinate, and model these domains. Finally, DNP students design, lead, and generate expertise and knowledge for these domains. When developing outcomes for graduate programs, faculty need to additionally consider the specific competencies required for each specialty certification as these delineate one specialty from another.

TABLE 13.2 DEVELOPING PROGRAM OUTCOMES

Current End-of-Program Outcome	Suggested Revision	AACN *Essential* Domain Descriptor
Participate in the advancement of the profession to improve healthcare for the betterment of the global society.	Participate in the advancement of the profession to improve healthcare and equitable population health outcomes, spanning from prevention to management of disease through collaboration in both traditional and nontraditional partnerships with affected communities, industry, local government entities, and others for the betterment of an increasingly diverse and global society.	"Domain 3: Population Health: Population health spans the healthcare delivery continuum from public health prevention to disease management of populations and describes collaborative activities with both traditional and non-traditional partnerships from affected communities, public health, industry, academia, health care, local government entities, and others for the improvement of equitable population health outcomes" (AACN, 2021, p. 11).

Source: American Association of College of Nursing. (2021). *The Essentials: Core competencies for professional nursing education* (p. 11). AACN. https://www.aacnnursing.org/Portals/0/PDFs/Publications/Essentials-2021.pdf

Copyright Gerry Altmiller, 2024. Reprinted by permission, 2024.

Curriculum Mapping for Competency-Based Education

Traditional curriculum mapping sought to answer four overarching questions: what is taught, how it is taught, when it is taught, and how it is evaluated (Harden, 2001). From that, educators could arrive at conclusions about whether the curriculum was complete or needed strengthening, and where gaps existed, or material was redundant (Linton, 2019). Curriculum mapping for CBE has a different focus in that the mapping should identify where opportunities for demonstrating competency are present and whether there is adequate layering for the learner to develop competency over time (Altmiller, 2023). Different from the teacher-centered approach of placing checkmarks where content is presented, mapping for competency requires learner-centered objective data that clarify what learners do with the knowledge they have gained. Activities should be clearly described so that faculty can see how competency is layered and developed as the learner moves through the program.

Many mapping tools are available to faculty. Mapping is best done in an Excel® file because it can hold a large amount of data. Whatever tool is chosen, the work should follow a process that creates transparency as curricular decisions will be based on the findings of the mapping. Individual course mappings should be reviewed in teams as a verification strategy. Eventually, all course mappings should be placed into one master document so that each standard that the curriculum is mapped against can be analyzed for presence and intensity of opportunities for learners across the curriculum to develop competency. Areas not well represented by competency-based activities (gaps) in the mapping should become the focus of faculty efforts to increase opportunities for learners to build knowledge, skills, and attitudes.

After the initial mapping is completed, a report identifying strengths and weaknesses as well as the mapping document itself should be shared with faculty and be used to guide curricular changes. Additionally, a meeting with practice partners, particularly those managing nurse residency programs for undergraduate students and those managing clinic personnel for graduate students, can yield meaningful data that can be coupled with the mapping analysis to guide curricular redesign. Two brief questions: (a) What practice gaps do you see in the abilities of the nurses/APRNs being hired? and (b) What strengths would you like to see in the nurses/APRNs being hired that you are not seeing? can yield data to provide additional impetus for supporting the development of competency-based activities for learners.

The curriculum mapping serves as a living document to house the evidence for CBE across the curriculum. It should be updated every 12 to 18 months as faculty make incremental changes to course activities and assessments over time to build a stronger competency-based program. Continued maintenance of the mapping helps to ensure the fidelity of the curricular plan and adherences to standards, while capturing the continuing development of competency-based learning activities and assessments over time.

Course Outcomes as Competency Statements

Developing course outcomes should be done after the curriculum mapping analysis is complete because redundant courses may be removed from the program, and some deficits may be addressed across courses, thus requiring the development of corresponding course outcomes. Competency-based outcomes are practice driven in nursing education, clearly stating what the learner will be able to do on completion of the program or course that enable that person to perform in their professional context (Gosselin, 2019). This differs from content-driven outcomes that describe the knowledge that will be obtained by the end of a course or program. Descriptors such as list, discuss, describe, explore, discover, and identify are knowledge based. In CBE, course outcomes are competency statements that articulate measurable and observable behaviors to be achieved by the end of the course. The subcompetencies of the *Essentials* can guide the development of course outcomes, but it is important to ensure those subcompetencies are met in multiple courses and contexts and are evaluated by multiple assessors over time.

Consider a course outcome that indicates learners will discover how social determinants impact health. When revising course outcomes from a knowledge focus to a competency-based statement, educators need to determine what they want the learner to do with whatever they "discover." Is it to address needs based on inequities? To assess for inequities based on socioeconomic factors? To teach patients strategies to overcome some of these factors? In CBE, it is not enough to "know" or "discover" something. Learners must "do" something with what they learn. The "do" should be determined by the faculty member in the course and be directed by the course outcomes. Table 13.3 demonstrates the difference between knowledge-based and competency-based course outcomes. A structured worksheet (Appendix B) that considers current knowledge-based outcomes and what learners are expected to "do" to achieve competency may be helpful in organizing the work to formulate competency-based course outcomes.

TABLE 13.3 COMPARISON OF KNOWLEDGE-BASED COURSE OUTCOMES AND COMPETENCY STATEMENTS AS COURSE OUTCOMES

Course Outcome With Knowledge Focus	Course Outcome as Competency Statement
Identify pertinent resources to answer clinical questions and explain how these can be used.	Use appropriate search strategies to locate the best evidence to answer clinical questions.
Discuss learning attitudes and behaviors that support success and strong performance.	Use standardized learning self-assessment tools and, from the data, develop an academic success plan.
Describe effective strategies for leveling evidence used to guide practice.	Develop tables of evidence based on peer-reviewed articles on a clinical topic.
Explore treatment options for an older adult diagnosed with depression.	Integrate evidence-based best practices into a plan of care for an older adult diagnosed with depression.
List the components of a comprehensive physical assessment for a neonate.	Demonstrate a comprehensive physical assessment for a neonate.

Copyright Gerry Altmiller, 2024. Reprinted by permission, 2024.

Managing Curricular "Drift"

Frequently in academia, faculty are assigned to teach courses they are unfamiliar with and as a result, make changes to the content, the assignments, and sometimes the course learning outcomes. This is known as curricular drift where educators unintentionally make changes that affect the overall program plan. Therefore, once the infrastructure for CBE and assessment are in place within a curriculum, policies to prevent curricular drift need to be developed to ensure significant changes to courses are approved through the appropriate curriculum committee. The role of these committees should not be to restrict innovation but should be focused on providing guidance to ensure that courses remain true to their purpose within the overall curriculum and maintain key activities and assessments that support CBE. This does not mean that faculty cannot make changes to courses; it means that significant changes require discussion with the appropriate curriculum committee to ensure fidelity to the curriculum plan and CBE as evidenced in the curriculum mapping document.

STRATEGIES TO ENHANCE COMPETENCY-BASED EDUCATION

Building a competency-based curriculum aligned with specific standards such as the AACN *Essentials* or the QSEN Competencies requires educators to ascertain that learning opportunities to develop competency are provided across the curriculum in a systematic way that layers activities and assessments and prevents duplication and redundancy. Backward design is not only used in building competency within courses but can be used to build competency across the curriculum. Table 13.4 demonstrates how the AACN *Essentials* Competency 4.2 Use the Best Evidence in Practice might be implemented across the curriculum with each activity building on the previous activity.

Competency is the result of planned and repeated practice. Required lab practice hours for students in each clinical course is a strategy that supports competency development in multiple contexts. The requirement could be implemented by creating stations in the laboratory for learners to practice skills appropriate to their current clinical course. Some schools have student work programs that may support the hiring of several senior nursing students to oversee the laboratory practice. This structure has the added benefit of creating an opportunity for more advanced nursing students to share expertise with lower level students (e.g., seniors guiding learning of juniors). To monitor attendance, the creation of a QR code that connects to a Qualtrics® report can easily provide a monthly report that tracks student visits to the lab. Students would scan the QR code with their phone when entering the lab to practice. Faculty determine the number of hours per semester and should be careful to break down the requirement by months so that students do not overwhelm the lab at the end of the semester. An important caveat is that only 1 hour of practice is permitted in a single visit to ensure repeated practice over time. Syllabi should state the required number of hours per month and mandate that all lab practice hours must be completed before the final clinical evaluation to support learners in transferring skill acquisition into competency in the clinical practice setting.

Simulation approximates the "real work" of nursing and has been shown to be effective in developing competency in multiple formats including virtual simulation (Brown et al., 2021), screen-based simulation (Altmiller et al., 2023), online

TABLE 13.4 IMPLEMENTATION OF AACN *ESSENTIALS* COMPETENCY 4.2 USE THE BEST EVIDENCE IN PRACTICE

Subcompetency	Learning Activity/Assessment
Beginning 4.2a Evaluate clinical practice to generate questions to improve nursing care.	Write a paper about process improvement to decrease variation and improve care.
Middle 4.2b Evaluate appropriateness and strength of evidence. 4.2c Use best evidence in practice.	Submit a table of evidence with a minimum of 5 studies or peer-reviewed articles on a clinical topic.
End 4.2d Participate in the implementation of practice change to improve nursing care. 4.2e Participate in the evaluation of outcomes and their implications for practice.	Participate in practice change to improve nursing care at the clinical site. Provide the rationale to clinical faculty for why a particular nursing intervention is chosen.
Advanced Nursing Specialty 4.2f Use diverse sources of evidence to inform care. 4.2g Lead the translation of evidence into practice.	Conduct a project to develop, lead, and evaluate a practice change to improve care.

Source: Subcompetencies from the American Association of College of Nursing. (2021). *The Essentials: Core competencies for professional nursing education* (p. 38). AACN. https://www.aacnnursing.org/Portals/0/PDFs/Publications/Essentials-2021.pdf
Learning Activities/Assessments developed by Gerry Altmiller. Copyright Gerry Altmiller, 2024. Reprinted by permission, 2024.

standardized patient simulation (Orr et al., 2022), and in-person standardized simulation (Perry et al., 2022). Simulations designed for component complexity focus on a specific aspect of work, such as assessing a patient with asthma and prescribing the appropriate treatment. Simulations with component complexity serve as a "check in" to observe the learner is mastering required content and to provide feedback for improvement. As learners move through the program and gain increasing competency, simulations can be designed for coordination complexity such as presenting a patient with an undetermined diagnosis and having the learner conduct an assessment, prioritize the patient's health problems, and develop a plan of care with the patient. This higher complexity simulation requires more refined knowledge, skills, and attitudes to demonstrate competency.

How competencies are implemented across the curriculum is decided by faculty. Gaps evidenced in the curriculum mapping can be addressed through incremental changes to course activities and classroom learning. Working through unfolding case studies or participating in role play are forms of experiential learning. Having learners use standardized communication processes in class such as simulating a patient hand-off or a call to a prescriber using **s**ituation, **b**ackground, **a**ssessment, and **r**ecommendation (SBAR) supports the development of communication competency. Ask Me 3® is a 3-question process for patient teaching from the Institute for Healthcare Improvement (IHI, 2019). Including these three questions at the end of each class provides an opportunity for learners to formulate a teaching plan for patients about what they have learned:

1. What is my main problem?

2. What do I need to do? and

3. Why is it important for me to do this?

Students can use these questions to make complicated health information understandable for patients and families and enhance their own competency in promoting the patient's ability to manage health problems.

Artificial Intelligence

As faculty seek innovative ways to implement CBE and assessment, artificial intelligence (AI) can provide ideas and ease the workload. AI can be useful in building rubrics for assignments and simulations. Although faculty are concerned that learners may use AI for completing assignments, faculty can help learners use it responsibly. For instance, an assignment might have learners use AI to create a plan of care based on a patient's comorbidities and cultural considerations and then require the student to critique the plan of care and provide rationales to support their work. Faculty can harness the power of AI to develop activities that support learners in developing competency in specific areas of practice. Exhibit 13.1 demonstrates the results of an AI search for active learning strategies to address systems-based practice. The question asked was: "How can learners develop competency for incorporating cost-effectiveness in patient care?"

ROLE OF THE EDUCATOR IN COMPETENCY-BASED EDUCATION

In traditional education models, the instructor leads the class through course content, explaining concepts, providing examples, and assessing for knowledge development. In CBE, the instructor's role changes to one of coach and facilitator of learning. Learners are expected to assume greater responsibility for their learning, with educators guiding the class while also supporting a personalized plan for individual development. Examples of this might be encouraging learners to choose

---

EXHIBIT 13.1 Results of AI Search for Active-Learning Strategies to Incorporate Cost-Effective Care

Role-playing scenarios where students consider cost implications of care options
Case studies analyzing the cost–benefit tradeoffs of different interventions
Student debates arguing for or against costly new treatments based on evidence
Games or simulations requiring students to allocate limited resources
Reflective writing assignments about providing quality care on a budget

---

AI, artificial intelligence.
Copyright Gerry Altmiller, 2024. Reprinted by permission, 2024.

clinical assignments that expand their knowledge base and introduce learning experiences they have not yet had or having learners maintain portfolios that can be used to provide evidence of competency and serve as supportive documentation during their summative clinical evaluation.

Faculty plan coursework based on the expected course outcomes, providing opportunities for individuals to enlist varied resources that align best with their learning style and pace. Formative feedback is an essential part of informing the learner of progress toward competency and therefore should be frequent. Learners need to understand the role feedback plays in their learning and be open to accepting it, reflecting on it, and integrating it to adjust practice and improve performance. Faculty need to provide feedback in a way that builds confidence and provides learners with options for improvement. Beginning feedback with a caring statement that conveys the instructor's motivation as helping the learner achieve goals may support learners to be more open to receiving feedback (Altmiller, 2016). Providing feedback using this mnemonic may serve as a standardized process and be a helpful strategy in delivering feedback:

- I saw (provide objective data),
- I think (state faculty concern related to the impact on the patient or sometimes the team), and
- I wonder (provide an open invitation for the learner to share his or her the learner's thinking).

FUTURE DIRECTIONS FOR COMPETENCY-BASED EDUCATION IN NURSING EDUCATION

As faculty integrate CBE and assessment into nursing curricula, conducting research to provide evidence of its efficacy is paramount to its sustainability. A backward design framework can be used to evaluate and better understand the innovative teaching strategies and assessment instruments that are developed to support CBE in nursing. Backward design in education research is a process patterned after backward curricular design whereby the researcher first identifies the goal of the research project, particularly asking what is learned and why and identifying the desired result (Jensen et al., 2017). The next step is developing a measure that provides acceptable evidence; for example, what is learned can be answered by a score on a project and why it is effective can be answered by asking motivational questions. The final step is designing the learning experiences and teaching materials that facilitate learner mastery. Conducting research to better understand what strategies work in CBE and why will contribute to building scholarship of teaching and learning.

Other important considerations are the development of policies within academic institutions to support the implementation of CBE. This includes faculty and administrators determining progression standards and testing methods. The opportunity for faculty to create a trajectory for their research and professional development will be expanded as nursing education at all levels requires valid and reliable methods of evaluation to measure clinical competency as well as to evaluate the more difficult constructs associated with attitudes and professionalism to ensure practice-ready nurses.

SUMMARY

National nursing organizations are calling for and supporting the transition of nursing education to a competency-based framework as a means to better prepare the nursing workforce and promote practice readiness. The transition to CBE is challenging for faculty as the focus of nursing education has been traditionally on content and knowledge development and with CBE, the focus is on the outputs of education demonstrated by the learner as competencies. While strategies for implementation, assessment, and tracking are needed, opportunities for creativity in teaching and conducting education research set the stage for an extraordinary time of innovation and advancement for nurse educators.

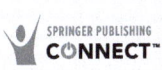

A robust set of instructor resources designed to supplement this text is located at http://connect.springerpub.com/content/book/978-0-8261-8892-2. Qualifying instructors may request access by emailing textbook@springerpub.com.

REFERENCES

Altmiller, G. (2016). Strategies for providing constructive feedback to students. *Nurse Educator, 41*(3), 118–119. https://doi.org/10.1097/NNE.0000000000000227

Altmiller, G. (2019). Content validation of Quality and Safety Education for Nurses (QSEN) pre-licensure clinical evaluation instruments. *Nurse Educator, 44*(3), 118–121. https://doi.org/10.1097/NNE.0000000000000656

Altmiller, G. (2023). Curriculum mapping for CBE: Collecting objective data. *Nurse Educator, 48*(5), 287. https://doi.org/10.1097/NNE.0000000000001462

Altmiller, G., Jimenez, F., & Wilson, C. (2023). Screen-based patient simulation: An exemplar for developing and assessing competency. *Nurse Educator, 49*(4),179–183. https://doi.org/10.1097/NNE.0000000000001585

American Association of College of Nursing. (2021). *The essentials: Core competencies for professional nursing education.* AACN. https://www.aacnnursing.org/Portals/0/PDFs/Publications/Essentials-2021.pdf

Association of American Medical Colleges. (2014). *Core Entrustable Professional Activities for entering residency.* https://www.aamc.org/about-us/mission-areas/medical-education/cbme/core-epas

Bloom, B. S. (1956). *Taxonomy of educational objectives: The classification of educational goals* (1st ed.). Longman Group

Brown, K. M., Swoboda, S. M., Gilbert, G. E., Horvath, C., & Sullivan, N. (2021). Integrating virtual simulation into nursing education: A roadmap. *Clinical Simulation in Nursing, 72*, 21–29. https://doi.org/10.106/j.ecns.2021.08.002

Corrigan, C., Moran, K., Kesten, K., Conrad, D., Manderscheid, A., Beebe, S., & Pohl, E. (2022). Entrustable professional activities in clinical education: A practical approach for advanced nursing education. *Nurse Educator, 47*(5), 261–266. https://doi.org/10.1097/NNE.0000000000001184

Covert, H., Sherman, M., Miner, K., & Lichtveld, M. (2019). Core competencies and a workforce framework for community health workers: A model for advancing the profession. *American Journal of Public Health, 109*(2), 320–327. https://doi.org/10.2105/AJPH.2018.304737

Frank, J. R., Snell, L. S., Cate, O. T., Holmboe, E. S., Carraccio, C., Swing, S. R., Harris, P., Glasgow, N. J., Campbell, C., Dath, D., Harden, R. M., Iobst, W., Long, D. M., Mungroo, R., Richardson, D. L., Sherbino, J., Silver, I., Taber, S., Talbot, M., & Harris, K. A. (2010). Competency-based medical education: Theory to practice. *Medical Teacher, 32*(8), 638–645. https://doi.org/10.3109/0142159X.2010.501190

Gosselin, D. (2019). Competencies and learning outcomes. *Integrate: Interdisciplinary teaching about Earth for future sustainability.* https://serc.Carleton.edu/integrate/programs/workforceprep/competencies_and_LO.html

Harden, R. M. (2001). AMEE Guide No.21: Curriculum mapping: A tool for transparent and authentic teaching and learning. *Medical Teaching, 23*(2), 123–137. https://doi.org/10.1080/01421590120036547

Humphrey-Murto, S., Wood, T. J., Ross, S., Tavares, W., Kvern, B., Sidhu, R., Sargeant, J., & Touchie, C. (2017). Assessment pearls for competency-based medical education. *Journal of Graduate Medical Education, 9*(6), 688–691. https://doi.org/10.4300/JGME-D-17-00365.1

Institute for Healthcare Improvement. (2019). *Patient safety essentials toolkit: Ask Me 3®.* https://www.ihi.org/sites/default/files/SafetyToolkit_AskMe3.pdf

Institute of Medicine. (2003). *Health professions education: A bridge to quality.* National Academies Press.

Jensen, J. L., Bailey, E. G., Kummer, T. A., & Weber, K. S. (2017). Using backward design in education research: A research methods essay. *Journal of Microbiology & Biology Education, 18*(3), 1–6. https://doi.org/10.1128/jmbe.v18i3.1367

Kavanagh, J. M., & Sharpnack, P. A. (2021). A crisis in competency: A defining moment in nursing education. *Online Journal of Issues in Nursing, 26*(1), 1. https://doi.org/10.3912/OJIN.Vol26No01Man02

Kavanagh, J. M., & Szweda, C. (2017). A crisis in Competency: The strategic and ethical imperative to assessing new graduate nurses' clinical reasoning. *Nursing Education Perspectives, 38*(2), 57–62. https://doi.org/10.1097/01.NEP.0000000000000112

Linton, M., Knecht, L., Dabney, B., & Koonmen, J. (2019). Student-centered curricular revisions to facilitate transition from associate degree in nursing to bachelor of science in nursing education. *Teaching and Learning in Nursing, 14*(4), 279–282. https://doi.org/10.1016/j.teln.2019.06.008

Miller, G. E. (1990). The assessment of clinical skills/competence/performance. *Academic Medicine, 65*(Suppl. 9), S63–67. https://doi.org/10.1097/00001888-199009000-00045

National League for Nursing. (2023). *NLN vision statement: Integrating competency-based education in the nursing curriculum.* https://www.nln.org/docs/default-source/default-document-library/vision-series_integrating-competency-based-education-in-the-nursing-curriculumd6eb0a1e-1f8b-4d60-bc4f-619f5e75b445.pdf

Oermann, M. H. (2022). Some principles to guide assessment of competencies. *Nurse Educator, 47*(1), 1. https://doi.org/10.1097/NNE.0000000000001143

Orr, Z., Machidawa, E., Unger, S., & Romem, A. (2022). Enhancing the structural competence of nurses through standardized simulation. *Clinical Simulation in Nursing, 62,* 25–30. https://doi.org/10.1016/j.ecns.2021.09.005

Perry, J., Powers, S. C., Haskell, B., & Plummer, C. (2022). Simulated home visit to promote chronic disease management competencies in prelicensure nursing students. *Nurse Educator, 47*(6), E132–E135. https://doi.org/10.1097/NNE.0000000000001229

QSEN Institute. (2022). *Competencies.* https://www.qsen.org/competencies

Rotthoff, T., Kadmon, M., & Harendza, S. (2021). It does not have to be either or! Assessing competence in medicine should be a continuum between an analytic and holistic approach. *Advances in Health Sciences Education, 26*(5), 1659–1673. https://doi.org/10.1007/s10459-021-10043-0

ten Cate, O. (2013). Nuts and bolts of entrustable professional activities. *Journal of Graduate Medical Education, 5*(1), 157–158. https://doi.org/10.4300%2FJGME-D-12-00380.1

Wittmann-Price, R. A., & Gittings, K. K. (2021). *Fast facts about CBE in nursing.* Springer Publishing Company

Curriculum Development and Course Design in Nursing Education

14

Stephanie Stimac DeBoor

OBJECTIVES

1. Analyze the processes of curriculum development and revision and related role of the nurse educator
2. Evaluate the major components of an existing curriculum, their interrelationships, and how they influence the implementation and evaluation of the curriculum
3. Explore the development of a course and their relationship to the overall curriculum

INTRODUCTION

When developing curriculum for a nursing program, it is vital that nurse educators consider the context in which teaching takes place. The curriculum provides that context with an overview of the mission or purpose of the program, its vision for the future, the values or philosophy that relate to its mission, and the ultimate goals for the program. Nurse educators and learners participating in the program should be familiar with the curriculum to appreciate the end goal and ensure the integrity of its mission.

This chapter describes the components and processes for curriculum development or revision for schools of nursing and for educational programs related to professional education in healthcare settings; reviews the factors that influence educational programs and curricula; and provides educators with guidelines for collecting and analyzing data to make informed decisions about revising or developing curricula. Finally, the chapter provides an example of course design based on the framework of using backward design.

To gain an appreciation of the connection of teaching to the curriculum or educational program, the components of the curriculum are described. The influence of the components on the teacher, student/learner, courses or classes, and related learning activities are considered. Included is the importance of program and student learning outcomes (SLOs) and how they direct subsequent instructional strategies and ongoing evaluation of the program. Though the setting can vary according to the type of educational program (e.g., schools of nursing or healthcare agencies), the same processes and components of the curriculum apply.

BACKGROUND

Prior to, but certainly since the pandemic, nursing education is changing in response to newer trends in healthcare and education, online and distance delivery, emphasis on patient-centered care that includes quality and safety, interprofessional collaboration, a focus on learner-centered strategies, and the influences of technology and simulated learning experiences. These forces call for curriculum transformation to change from the traditional content-laden program to concept-based frameworks for the preparation of professionals capable of critical thinking when providing competent and compassionate care. The American Association of Colleges of Nursing (AACN, 2021) and the National League for Nursing (NLN, 2023) call for schools of nursing to incorporate competency-based education within the nursing curriculum. *The Future of Nursing 2020–2030: Charting a Path to Achieve Health Equity* examines challenges facing healthcare providers (National Academy of Medicine [NAM], 2021). One of the key components of this consensus study is the education and competency development needed to prepare nurses, including advanced practice nurses, to practice outside of acute care settings and lead efforts to build a culture of health and health equity.

Often, rather than focusing on concepts, competency-based teaching, and learning strategies, both new and experienced teachers focus on the specific content of the classes or sessions they teach and lose sight of the course objectives and how they relate to the overall program and curriculum. The temptation is to adjust these objectives and content to the individual teacher's personal interests and expertise. Such changes can result in the loss of the program's intent and planned SLOs. If a teacher identifies the need to update the content of a class and thus the objectives, it is important to compare the proposed change to the overall curriculum and accreditation standards to discover its impact on the total program. One significant way to avoid this issue is to change the typical course design by implementing a backward design framework for course/content development. This option keeps the emphasis on the intended learning outcomes and learning needs of the student, rather than the faculty's interests. Additionally, one can create crosswalk tables to ensure that accreditation standards and competency goals are maintained when there are changes to the course content. Such changes can involve revision of the curriculum and, depending on the setting, include other members of the educational team. In the case of major changes, approval processes for the revisions might be necessary through the hierarchical structures in the involved nursing program or healthcare setting. These processes focus on curriculum revision. However, if the need is for a new curriculum or educational program, the processes become that of curriculum development.

NEEDS ASSESSMENT

Developing a new educational program or revising an existing one calls for a needs assessment; that is, there must be compelling factors to cause the change or to create a new one. For the purposes of this text, a brief review is provided of possible factors that influence change or the development of new programs in academic or healthcare settings. DeBoor (2023) discusses in detail Keating's (2005) external and internal frame factors that influence curriculum development and offers outlines for collecting and analyzing relevant data for making decisions related to this activity. Figures 14.1 and 14.2 present models of these external and internal factors.

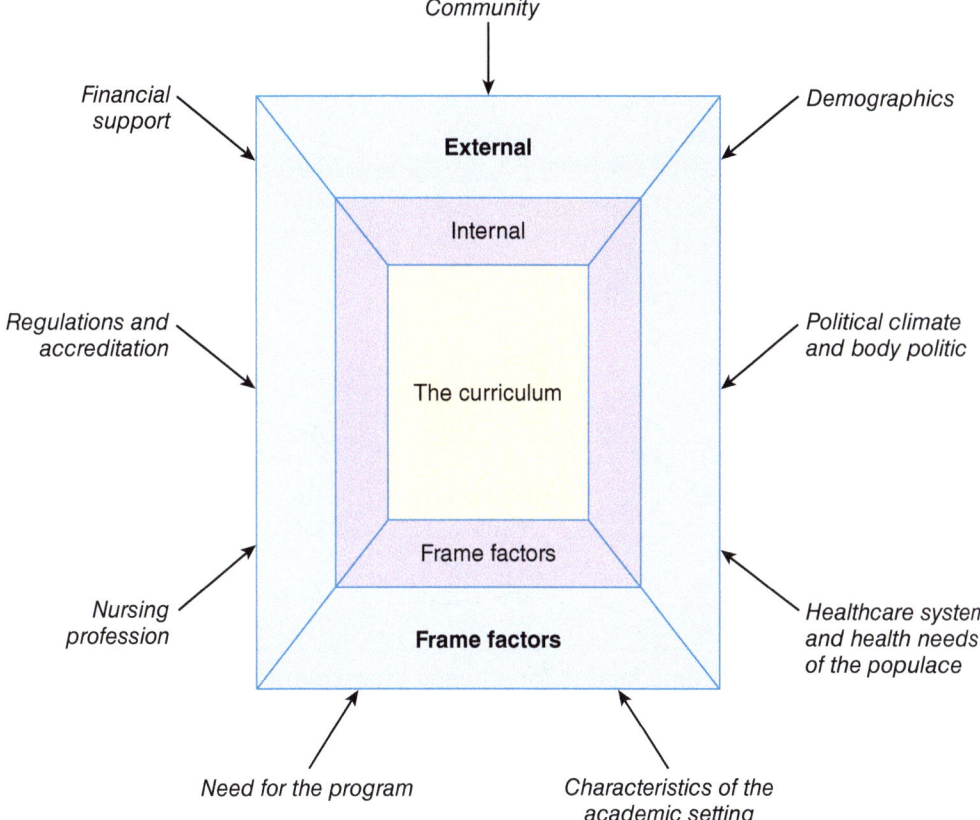

FIGURE 14.1 External frame factors for a needs assessment for curriculum development in nursing.
Source: Adapted from Johnson, M. (1977). *Intentionality in education.* Center for Curriculum Research and Services. From Keating, S. B. (2005). Needs assessment: The external and internal frame factors. In S. DeBoor (Ed.), *Keating's curriculum development and evaluation in nursing education* (5th ed., pp. 49–69). Springer Publishing Company.

Faculty members in the academic setting and changes in accreditation standards are often the catalyst for revision or the development of new programs in schools of nursing. While the major functions of faculty may be those of teaching, research and scholarly activities and service to the institution and community are also expectations. Service to the institution includes membership on curriculum committees and participation in level and course meetings that may lead to revision of the program. Members of committees, level and course coordinators, other teachers, and administrators may identify the need for change to bring the curriculum up to date or to adjust learning objectives to improve SLOs. These educators may also be aware of changes in nursing education or the healthcare system that call for new programs to meet the demands of the profession and needs of the population. In such instances, there is a suggestion for development of a new program.

Nurse educators in healthcare settings experience the same indicators for the need to change educational programs or create new ones in either staff

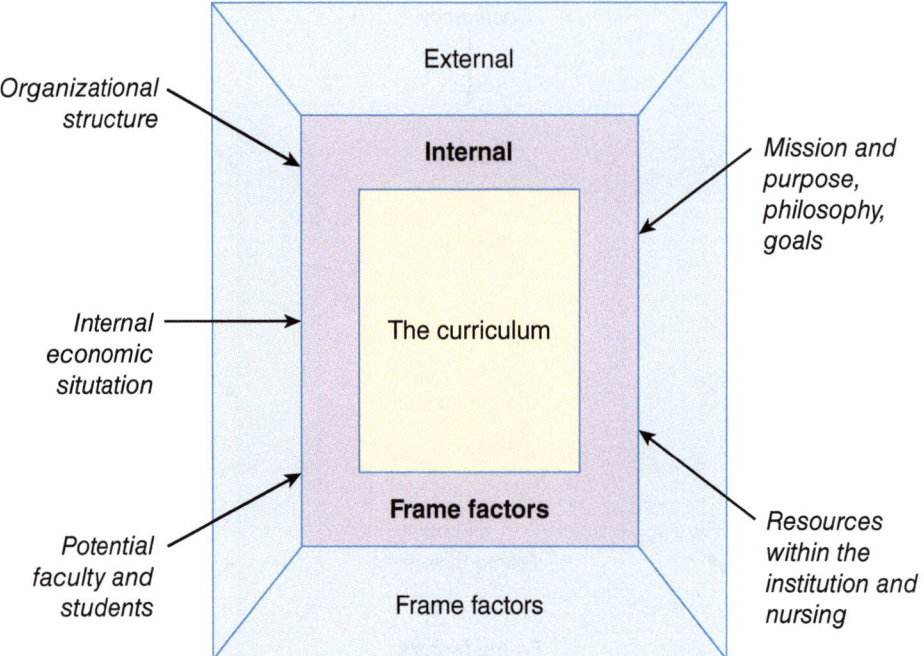

FIGURE 14.2 Internal frame factors for a needs assessment for curriculum development in nursing.

Source: Adapted from Johnson, M. (1977). *Intentionality in education*. Center for Curriculum Research and Services. From Keating, S. B. (2005). Needs assessment: The external and t frame factors. In S. DeBoor (Ed.), *Keating's curriculum development and evaluation in nursing education* (5th ed., pp. 49–69). Springer Publishing Company.

development or patient education. While their central role may be teaching staff or patients, at the same time, they often recognize the need for new programs to update staff knowledge and skills or to educate patients on the newest treatment protocols and preventive healthcare strategies. The organizational structure is different from academic settings, but nurse educators in healthcare agencies also revise or create new programs and consult with other members of the organization, such as nurse administrators and managers, and other members of the multidisciplinary team.

EXTERNAL FRAME FACTORS

No matter what the setting, the need for creation of new programs or revision of existing ones, the process for change is much the same. There are factors that influence the educational program and curriculum and indicate that a needs assessment is in order. External frame factors are those that are outside of the parent institution in which the program is housed; for example, the healthcare system and changes, nursing profession, community and population served by the institution, competitive schools or agencies, government and political bodies, and accrediting and program approval agencies. Table 14.1 provides examples of external frame factors influencing educational programs in academic and healthcare settings.

TABLE 14.1 SAMPLE EXTERNAL FRAME FACTORS INFLUENCING EDUCATIONAL PROGRAMS IN ACADEMIC AND HEALTHCARE SETTINGS

External Frame Factor	Academic Settings	Healthcare Settings
Healthcare system and internal changes	New technologies Changes in delivery of care (primary, acute, chronic care)	Novel illnesses (e.g., coronavirus pandemic) New technologies Healthcare demands: primary, secondary, tertiary
Nursing profession	National Academy of Medicine (formerly known as the Institute of Medicine) calls for higher education Certification for advanced practice and leadership roles Degree level for entry to practice Competency-based education	Orientation needs Skills and EBP updates Continuing education requirements Role of nurse educators in patient education
Community and population served	Role of school of nursing in providing nursing workforce locally, regionally, and nationally Population healthcare needs; e.g., geriatrics, major causes of morbidity and mortality, health promotion and maintenance, etc.	Rural, suburban, urban Type of services (acute, tertiary, extended care, nursing home, rehabilitation, public health, home care, hospice, etc.) Population healthcare needs; e.g., geriatrics, major causes of morbidity and mortality, prevention
Competitive schools or agencies	Levels of nursing programs in direct competition Programs articulating with each other (e.g., associate degree leading into baccalaureate or master's programs) Other programs in direct competition for clinical sites (e.g., medical school, physician assistant program, social work) Possibilities of collaboration	Competitive agencies in the region Specialty units Possibilities for collaboration

(continued)

TABLE 14.1 SAMPLE EXTERNAL FRAME FACTORS INFLUENCING EDUCATIONAL PROGRAMS IN ACADEMIC AND HEALTHCARE SETTINGS (*continued*)

External Frame Factor	Academic Settings	Healthcare Settings
Government and political bodies	Involvement in political activities that support higher education Awareness of financial programs that support student financial aid, program development, and research	Regulations governing healthcare services at state and national levels Medicare and Medicaid reimbursement policies Health insurance and other payers for healthcare services Regulations affecting professional practice
Accrediting and program approval agencies	Commission on Collegiate Nursing Education, Accreditation Commission for Education in Nursing, or Commission for Nursing Education Accreditation Regional accreditation Specialty accreditation Board of nursing approval	The Joint Commission Community-based accreditation and by specialty Specialty certifications (e.g., Chest Pain, Stroke, Center of Excellence, Magnet®) Board approval Government regulations

EBP, evidence-based practice.

INTERNAL FRAME FACTORS

Internal frame factors are those that come from within the institution housing the educational program. Like external frame factors, these influence the need for change or the creation of new programs. Nurse educators in an academic setting, as contributing members to the school of nursing, participate on curriculum committees and other governance bodies within the school and the various levels of the institution such as department, division, or university-wide curriculum committees. Even faculty senates have influence and approval powers for curricula and their creation, revision, and/or discontinuance. The administrators of the institution also have influence; these persons may include the president, vice president(s), provost, dean, associate deans, and chairs or directors of academic programs. All new programs must go through the appropriate echelons of approval bodies from the school or department faculty to the chief administrative officer.

Major revisions experience the same approval processes as new programs. However, depending on the extent of the revision, such as minor changes to course content to meet student learning objectives, approval at higher levels may not be necessary. These types of revisions require discussion and approval with faculty and/or the school's curriculum committee. Internal frame factors in the academic setting include organizational and administrative structures, physical plant and

14. CURRICULUM DEVELOPMENT AND COURSE DESIGN IN NURSING EDUCATION

resources, budget, faculty and staff numbers and qualifications, faculty governance, and the student body and its characteristics.

Internal frame factors that influence healthcare settings are similar to those in academic settings. The cost and benefits of educational programs for patients and staff development influence the creation and revision of the curricula. Other factors are the type of organization (e.g., public or private, religion-based or nonsectarian, profit or nonprofit); administrative structure; physical plant; budget; nature of the staff, both professional and nonprofessional; governance; and characteristics of the population served. Table 14.2 provides examples of internal frame factors influencing academic and healthcare settings.

TABLE 14.2 SAMPLE INTERNAL FRAME FACTORS INFLUENCING EDUCATIONAL PROGRAMS IN ACADEMIC AND HEALTHCARE SETTINGS

Internal Frame Factor	Academic Settings	Healthcare Settings
Organizational and administrative structures (public or private; religion based or nonsectarian)	Place of nursing program within the institution (layers of decision-making) Sources of funding (e.g., state, tuition, endowments)	Place of education within agency, power structure, person(s) to whom the educator reports Agency structure (e.g., independent, part of a healthcare system, governmental agency) Funding sources
Physical plant and resources	Faculty offices, classroom, labs and simulation suites, conference rooms, media supplies, and services Library services Technology and other support	Audiovisual materials, learning labs/simulation suites, classrooms, conference rooms, internet access and support Supplies and services
Budget	Legislative influences and budgetary cuts (state and federal funding) Control for forecasting needs and expenditures External funding resources Scholarship and research support	County, state, and federal funding Cost of program and benefit analysis Control for forecasting needs and expenditures
Governance	Faculty involvement (within the school of nursing and university level) Student representation	Place of educational program in the agency Educator involvement in governance

(continued)

TABLE 14.2 SAMPLE INTERNAL FRAME FACTORS INFLUENCING EDUCATIONAL PROGRAMS IN ACADEMIC AND HEALTHCARE SETTINGS (continued)

Internal Frame Factor	Academic Settings	Healthcare Settings
Nature of the staff both professional and nonprofessional	Faculty numbers and qualifications Support-staff adequacy	Qualifications and experience of educators Staff support adequacy
Characteristics of the population served	Student body Community served by the students and faculty	Patient population Staff; e.g., nursing and other providers of care
Internal program approval	Periodic review by institution; frequency	Administrators Advisory board

Nurse educators should be aware of the environment in which they teach. Identification and implementation of new educational programs, along with those who teach in the programs, must be part of the processes for conducting a needs assessment and developing a curriculum. While teaching dominates their activities, educators' involvement in the assessment contributes to dynamic, evolving, and quality programs.

COMPONENTS OF THE CURRICULUM

When developing or revising curricula, the importance of involving key stakeholders in the process so that schools and healthcare agencies respond to the healthcare needs of the community cannot be overemphasized. Four major statements—the mission, vision, values (philosophy), and goals—provide an overview of the educational program and directions for its implementation. The process comes full cycle by using the content in the statements as guidelines for continuous quality improvement and summative evaluation on how well the program is performing. In reviewing the literature of these four major statements, whether for higher education or healthcare organizations, the definitions are similar across the board. Gurley et al. (2015) provided clear definitions that remain consistent today from their review of the literature related to the mission, vision, values, and goals of an educational program. There are four guiding statements of the curriculum that are useful to faculty in the process of revision or development.

Briefly, the four major statements are:

1. The *mission statement* declares the purpose of the program.
2. The *vision statement* encompasses the future expectations of the graduates of the school or the healthcare agency's role in healthcare.
3. The *values (philosophy) statement* describes the faculty/educators' philosophy about teaching and learning, healthcare, the profession, diversity, social justice, and so on.
4. The *end-of-program goals* describe the final product (graduate) of the program based on the mission, vision, and values of the program.

A conceptual or organizational framework follows the four statements; integrates the beliefs, theories, and concepts described in the statements; and delineates the learning outcomes to meet the specified program goals. Measurable objectives within the learning outcomes lead to an implementation plan that includes a list of courses or learning sessions. These courses or sessions start with objectives that serve as guidelines to measure learning outcomes derived from the goals of the program. To implement the curriculum, teachers further develop the courses and sessions into course content, learning activities, and assessment and evaluation activities to measure learning outcomes according to the objectives.

Both organizations and academic institutions have a hierarchical process for review and approval of new and updated curriculum. This usually consists of multiple members that represent different departments or academic units and are knowledgeable about how a curricular proposal may affect the workings for the organization or academic setting. For example, if a telemetry unit of a hospital holding chest pain certification wanted to make a change in the onboarding of new employees, members of the curriculum committee would review the curricular proposal in relation to effects on other departments' (emergency department and critical care units) onboarding processes and provide their decision for approval, denial, or further recommendations. In an academic setting, the proposal may start within a specific unit and follow many steps for technical review from admissions and records, departmental review, the university SLO and core objectives committees, information resource assessment, university courses and curriculum committee, the provost's office, and a final review by admissions and records. It is important to know the process and put forward a proposal that contains all of the components necessary for review.

Content Considerations

When developing courses for the curriculum, educators may consider concepts and content that will be woven throughout the program of study. Scaffolding, a term first coined by Wood et al. (1976), is a constructivist way of assisting the learner to develop a beginning understanding of content and advancing to independence based on exposure to information and experiences. Material can be broken down into smaller content and skills, moving up Bloom's taxonomies toward the independent practitioner. Figure 14.3 provides an example of scaffolding for social justice content in a baccalaureate nursing program, beginning with the content delivered in a prerequisite sociology course and continued throughout the curriculum.

Course Development

For course development, some schools of nursing use accreditation standards as organizational frameworks. These include the Accreditation Commission for Education in Nursing (ACEN, 2023), Commission on Collegiate Nursing Education (CCNE, 2018; in effect through December 31, 2024); and the National League for Nursing Commission for Nursing Education Accreditation (2021) standards and criteria. Accreditation is discussed in Chapter 18. Many baccalaureate and higher degree programs integrate the AACN's *The Essentials: Core Competencies for*

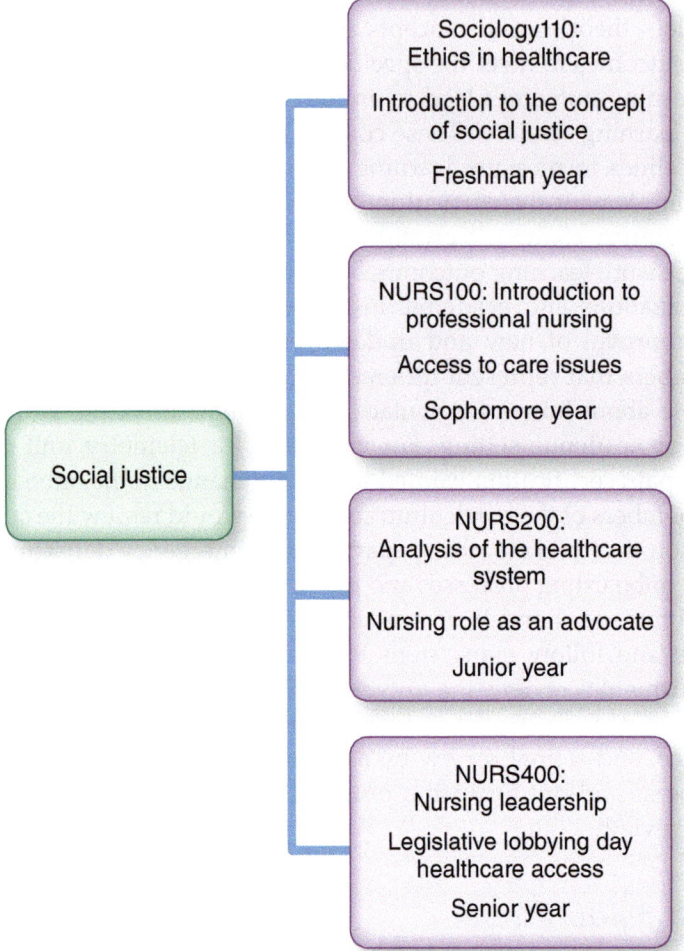

FIGURE 14.3 Sample scaffolding of social justice content in a baccalaureate nursing curriculum.

Professional Nursing Education (2021). Organizational frameworks, in addition to providing guidelines for the program, also provide a framework for assessment of the terminal SLO and evaluation of the program.

Based on the mission and/or vision, the philosophy/values statements, purpose of the program, and overall goals set the stage for defining the practice-ready program outcomes, SLO, objectives, or competencies that the curriculum or educational program purports to achieve. The literature uses many terms to signify educational goals or aims, objectives, and the steps for completing them. Most nurse educators express the steps toward achieving desired learning outcomes in behaviorally stated objectives. Breaking the mold of a typical course design, many nursing programs and educators have implemented the backward design framework (Wiggins & McTighe, 1998) for course/content development. The advantage to this format is that it blends well with competency-based learning, and educators need to intentionally consider the learning outcomes of the overall curriculum before determining any other step in the process.

IMPLEMENTATION PLAN

To carry out the educational program or the curriculum, one organizes an implementation plan according to the terminal program goals or practice-ready program outcomes. To reach these outcomes, a series of steps is necessary to assist the learner to progress through the program and reach the ultimate goals. A familiarity with educational taxonomies is helpful when assessing or developing objectives to fit the level of learner. Course objectives are sequenced to meet the identified level objectives. This becomes the plan or program of study.

There are three stages used in backward design:

1. identify desired results,
2. determine acceptable evidence, and
3. plan learning experiences and instruction (Wiggins & McTighe, 2005).

In Stage 1, the educator first reviews the program goals or outcomes as defined for the curriculum and considers the learning goals for the course. Wiggins and McTighe (2005) recommend that while focusing on the student learning goals, educators should ask themselves the following questions:

- What do we want the student to learn?
- What knowledge, skills, and abilities must be taught for the student to achieve mastery of the content?
- What content will yield retention of knowledge years later?

Answering these questions will help to develop the specific content for achieving the SLOs and identification of the desired results.

In Stage 2, the educator considers methods of assessment and evaluation to ensure learning is occurring. Examples of these methods may include group projects, tests and quizzes, a course paper, poster, portfolio, case studies, clinical observation, and concept mapping. The educator should choose the best tool for evaluating each assignment. Examples may include rubrics, self-assessments, peer grading, or classroom polling.

In Stage 3, the educator creates meaningful experiences through active teaching and learning strategies to achieve student outcomes. Tables 14.3 and 14.4 are modified examples of an undergraduate and a graduate course using a backward design framework.

SYLLABUS DEVELOPMENT

In the academic setting, each course requires a syllabus. The syllabus provides an outline of what the student can expect in learning outcomes, content, and evaluation throughout the semester. Each institution may have specific requirements, but most have similarities across institutions. The syllabus should begin with the title of the course and the semester provided, faculty information, a course description, pre-/corequisites, required texts and equipment, SLOs, course procedures, grading for the activities being provided, policies, and a course calendar. The course calendar should include the week/date(s), learning modules, focused readings and preparatory materials, and in-class activities. Parallel descriptions for courses apply to the healthcare setting educational sessions as well. At the very least, the session

TABLE 14.3 SAMPLE OF UNDERGRADUATE COURSE INTEGRATING BACKWARD DESIGN*

NURS 301: Health Assessment of the Individual

Course Description: Foundations of health assessment which include gathering, analyzing, synthesizing, communicating and documenting data to make nursing clinical judgments

Practice Ready Program Outcomes (PRPOs)
1. Apply quality improvement principles, standards, methods, and strategies to identify health and systems problems and support evidence-based change in practice settings.
2. Implement a safe, systematic process across settings using evidence-based strategies and standards, to promote a just culture of safety and to prevent or minimize risk to self, patients, and environment.
3. Demonstrate communication strategies, leadership, and teamwork to intentionally collaborate with interprofessional teams, individuals, groups, and populations across a range of sociocultural settings and to advocate for diverse, equitable, and inclusive care in professional environments.
4. Use a systematic approach to clinical reasoning based on best evidence, research, and knowledge from nursing and other disciplines to make decisions which optimize the health of populations, the delivery of care across a range of sociocultural settings, and the advancement of the nursing profession.
5. Deliver person- and population-centered care that is respectful of differing sociocultural needs based on best evidence, clinical judgment, and sound legal/ethical principles to promote plans of care and maximize health for diverse individuals, groups, and populations
6. Model a professional identity through personal and professional advocacy that promotes the needs of self, individuals, groups, populations, and the nursing profession while improving the healthcare system.
7. Use health care technology, data, and information literacy, while considering risks and ethical requirements, to plan, implement, and evaluate person and population-centered care and assist in system-wide best practice decisions in a variety of settings.

Student Learning Outcomes (SLOs)
1. Recognize assessment techniques that collect objective and subjective data pertinent to the individual's health or situation.
2. Evaluate clinical situations and patient conditions to choose the correct type of assessment and select prioritized assessment techniques.
3. Interpret patterns found in data collection and assessment findings to inform care and evaluate patient outcomes.
4. Describe how therapeutic communication establishes and maintains the nurse-client relationship.
5. Identify how healthcare information technologies are used in health assessment.
6. Use appropriate medical terminology to describe assessment findings in communicating with the interprofessional healthcare team

Module and Topic Title	Practice-Ready Program Outcomes/Alignment	Student Learning Outcomes (Course Level)-Alignment	Module Outcomes	Content	Assessment (e.g., discussion, paper)	Learning Materials (textbook readings, articles, videos, etc.)	Simulation
Module 4: Cardiovascular	PRPO 3: Demonstrate communication strategies... PRPO 4: Use a systematic approach to clinical reasoning based... PRPO 5: Deliver person- and population-centered care... PRPO 7: Use healthcare technology, data....	SLO 1: Recognize assessment techniques SLO 2: Evaluate clinical situations and patient conditions SLO 3: Interpret patterns found in data collection... SLO 4: Describe how therapeutic communication... SLO 5: Identify how healthcare information technologies... SLO 6: Use appropriate medical terminology to describe...	1. Interpret labs and diagnostics to identify patterns and individualize patient assessment (SLO 3) 2. Identify focused cardiovascular subjective questions to understand the patient's history, present illness (SLO 1,3) 3. Apply Acute Coronary Syndrome algorithm to adequately respond to new onset chest pain (SLO 2) 4. Differentiate between heart attack (MI), cardiac arrest, and heart failure (SLO 6) 5. Determine correct technique and order of the cardiovascular assessment (SLO 1)	Data Collection: Troponin CK-MB BNP Total Cholesterol, HDL, LDL Clotting (aPTT, Factor Xa, PT/INR) 5-lead EKG 12-lead EKG Transthoracic Echo Transoesophageal Echo Stress test Venous/arterial ultrasound Subjective: Chest pain ED drugs and nitroglycerine Weight gain Objective Pulse and heart rate Apical pulse Blood pressure JVD Carotid artery assessment 7 Ps	Adaptive Learning Pre- and Postclass Quizzes Entrance Ticket on A&P and Medical Terminology Participation Activities Patient Z Case Study (A-fib RVR, Chest pain r/o ACS) Time to Climb game Next Generation Case Study: DVT and PE	Readings: Chapters 17 and 18 Lecture Asynchronous Lecture and Materials In Class Demonstration	Virtual Simulation: Patient A Content Reinforced: Pneumonia and DVT Virtual Simulation: Patient B Content Reinforced: Osteoarthritis with Total Knee arthroplasty and A-fib

(continued)

TABLE 14.3 SAMPLE OF UNDERGRADUATE COURSE INTEGRATING BACKWARD DESIGN (continued)

Module and Topic Title	Practice-Ready Program Outcomes/ Alignment	Student Learning Outcomes (Course Level)- Alignment	Module Outcomes	Content	Assessment (e.g., discussion, paper)	Learning Materials (textbook readings, articles, videos, etc.)	Simulation
			6. Synthesize data from chart review, subjective assessment, and objective assessment to identify patterns or altered concepts, recognize cues and generate solutions/take action (SLO 3) 7. Describe normal and abnormal findings using appropriate medical terminology (SLO 6)	APE to man Regurgitation vs. stenosis murmurs S3 and S4 sounds Special populations with: Pacemaker Cardioversion Concepts Perfusion Inflammation Fluid and Electrolyte balance Exemplars Symptomatic bradycardia ACS Atrial fibrillation PAD Pericarditis DVT Hyperkalaemia/hypokalaemia Heart failure PVD	Content Reinforced in Exam 1 Review Exam, Final Review Exam Exam 1, 2, Final Traditional Question Portions Next Generation Portion of Exam 1: Heart Failure Next Generation Portion of Exam 2: DVT		

7 Ps, pain, pallor, paraesthesia, paralysis, polar temperature, puffiness, pulselessness; A & P, anatomy and physiology; ACS, acute coronary syndrome; A-fib, atrial fibrillation; A-fib RVR, atrial fibrillation with rapid ventricular response; APE to man, acronym for heart valves, aortic, pulmonic, Erb's point, mitral; aPTT, partial thromboplastin time, activated; BNP, B-type natriuretic peptide; CK-MB, creatine kinase-myocardial band; DVT, deep vein thrombosis; EKG, electrocardiogram, echo, echocardiogram; ED, emergency department; exam, examination; Factor Xa, activated factor X, clotting protein; HDL, high-density lipoprotein; JVD, jugular vein distention; LDL, low-density lipoprotein; PAD, peripheral artery disease; PE, pulmonary embolism; PT/INR, prothrombin time and international normalized ratio; PVD, peripheral vascular disease; r/o, rule out; S3, third heart sound; S4, fourth heart sound.

Source: Created by Haley McNeil, MSN, RN

14. CURRICULUM DEVELOPMENT AND COURSE DESIGN IN NURSING EDUCATION

TABLE 14.4 SAMPLE OF GRADUATE COURSE INTEGRATING BACKWARD DESIGN*

Course Name: N700 Populations and Aggregate Health Issues
Evaluation Code: Exam= E, Quiz =Q, Presentation = P, Simulation = SI, Clinical Encounter Notes = CE, Case Study = CS, Manuscript = M, Clinical = CL, Discussions=D, Concept Map=CM, Other="Short Explanation"

Course Student Learning Objective	Essentials Subcompetency	Essentials Subcompetency Description	Assessment/ Measurement	Module for Assignment Location
Analyze the roles/responsibilities of advanced practice nursing in inter professional health care.	1.1e	Translate evidence from nursing science as well as other sciences into practice.	D	Developing Health Promotion Programs
	1.1g	Integrate an understanding of nursing history in advancing nursing's influence in healthcare.	D	Historical Look at Nurses' Roles in Population Health and Care Models
	1.2h	Employ ethical decision-making to assess, intervene, and evaluate nursing care.	Q	Care of Vulnerable Populations
	1.2i	Demonstrate socially responsible leadership.	D and Other: Course Project	Collaboration and Community Partnerships
	4.2g	Lead the translation of evidence into practice.	D	Developing Health Promotion Programs
	6.1j	Role-model respect for diversity, equity, and inclusion in team-based communications.	Q and Other: Course Project	Care of the Vulnerable Populations

*Subcompetencies (and numbers) from the American Association of Colleges of Nursing. (2021). *The essentials: Core competencies for professional nursing education*. https://www.aacnnursing.org/Portals/0/PDFs/Publications/Essentials-2021.pdf

Source: Created by Theresa Watts, PhD, MPH, RN, CPH.

> **EXHIBIT 14.1 Syllabus Template**
>
> **Course number and title**, which should clarify its unique focus
>
> **Description** of the course, which should be an informative but succinct description that provides an overview of the intent of the course and addresses both theory and clinical components but does not outline specific teaching strategies or evaluation methods used
>
> **Prerequisites** or specific courses on which this one is built
>
> **Corequisites** or courses that must be taken concurrently with this one
>
> **Course instructor**
>
> **Course credits** how those credits are allocated among theory, clinical, and laboratory components, with the hours-to-credit ratio
>
> **Policies (including information on academic accommodations)**
>
> **Course objectives (SLO)**, which should reflect the curriculum concepts, be appropriate for the level of the learners, and build on previous knowledge. Each of these might also be linked to the appropriate core curriculum concept
>
> **Teaching methods**
>
> **Textbooks and other key resources**
>
> **Evaluation'** with the percentage of final course grade for each specified and due dates of assignments and tests
>
> **Grading scale**
>
> **Outline of the topics** to be addressed in the course and the sequence of those discussions

SLO, student learning objectives.

should include the title, a brief description, the expected learning outcomes/objectives, a topical outline, the time frame, and a description of the learning activities such as demonstration, practice, lecture, and group work. A statement on measurement of the outcomes and evaluation of the session should be mentioned, such as a quiz or ratings, according to objectives and teaching effectiveness.

An example of a syllabus template is provided in Exhibit 14.1.

CURRICULUM, CONCEPT, OR CONTENT MAPPING

When developing courses for the curriculum, it is helpful for educators to review the curriculum and program as a whole to ensure that key concepts and content are included in the courses. To accomplish this task, it is useful to create curriculum or content maps that trace the concepts throughout the program. Levin and Suhayda (2018) identify curriculum mapping as a way for faculty to assess unification of accreditation standards, SLOs, and curriculum. In addition, it is a way to build collaboration among colleagues. When mapping accreditation standards to current courses, if using the AACN *Essentials*, not all domains, competencies, and subcompetencies need to be included in each individual course. Mapping identifies how each course fits with others in the program and provides a clear delineation of where the domains, competencies, and subcompetencies reside and which, if any, are missing. Using a table or spreadsheet can prove beneficial in identifying any missing information. For example, the educator can list the course and SLOs within the course down

TABLE 14.5 SAMPLE PORTION OF CURRICULUM MAPPING/CROSSWALK*

Course and SLO	Domains									
	1	2	3	4	5	6	7	8	9	10
700-1					5.3f	6.2g, h, j 6.4g, h 6.1l			9.5g	10.1d
700-2	1.1e, f		3.1j 3.2k, l							

*Domains and numbers from the American Association of Colleges of Nursing. (2021). *The essentials: Core competencies for professional nursing education.* https://www.aacnnursing.org/Portals/0/PDFs/Publications/Essentials-2021.pdf

SLO, student learning objectives.

the vertical axis and the domains along the horizontal axis. The subcompetencies under each domain can then be mapped to the course SLO as depicted in Table 14.5.

BUDGETARY CONSIDERATIONS

Budgets in the Academic Setting

Curriculum development or revision also requires consideration of the impact to the overall budget. While faculty are not directly involved in the process of budget planning or management, they should have an appreciation for its place in developing and revising educational programs and curricula. In an academic setting, the dean or director of the school, college, or department of nursing usually has control over budget development and requests for funds to offer the program. The dean or director also estimates additional budget items to supplement normal expenditures. The everyday costs to implement a curriculum include faculty and staff salaries; equipment and supplies; technology; computer hardware and software for faculty, staff, and classroom support; simulation and other skills lab equipment and supplies; faculty development activities, including research, scholarly activities, and travel; and the physical facilities such as offices, classrooms, conference rooms, labs, and so on. Additional funding beyond the usual includes the costs associated with program development and revision, such as release time for faculty members involved in the process and additional office supplies to support the development activities. Periodic program approval and accreditation expenses are part of the budget as well, including accreditation fees, release time for faculty and staff, and costs related to completing the accreditation self-study. These are some examples of the costs for maintaining a nursing program in the academic setting and are not necessarily complete.

Forecasting budget needs for the future and decisions about the expenditures and maintenance of the budget are usually within the prerogative of the dean or director; however, these functions can differ according to the organizational structure and culture of the institution. The size of the program also influences administration of the budget; for example, in small programs, the dean or director may be solely responsible for planning, requesting, expending, maintaining, and reporting on the budget. Larger programs may have an administrative assistant or staff to whom the dean delegates budget responsibilities.

Sources of funding are critical to the life of the program and the assurance of the quality of the program. In large multipurpose colleges and universities, nursing programs are often targeted as expensive owing to the clinical nature of the program and low student-to-faculty ratio required for safe clinical supervision of students. Nursing's reply to these challenges usually points out that the prerequisite courses from the sciences and liberal arts that are part of the nursing program provide many full-time equivalents (FTEs) for the other disciplines.

Funding for the nursing program is dependent on the nature of the parent institution; for example, legislative decisions about income from general funds and tuition if state-supported and use of tuition and endowment funds for private schools. Not all programs, whether state-funded or private, can rely solely on these sources of funds. Often sought are grants, donations in the form of endowments and scholarships, and revenue-generating opportunities. Faculty members are involved in activities such as grant writing, with release time for research and program development when grants are funded. Revenue-generating programs include faculty practice clinics with Medicare, Medicaid, and healthcare insurance reimbursement funding. Charging student laboratory, technology, and online fees to cover costs and special program differential tuition are additional sources of funds that pay for supplies, services, and faculty and staff salaries.

All of these factors point out the need for faculty members to be aware of the sources of funding and costs to run the nursing program. Many deans and directors share budget planning and spending with faculty to involve them in the process and seek their input on cost savings and revenue generation. Such activities contribute to an appreciation of the budget and its influence on the implementation and quality of the program.

Budgets in the Healthcare Setting

Financial support for professional nursing education or patient education varies widely in healthcare agencies. Depending on the size of the institution, its purpose, and its sources of funding, the budget for educational services may be set aside separately or as part of another department within the agency. Large medical centers and academic health science centers usually have an educational department staffed by nurses and other specialty educators who have expertise in developing programs and teaching. Services include staff development, orientation of new staff, and patient education. A nurse or health educator may serve as the educator and coordinator for these programs with staff nurses, physicians, and other healthcare professionals providing content within their areas of expertise. The budget for this type of structure is usually within the agency's overall budget or set aside to target specific educational services. In larger institutions, the education department may be composed of several staff members and coordinated by a manager who has administrative support staff. Budget responsibilities fall to the manager of the program, who accounts for staff salaries and benefits, office supplies and services, media and computer hardware and software, and associated facilities such as conference rooms, classrooms, and laboratories.

The educator's role is to make the case for educational needs in the agency and the associated costs for their delivery. Often orientation of new employees and ongoing education to meet accreditation standards are the most common educational programs provided in the healthcare organization. A well-prepared and supported new nurse can result in employee satisfaction and reduction of turnover, which can prove quite costly. On average, turnover of a bedside RN can cost an organization just over $52,000 (NSi Nursing Solutions, 2023). Cost savings realized by the implementation of educational programs for staff and patients provide a significant rationale for the existence of the program. Larger institutions may have several educators on staff with administrative assistant support. Smaller institutions depend on an individual staff member's identification of educational needs, development of programs, and program implementation. Costs associated with these activities are absorbed into the time spent in delivering the services as a part of the care provided. Health departments and other governmental agencies use general funds to pay for educational programs. Again, depending on size, there may be dedicated nurses or health educators to provide patient education services and professional development and orientation. If it is a large department within the healthcare agency, the director or manager of the education department is responsible for the budget, while smaller agencies may depend on separate requests to the agency administrator for the educational program. Nonprofit agencies in the community also provide patient education services. These agencies often rely on donations, endowments, and to some extent fees for services. The agencies may employ nurses or health educators or integrate the services into the specific care services that they provide.

As with academic settings, it is necessary for the nurse educator to document the need for education, justify its expense, and manage provided funds. While educational services in healthcare settings are vital to maintain a competent staff and provide preventive and health maintenance educational services for patients, the importance of education is sometimes lost. Nurses in these settings have a responsibility to bring the need to the attention of the administrators and the public so that budgets for the services can be developed that are reasonable in cost, justify their need, result in cost savings and improved quality of patient care, and are sustainable over time.

SUMMARY

This chapter reviewed the role of educators in schools of nursing and healthcare agencies in the context of the educational programs in which they teach. It compared the differences between curriculum development and revision and pointed out the necessity for examining the external and internal frame factors that influence change or the creation of a new program. The chapter examined the major components of the curriculum, their interrelationships, and the implementation of course design within the curriculum and its evaluation. Mapping illustrated how nurse educators can track concepts or content throughout the curriculum to ensure their presence in levels of the program and the program's alignment with accreditation standards. The chapter also included a brief overview of the budget process for programs in both academic and healthcare settings.

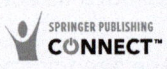 A robust set of instructor resources designed to supplement this text is located at http://connect.springerpub.com/content/book/978-0-8261-8892-2. Qualifying instructors may request access by emailing textbook@springerpub.com.

REFERENCES

Accreditation Commission for Education in Nursing. (2023). *Accreditation manual-2023 standards and criteria. Section III, Standard 4, Curriculum.* https://resources.acenursing.org/space/SAC/1825603752/STANDARD+4+-+Curriculum

American Association of Colleges of Nursing. (2021). *The essentials: Core competencies for professional nursing education.* https://www.aacnnursing.org/Portals/0/PDFs/Publications/Essentials-2021.pdf

Commission on Collegiate Nursing Education. (2024). *Standards, procedures & guidelines.* https://www.aacnnursing.org/ccne-accreditation/accreditation-resources/standards-procedures-guidelines

DeBoor, S. S. (2023). Needs assessment: The external and internal frame factors. In S. S. DeBoor (Ed.), *Keating's curriculum development and evaluation in nursing* (4th ed., pp. 49–69). Springer Publishing Company.

Gurley, D. K., Peters, G. B., Collins, L., & Fifolt, M. (2015). Mission, vision, values, and goals: An exploration of key organizational statements and daily practice in schools. *Journal of Educational Change, 16,* 217–242. https://doi.org/10.1007/s10833-014-9229-x

Johnson, M. (1977). *Intentionality in education.* Center for Curriculum Research and Services.

Keating, S. B. (2005). Needs assessment: The external and internal frame factors. In S. B. Keating (Ed.), *Curriculum development & evaluation in nursing.* Lippincott, Williams & Wilkins.

Levin, P. F., & Suhayda, R. (2018). Transitioning to the DNP: Ensuring integrity of the curriculum through curriculum mapping. *Nurse Educator, 43*(3), 112–114. https://doi.org/10.1097/NNE.0000000000000431

National Academy of Medicine. (2021). Educating nurses for the future. In M. K. Wakefield, D. R. Williams, S. Le Menestrel, & J. L. Flaubert (Eds.), *The future of nursing 2020–2030: Charting a path to achieve health equity* (pp.189–233). The National Academies Press.

National League for Nursing. (2023). *NLN publishes new vision statement: Integrating competency-based education in the nursing curriculum.* https://www.nln.org/detail-pages/news/2023/02/09/nln-publishes-new-vision-statement-integrating-competency-based-education-in-the-nursing-curriculum

National Leage for Nursing Commission for Nursing Education Accreditation. (2021). *Accreditation standards for nursing education programs.* https://irp.cdn-website.com/cc12ee87/files/uploaded/CNEA%20Standards%20October%202021-4b271cb2.pdf

NLN Commission for Nursing Education Accreditation (CNEA) (2021). Accreditation standards for nursing education programs. Retrieved from https://irp.cdn-website.com/cc12ee87/files/uploaded/CNEA%20Standards%20October%202021-4b271cb2.pdf

NSi Nursing Solutions. (2023). *2023 NSI national health care retention & RN staffing report.* https://www.nsinursingsolutions.com/Documents/Library/NSI_National_Health_Care_Retention_Report.pdf

Wiggins, G., & McTighe, J. (1998). Backward design. *Understanding by design* (pp. 13–34). Association for Supervision and Curriculum Development.

Wiggins, G., & McTighe, J. (2005). Backward design. *Understanding by design* (2nd ed., pp. 14–20). Association for Supervision and Curriculum Development.

Wood, D., Bruner, J., & Ross, G. (1976). The role of tutoring in problem solving. *Journal of Child Psychology and Child Psychiatry, 17,* 89–100. https://doi.org/10.1111/j.1469-7610.1976.tb00381.x

V

Evaluation of Learner and Program

Assessment Methods

Marilyn H. Oermann

OBJECTIVES

1. Compare assessment, evaluation, and grading processes
2. Describe methods for assessment and examples of their use in nursing education

INTRODUCTION

Assessment is the process of collecting information about student learning and performance to identify further learning needs, plan learning activities to meet those needs, and evaluate the outcomes and competencies met by the students. Students assess their own learning and performance to identify areas in which they need more practice. Assessment also provides information on the quality of the teaching, courses, practice experiences, curriculum, and other aspects of the educational program.

This chapter explains assessment, evaluation, and grading in nursing education. Methods are described for assessing learning, and examples are provided for many of these methods. Tests are a common assessment method used in nursing education, and various types of test items are described in Chapter 16. There is a separate chapter (Chapter 17) on clinical evaluation, and methods such as rating scales and rubrics are presented in that chapter.

ASSESSMENT

Assessment is the collection of information about student learning and performance. Assessment that provides information about the student's progress in the course and further learning needs is diagnostic: This is feedback for the educator and students to identify gaps in learning and plan relevant learning activities. Assessment also is used at designated times in the course such as at midterm and the end of the course to measure the outcomes of learning and determine students' grades. The data collected through assessment provide the basis for students' grades.

Assessment also provides information about the quality of teaching in a course. At the end of a course, students typically evaluate the effectiveness of the teacher and quality of the instructional methods, feedback to students, interactions with them, availability, and other areas related to the course. Students, graduates, and alumni assess the nursing program as part of program evaluation. Other uses of assessment are to select students for admission to the educational institution and school of nursing.

There are five principles the teacher should use when assessing student learning:

1. *Identify the competencies, outcomes, or objectives to be assessed.* Another way of thinking about this is: What is being assessed?
2. *Select appropriate assessment methods.* The methods for assessing learning (e.g., a test or written assignment) should provide information about the specific competency, outcome, or objective being assessed.
3. *Meet students' needs.* The assessment should provide feedback to individual students about their progress. The most important role of assessment is identifying where further learning is needed and planning appropriate strategies to help students learn and improve their performance.
4. *Use multiple assessment methods.* Decisions about learning and performance are often high stakes, having serious consequences for students, and should not be based on one test or assignment. Multiple assessment methods are needed to provide data for determining if the outcomes of a course were met and students have developed the essential competencies.
5. *Recognize the limitations of assessment when making decisions about students.* One teacher-made test, for example, may not be a true measure of the student's learning about that content. The test may have flaws in its design and other factors may influence the results (Brookhart & Nitko, 2019).

EVALUATION

While assessment is done *for* learning, evaluation *of* learning determines whether students developed the essential competencies and achieved the outcomes of the course (Oermann, 2022). The educator analyzes test scores, collects other assessment data, and then makes a value judgment about student learning and performance. There are two types of evaluation: formative and summative. In formative evaluation, the teacher assesses learning, gives feedback to students about gaps in learning, and plans further instruction to guide their learning. Giving prompt, specific, and instructional feedback is critical to the learning process and a characteristic of good teaching. Data collected through formative evaluation should not be graded because this feedback is intended to help students learn (Oermann et al., 2025).

Summative evaluation determines what students have learned. This is evaluation at the end of a point in time (e.g., at midterm and the end of a course) for determining grades.

GRADING

A grade is a symbol (e.g., A through F, pass–fail) that represents the student's achievement in a course. Grades are for summative evaluation, indicating how well the student performed in individual assignments, clinical practice, the skills laboratory, simulation, and the course as a whole.

There are different grading systems that can be used. A common grading system is with letters (A, B, C, D, E or A, B, C, D, F), sometimes combined with + and –. Grades also can be represented by percentages (100, 99, 98, . . .), which, in turn, can be used to assign a letter grade, for example, A = 90% to 100%. Two-dimensional systems such as pass–fail and satisfactory–unsatisfactory are used frequently for grading in clinical courses.

The grade is based on the data collected through the various assessment methods in the course. Each of these methods should be weighted in the overall course grade based on the emphasis of the outcomes and content evaluated by them in the course. For example, a unit examination in an adult health nursing course should count more in the course grade than a short assignment.

NORM- AND CRITERION-REFERENCED INTERPRETATION

There are two main ways of interpreting test scores and other assessment data. When tests are scored and papers and other assignments are graded, the result is a number. The number itself, however, has no meaning. For example, if the teacher tells students their scores on a test are 20 or 22, what does that mean? Scores need to be referenced or compared to some standard or to other students' scores. A score of 22 might be the highest score possible on the test or the highest score among the students who took it. To interpret a score, there needs to be a reference to compare the score against.

Test scores and the scores resulting from other types of assessment can be interpreted using norm- or criterion-referenced standards. In norm-referenced interpretation, each student's score is compared to those of a norm group. The norm group is often other students' test scores: Students who perform better than their peers receive higher scores (Brookhart & Nitko, 2019). Grading on a curve is an example of norm-referenced interpretation. Students' scores are rank ordered from highest to lowest, with grades based on where a student's score falls in the ranking. For example, the top 10% of students might receive an A and the lowest 10% an F.

In clinical practice, a tool on which student performance is rated on a scale of below to above average is norm-referenced: Each student's clinical performance is compared to the group of learners. Norm-referenced interpretation does not indicate what a student can and cannot do; it reflects instead if the student's performance is better or worse than other students in the clinical group (Oermann et al., 2025).

In criterion-referenced interpretation, students' tests and other scores from an assessment are compared to preset criteria, not to how well they performed in relation to other learners. The grades are based on what the student has learned and can do. With criterion-referenced interpretation, the teacher might indicate the percent of items answered correctly on a test. In clinical evaluation with criterion-referenced tools, students are evaluated on whether they could perform the competencies specified on the tool or designated for achievement at this point in the program.

COMPETENCIES AND OUTCOMES FOR ASSESSMENT

The competencies to be achieved in a nursing course and program and other learning outcomes provide the basis for planning instruction, teaching students in varied settings, and assessing their learning and performance. Competencies are the *observable abilities* of students or healthcare providers (Oermann, 2022). Because they are observable, teaching strategies can be planned to promote their development over time, and their performance can be assessed. Altmiller (2023) explained how to map the competencies across the curriculum to assess the adequacy of learning activities and identify gaps and redundancies in the curriculum. Competency-based education was described in depth in Chapter 13.

Nursing programs also may specify the student learning outcomes or the objectives for a course and program. An outcome is a statement that describes the knowledge, skills, and values that students should attain at the end of a unit or module, a course, or the program. Outcomes reflect expected student learning, not necessarily performance. Objectives are typically more specific behaviors the learner is expected to achieve at the end of the instruction. There are many different definitions of competencies, outcomes, and objectives in the literature. Faculty in a school of nursing should use consistent terminology for their courses and throughout the program.

The assessment methods and the evaluation that is done in a course and program are based on the competencies or outcomes to be met by students. These may be written in three domains of learning, although generally they involve an integration of these domains: the knowledge and higher level cognitive skills to be acquired (cognitive domain), values to be developed (affective domain), and skills to be performed (psychomotor domain). Each of these domains has its own taxonomy that levels the learning that can occur. The cognitive taxonomy has six levels increasing in complexity: remembering, understanding, applying, analyzing, evaluating, and creating (Anderson & Krathwohl, 2001; Bloom et al., 1956). These are defined in Exhibit 15.1 with an example of an objective written at each level. The taxonomy of the cognitive domain is valuable in planning the assessment because it helps the teacher focus the test item or other assessment method on a particular cognitive level (Oermann et al., 2025). If the outcome relates to application, the assessment should determine if students can apply what they are learning to a new situation or in a new context. By using the taxonomy, the teacher can avoid assessment methods that focus on recall of facts and memorization when the intended outcomes of learning are at a higher level.

The affective domain taxonomy levels values, attitudes, and beliefs from knowing them to internalizing them as a basis for decisions. The psychomotor domain focuses on the development of motor skills and the phases that learners progress through as they gain expertise in skill performance.

EXHIBIT 15.1 Cognitive Domain Taxonomy and Examples

1. *Remembering*: Recall of facts and specific information
   Example: List two symptoms of congestive heart failure.
2. *Understanding*: Comprehension and ability to explain material
   Example: Describe classes of heart failure based on functional capacity.
3. *Applying*: Use of information in a new situation
   Example: Apply clinical practice guidelines to care of patients with heart failure.
3. *Analyzing*: Ability to break down material into its parts and identify the relationships among them
   Example: Compare psychometric properties of instruments for measuring the quality of life of patients with heart failure.
4. *Evaluating*: Ability to make value judgments based on internal and external criteria
   Example: Evaluate the strength of the evidence related to follow-up care of patients with heart failure.
5. *Creating*: Ability to combine elements to develop a new product
   Example: Develop a plan for managing patients with acute decompensated heart failure.

ASSESSMENT METHODS

Tests are a common assessment method for determining students' learning in a course and certifying nurses' knowledge in the clinical setting; for example, competency tests during orientation. While tests are used frequently, they are not the only assessment method to be considered. Other assessment methods are listed in Exhibit 15.2. Some of these are used predominantly for assessment in the classroom or online environment, such as tests and papers, and others are designed for assessing learning and performance in a practice environment, such as observation with a rating scale.

Test

A test is a set of items to which students respond in written or sometimes oral format. Tests are typically scored based on the number of correct answers, are administered in the same way to all students, and are usually timed. Tests may be used for admission to a college or university and to the nursing program. In many prelicensure nursing programs, students take tests as they progress through each level and at the end of the program to identify gaps in learning, assess their risk for not passing the National Council Licensure Examination (NCLEX®), and provide feedback to students and faculty for developing a learning plan for students to be successful in the nursing program and on the NCLEX. Another use of tests is for evaluating student learning and performance at the end of a nursing program for program evaluation rather than indicating what students have learned in a particular course. The educator can integrate short informal quizzes in a class or as a preclass assignment to gauge student learning and identify where further instruction may be needed.

There are many types of test items that can be used for assessment of learning in nursing courses. Chapter 16 describes different types of test items, principles for writing each of those items, and test and item analysis.

EXHIBIT 15.2 Assessment Methods

Test
Quiz
Paper and other written assignments
Concept map
Case (scenario, unfolding case, case study)
Media clip
Electronic portfolio
Discussion
Conference
Group project
Simulation
Standardized patient
Objective structured clinical examination
Observation with rating scale
Self-evaluation

Papers and Other Written Assignments

Papers and other types of written assignments enable students to search for literature and resources, apply evidence to practice, build higher level thinking skills, and for some assignments, improve writing skills (Oermann et al., 2025). All too often, however, students complete assignments that are not geared to any particular competency or goal of the course; these assignments may have been in a course for years but are no longer relevant for the aims of the current course. Written assignments should be carefully selected based on the competencies or outcomes to be met. If an outcome relates to identifying resources for evidence-based practice, students could prepare a paper comparing clinical point-of-care tools, Cochrane Library reviews, and other sources of evidence for use in the practice setting. In this way the paper is designed to assess if students can identify relevant resources for evidence-based practice in nursing—the objective of the assignment.

Faculty members should periodically review the papers and other written assignments in courses to confirm that they are still relevant, meet specific competencies or outcomes of the course, are not "busywork," are not too repetitive, and build on one another across different courses. While some repetition is important to develop knowledge and cognitive and writing skills, once students have mastered writing certain types of papers, the teacher might transition to a new assignment.

Formal Paper for Improving Writing Skill

Students at all levels of nursing education need to write effectively, but many students lack these skills. Term papers and other formal papers, which include drafts, feedback from the teacher on the substance of the paper and the quality of the writing, and revisions based on that feedback, enable students to develop their writing ability. There are many types of formal papers students can write in a course, such as term papers, literature reviews, research reports, and papers analyzing concepts and their application to patient care, among others. Exhibit 15.3 lists examples of formal papers for assessment in a nursing course.

EXHIBIT 15.3 Examples of Formal Papers for Assessment

Term paper
Development of research proposal
Research reports
Literature, integrative, and other types of reviews
Paper in which students critique and synthesize evidence and report on its application to clinical practice
Paper analyzing concepts and their use in patient care
Paper comparing different interventions and their evidence base
Concept analysis paper
Critical analysis paper in which students analyze issues, compare options, and develop arguments for a position

---

Source: Adapted from Oermann, M. H., Gaberson, K. B., & De Gagne, J. C. (2025). *Evaluation and testing in nursing education* (7th ed., p. 160). Springer Publishing Company. Reprinted with permission of Springer Publishing.

Reflective Journal

Reflective journals encourage students to reflect on their experiences and think critically about them. Reflective journals also provide opportunities to better understand patients' perspectives and the clinical environment, evaluate their own responses, develop clinical judgment skills, and cope with the stress of an unexpected clinical situation (Mumba et al., 2022; Murillo-Llorente et al., 2021; Nelms Edwards et al., 2019; Oermann et al., 2025; Yang et al., 2022). For assessment, journals allow faculty to provide feedback and respond to possible difficulties students might be encountering in the clinical setting. While some teachers assess journals for summative evaluation and grading, when the aim of the journal is to reflect on experiences and gain meaning from them, journals should be used for feedback purposes only and not graded.

Short Written Assignment

Another type of written assignment for assessment is a short paper that focuses on a specific content area or outcome (Oermann et al., 2025). For example, students might write a one-page paper that compares two similar patient problems and how to differentiate them in an assessment; a paragraph that describes using SBAR (situation, background, assessment, and recommendation) for bedside handoff; and a two-page paper that examines nursing interventions and supporting evidence for a patient with a particular health problem. Short assignments provide an opportunity for teachers to give quick feedback on students' knowledge, higher level thinking skills, and sometimes also writing skills. Short assignments can be completed by students individually or as a small group activity and can be used for formative and summative evaluation.

Assessment of Papers and Other Written Assignments

For any written assignment, the teacher needs to have specific criteria for assessment, which should be shared with students prior to beginning the paper. The criteria depend on the type of assignment. For formal papers, the quality and comprehensiveness of the content, use of relevant and current literature, organization of the paper, writing style, and reference style would be considered. For other types of written assignments, some of these criteria would not be appropriate.

The educator should develop a rubric for evaluating the paper. A rubric is a scoring guide, specifying the criteria to be assessed and points allotted to each criterion. Students should have the rubric ahead of time so they can prepare the paper accordingly. A rubric is useful for both instructional purposes and assessment because it guides students in writing the paper and teachers in assessing it (Brookhart & Nitko, 2019). Table 15.1 provides an example of a rubric for scoring a formal paper in a nursing course.

Following are principles for assessing papers and other written assignments:

1. Written assignments should be planned to guide students in achieving specific competencies and outcomes of the course, and the criteria for assessment should address those.

2. The number of required papers in a course should be reasonable. If the aim is to improve writing, students need to complete drafts and receive feedback on content and writing. The number of drafts should be considered in decisions about written assignments in a course.

TABLE 15.1 EXAMPLE OF A RUBRIC FOR SCORING A FORMAL PAPER IN A NURSING COURSE

CONTENT		
Content relevant to purpose of paper, comprehensive, and in depth	Content relevant to purpose of paper	Some content not relevant to purpose of paper, lacks depth
10 9 8	7 6 5 4	3 2 1
Content accurate	Most of content accurate	Major errors in content
10 9 8	7 6 5 4	3 2 1
Sound background developed from concepts, theories, and literature	Background relevant to topic but limited development	Background not developed, limited support for ideas
20–15	14–7	6–1
Current research synthesized and integrated effectively in paper	Relevant research summarized in paper	Limited research in paper, not used to support ideas
10 9 8	7 6 5 4	3 2 1
ORGANIZATION		
Purpose of paper/thesis well developed and clearly stated	Purpose/thesis apparent but not developed sufficiently	Purpose/thesis poorly developed, not clear
5	4 3 2	1
Ideas well organized and logically presented, organization supports arguments and development of ideas	Clear organization of main points and ideas	Poorly organized, ideas not developed adequately in paper
10 9 8	7 6 5 4	3 2 1
Thorough discussion of ideas, includes multiple perspectives and new approaches	Adequate discussion of ideas, some alternate perspectives considered	Discussion not thorough, lacks detail, no alternate perspectives considered
10 9 8	7 6 5 4	3 2 1

(continued)

TABLE 15.1 EXAMPLE OF A RUBRIC FOR SCORING A FORMAL PAPER IN A NURSING COURSE (*continued*)

ORGANIZATION (*continued*)

Effective conclusion and integration of ideas in summary	Adequate conclusion, summary of main ideas	Poor conclusion, no integration of ideas
5	4 3 2	1

WRITING STYLE AND FORMAT

Sentence structure clear, smooth transitions, correct grammar and punctuation, no spelling errors	Adequate sentence structure and transitions; few grammar, punctuation, and spelling errors	Poor sentence structure and transitions; errors in grammar, punctuation, and spelling
10 9 8	7 6 5 4	3 2 1
Professional appearance of paper, all parts included, length consistent with requirements	Paper legible, some parts missing or too short/too long considering requirements	Unprofessional appearance, missing sections, paper too short/too long considering requirements
5	4 3 2	1
References used appropriately in paper, references current, no errors in references, correct use of APA style for references	References used appropriately in paper but limited, most references current, some citations or references with errors and/or some errors in APA style for references	Few references and limited breadth, old references (not classic), errors in references, errors in APA style for references
5	4 3 2	1
Total Points _____ (sum points for total score)		

APA, American Psychological Association.
Source: Adapted from Oermann, M. H., Gaberson, K. B., & De Gagne, J. C. (2025). *Evaluation and testing in nursing education* (7th ed., pp. 164–165). Springer Publishing Company. Reprinted with permission of Springer Publishing.

3. Written assignments should foster students' higher level thinking about the content rather than summarizing what they read unless summarizing was the objective of the assignment.
4. The directions about the purpose and format of the paper should be clear; students should know the dates when drafts and the final paper are due; and they should have the rubric ahead of time.
5. In evaluating papers in which students analyze issues, the criteria should focus on the rationale for the position, not the specific position.
6. The teacher should read papers anonymously (to avoid potential bias); read each paper twice before scoring (to gain an overview of how students approached the topic, as the rubric may need to be modified if no students addressed a particular content area); and grade papers in random order (to avoid bias, as papers read first may be scored higher than those at the end).
7. If unsure about a grade on a paper or other assignment, the teacher should have a colleague read the paper, also anonymously (Oermann et al., 2025).

Concept Map

A concept map is a graphical presentation of concepts and how they relate to one another (Van Rensburg et al., 2023). Concept maps enable students to apply theory to practice, gain new knowledge, and improve critical thinking and clinical judgment (Innis et al., 2023). In clinical practice, concept maps can help students plan their care for a patient, organize information, and visualize how the assessment data, problems, treatments, medications, and other information are interrelated. Students can develop a concept map as part of their planning for clinical practice and then revise the map after caring for the patient. While concept maps are typically assessed for formative purposes, they also can be graded if students explain the relationships among concepts in the map. An example of a concept map is in Figure 15.1.

Cases

Cases—clinical and other scenarios that students analyze and answer questions about—allow students to apply concepts and readings to clinical situations, identify problems and interventions, and weigh possible actions. Depending on how the case and questions are written, cases develop students' problem-solving, decision-making, and clinical judgment skills (Hensel & Billings, 2020; Pence, 2023). Cases are useful for assessing those outcomes if the questions focus on the process of clinical judgment and reasoning (Fink & Martyn-Nemeth, 2023).

Cases typically present a clinical scenario that integrates various concepts, followed by questions about that scenario. Hensel and Billings (2020) recommended including multiple pieces of information in the scenario. Often the scenarios are short to avoid directing students' thinking in advance. Questions can ask students what they noticed in the situation, to decide what is likely wrong with the patient, to identify additional data to collect, to propose actions that are appropriate or if no actions are needed, and to reflect on how patients might respond to those actions.

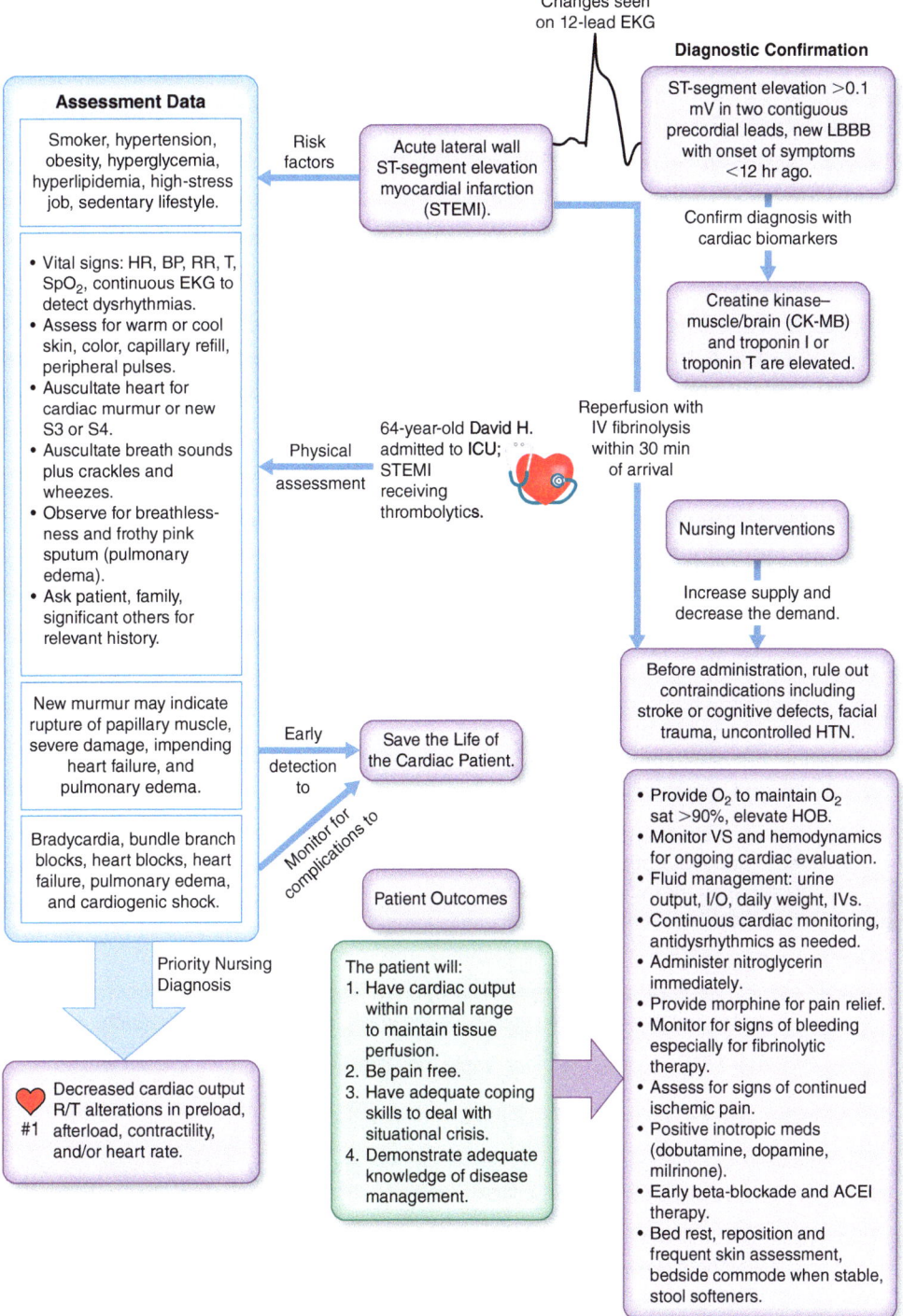

FIGURE 15.1 Example of a concept map.

ACEI, angiotensin-converting enzyme inhibitors; BP, blood pressure; HOB, head of bed; HR, heart rate; HTN, hypertension; I/O, intake/output; RR, respiratory rate; R/T, related to; SpO2, oxygen saturation; T, temperature; VS, vital signs.

Source: Developed by Deanne A. Blach, MSN, RN, CNE, NPD-BC, 2024. Reprinted with the permission of Deanne A. Blach, 2024.

Unfolding cases simulate a changing scenario similar to what might occur in actual clinical practice. With this method the case unfolds to reveal new information about the situation, and students make decisions about the relevance and meaning of these new data. Unfolding cases are valuable for assessing students' understanding of the clinical situation and their clinical judgment and other cognitive skills (Ellis et al., 2023; Hekel et al., 2023; Liu, 2023; Pence, 2023). Case studies are longer and provide background information about the patient, family, community, or other context. In their analysis of a case study, students can cite related literature and provide a rationale for their analysis and any decisions they made.

Cases can be analyzed by students individually or in small groups in class, online, or in postclinical conferences. With this method, the teacher can provide feedback on the content and thought process used by students to arrive at their answers. Typically, cases are used for instruction and not for grading. However, if the teacher wanted to grade student responses to cases, they would be evaluated similarly to a written assignment or an essay item (establishing criteria for grading, developing a rubric, scoring answers to the questions using the rubric, and following other principles for scoring essay items). Exhibit 15.4 provides an example of a short integrative case, an unfolding case, and a case study.

EXHIBIT 15.4 Examples of Cases for Assessment

Case
Your patient fell at home and was admitted yesterday with a hip fracture. She is scheduled for surgery today. At shift report the nurse says the patient had lab work done on admission, but does not know the results. Later you find that the patient's hemoglobin is 5.0 g/dL and hematocrit is 16%.

1. What were unsafe practices in this situation?
2. Which National Patient Safety Goals were not met? What are the implications of this situation for the patient's care?
3. What should have been done?

Unfolding Case
Your 93-year-old patient in a long-term care facility has a Stage I pressure ulcer at her sacrum. The patient is also coughing and tells you she is too weak to get out of bed for lunch.

1. Describe what the pressure ulcer would look like. What other data should you collect? Why?
2. Develop a plan of action for this patient, with a rationale.

The following day the patient is coughing more, has shortness of breath, and is more fatigued. A nurse tells you in report it looks like the patient has a blister on her sacrum.

1. What does this new information mean?
2. What are some possible problems of this patient? List them in priority and provide a rationale for your prioritization.
3. What information will you report to the nurse at handoff using SBAR?

The patient's daughter comes to find you on the unit and tells you she is angry that a nurse moved her mother to a chair.

1. What would you say to her? Why?
2. How can you provide patient-centered care in this situation?
3. If the patient's pressure ulcer is worsening, what observations would you expect to make? Based on those observations, what interventions should be implemented now?

(continued)

> **EXHIBIT 15.4 Examples of Cases for Assessment (*continued*)**
>
> **Case Study**
> A patient comes to the ED with severe abdominal pain and diarrhea. The patient has lost 12 pounds in the past 2 weeks and has no appetite. The nurse does not detect any masses, but there is abdominal tenderness and pain. The patient's wife indicates the patient has been healthy except for this "flu," which has lasted for 2 weeks. She says the patient travels frequently and was recently in Portugal and Canada. The patient does not smoke or drink alcohol. The wife explains that last year the patient was treated for depression but is fine now and has no prior health problems. They have two children, and the grandparents are currently watching them.
>
> 1. What are possible problems that the patient might have? What information in this case supports your tentative problem list?
> 2. List two questions you would ask the wife next and explain why this information is important.
> 3. What laboratory tests would you expect to be ordered? Why?
> 4. Add laboratory values to the case and discuss with a peer how that information would influence decisions about the patient's problems or treatments.

Media Clip

Short segments of a digital recording, a video from YouTube, and other media clips can also be used for assessment. Media clips allow students to visualize the clinical situation and get a sense of what the experience is like for patients, families, and providers. Questions can be developed by the teacher related to the multimedia for students to answer, either for formative or summative purposes.

Electronic Portfolio

In an electronic portfolio, students collect materials they have developed in the course that provide documentation that they have achieved the competencies and met the outcomes of the course. Portfolios also can be used for program evaluation, job applications, and career development. Nurses can continue to add materials and documentation of their accomplishments to their portfolios. In this way the portfolio represents the continued development of a student's expertise and accomplishments over a period of time.

There are two types of portfolios: best work and growth (Brookhart & Nitko, 2019). Best-work portfolios contain examples of students' "best" products of learning; when used for assessment, these products provide evidence that students have achieved the competencies and outcomes of the course. Growth portfolios are portfolios in process for faculty to provide feedback to students (formative evaluation) and for students to reflect on their progress in the course or program.

The contents of the portfolio depend on the competencies and outcomes to be assessed. Students can select papers and projects they completed in the course, group projects, self-reflections on clinical and other experiences, and other products they developed that demonstrate their learning and achievement. When portfolios are graded, a rubric should be used for the evaluation. There are many free software programs that students can use to develop an electronic portfolio.

Discussions and Conferences

Discussions are an exchange of ideas between two or more people (Oermann et al., 2025). These are often informal but may also be planned discussions about a particular topic. In a discussion the teacher can assess students' knowledge of a topic, explore decisions made and the reasoning underlying those decisions, and provide feedback to learners. Open-ended questions rather than ones answered with a "yes–no" response encourage students' higher level thinking and promote discussion about alternate perspectives and approaches. Questions are an effective method for assessing students' thinking because the teacher can ask them to discuss options they considered and explain how they arrived at their decisions.

Questions should be sequenced from a low to a high level. The teacher can begin with factual questions to assess students' knowledge and understanding, and then can explore the process used to think through a situation, analyze problems, and arrive at actions to take. The learning environment has to be one that values discussion about alternate views so students are comfortable in sharing their thinking. Merisier et al. (2018) emphasized that finding the correct answer is not the most important part of questioning, but instead the focus should be on the rationale. An advantage of using questions for assessment is the teacher can carefully plan questions to lead students through the clinical judgment process and share their thinking about the data, significant cues, potential problems, multiple interventions that might be used, and outcomes to evaluate.

Conferences are planned discussions on a topic. These include pre- and postclinical conferences, interprofessional conferences, and other types of seminars in which the student participates. In a conference, students develop their oral communication skills and ability to lead and engage others in a discussion. Assessment of student participation in a conference is typically best for formative evaluation because the teacher can provide feedback to students as a group and individually during the discussion. This feedback can encourage students to consider other points of views and think more broadly about a topic. Educators also can clarify any misunderstandings and share how they would analyze a situation and arrive at a decision. However, conferences can be evaluated for summative purposes, including how well a student led a conference and the quality of students' participation in it. If conferences are assessed for grading purposes, specific criteria need to be established and shared with students prior to their leading or participating in the conference. These criteria include how well the student led the group discussion, presented ideas to the group, and encouraged peers to participate in the discussion. The criteria should also address the student leader's knowledge of the topic and preparation for the conference.

Group Projects

Group projects encourage cooperative learning and development of skills in teamwork and collaboration. Some group projects are short term with students meeting in class, online, or outside of class for the time it takes to develop the product, such as a poster or group presentation. Other groups, however, are long term, for example the length of the course for cooperative learning purposes. With either type of group, the group product and individual student participation in the group can be assessed.

The difficulty with group projects is grading them, especially when students contribute unequally to the group work. Varied strategies for grading can be used. One strategy is to give a group grade—all students in the group get the same grade for the project regardless of the contributions and quality of the work of individual students in the group. Another strategy is for each student to describe what they did as part of the group project, with the teacher evaluating these individual parts and assigning each student a separate grade. The grade for the individual student might be only the individual student's score, or a group grade can be given in addition. One final strategy is for students to prepare both a group and an individual product, both of which are graded.

When group projects are assessed, the teacher needs a rubric developed specifically for evaluating that project (Brookhart & Nitko, 2019). The rubric should include criteria related to the substance of the group project, the quality of the presentation, and how well the students worked together as a team.

Simulation

Chapter 9 examined the use of simulations in teaching and assessment. With simulations, students can analyze scenarios, make decisions about problems and actions to take, carry out interventions, demonstrate techniques and skills, and evaluate the effects of their decisions. In simulations students can engage in the deliberate practice of skills, improving their performance. Simulations provide for learning and practice both individually and as a team (intra- and interprofessional).

Simulations can be used for both formative and summative evaluation. For formative evaluation, in the debriefing session teachers can provide feedback to students to further develop their understanding and guide them in transferring learning to clinical practice, among other outcomes (Kim et al., 2023). The debriefing provides an opportunity to explore different perceptions of what occurred in the simulation, examine actions taken or not taken and other possible approaches, and analyze each student's role. When simulation is used for summative evaluation, the aim is to verify if the student can perform specific competencies. Summative evaluation is high stakes for participants, and simulations must meet rigorous standards (Buléon et al., 2022). There should be standardization in setting up and conducting the simulation so there is consistency with the evaluation; the tools must be valid and reliable; the evaluator needs to be trained in the process, use of the tools, and scoring; and if the evaluation is high stakes (used for making critical decisions about the student, for example, students need to pass the evaluation to pass the course), more than one rater should be used (Oermann et al., 2025). These decisions are too important to be based on only one person's observations and judgment.

Standardized Patient

Standardized patients (SPs) are actors trained to portray the role of a patient, family member, or another individual. With SPs, students can gain knowledge, refine their clinical and communication skills, and increase their confidence (Chua et al., 2023). SPs are often used for formative evaluation, with the SP providing feedback to the student. The encounter with the SP may be video recorded for self-evaluation by the student and evaluation by the faculty member. Because SPs recreate the same clinical situation each time they are with a student, providing for consistency in the assessment, they also can be used for summative evaluation and high-stakes decisions.

Objective Structured Clinical Examination

Another assessment method is an objective structured clinical examination (OSCE). With OSCEs, students rotate through stations where they perform a skill or activity, analyze cases, or demonstrate other competencies. At each station in the OSCE, students are evaluated on their performance, often with rating scales or checklists. OSCE are effective for assessing a wide range of competencies and are valid and reliable (Goh et al., 2019, 2022).

When setting up an OSCE for formative or summative evaluation:

- An examination blueprint should be developed that specifies the skills and other competencies to be assessed and types of scenarios to be used. Case scenarios should be written based on this blueprint and by faculty members who have expertise in the content and competencies.
- Multiple OSCE scenarios can be developed to provide more than one assessment of students' knowledge and performance.
- The content validity of the scenarios should be established prior to using them for an OSCE.
- SPs should be trained to portray the patient diagnosis or situation related to the skills of the student to be assessed.
- Rating scales, checklists, and other tools used for evaluation must be valid and reliable, including interrater reliability. The validity and reliability of the tools should be established prior to using them for summative evaluation.
- Evaluators, and SPs if their role includes giving feedback to students and rating their performance, need to be trained on the expected performance and proper use of the tools.
- If OSCEs are used for summative purposes, a standard needs to be set as to the score that differentiates students who pass from those who do not.

Observation and Rating Scale

The predominant strategy used to evaluate the performance of students is observing them in clinical practice, simulation and learning laboratories, and other settings, and rating their performance on a checklist (for skills) or rating scale (for a broader assessment). Educators observe students carry out patient care individually or as a team and make a judgment about the quality of that performance. The rating scale, also called clinical evaluation tool or form, lists the competencies and other behaviors to be demonstrated by students and a scale (for example, pass-fail) for rating their performance of them. Observation and rating scales are discussed in Chapter 17.

Self-Evaluation

An important outcome of a nursing education program at all levels is the ability of students to evaluate their own learning and performance. With this self-reflection, students can identify areas in which continued learning and development need to occur. Self-evaluation is a developmental process. With a positive teacher–student environment, students will be more likely to share reflections and own assessment with their teachers than in an environment that is punitive and viewed as not facilitating their learning. Self-evaluation is for formative evaluation only and should not be graded.

SUMMARY

Assessment is the collection of information about student learning and performance. It is critical in determining the student's grade in a course because assessment provides the data on which the grade is based. Assessment also reveals gaps in learning and performance and the need for further instruction. When the teacher adds a value judgment about the quality of learning and performance, the process is evaluation. Formative evaluation occurs throughout the instructional process and provides feedback to students. Summative evaluation "summarizes" what students have learned. This is evaluation at the end of a point in time (e.g., midterm and the end of a course) for determining a course or clinical grade.

A grade is a symbol (A through F, pass–fail) that represents the student's achievement in a course and clinical practice. Grades are for summative evaluation, indicating how well the student performed in individual assignments, practice settings, and the course as a whole. Test scores and the scores resulting from other types of assessment can be interpreted using norm- or criterion-referenced standards. In norm-referenced interpretation, each student's score is compared to those of a norm group. In contrast, in criterion-referenced interpretation, students' tests and other scores from an assessment are compared to preset criteria, not to how well they performed in relation to other learners. Clinical courses can be graded with letter grades, such as A through F, or as pass–fail and other two-dimensional systems.

There are many methods teachers can use to assess students' learning in a course and their performance skills. Tests are a common method in nursing education. Another assessment method used frequently in courses is written assignments. Students can prepare formal papers such as term papers, reflective journals, short papers, concept maps, and other written assignments that assess student learning.

With integrative cases, unfolding cases, and case studies, students can apply knowledge to practice situations and develop their higher level thinking skills. These are also appropriate for assessment. Cases typically present a clinical scenario that integrates various concepts followed by questions about that scenario. Students analyze the scenario and might identify patient problems, possible interventions, and alternate ways of approaching the situation. Rather than describing the scenario in print form, short segments of a digital recording, a video from YouTube, and other media clips can also be used to present the scenario.

In an electronic portfolio, students collect materials they have developed in the course that provide documentation that they have met the course outcomes. Portfolios are valuable for assessment because they contain the evidence for judging if students have met the outcomes of the course.

Discussions are an exchange of ideas between two or more people. Educators engage in many discussions with students, one-to-one and in small groups, for teaching and for providing feedback to students. Conferences are planned discussions about a topic. These include pre- and postclinical conferences, interprofessional conferences, and other types of seminars in which the student participates. In a conference, students can develop their oral communication skills and ability to lead and engage others in discussing an issue or a problem and deciding on actions to take.

Group projects encourage cooperative and active learning, teamwork, and communication, among other outcomes. Some group projects are short term, with students meeting in class, online, or outside of class for the time it takes to develop the product such as a poster or group presentation. Other groups are long term; for example, the length of the course, for cooperative learning purposes.

With simulations, students can analyze scenarios and make decisions about actions to take, demonstrate techniques and skills, and implement care individually and as a team including an interprofessional team. These activities and others completed in a simulation can be assessed for feedback to students and for summative evaluation. SPs are actors trained to portray the role of a patient with a specific condition. With SPs, students can be assessed on interpersonal and communication skills, history and physical examination techniques, and other competencies. Another assessment method is an OSCE. With OSCEs students rotate through stations where they are evaluated on their competencies.

The predominant strategy used to evaluate the performance of students is observing them in practice and rating their performance on a checklist or rating scale, discussed in Chapter 17. An important outcome of a nursing education program at all levels is the ability of students to evaluate their own learning and performance. With this self-reflection, students can identify areas in which further learning and development need to occur.

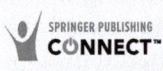

A robust set of instructor resources designed to supplement this text is located at http://connect.springerpub.com/content/book/978-0-8261-8892-2. Qualifying instructors may request access by emailing textbook@springerpub.com.

REFERENCES

Altmiller, G. (2023). Curriculum mapping for competency-based education: Collecting objective data. *Nurse Educator, 48*(5), 287. https://doi.org/10.1097/NNE.0000000000001462

Anderson, L. W., & Krathwohl, D. R. (Eds.). (2001). *A taxonomy for learning, teaching, and assessing: A revision of Bloom's taxonomy of educational objectives*. Longman.

Bloom, B. S., Englehart, M. D., Furst, E. J., Hill, W. H., & Krathwohl, D. R. (1956). *Taxonomy of educational objectives: The classification of educational goals. Handbook I: Cognitive domain*. Longman.

Brookhart, S. M., & Nitko, A. J. (2019). *Educational assessment of students* (8th ed.). Pearson.

Buléon, C., Mattatia, L., Minehart, R. D., Rudolph, J. W., Lois, F. J., Guillouet, E., Philippon, A. L., Brissaud, O., Lefevre-Scelles, A., Benhamou, D., Lecomte, F., Group, T. S. A. W. S., Bellot, A., Crublé, I., Philippot, G., Vanderlinden, T., Batrancourt, S., Boithias-Guerot, C., Bréaud, J., . . . Chabot, J. M. (2022). Simulation-based summative assessment in healthcare: An overview of key principles for practice. *Advances in Simulation (London, England), 7*(1), 42. https://doi.org/10.1186/s41077-022-00238-9

Chua, C. M. S., Nantsupawat, A., Wichaikhum, O. A., & Shorey, S. (2023). Content and characteristics of evidence in the use of standardized patients for advanced practice nurses: A mixed-studies systematic review. *Nurse Education Today, 120*, 105621. https://doi.org/10.1016/j.nedt.2022.105621

Ellis, M., Hampton, D., Makowski, A., Falls, C., Tovar, E., Scott, L., & Melander, S. (2023). Using unfolding case scenarios to promote clinical reasoning for nurse practitioner students. *Journal of the American Association of Nurse Practitioners, 35*(1), 55–62. https://doi.org/10.1097/JXX.0000000000000806

Fink, A. M., & Martyn-Nemeth, P. (2023). Socratic inquiry, syllogism, schematic cases, and symbolism: Critical thinking strategies for nursing education. *Nurse Educator, 48*(3), 125–130. https://doi.org/10.1097/NNE.0000000000001324

Goh, H. S., Ng, E., Tang, M. L., Zhang, H., & Liaw, S. Y. (2022). Psychometric testing and cost of a five-station OSCE for newly graduated nurses. *Nurse Education Today, 112*, 105326. https://doi.org/10.1016/j.nedt.2022.105326

Goh, H. S., Zhang, H., Lee, C. N., Wu, X. V., & Wang, W. (2019). Value of nursing objective structured clinical examinations: A scoping review. *Nurse Educator, 44*(5), E1–E6. https://doi.org/10.1097/nne.0000000000000620

Hekel, B. E., Pullis, B. C., Edwards, A. P., & Alexander, J. (2023). Teaching social determinants of health through an unfolding case study. *Nurse Educator, 48*(3), 137–141. https://doi.org/10.1097/NNE.0000000000001333

Hensel, D., & Billings, D. M. (2020). Strategies to teach the national council of state boards of nursing clinical judgment model. *Nurse Educator, 45*(3), 128–132. https://doi.org/10.1097/NNE.0000000000000773

Innis, J., Johnston, S., & Cambly, E. (2023). Concept mapping in simulation within nursing education: A scoping review protocol. *Nursing Reports, 13*(1), 109–113. https://doi.org/10.3390/nursrep13010011

Kim, G., Issenberg, S. B., & Roh, Y. S. (2023). Factors affecting nursing students' reflective thinking during simulation debriefing. *Nurse Educator, 49*(3), E120–E125. Advance online publication. https://doi.org/10.1097/NNE.0000000000001560

Liu, W. (2023). Effect of unfolding case-based learning on clinical judgment among undergraduate nursing students. *Nurse Educator, 49*(3), 141–146. Advance online publication. https://doi.org/10.1097/NNE.0000000000001526

Merisier, S., Larue, C., & Boyer, L. (2018). How does questioning influence nursing students' clinical reasoning in problem-based learning? A scoping review. *Nurse Education Today, 65*, 108–115. https://doi.org/10.1016/j.nedt.2018.03.006

Mumba, M. N., Kaylor, S. K., Townsend, H., Barron, K., & Andrabi, M. (2022). Improving confidence in clinical assessment skills through service-learning experiences among nursing students. *Journal of Nursing Education, 61*(5), 272–275. https://doi.org/10.3928/01484834-20220303-02

Murillo-Llorente, M. T., Navarro-Martínez, O., Valle, V. I., & Pérez-Bermejo, M. (2021). Using the reflective journal to improve practical skills integrating affective and self-critical aspects in impoverished international environments. A pilot test. *International Journal of Environmental Research and Public Health, 18*(16), 8876. https://doi.org/10.3390/ijerph18168876

Nelms Edwards, C., Mintz-Binder, R., & Jones, M. M. (2019). When a clinical crisis strikes: Lessons learned from the reflective writings of nursing students. *Nursing Forum, 54*(3), 345–351. https://doi.org/10.1111/nuf.12335

Oermann, M. H. (2022). Some principles to guide assessment of competencies. *Nurse Educator, 47*(1), 1. https://doi.org/10.1097/NNE.0000000000001143

Oermann, M. H., Gaberson, K. B., & De Gagne, J. C. (2025). *Evaluation and testing in nursing education* (7th ed.). Springer Publishing Company.

Pence, P. (2023). Nursing students' perceptions of learning with NGN-style case studies. *Nurse Educator, 48*(2), 103–107. https://doi.org/10.1097/NNE.0000000000001292\

Van Rensburg, G. H., Botma, Y., & Roets, L. (2023). Educators' ability to use concept mapping as a tool to facilitate meaningful learning. *Contemporary Nurse, 59*(3), 238–248. https://doi.org/10.1080/10376178.2023.2223714

Yang, K. H., Chen, H., Liu, C. J., Zhang, F. F., & Jiang, X. L. (2022). Effects of reflective learning based on visual mind mapping in the fundamentals of nursing course: A quasi-experimental study. *Nurse Education Today, 119*, 105566. https://doi.org/10.1016/j.nedt.2022.105566

Developing and Using Tests

16

Desirée Hensel

OBJECTIVES

1. Explain how assessment validity and reliability affect test quality
2. Describe general rules for writing test items to measure desired learning outcomes
3. Apply specific rules for writing test items of various types
4. Discuss test design and administration practices that may affect the reliability of test scores

INTRODUCTION

A test is a measurement instrument designed to assess learners' knowledge and cognitive abilities. Teachers use test results to make important educational judgments and decisions that affect learners, teachers, patients, future employers, and the educational program. Like every measurement instrument, a test must produce relevant and consistent results to form the basis for sound inferences about what learners know and can do. Good planning, careful test construction, proper administration, accurate scoring, and sound interpretation of scores are essential for producing useful test results. This chapter presents a brief discussion of assessment concepts that influence the quality of test results, and then describes the process of planning, constructing, administering, scoring, and analyzing tests.

ASSESSMENT QUALITY OF TESTS

Like any measurement instrument, a test should produce relevant, accurate results. A teacher who constructs a test or decides to use an existing test needs confidence in its assessment quality. Two main considerations of the quality of a test are assessment validity and reliability.

Assessment Validity

While traditional perspectives of validity emphasized whether a test measured its intended concepts and constructs, contemporary viewpoints focus on the accuracy or appropriateness of inferences about test results and how those results are used. This understanding of assessment validity therefore focuses on the consequences of testing: Do teachers draw relevant, meaningful conclusions about learners' knowledge and abilities based on their test scores, and what are the intended and unintended consequences of those conclusions (Brookhart & Nitko, 2019; Oermann et al., 2025)? Teachers can have greater confidence in the validity of their interpretation and use of test scores when they collect evidence of four major considerations for validation: content, construct, assessment–criterion relationships, and consequences (Miller et al., 2013).

The purpose of *content validation* is to determine the extent to which test items accurately represent a particular content domain. A test contains only a sample of all possible items about a content domain that could be written, but teachers usually want to generalize from that sample to the universe of items. Thus, if a student correctly answers 89% of items on a community health nursing test, the teacher usually infers that the student would answer correctly 89% of all items related to that content domain (Oermann et al., 2025). However, it is difficult to judge if a single test truly represents all aspects of the larger domain.

Construct validation concerns the extent to which it is possible to make inferences from test results to more general abilities and characteristics. A construct is a theoretical construction that can be inferred from an observed behavior (e.g., clinical judgment). Construct validation involves two fundamental issues: construct representation and construct relevance (Miller et al., 2013). If test items do not adequately represent important elements of the construct, assessment validity is decreased. Tests that additionally measure abilities unrelated to the construct of interest, such as familiarity with cultural colloquialisms, spelling skill, or writing ability, introduce construct irrelevance variation that also decreases assessment validity. Evidence of construct representation and relevance should be collected during the test development process by clearly defining the meaning of the construct. Correlating test results with other measures of the same construct is another way to obtain construct validation (Miller et al., 2013).

Assessment–criterion relationship considerations focus on the extent to which test results (the assessment) predict performance on another assessment (the criterion measure), either in the future (predictive) or at the same time (concurrent). Nursing faculty often use scores from standardized comprehensive exams at the end of a program to predict performance on high-stakes tests such as the National Council Licensure Exam (NCLEX®) and certification exams, but they rarely have use for concurrent validity evidence for teacher-made tests (Oermann et al., 2025).

Consideration of consequences is important because testing has both intended and unintended consequences. Use of standardized testing programs can have the intended effect of identifying students who are likely to pass licensure or certification exams. The unintended effect might be to increase student anxiety (Oermann et al., 2025), and some students may retain false information after testing based on interpretations of incorrect answer options (Cox, 2019).

Multiple factors influence test validity. Some characteristics of the test itself, such as clerical errors, unclear directions, too few test items, and a noticeable pattern of correct responses, might decrease the validity of inferences made about the test scores. Student factors, such as lack of motivation to perform well, test anxiety, illness, or an emotionally upsetting experience, might also affect students' performance on tests and thereby decrease measurement validity. Finally, factors associated with the administration and scoring of tests can lower assessment reliability. Such factors include allowing insufficient time for testing, errors in scoring, variability in the amount of aid to students who ask questions during an examination, and failing to follow the protocol for administering a standardized test (Oermann et al., 2025).

Assessment Reliability

Reliability concerns the consistency, stability, or reproducibility of test scores. Measurement reliability boosts the teacher's confidence in assessment results. However, perfect consistency is not possible due to the influence of many extraneous factors. Inconsistency introduces an unknown amount of error into every assessment result. Reliability estimates therefore gauge the amount of measurement error present under varying conditions. The smaller the measurement error, the greater the assessment reliability (Miller et al., 2013). Assessment reliability is an essential condition for assessment validity. However, highly consistent results do not guarantee a high degree of validity, because the assessment might be reliably measuring the wrong construct. Assessment reliability only provides the consistency that makes valid inferences possible.

Because of different types of consistency, there are different methods of determining assessment reliability:

- Stability: consistency over time
- Equivalence: consistency among different forms of the assessment
- Internal consistency: consistency within the assessment itself
- Interrater reliability: consistency of judgments among different raters (Oermann et al., 2025)

For teacher-made tests, internal consistency methods are the most appropriate methods of estimating reliability. The split-length or split-half internal consistency method shows the degree to which very similar results are obtained from both halves of the same test. Longer tests tend to yield higher reliability estimates because they sample the content domain more fully. Consequently, split-half methods typically underestimate the true reliability of the whole test. However, this underestimation can be corrected statistically. An alternative approach is to calculate the intercorrelation among items using a Cronbach's alpha or Kuder-Richardson (KR) coefficient to look at how individual items relate to the entire test. The difference between those statistics is that the KR is used with dichotomously scored items while a Cronbach's alpha can be used with either dichotomous or polytomous scoring methods (Hensel & Cifrino, 2022).

It is important to remember that a reliability estimate is not a stable property of the test itself; it will fluctuate each time the test is used with different groups of students. Various factors affect assessment reliability, arising from three main sources:

- The test itself: test length, homogeneity, and technical quality of test items
- The test-taker: heterogeneity of student ability, number of students, test-taking skill, motivation
- Testing conditions: test security (prevention of cheating), adequacy of time (Oermann et al., 2025)

The desired degree of reliability depends on factors such as the importance of the decisions made based on test scores, the consequences of such decisions, and whether it is possible to reverse the decision later. For most teacher-made tests, a reliability coefficient of .60 to .85 is desirable (Miller et al., 2013).

TEST PLANNING

Adequate planning for test construction is essential for tests to produce reliable results that can be used to make valid judgments about how much students know about a content domain. This section of the chapter describes the steps involved in planning for test construction.

Purpose of the Test and Students to Be Tested

Decisions involved in planning a test should be based on the purpose of the test and characteristics of the students to be tested. If a test is intended to measure the degree to which students have met course learning objectives, and the test score will be used to determine a grade, the purpose is summative. A test designed to provide feedback to staff nurses about how much they learned during a continuing education program has a formative purpose. Understanding the characteristics of the learners to be tested helps a teacher determine which test item format to use, how many items to include, and how to score the test. Student factors that might influence these decisions include English language literacy, academic program level, and previous testing experience, among others (Oermann et al., 2025).

Test Length

The ideal length of a test (i.e., the number of test items or total possible points) depends on several variables, including the test's purpose, ability level of the students, available testing time, and desired reliability of test results. As noted earlier, longer tests usually produce more reliable results because they sample the content domain more fully. Most students working at their normal pace should be able to complete a test of the appropriate length within the allotted time (Brookhart & Nitko, 2019; Miller et al., 2013). The number of test items that can be completed in a fixed time period should take into account the nature of the assessment tasks. Items with complex assessment tasks, such as analyzing patient data, take more time to complete; therefore, fewer items of those types can be included on a test with a fixed administration time.

Item Formats

Item types fall within two broad categories of either selected response or constructed response. Selected response items can further be classified as conventional or technology-enhanced items (TEI) which make use of different formats to broaden ways to measure students' knowledge and skills (Bryant, 2019). Table 16.1 provides an overview of item types.

A test that contains several item formats gives students greater opportunity to demonstrate their competency than tests with only one item format (Betts et al., 2019; Brookhart & Nitko, 2019). Each item format has advantages and disadvantages. Some desired learning outcomes are better measured with certain item formats. For

TABLE 16.1. COMPARING TEST ITEM TYPES

Item Category	Key Features	Examples
Selected Response Conventional	<ul><li>Paper-pencil or computer delivery</li><li>Objective scoring methods</li><li>Limited ability to measure complex thinking</li><li>Highest risk of passing through guessing</li></ul>	<ul><li>True/false</li><li>Matching</li><li>Multiple choice</li><li>Multiple response</li></ul>
Selected Response TEI	<ul><li>Computer delivery</li><li>Objective scoring methods</li><li>Broadens ways to measure complex thinking</li><li>Use is driven by the testing platform</li></ul>	<ul><li>Drag-and-drop</li><li>Drop-down</li><li>Matrix</li><li>Hotspot/highlight</li></ul>
Constructed Response	<ul><li>Paper-pencil or computer delivery</li><li>Mostly subjective scoring (completion can be objective)</li><li>Allows for demonstration of complex thinking</li><li>Subjective scoring requires hand grading</li></ul>	<ul><li>Short answer</li><li>Fill-in-the-blank</li><li>Essay</li></ul>

TEI, technology-enhanced items.

example, an essay format would be more suitable than a multiple-choice item to measure the desired learning outcome of "discuss the comparative advantages and disadvantages of wet-to-dry and autolytic dressings for Stage III pressure injuries."

Students should have adequate practice with the item format types that a teacher will use on tests; this might be accomplished by using various item formats in classroom exercises (Hensel et al., 2024). Many prelicensure nursing programs have increased their use of TEI formats on examinations to prepare students for item types they will experience on the NCLEX. However, writing these items can be challenging, and even NCLEX® uses instructional design specialist to help format questions written by faculty content experts into TEI items (Betts et al., 2019). It is also important to understand that at this time there are no data to support requiring a certain percentage of TEI items on teacher-created examinations (Hensel et al., 2024). Thus, the desired learning outcomes, the specific competency to be assessed, students' ability level, options available in the testing platform, and faculty skills with writing complex item types should determine the teacher's choice of item formats.

Scoring Procedures

The choice of item format affects the choice of test scoring procedures. Dichotomous scoring counts an item as correct or incorrect and is best used when items have a single correct answer. When an item has a multiple-response structure, dichotomous scoring methods provide a less precise measurement of a student's abilities and are associated with lower examination scores compared to polytomous methods that award partial credit (Betts et al., 2022; Harding & Bonaduce, 2023).

There are several different approaches to awarding partial credit (Oermann et al., 2025). One approach is to award points for every correct response, a method referred to as 0/1 scoring. This method works best when students are instructed to select limited responses. Another approach is to use a +/- method and award points for correct responses while also subtracting points for incorrect selections. This method is ideal when students are instructed to "select all that apply" because it prevents students from getting the maximum score on an item by selecting all options. Still another approach is to award points based on how many correct linked responses are selected. NCLEX uses different partial scoring methods for different item types (National Council of State Boards of Nursing [NCSBN], 2021a), but not all testing platforms have the capability to use multiple methods. Therefore, faculty should select partial scoring methods that are transparent, work well with a given testing platform, and can be consistently applied (Hensel, 2022).

TEST BLUEPRINT

The best way to ensure that a teacher will be able to make valid judgments about the meaning of test scores is to construct a test blueprint before beginning to choose or write test items. A test blueprint, also called a test plan or table of specifications, guides the teacher to write items at the appropriate level to test the desired content areas. Without a test blueprint, teachers often rely on ease of construction in writing items. This often results in tests with a limited sample of assessment tasks that might omit outcomes that are more important but more difficult to assess (Miller et al., 2013).

Essential elements of a test blueprint include (a) a list of major topics or learning outcomes (or both) that the test will assess, (b) the level of complexity of assessment tasks, and (c) the emphasis that each topic or learning outcome will have, as indicated by the number or percentage of items or points (Oermann et al., 2025). Figure 16.1 is an example of a blueprint for a unit test on preoperative nursing care. The row headings along the left margin are the main topic areas to be tested; in this case, they comprise a general outline of content. A more detailed content outline, a list of relevant learning outcomes, or both can be used instead. The column headings across the top for this blueprint were selected from an updated taxonomy of cognitive objectives (Anderson & Krathwohl, 2001). The teacher who prepared this blueprint chose not to use all the cognitive levels, but other teachers might use all levels or even a different taxonomy.

The body of the blueprint is a grid formed by the intersections of topic areas and cognitive levels. The cells in the grid represent one or more test items to be developed related to that content area and cognitive level, and the numbers represent the number of points allotted to that cell. The teacher should judge the appropriate emphasis and balance of content areas and cognitive levels to determine which cells should be filled and by how many points; some cells can remain blank, as in this example (Oermann et al., 2025).

A test blueprint is a useful tool for guiding a teacher to select or write test items at the appropriate level to assess important content areas and learning outcomes. It also

	Cognitive Level				
Content	R	U	Ap	An	Total Points
I. Preoperative nursing assessment		4	6	5	15
II. Patient safety	2	3	1	2	8
III. Legal and ethical issues		2	2	2	6
IV. Planning nursing care		3	2	3	8
V. Patient and family teaching		2	4		6
VI. Documentation	2	3	4	4	13
Total points	4	17	19	16	56

Figure 16.1 Example of a test blueprint for a unit test on preoperative nursing care.
An, analyzing; Ap, applying; R, remembering; U, understanding

should be used to inform students about the nature of the test and how to prepare for it. Although they might have a general idea of what content areas will be tested, students often are unaware of the cognitive levels at which they will be assessed. Although the objectives or outcomes should inform students of the expected level of performance, students might not be able to interpret these accurately. Some teachers worry that sharing the test blueprint with students will encourage them to study only the content areas that will be tested, but this is not a harmful outcome: With knowledge of the content areas to be emphasized most heavily, students can focus their time and energy on studying those content areas and preparing for assessment tasks at the appropriate levels. Teachers should also understand that blueprints are different than detailed study guides that might include specific information about each question.

WRITING THE TEST ITEMS

When teachers are ready to begin constructing the test, they should select or write test items that correspond to each numbered cell in the test blueprint. Regardless of item format, teachers should consider the following general rules that contribute to the quality of test items:

1. *Every item should measure something important.* Items should be written to test students' competency with important content instead of testing trivial or obscure content with the intent of determining which students have read the assigned material. This important content should be reflected in the test blueprint. There

is no reason to set a fixed number of items or points on all tests, other than for ease of calculating a percentage score. It is better to have a smaller number of test items that assess knowledge of important content than to add meaningless items that serve only to increase test-taking time and that might make valid interpretation of scores more difficult (Oermann et al., 2025).

2. *Every item should have a correct answer.* "Correct" means that experts would agree on the answer (Miller et al., 2013). Citing a specific authority in the item, such as "according to the AORN Guidelines for Perioperative Practice," prevents students' arguing a response other than the expected answer. Items that ask students to state an opinion on an issue and support that position with evidence should not be scored as correct or incorrect, but with variable credit based on the rationale given and soundness of reasoning.

3. *Use simple, clear, concise, grammatically correct language.* Clear wording of test items is essential for students' understanding of the assessment task required. The goal is to include enough detail to communicate the intent of the test item but to avoid extraneous words and complex syntax that only increase reading time and that might confuse nonnative English speakers. Linguistic simplification in tests has been shown to benefit even native English speakers by decreasing reading time (Moore & Clark, 2016).

4. *Avoid jargon, slang, and unnecessary abbreviations.* Although healthcare professionals frequently use jargon and acronyms informally in the practice environment, informal language in a test item might fail to communicate accurately the meaning of the item. Many students are at least somewhat anxious when taking tests, and they might not interpret an abbreviation correctly in terms of the context in which it is used. For example, in a healthcare setting, SOB can mean short of breath or side of bed. As noted, slang, jargon, acronyms, and abbreviations contribute to linguistic complexity for nonnative English speakers. Also, given growing concern about healthcare errors attributed to poor communication, nurse educators should use only those abbreviations approved for use in clinical settings.

5. *Use positive wording.* Avoid using words like *no*, *not*, and *except* in test items. Negative wording is particularly difficult for nonnative English speakers to understand, but test-anxious students also might not read such sentences accurately. Negative forms are particularly confusing in true–false items. Teachers should avoid asking students to identify the incorrect alternative as the correct response to the item, as in this example of a multiple-choice stem: "Which of the following is NOT an indication for high-level disinfection of surgical instruments and equipment?" This wording tends to reinforce the incorrect alternative, and it might cause confusion when students try later to recall the correct information.

6. *Items should not contain irrelevant cues to correct answers.* Flaws in item construction can allow test-wise students to improve their chances of guessing the correct answer when they do not know it, interfering with valid interpretations of their scores (National Board of Medical Examiners [NBME], 2021). Irrelevant cues include:

    - A multiple-choice stem that is grammatically inconsistent with one or more alternatives.

- Repeating important words from the stem in only the correct answer.
- Using qualifiers such as "never" and "always" in incorrect alternatives and "usually" or "often" in correct options.
- Having a consistent pattern of correct answers being longer than incorrect alternatives or true statements being longer than false statements.
- Using the same response position consistently for correct answers.

7. *No item should depend on another item for meaning.* Items should not be linked such that students who answer one item incorrectly will likely answer the related item incorrectly. An example of such linking is:

   1. Which drug should be available in case of malignant hyperthermia? _____
   2. What solvent should be used to mix the drug in Item 1? _____

   However, a series of items that relate to a particular context such as a diagram, case study, or graphic are called interpretive or context-dependent items. This is not a violation of the rule because the items relate to a common context, not to each other (Oermann et al., 2025), nor is it a violation in a rationale question designed to test understanding of relationships (Petersen et al., 2020).

8. *Eliminate unnecessary information.* Including fictitious patient names or initials in test items increases reading time unnecessarily, might be a distraction from the item's intent, and might introduce cultural bias. If the purpose of an item is to assess whether students can evaluate the relevance of clinical data and use only relevant information to arrive at the correct answer, extraneous data other than patient names can be included (Oermann et al., 2025).

9. *Request peer critique of the test item.* Colleagues who teach the same content or who are skilled in the technical aspects of item writing are the best critics of newly written test items.

10. *Prepare more test items than the test blueprint calls for.* This will permit replacement of items discarded in the critique process. Unused extra test items can be kept in a test item bank for future use.

ITEM-WRITING PRINCIPLES FOR SPECIFIC ITEM FORMATS

In addition to the general item-writing rules previously described, there are specific principles for writing test items of each item format. The following discussion offers helpful suggestions for writing effective test items of various types. For a more in-depth discussion and specific guidelines for developing items of each type, see Oermann et al. (2025).

True–False

A true–false item comprises a statement that the student must judge as true or false. True–false items are most effective for testing recall of specific information or for understanding a principle or concept. These work well as quizzes to determine if readings have been done, but they are not useful for testing complex thinking and

> **EXHIBIT 16.1 Examples of True–False Items**
>
> T F According to the AORN Guideline for Surgical Attire, the scrub top should be donned before the cap. (F)
>
> T F The circulating nurse should check the position of the patient's feet before surgical drapes are applied. (T)
>
> T F The ordered preoperative antibiotic dose should be repeated if the procedure lasts 2 hours or more. (T)

Note: Correct answers are in parentheses.

reasoning. Because these items require relatively little time to read, students can respond to several of them in a short period of time, allowing the teacher to sample a broad content area. The main disadvantage of true–false items is the 50% probability of guessing the correct answer. Examples of true–false items are in Exhibit 16.1. Important principles to follow when constructing these items are:

- Avoid testing the recall of trivial information.
- Each statement should be unconditionally true or false without qualification.
- Each item should include only one idea to be tested; multiple ideas often result in part of the statement being true and part being false.
- Attempt to make all true–false items similar in length.
- Use approximately the same number of true statements and false statements, or include slightly more false than true items, because false statements tend to have higher discrimination power (Brookhart & Nitko, 2019).
- Avoid ordering true–false items in a noticeable pattern, such as TTFF or TFTF.

Matching Exercises

Matching exercises comprise a series of homogeneous items (premises) with the same set of responses. They are most appropriate for assessing students' ability to classify and categorize information such as definitions of terms, generic and trade names of medications, or pharmacologic classifications (Miller et al., 2013). A sample matching exercise is in Exhibit 16.2. Important principles to follow when constructing matching exercises are:

- Keep the lists of premises and responses short. Miller et al. (2013) recommended four to seven items in each column.
- Directions for each matching exercise should state the basis on which premises and responses should be matched, and whether each response can be used once, more than once, or not at all.

Multiple-Choice and Multiple-Response

Multiple-choice (MC) and multiple-response (MR) items can be used to assess many types of desired learning outcomes at various levels of the cognitive taxonomy,

> **EXHIBIT 16.2 Sample Matching Exercise**
>
> Directions: For each description of a pressure injury in Column A, select the appropriate stage from Column B. Responses in Column B can be used once, more than once, or not at all.
>
> | Column A | Column B |
> |---|---|
> | 1. Base of the lesion is covered by slough or eschar or both (e) | a. Stage I |
> | 2. Exposed bone or tendons are visible or directly palpable (d) | b. Stage II |
> | | c. Stage III |
> | 3. Shiny or dry shallow lesion without sloughing or bruising (b) | d. Stage IV |
> | | e. Unstageable |
> | 4. Visible subcutaneous fat without exposure of bone or muscle (c) | |

especially application and analysis. Well-written MC and MR items include new information in the stem and require students to apply concepts and principles or use analytical thinking to respond to the item.

Each MC or MR item comprises three parts: stem, correct answer, and distractors. The stem is a question or incomplete sentence that must be answered or completed by one or more of the alternatives. The alternatives or options include the correct answer and several distractors (incorrect options). The correct or best answer is also called the keyed response because it is the alternative marked on the answer key often indicated with an asterisk. Distractors should appear plausible to students who are unsure of the correct answer. Examples of multiple-choice and multiple-response items are in Exhibit 16.3.

Whether the stem is a question or incomplete statement, it must clearly communicate the intent of the item. The stem should present a problem or issue that relates to an important learning outcome. The stem may include a clinical scenario or medical record to add context for testing interpretations of data or decision-making

> **EXHIBIT 16.3 Examples of Multiple-Choice and Multiple-Response Items**
>
> 1. According to the Surgical Care Improvement Project, prophylactic antibiotics other than vancomycin should be administered:
>   a. For at least 24 hours preoperatively
>   b. For at least 72 hours postoperatively
>   c. Up to 2 hours before incision
>   d. Within 1 hour of incision*
> 2. Which adverse medication reactions are common in older surgical patients? Select all that apply.
>   a. Confusion*
>   b. Dry mouth*
>   c. Headache
>   d. Nausea and vomiting*
>   e. Respiratory depression

(Betts et al., 2019; NBME, 2021). The student should be able to read the stem and know what type of response the teacher expects (Brookhart & Nitko, 2019). Guidelines for writing the stem include:

- Clearly present sufficient information for the problem to be solved. As a test of clarity and completeness, the item writer should cover the alternatives and judge whether the stem alone specifies what to look for in the alternatives.
- Avoid including extraneous information unless the purpose of the item is to assess students' ability to differentiate relevant from irrelevant data. Humorous content should be avoided because it can be confusing to nonnative English speakers.
- Do not use the stem to teach. The goal of testing is to assess learning, not to teach or reinforce information.
- Eliminate key words from the stem that would provide a clue to the correct answer, such as a word in the stem that can relate to the same concept as a word used in the answer; for example, *aging* and *elderly*.
- Avoid negative wording; ask for the correct or best answer rather than the only incorrect response, as previously discussed. If there is no acceptable alternative wording, consider revising the stem to a true–false, completion, or multiple-response format.
- Avoid ending a stem in the form of an incomplete sentence with "a" or "an" because these words provide clues as to whether the correct answer begins with a consonant or a vowel. Ending the stem with "a/an" is not a good remedy because students then must read each alternative with "a" and then again with "an."
- If the stem is an incomplete sentence, the alternatives should complete the statement at the end of the sentence. A blank in the middle of the sentence, which the correct answer is supposed to fill, acts as a barrier to reading comprehension (Brookhart & Nitko, 2019; Oermann et al., 2025).

Alternatives are listed under the stem and can vary in number. The more options, the more discriminating the item, if all options are plausible. Most standardized tests use four alternatives for MC tests, and NCLEX® will use up to 10 for MR items (Petersen et al., 2020). However, it is not necessary for teacher-made tests to have the same number of alternatives for every item. If the teacher can construct only two plausible distractors for one correct answer, a three-option item is certainly acceptable (Raymond et al., 2019). Good alternatives should be free of technical flaws that add unnecessary difficulty and cues that benefit savvy test takers (NBME, 2021). Guidelines for writing alternatives include:

- Make all alternatives similar in length, detail, and complexity. Test-wise students look to find longer options knowing that the teacher may include more details on correct options which typically are written first.
- Each alternative should contain the same number of parts. If the correct answer contains two parts so should the distractors.
- Alternatives should be grammatically consistent with each other and with the stem (if it is an incomplete sentence).

- All alternatives should sample the same content domain, such as nursing interventions, diagnostic test results, or assessment findings.
- Avoid including opposite responses in the alternatives because this is often a clue that the correct answer is one of the opposites.
- If words are repeated in each alternative, move them to the stem to decrease reading time.
- If the stem is a complete sentence or question, end it with the appropriate terminal punctuation and begin each alternative with a capital letter. If the alternatives complete an incomplete sentence in the stem, end the stem with a comma or colon as appropriate, begin each alternative with a lower-case letter, and use terminal punctuation at the end.
- Alternatives with ranges of numerical values should not overlap with each other.
- Place each alternative on a separate line and all lines in one column under the stem.
- Avoid using *none of the above* and *all of the above* as alternatives. If a student knows that at least one of the other options is true, *none of the above* can be eliminated
- If students are required to choose the best rather than the correct answer, the best answer should be supported by evidence (Oermann et al., 2025).

MR items allow students to select one or more options as the correct or best answers. Instructions might indicate to select all that apply, to select a certain number of items (referred to as select N for which N means number), or in TEI variations to select options from a group (Betts et al., 2022). The preferred response method for MR items is to have students indicate every correct alternative directly on the examination or score sheet. Teachers should avoid using complex multiple-choice or combined-response forms where students select from assembled answer combinations, such as a & b and b, d, e, because these items tend to provide more cueing (Butler, 2018).

Matrix

Matrix items are a TEI format that requires students to categorize answer options by selecting the appropriate cells in a table (Oermann et al., 2025). A multiple-choice matrix allows selection of a single correct response per row. Those items might ask if a treatment is indicated or not indicated; if a finding shows a client is improving, staying the same, or declining; or if teaching is understood or not understood. A multiple response matrix uses overlapping categories of findings or interventions allowing the student to select more than one option per row. Exhibit 16.4 provides examples of matrix items.

Considerations for writing matrix questions include:

- Avoid using matrix questions for grading unless answers can be directly entered on the table. Work-arounds that place numbers in cells and require students to look in multiple places to answer questions increase risk of transposition errors and disadvantage students with learning differences (Hensel, 2022).

EXHIBIT 16.4 Examples of Matrix Items

1. The nurse teaches a client about prescribed ciprofloxacin to treat their pneumonia. Click to specify if each client statement indicates understanding or no understanding of the medication teaching. Each row must have one selection.

Client statement	Understanding	No understanding
"I can take ciprofloxacin with milk if it upsets my stomach."	○	○ *
"I should immediately stop taking my ciprofloxacin if I develop pain or swelling around my joints."	○ *	○
"I need to make sure I drink at least 2 liters of water a day while taking ciprofloxacin."	○ *	○
"I will need to return to have my ciprofloxacin level drawn."	○	○ *

2. The nurse assesses a 6-year-old female in the emergency department with a history of sickle cell disease. For each finding, click to indicate if the finding is consistent with vaso-occlusive crisis, acute chest syndrome, or splenic sequestration. Each finding may support more than one condition. Each column must have at least one response option selected.

Findings	Vaso-occlusive crisis	Acute chest syndrome	Splenic sequestration
Pain only in lower legs	☐ *	☐	☐
Crackles in lung bases	☐	☐ *	☐
Respiratory rate 32 bpm	☐ *	☐ *	☐ *
Pulse oximeter 90% on room air	☐ *	☐ *	☐ *
Soft abdomen	☐ *	☐ *	☐
Blood pressure 108/70	☐ *	☐ *	☐

- Review the platform's rules for how many cells can be used to create the matrix. The platform may have rules for maximum rows and or columns.
- Clearly specify in the instructions if students are to select one or more items per row. Additional instructions should be included if there must be at least one item selected in a category.
- Determine point values for the matrix, how the item will be graded, if items will be scored by columns or rows, and if a guessing penalty will apply. One method is to consider awarding one point per correct option selected.

> **EXHIBIT 16.5 Example of a Drop-Down Item**
>
> In a client with cirrhosis and ascites who develops confusion, the nurse anticipates administering
>
> [select] to [select]
>
> *After clicking* select *the following options appear.*
>
> | lactulose * | to | decrease ammonia* |
> | phenobarbital | | improve cognition |
> | risperidone | | prevent seizures |

Drop-Down

A drop-down item is a TEI short answer format that appears as a drop-down menu used to complete missing information in a sentence, paragraph, or table (Oermann et al., 2025). The word *select* typically appears for the missing information. After clicking on *select*, the answer options appear. Some test items may have a single drop-down while others may use several related drop-down menus to measure students' understanding of relationships. For instance, a rationale version of a drop-down item, as shown in the example in Exhibit 16.5, requires the student to identify the correct medication and then justify the reason for giving that medication.

Considerations for writing drop-down items include:

- For items with multiple drop-downs, use the same number of answer options in all drop-down menus. This is typically 3 to 5 options (Petersen et al., 2020).
- Keep all answer options within a drop-down short and similar in format.
- Pay particular attention that there are no grammatical clues such as "a" or "an" that cue the test taker.
- Determine the scoring procedures for items with multiple drop-down menus.

Drag-and-Drop

The TEI drag-and-drop format involves moving a "token" (answer option) to a "target" (blank). The drag-and-drop format is flexible and can be used to measure a wide variety of cognitive levels and thinking skills (Oermann et al., 2025). Ordered response variations require students to arrange options in a specific order such as high to low priority. Other drag-and-drop item variations resemble multiple response items by requiring that the student move all correct options from a list on the left to an answer space or categories on the right. Still other drag-and-drop variations use

> **EXHIBIT 16.6 Example of a Drag-and-Drop Item**

1. Drag the most appropriate options from the choices below to complete the sentence.

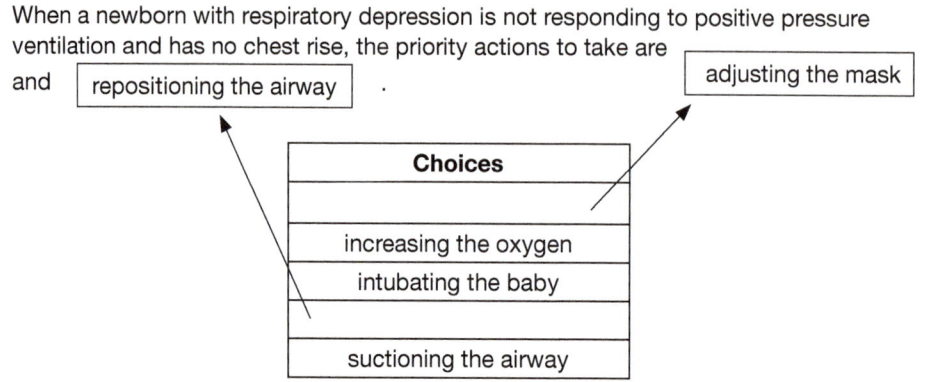

Note: Once selected, the token (answer option) moves to fill in the empty target.

tokens as short answers to complete sentences, paragraphs, tables, or diagrams (see Exhibit 16.6). Considerations for writing drag-and-drop items include:

- Drag-and-drop items require use of fine motor skills to manipulate a computer mouse.
- How drag-and-drop items display varies widely per testing platform.
- Not all testing platforms can autograde drag-and-drop items if the order that items are arranged matters.

Highlight

Highlight items, also called hotspots, require students to select parts of a text, table, or graphic to answer a question. Items might ask students to identify areas on a graphic, such as indicating where to assess the fetal heart rate on a diagram of a maternal abdomen. Other formats require students to select words, phrases, or lines directly from a medical record to answer the question. Such items are considered more authentic assessments of nursing practice than selecting answers from lists of options. The item might ask what findings need immediate follow-up, what orders to implement first, or what findings indicate the treatment plan is working. While highlight items can be hand graded on paper-pencil test, they are most often used in the TEI format. Instructions may include the phrase "click to highlight." Tokenizing words, phrases, lines, or areas in advance makes them selectable to highlight (Petersen et al., 2020). Hovering over the text with a mouse will show what is selectable. Clicking the tokenized area applies the highlight to the phrase. Like a multiple response item, highlight items contain correct and incorrect tokenized options (Petersen et al., 2020).

Exhibit 16.7 displays an example of a highlight item. A good deal of preplanning and knowledge of the testing platform's capabilities are required to write a good

EXHIBIT 16.7 Example of a Highlight or Hotspot Item

1. The nurse reviews the laboratory findings of a client with end stage renal disease. Click to highlight the findings that suggest the client is developing peritonitis.

Laboratory Report

Lab results		Reference range
BUN	50 mg/dL	10–20 mg/dL
Creatinine (Serum)	9.7 mg/dL	0.9–1.4 mg/dL
C-Reactive Protein	60.5 mg/L.	<1.0 mg/dL
Potassium (Serum)	5.96 mEq/L	3.5–5 mEq/L
Phosphorus	6.1 mg/dL	2.8–4.5 mg/dL
White Blood Cells (Serum)	13.44 × 10^3 cells/mm^3	4.5–10.5 × 10^3 cells/mm^3
Neutrophils (Serum)	85.8%	55%–70%

Hovering over text shows what is selectable. Clicking applies the highlight.

Laboratory Report

Lab Results		Reference range
BUN	50 mg/dL	10–20 mg/dL
Creatinine (Serum)	9.7 mg/dL	0.9–1.4 mg/dL
C-Reactive Protein	60.5 mg/L.	<1.0 mg/dL
Potassium (Serum)	5.96 mEq/L	3.5–5 mEq/L
Phosphorus	6.1 mg/dL	2.8–4.5 mg/dL
White Blood Cells (Serum)	13.44 × 10^3 cells/mm^3	4.5–10.5 × 10^3 cells/mm^3
Neutrophils (Serum)	85.8%	55%–70%

---

highlight question. In developing these items, the teacher should consider these principles:

- All information the test taker needs to select must be in one area. If an interactive medical record is used the item should only address one page of the record.
- Some testing platforms may have difficulty capturing tokenized phrases that are not on one line because the token will need to have a zig-zag shape. Highlighting is made easier if there is one order or lab value per line.
- Students with certain visual impairments may have difficulty with some colors in highlight items.

> **EXHIBIT 16.8 Examples of Short-Answer Items**
>
> 1. A patient weighs 220 lbs. You need to prepare an initial dose of 2.5 mg/kg of dantrolene sodium. What is the correct dose in milligrams? _____ Show your work:
> _____
>
> 2. According to Spaulding classification, what level of items should receive a minimum of high-level disinfection? _____

Short-Answer

Short-answer items require a word, phrase, or number as an answer. These occur in two formats: question and completion (also known as fill-in-the-blank). These items are best used to assess the recall of specific information and ability to perform calculations. Short-answer items might ask students to label a diagram, identify specific items, or provide correct abbreviations for medical terms. Completion items, also called cloze items, consist of a statement with a key word or phrase missing; the student must supply the missing material. Examples of short-answer items are in Exhibit 16.8.

Guidelines for writing these items include:

- Do not use verbatim material from textbooks and other readings; doing so can result in assessing only recall of information without comprehension.
- Construct the item so that only one unique word, phrase, or number will correctly complete the item.
- Write items that are specific enough that they can be answered briefly. Think of the correct answer first and then write a question or statement to elicit that response. If more than one response could be correct, list all possible correct answers on the answer key.
- Items requiring mathematical calculations should specify the nature of the desired response and degree of specificity including what decimal place to round to.
- For fill-in-the-blank items, place the blank at or near the end of the statement to make it easier for students to discern the intent of the item after reading it only once. Avoid giving grammatical clues such as "a" or "an" and singular or plural forms just before the blank. If more than one blank is used, blanks should be equal in length to avoid giving a clue to desired length of response.
- Direct students where to record their answers.

Essay

Essay items are useful for assessing complex learning outcomes. Essay items are appropriate for assessing students' abilities to analyze (patient data, clinical situations, ethical issues); critique (scientific evidence, approaches to solving a problem, arguments for and against a position or decision); and develop (teaching plans, protocols). Examples of essay items are in Exhibit 16.9. Although responses to essay items require students to compose and write responses, the quality of their writing should not influence the evaluation of their responses which should reflect nursing knowledge or practice.

> **EXHIBIT 16.9 Examples of Essay Items**
>
> 1. Give three examples of circumstances in which perioperative personnel should wear personal protective equipment when handling used instruments and equipment. (3 points)
> 2. Critique arguments for and against the practice of suspending Do Not Resuscitate status when patients undergo surgery. Based on your critique, state which position you believe is the strongest and provide a rationale supporting your choice. (7 points)

Essay items can assess depth of knowledge, but not breadth of a content domain. Teachers usually can include only a few of them on a test because of the time needed to organize and write responses. Some teachers allow students to choose a subset of essay items to respond to. For example, from a set of six essay items, students are allowed to choose which four they want to answer. Miller et al. (2013) advised against this practice because, when students choose which items to answer, they actually are taking different tests, which affects measurement validity.

In writing essay items, the teacher should: (a) develop items that require analysis, integration, and synthesis rather than summary of the content; (b) use clear wording to direct students to the intended response; (c) prepare students for an essay test by asking questions in class, clinical practice, and online that require clinical reasoning, synthesis of content from various sources, critique of opposing views, and comparison of approaches; (d) indicate the point value of each essay item and/or an approximate amount of time students should allot to answering it; and (e) write an ideal answer to each essay item while drafting it to determine whether it is clearly stated and could be answered in a reasonable time frame. The teacher can save this ideal response to use when constructing a scoring rubric.

Essay items can be scored by two methods, holistic and analytic. *Holistic scoring* involves reading the entire response and judging its overall quality. This can be done by comparing each student's response with those of other students and ranking them by degrees of quality. Answers are read to assess the overall quality of response (sometimes by comparing them to a model answer), and then sorted into piles representing different degrees of quality; each pile then receives a particular score. For *analytic scoring*, the teacher identifies the content that should be included in the answer and assigns possible points for each content area. A scoring rubric can be developed that describes how points should be assigned for various degrees of completeness, logic, organization, and accuracy. Use of an analytic rubric also provides feedback to students about the quality of their essay responses (Oermann et al., 2025).

There is a great deal of subjectivity in grading essay questions and responses can be scored differently by different teachers or by the same teacher at different times. Essay items that are highly structured and focused tend to produce greater reliability in scoring. To limit bias one can:

- Evaluate all student responses to one essay item before reading responses to the next one. This limits the carryover effect in which the teacher develops an impression about the student's knowledge and ability from one answer and tends to expect the same quality of response for the next essay item.
- Mask the identity of the students until all responses are scored. This limits the influence by general impressions of or by feelings about students when evaluating essay responses.

- Focus on the substance of essay responses. This helps decrease judgments based on the students' writing abilities.
- Read essay responses in random order, rearrange the order before scoring another item, and read each response twice before computing a score. This prevents "rater drift" that leads to lower scoring caused by teacher fatigue and time constraints.

Context-Dependent Item Sets

A context-dependent item set (also known as an interpretive exercise) is a group of test items that relate to the same introductory material. The introductory material might be a description of a clinical situation, a set of patient assessment findings or laboratory test results; a diagram; a graph; a table; a photograph; or excerpts from healthcare records, textbooks, or research reports. Students read, interpret, and analyze the introductory material and then respond to each test item related to it. The test items in the interpretive exercise can be in any item format, but all items in the same set should be the same format.

Context-dependent item sets are most appropriate for assessing higher level learning outcomes such as application of knowledge to novel situations, solving problems, making decisions, synthesizing information, and creating or developing new approaches. Interpretive items are also included in licensure, certification, and other standardized tests, so students should have some experience with this type of test item during their academic program. A sample context-dependent item set is provided in Exhibit 16.10.

Suggestions for developing these item sets are:

- The introductory material or context should provide enough information for analysis without limiting or directing students' thinking or creativity. One approach is to draft the test items first and then construct introductory material that includes the essential information needed to respond to the items.
- The introductory material can include irrelevant as well as relevant information if the intent of the exercise is to assess the student's ability to select relevant data on which to base judgments. All information included, however, should appear logical and pertinent to the situation.
- All items in the set should relate directly to the introductory material; students should not be able to arrive at a correct or best answer without reading and analyzing the context.
- The length of the context should correspond to the number of items that relate to it. It is a waste of students' time to read a lengthy scenario before responding to only two test items related to it.
- Arrange the context-dependent item set so that it is clear to the students which items relate to the introductory material. Use a heading to indicate the item numbers in the set (e.g., "Items 34 to 38 relate to the following patient assessment findings") and consider centering the introductory material horizontally on the page so that it is more visible (Oermann et al., 2025).

> **EXHIBIT 16.10 Sample Context-Dependent Item Set**
>
> Items 1 to 4 relate to the following situation:
>
> An 82-year-old woman is scheduled for an open reduction and internal fixation of her right femur. She rates her pain at 4 on a 1 to 10 scale and has not received any preoperative sedation. Three days ago, on admission, an indwelling urinary catheter was inserted, and it is now draining clear, light yellow urine. While transferring the patient to the OR bed, the perioperative RN notices a reddened area on her sacrum, approximately the size and shape of a silver dollar; the skin is intact with no blistering apparent and it feels warm to touch. The patient is positioned supine on the fracture OR bed with the left leg supported in a padded stirrup. Her right arm is positioned over her chest in a sling and the left arm is on a padded arm board.
>
> T F 1. According to the National Pressure Ulcer Advisory Panel's definitions of pressure injuries, the perioperative RN should document the lesion on the patient's sacrum as Stage I. (T)
>
> T F 2. This patient is at an increased risk for inability to give informed consent for the surgical procedure. (F)
>
> T F 3. The patient's position on the OR bed increases her risk of compression and stretch injury to the left sciatic nerve. (T)
>
> T F 4. According to the National Guideline Clearinghouse's guideline for prevention of catheter-associated urinary tract infections, this patient has an increased risk of such an infection. (T)

NEXT GENERATION NCLEX®

Faculty in prelicensure programs frequently strive to write test items in a format that students will experience on the licensure examination; this is referred to as writing "NCLEX-style" items. The National Council Licensure Examination or NCLEX® is a computer-adaptive examination that includes stand-alone items and case studies to measure knowledge of client needs and clinical judgment skills (Betts et al., 2022). The revised version of the examination, known as Next Generation NCLEX® (NGN), includes item formats used on previous versions of the examination and new TEI response types with multiple variations (Betts et al., 2022). Except for calculation questions, all items use a selected response format. The new item response types are:

- Extended multiple response: Select all that apply, Select N, Multiple response grouping
- Matrix/Grid: Multiple response, Multiple choice
- Drag-and-drop: Cloze, Rationale
- Drop-down: Cloze, Rationale, In table
- Highlight: In text, In table
- Bow-tie
- Trend

Case studies and stand-alone bow-tie and trend items are used to evaluate clinical judgment (Betts et al., 2022). These questions are designed to test contextual decision-making based on the six steps of the NCSBN Clinical Judgment Measurement Model (NCJMM). In order those six steps are:

- Recognize cues
- Analyze cues
- Prioritize hypotheses
- Generate solutions
- Take action
- Evaluate outcomes

Brief explanations of how to write clinical judgment items follow. Greater details on writing case studies, and specific-item variations can be found in *Evaluation and Testing in Nursing Education* (Oermann et al., 2025) and in the *Next Generation NCLEX News* publications series on the NCSBN website (https://www.ncsbn.org).

Case Studies

Case studies are six-question context sets that test in order the six sequential steps of the NCJMM (Betts et al., 2022). Cueing clearly indicates that items belong to a six-item case study and specifies the sequential number of the question. Case studies are based on a clinical scenario displayed as an interactive medical record (NCSBN, 2020). They begin with an overview sentence that briefly explains the context of the scenario typically including the client age, gender, and care setting. The overview sentence is followed by an interactive medical record with one or more pages referred to as *tabs*. Tabs might include nurses' notes, history and physical, admission notes, vital signs, intake and output, orders, medication administration, flowsheets, progress notes, laboratory reports, or diagnostic reports (NCSBN, 2021).

Unlike traditional context-related sets, case studies may unfold with updated data being added to the medical record at any point. Like a real medical record once data have been added, the record remains available throughout the rest of the scenario. Building a medical record that conveys essential information without becoming overly complicated can be one of the most challenging aspects for faculty of building a case study (Hensel & Billings, 2023). Teachers need to understand the limitations of their testing platforms as they build medical records to ensure students can access information throughout the case without navigating backward.

The question follows the medical record. On the NCLEX the medical record is displayed on the left side of the computer screen and the question on the right. An additional sentence may appear before the question stem to cue the test taker if more data have been added to the medical record, to clarify what the nurse has done or is doing, or to illuminate an aspect of the client's status. Case studies include a variety of item response formats (Betts et al., 2022). Once an item is answered, backward navigation is not permitted. The process of listing the item number, overview sentence, medical record, and question is repeated for each clinical judgment step until the case ends with a question pertaining to the evaluation of outcomes. Developing a case study is very time consuming and requires a great deal of faculty skill (Oermann et al., 2025). When deciding to include case studies on a test, faculty should consider that as yet there is no evidence to support whether graded case studies are better than nongraded cases for preparing students for NCLEX (Hensel et al., 2024)

Stand-Alone Clinical Judgment Items

The term *stand-alone item* means that a question is complete by itself and does not need to appear in a specific order within an examination. Stand-alone clinical judgment items may be one of two types: bow-tie or trend (NCSBN, 2021b). Bow-tie and trend items are designed to evaluate multiple components of the NCJMM in a single question for a single client with a known or implied diagnosis. Stand-alone items will still display information in the form of a medical record; however, they will not unfold like a case study.

A bow-tie is a drag-and-drop item that essentially tests all NCJMM steps in a single question (NCSBN, 2021b). The test taker needs to read the medical record, identify key information, analyze the situation, and then place answer options into five spaces arranged in a configuration similar to a bow-tie. The test taker selects the condition the client is most likely experiencing from a list of four answer options and places it in the middle of the diagram. Based on the selected condition, the test taker places two actions to take, chosen from a list of five options, on the left side of the diagram. Finally, they complete the right side of the diagram with two parameters to monitor the client's progress, selected from a list of five options. Teachers desiring to use bow-tie items on examinations must understand their testing platform's capabilities as this item type is not widely available in all testing platforms.

Trend items require the test taker to review a series of time stamped data displayed in a medical record and make one or more clinical decisions. These items can test one or more clinical judgment steps and can use any response format other than bow-tie (NCSBN, 2021b). The trend data can reflect improved, declined, or unchanging client status. Using a narrative with different time points, multiple vital signs over the course of a day, or serial laboratory values are all ways to show trend data. Compared to bow-ties and case studies, trend items tend to be easier to write. This is especially true since many faculty already include questions about client changes on examinations. While the NCSBN does not specify the number of time points needed to make a trend item, faculty might consider that using at least three time points all with similar types of data is more likely to show a "trend" versus two time points that show just a "change."

ASSEMBLING THE TEST

The final appearance of a test and the way in which it is administered can affect measurement validity. Confusing directions, haphazard arrangement of components, and clerical errors all contribute to measurement error. Teachers can avoid such errors by following certain test design rules.

Arrange Items in a Logical Sequence

There are various methods for arranging items on the test: by order of expected difficulty, according to the sequence in which the content was learned, and a combination of the two. Using all item formats on a single test is not necessary nor recommended, but the longer the test, the greater variety of item formats can be included.

Within each item format, items can be arranged according to the order in which the content was presented in the course, which can help students recall essential information more easily. Finally, in the combination of item format and content sequencing, items can be arranged in order of expected difficulty, with easiest items first. Beginning each section with easier items can help anxious students relax so that they can demonstrate their best performance (Miller et al., 2013; Oermann et al., 2025). If case studies are used, they may be placed anywhere within the examination, but it is important that all questions related to a case are grouped together and appear sequentially.

Write Directions

The teacher should write a set of clear general directions for the test, including how and where to record responses, the amount of time permitted, and whether students may ask questions during the test (if given in person). Directions also may include signing a reaffirmation of a program's honor code because such codes have been shown to reduce cheating (Holden et al., 2021). A statement might express: "I confirm that I will not give nor receive any unauthorized help on this exam."

Avoid Crowding

Teachers should allow enough space between and around test elements so that each test item is distinct from the others. Tightly packing words on a page might minimize the amount of paper used, but it can also interfere with students' maximum performance by contributing to reading time and clerical errors.

Keep Related Material Together

In addition to grouping items of the same format together, the teacher should ensure that all parts of a test item appear on the same page, such as the stem and alternatives of a multiple-choice item and the directions and both columns of a matching exercise. As previously mentioned, the introductory material and all related context-dependent items should appear on the same page, if possible (Miller et al., 2013). Questions in case studies should appear sequentially.

Number Items Continuously

Although test items should be grouped according to format, the teacher should number them continuously from the beginning to the end of the test instead of starting each item format section with item number 1. This technique helps to prevent clerical errors when students record their answers on a separate answer sheet and helps students to recognize items they have skipped.

Proofread

To ensure optimum measurement reliability and validity, the test should be free of spelling, grammatical, and typing errors. The test designer often does not recognize their own errors, so a colleague who is familiar with the content should be asked to proofread a copy of the test before it is duplicated. Spell-check and grammar-check features of computer software are insufficient because they do not always recognize words that are spelled correctly but used in the wrong context, or structural errors such as giving two test items the same number.

Prepare an Answer Key

For both hand and electronic scoring, the teacher should prepare an accurate scoring key to provide a final check on the accuracy of the test items. This answer key should also be proofread by someone who did not prepare it, verifying that it is accurate. The teacher should also prepare ideal responses to short-answer items and prepare scoring rubrics for essay items.

ONLINE TESTING

The practice of administering online tests is now common in nursing programs that are offered through distance modalities or want students to gain practice testing in formats like their future licensure or certification examination. While students tend to prefer online testing, faculty are concerned with examination security, risk of cheating, and technical issues (Butler-Henderson & Crawford, 2020; Holden et al., 2021). There are several factors to consider when administering online examinations including the IT infrastructure that is in place, measures available to promote academic integrity, and design practices to help ensure the exam is fair and valid.

An adequate IT infrastructure is required to do secure online testing. Systems must be in place to deal with technological challenges that arise such as computer malfunctions, internet service interruptions, and testing platform issues. Some programs administer their online examinations in testing centers with live proctors on institutionally owned and supported computers; however, this method has scheduling considerations and may not be practical for distance accessible programs whose students live far from campus (Holden et al., 2021). Another consideration is whether to use a testing platform built into a program's learning management system (LMS) or to use a stand-alone testing platform, which involves additional licensing fees. Some platforms require an internet connection during examination administration, while others do not. If an internet connection is required and students will be testing in a group setting, the environment must have adequate bandwidth to transmit the volume of data.

Methods to decrease cheating can be technology based or assessment design and structure based. Assessment design methods include requiring a password, keeping the testing timeframe short, and displaying one question at a time. Two technology-based approaches teachers may employ to discourage cheating are lockdown browsers and remote proctoring systems (Butler-Henderson & Crawford, 2020; Holden et al., 2021). Lockdown browsers restrict students from opening other browser tabs during an examination but must be installed in advance. Remote proctoring technology involves the use of webcams and/or video surveillance to authenticate a student's identity and monitor their behavior during an examination. While created to be used when students are in remote locations, these programs can also be used as another layer of security when students test in large groups. Costs, concerns with data security, and student privacy are some barriers to using cheating detection programs (Holden et al., 2021).

Examination policies and procedures should be in place to guide when students will have access to their scores and what type of examination reviews will take place. Allowing students to immediately see their grades after submitting an online can be problematic. Those scores would not reflect any adjustments deemed appropriate following a test analysis. While some faculty may be hesitant to conduct post-test reviews of online tests with remote learners, exam reviews are an important part of the learning process. With consistent rules and careful planning faculty can lead reviews that preserve exam integrity even during a virtual review session of the test (Cobourne & Robb, 2022).

PREPARING STUDENTS TO TAKE TESTS

Teachers should create conditions under which students will be able to demonstrate their best performance on tests. One of these conditions involves adequate preparation of students to take tests (Brookhart & Nitko, 2019; Hensel et al., 2024; Miller et al., 2013).

Students need information about the test and need practice with item formats that will be used to prepare effectively for it. They should have sufficient time to prepare, so the date and time of the test should be announced well in advance. Although many teachers believe that unannounced or pop tests motivate students to study, no credible evidence supports this belief. Students also need to know about the testing conditions, including how much time will be provided; whether they will be able to use resources such as a calculator; number; and types of test items; and whether any items, such as cell phones, books, and papers, will be permitted in the testing room.

Students need to know which content domains will be assessed, the cognitive level at which they will be expected to perform, and the relative weights assigned to each content area. As previously discussed, teachers can communicate this information by sharing and discussing the test blueprint with students.

Test-Taking Skills

Students need adequate test-taking skills for the type of test to be administered. Skill in test taking is often called *testwiseness* (NBME, 2021), but this term more appropriately refers to the ability to use test-taking skills and experience, along with clues from poorly constructed test items to achieve a score higher than a student's true knowledge would predict. All students need adequate test-taking skills so that they are not at a disadvantage when their scores are compared with those of test-wise students. Some of these skills are:

- Following test directions
- Reading and understanding test items
- Recording responses accurately
- Using testing time wisely
- Getting adequate rest before a test (Oermann et al., 2025)

A common misconception is that students should not change their answers to test items because their first response is usually correct. However, research shows changing answers can lead to higher scores, and students should be encouraged to change answers any time they have a good reason for the change, such as later recalling necessary information (Coffey et al., 2023).

Test Anxiety

Teachers should prepare students to approach a test with helpful attitudes. Anxiety is a common response in testing situations, but test anxiety in nursing students has increased since the pandemic with estimates that 50% to 100% of undergraduate nursing students will experience test anxiety at least once (McCormick & Lamberson, 2024). The multidimensional state of worry and emotionality associated with test anxiety leads to physical and psychological symptoms that interfere with a student's critical thinking, results in more errors, and leads to decreased performance. Physical feelings and reactions associated with test anxiety relate to autonomic reactivity, producing symptoms such as perspiration, increased heart rate, and gastrointestinal upset, although not all test-anxious students have these reactions (Poorman et al., 2019).

Students whose text anxiety interferes with their test performance can benefit from treatment that addresses negative emotions (e.g., worry) and thoughts (e.g., distractibility, difficulty concentrating) as well as improvement of test-taking skills. Teachers who identify students who are affected by test anxiety should refer those students for treatment.

TEST AND ITEM ANALYSIS

Electronic scoring has the advantage of speed as well as the ability to generate test statistics and item analysis reports. Computer software for scoring scannable answer sheets and analyzing test results is widely available, and test analysis functions are built into most computer testing platforms. These applications provide useful information about how well the entire test functioned as a measurement instrument and about the effectiveness of each test item.

Test statistics usually include the range and distribution of scores, measures of central tendency (i.e., the average or typical score), measures of variability (e.g., standard deviation), and reliability estimates. These test characteristics help teachers to interpret the test results and make appropriate inferences about them.

To determine the effectiveness of each test item, teachers should review their difficulty and discrimination indexes or point biserial correlation coefficients. Item difficulty (or *p*-value) is calculated as the percentage of students who responded correctly to that item; values range from 0 to 1.00. When partial credit is awarded, item difficulty is determined by dividing the total points earned on an item by the points possible (Hensel & Cifrino, 2022). The difficulty level is commonly understood to mean that the higher the percentage, the easier the item. However, difficulty is not an intrinsic characteristic of a test item; different *p*-values can be obtained on the same item by students with different abilities or by students who were taught by more- or less-effective teachers. Difficulty level is also related to the probability of students' guessing the correct response. Thus, the probability of guessing the correct response to a true–false item is .50, whereas the probability of correctly guessing the answer to a five-option multiple-choice item is .20. Moderately difficult test items have *p*-values approximately halfway between the chance of blind guessing and 1.00.

The discrimination index, *D*-index, indicates how effectively each test item measures what the entire test measures. The *D*-index ranges from −1.00 to + 1.00. Negative values indicate that the item was answered correctly more often by students with low total test scores than by high-scoring students; this may indicate items that are flawed and should be revised. A *D*-index of .00 means that the item has no discriminating power because equal numbers of high- and low-scoring students answered it correctly. A positive *D*-index means that high-scoring students tended to answer the item correctly more often than low-scoring students.

Similarly, the point biserial correlation coefficient shows the association between a student's response to an item and their total exam score. It should be interpreted in the same way as the *D*-index; however, the use of a point biserial correlation coefficient is limited to items that are scored dichotomously (Hensel & Cifrino, 2022). A point biserial may be also calculated for each answer option to help identify specific areas of revision. For instance, if an item has a low *D*-index and one answer option has a negative point biserial, the teacher knows that answer option requires revision before the item could be used again on an examination.

Students often argue that if all or most of them answered an item incorrectly, that item should be deleted from the test, or that students who answered incorrectly should receive an extra point. Difficulty alone is an insufficient basis on which to delete a test item from scoring: The teacher should carefully review the item in question, and if it measures important content, was expected to be difficult for many students, and is not seriously flawed, it should remain. If there is a fatal flaw, such as omission of the correct answer from a multiple-choice item, that item should be eliminated, and the test rescored without it. Review of the discrimination index or point biserial correlation should help teachers determine whether a very difficult item effectively distinguished between high-scoring and low-scoring groups of students; if so, that item should be retained (Oermann et al., 2025).

SUMMARY

A test is a measurement instrument for assessing learners' knowledge and cognitive abilities. Test results allow teachers to make important educational decisions that affect learners, teachers, patients, future employers, and the educational program. A test must produce relevant and consistent results to form the basis for sound inferences about what learners know and can do. Good planning, careful test construction, proper administration, accurate scoring, and sound interpretation of scores are essential for producing useful test results. This chapter discussed assessment concepts that influence the quality of test results, and the process of planning, constructing, administering, scoring, and analyzing tests. Guidelines were presented for writing traditional selected response items, technology enhanced items, constructed response items, and context-dependent item sets. Items used on the NCLEX to measure clinical judgment were described. Finally, recommendations were made for online testing.

A robust set of instructor resources designed to supplement this text is located at http://connect.springerpub.com/content/book/978-0-8261-8892-2. Qualifying instructors may request access by emailing textbook@springerpub.com.

REFERENCES

Anderson, L. W., & Krathwohl, D. R. (Eds.). (2001). *A taxonomy for learning, teaching, and assessing: A revision of Bloom's taxonomy of educational objectives.* Longman.

Betts, J., Muntean, W., Kim, D., Jorion, N., & Dickison, P. (2019). Building a method for writing clinical judgment items for entry-level nursing exams. *Journal of Applied Testing Technology, 20*(S2), 21–36.

Betts, J., Muntean, W., Kim, D, & Kao, S. (2022). Next generation NCLEX®: Test design. *Next Generation NCLEX News.*

Brookhart, S. M., & Nitko, A. J. (2019). *Educational assessment of students* (8th ed.). Pearson Education.

Bryant, W. (2019). Developing a strategy for using technology-enhanced items in large-scale standardized tests. *Practical Assessment, Research, and Evaluation, 22*(1), 1. https://doi.org/10.7275/70yb-dj34

Butler-Henderson, K., & Crawford, J. (2020). A systematic review of online examinations: A pedagogical innovation for scalable authentication and integrity. *Computers & Education, 159*, 104024. https://doi.org/10.1016/j.compedu.2020.104024

Cobourne, K., & Robb, M. (2022). Virtual post-examination review: Strategies to promote student reflection. *Nurse Educator, 47*(5), 313–314. https://doi.org/10.1097/nne.0000000000001193

Coffey, J. S., Maruca, A. T., Polifroni, E. C., & Snyder, M. (2023). Changing test answers: A scoping review. *Nurse Education Today, 133*, 106052. https://doi.org/10.1016/j.nedt.2023.106052

Cox, C. W. (2019). Best practice tips for the assessment of learning of undergraduate nursing students via multiple-choice questions. *Nursing Education Perspectives, 40*(4), 228–230. https://doi.org/10.1097/01.nep.0000000000000456

Harding, M., & Bonaduce, S. (2023). NGN item type scoring in nursing course level examinations. *Teaching and Learning in Nursing, 19*(1), 16–19. https://doi.org/10.1016/j.teln.2023.05.007

Hensel, D. (2022). Fair testing and incorporating next generation NCLEX items into course examinations. *Nurse Educator, 47*(6), 352–353. https://doi.org/10.1097/NNE.0000000000001288

Hensel, D., & Billings, D. M. (2023). Creating a peer review process for faculty-developed next generation NCLEX items. *Nurse Educator, 48*(2), 65–70. https://doi.org/10.1097/nne.0000000000001322

Hensel, D., Billings, D. M., & Wiseman, R. (2024). Evaluation of the Maryland Next Gen Test Bank Project: Implications and recommendations. *Nursing Education Perspectives, 45*(4), 225–229. https://doi.org/10.1097/01.nep.0000000000001239

Hensel, D., & Cifrino, S. (2022). Item analysis and next-generation NCLEX. *Nurse Educator, 47*(5), 308–310. https://doi.org/10.1097/nne.0000000000001223

McCormick, S., & Lamberson, J. (2024). Interventions for test anxiety in nursing students: A literature review. *Teaching and Learning in Nursing, 19*(2), e404–e411. https://doi.org/10.1016/j.teln.2024.01.005

Miller, M. D., Linn, R. L., & Gronlund, N. E. (2013). *Measurement and assessment in teaching* (11th ed.). Prentice Hall.

Moore, B. S., & Clark, M. C. (2016). The role of linguistic modification in nursing education. *Journal of Nursing Education, 55*(6), 309–315. https://doi.org/10.3928/01484834-20160516-02

National Board of Medical Examiners. (2021). *NBME item writing guide.* Author.

National Council of State Boards of Nursing. (2020). Next generation NCLEX®: The case study. *Next Generation NCLEX News.* NCSBN.

National Council of State Boards of Nursing. (2021a). Next generation NCLEX®: Scoring models. *Next Generation NCLEX News.* NCSBN.

National Council of State Boards of Nursing. (2021b). Next generation NCLEX®: Stand-alone Items. *Next Generation NCLEX News.* NCSBN.

Oermann, M. H., Gaberson, K. B., & De Gagne, J. C. (2025). *Evaluation and testing in nursing education* (7th ed.). Springer Publishing Company.

Petersen, E., Betts, J., & Muntean, W. (2020). *Next Generation NCLEX® (NGN) Webinar.* NCSBN.

Poorman, S. G., Mastorovich, M. L., & Gerwick, M. (2019). Interventions for test anxiety: How faculty can help. *Teaching and Learning in Nursing, 14*(3), 186–191. https://doi.org/10.1016/j.teln.2019.02.007

Raymond, M. R., Stevens, C., & Bucak, S. D. (2019). The optimal number of options for multiple-choice questions on high-stake tests: Application of a revised index for detecting nonfunctional distractors. *Advances in Health Sciences Education, 24*(1), 141–150. https://doi.org/10.1007/s10459-018-9855-9

Clinical Evaluation

17

Marilyn H. Oermann

OBJECTIVES

1. Describe the clinical evaluation process, differences between formative and summative clinical evaluation, and guidelines for evaluating student performance
2. Describe methods for evaluating students in the clinical setting and guidelines for their use

INTRODUCTION

As students learn about nursing, they develop their knowledge base, higher level thinking skills, and a wide range of practice competencies essential for patient care. Learning concepts in a classroom or an online environment is not sufficient: Students need to apply those concepts and other knowledge to clinical situations and be proficient in carrying out care. Teachers guide student learning in the clinical setting and evaluate their performance in practice. This chapter describes the clinical evaluation process, the importance of giving prompt and specific feedback to students as they are learning, principles that are important when observing and rating performance, selected methods for clinical evaluation, and grading clinical practice.

WHAT COMPETENCIES SHOULD BE EVALUATED?

Each school of nursing establishes its own program and course outcomes or objectives, consistent with factors that were described in Chapter 14. Some of those outcomes relate to care of patients, families, and communities and are best met through clinical practice. In clinical practice, students develop multiple competencies that are essential to provide comprehensive, evidence-based care to patients with varied health problems and needs. In practice, students learn to apply their knowledge to clinical situations, transfer skills acquired in other settings to patient care, and develop their clinical judgment skills (Betts et al., 2024; Manetti, 2019, 2022; Sommer et al., 2021). They search for and use evidence to guide decisions, enabling them to learn about evidence-based practice and how it is implemented in patient care.

In clinical practice, students also learn about quality care and the nurse's role in improving healthcare quality and safety (Altmiller & Hopkins-Pepe, 2019; Cengiz & Yoder, 2020; Dolansky et al., 2024; Quality and Safety Education for Nurses [QSEN], 2022; Tarhan & Yıldırım, 2023; Young et al., 2021). With the goal of preparing students with the knowledge, skills, and attitudes for improving the quality of care,

QSEN developed competencies to be achieved by prelicensure and advanced practice nursing students, which are consistent with the American Association of Colleges of Nursing (AACN) *Essentials* (Dolansky et al., 2024).

Clinical practice allows students to continue to develop their psychomotor and technological skills, introduced in laboratory and simulation experiences; gain informatics competencies; collaborate with nurses and other health professionals and function on interprofessional teams (Interprofessional Education Collaborative Expert Panel [IPEC], 2016; Shorten et al., 2023); develop professional values; learn to accept responsibility for their own actions; and become self-directed learners. In clinical practice, students have an opportunity to care for a diverse patient population. These experiences are important in developing cultural competence and learning to provide equitable, quality, and patient-centered care (Charania & Patel, 2022; Foronda et al., 2022; Murray & Noone, 2022).

The outcomes of clinical practice can be stated as outcomes or objectives to be met in a clinical course, or as competencies to be developed by students. Regardless of the format, they provide the framework for the educator to plan clinical learning activities for students and for assessing their performance. A summary of competencies often developed in clinical practice is provided in Table 17.1. This table includes the core competencies needed by all healthcare professionals, such as patient-centered care, teamwork and collaboration, evidence-based practice, quality improvement, safety, and informatics (IPEC, 2016; QSEN, 2022), and an example of a competency (with related domain) from the AACN *The Core Competencies for Professional Nursing Education* (henceforth, Essentials) *Essentials* (2021). Not all

TABLE 17.1. COMPETENCIES DEVELOPED AND EVALUATED IN CLINICAL PRACTICE

Competencies	Related Domain in AACN *Essentials* With Sample Competency*
Apply concepts, theories, and other knowledge to clinical practice	1: Knowledge for Nursing Practice (1.2 Apply theory and research-based knowledge from nursing, the arts, humanities, and other sciences)
Use higher level thinking and clinical judgment in patient care	1: Knowledge for Nursing Practice (1.3 Demonstrate clinical judgment founded on a broad knowledge base)
Provide comprehensive and evidence-based care for patients with varied health problems and needs	Domain 2: Person-Centered Care (2.3 Integrate assessment skills in practice; 2.4 Diagnose actual or potential health problems and needs; 2.5 Develop a plan of care; 2.7 Evaluate outcomes of care)
Care for patients, families, and populations across the health continuum	Domain 3: Population Health (3.1 Manage population health)

(continued)

TABLE 17.1. COMPETENCIES DEVELOPED AND EVALUATED IN CLINICAL PRACTICE *(continued)*

Competencies	Related Domain in AACN *Essentials* With Sample Competency*
Use research and other evidence in clinical practice	Domain 4: Scholarship for the Nursing Discipline (4.2 Integrate best evidence into nursing practice)
Apply knowledge, skills, and values continuously improving the quality and safety of healthcare	Domain 5: Quality and Safety (5.1 Apply quality improvement principles in care delivery)
Communicate effectively with patients, families, communities, and interprofessional teams	Domain 2: Person-Centered Care (2.2 Communicate effectively with individuals) Domain 6: Interprofessional Partnerships (6.1 Communicate in a manner that facilitates a partnership approach to quality care delivery)
Demonstrate leadership skills within complex healthcare systems	Domain 7: Systems-Based Practice (7.1 Apply knowledge of systems to work effectively across the continuum of care)
Demonstrate competencies in psychomotor skills, information and communication technology, informatics, and other technologies	Domain 8: Informatics and Healthcare Technologies (8.2 Use information and communication technology to gather data, create information, and generate knowledge)
Demonstrate knowledge and values essential for providing care to a culturally and ethnically diverse patient population	Domain 9: Professionalism (9.6 Integrate diversity, equity, and inclusion as core to one's professional identity)
Accept responsibility for actions and decisions	Domain 9: Professionalism (9.3 Demonstrate accountability to the individual, society, and the profession)
Demonstrate continued learning and self-development	Domain 10: Personal, Professional, and Leadership Development (10.2 Demonstrate a spirit of inquiry that fosters flexibility and professional maturity)

*Some of these competencies are also integrated in other domains.
Source: American Association of Colleges of Nursing. (2021). *The essentials: Core competencies for professional nursing education*. AACN; Oermann, M. H., Gaberson, K. B., & De Gagne, J. C (2025). *Evaluation and testing in nursing education* (7th ed.). Springer Publishing Company. Reprinted by permission, Springer Publishing.

competencies are developed in every clinical course (e.g., some courses may not call for the acquisition of technological or delegation skills), but overall, most courses will move students toward achievement of these competencies as they progress through the nursing program.

CLINICAL EVALUATION PROCESS

In clinical evaluation, the teacher makes judgments about the quality of the students' performance in practice. These judgments indicate whether the student is meeting or has met the outcomes or objectives of the course and can perform the essential competencies to be developed. Clinical evaluation involves observing students' performance; assessing their understanding of the clinical situation through questions, discussions, and assignments completed by students; and collecting other data about student learning and performance. The teacher then uses these data to determine whether the student is progressing in the course, or at course end, has met each of the outcomes and can perform the competencies.

Clinical evaluation is a judgmental process (Oermann et al., 2025). The teacher's judgment influences the data collected through observations of students and other sources, and what those data mean; that is, decisions about the quality of the performance. First, in any clinical situation teachers can make varied observations of performance and collect different types of data on which to base the evaluation. For example, if two teachers observe a student in practice, one might collect information on how well the student interacted with the patient during a procedure, whereas the other focuses mainly on procedural skills, resulting in varied observations on which to judge the performance. Second, teachers can have different interpretations of how well the student performed. For this reason, it is important to have multiple sources of data and to collect data over a period of time before arriving at a conclusion about the quality of the student's performance.

Another issue is that the teacher's personal values, attitudes, beliefs, and biases can influence the observations made and decisions about the quality of the performance (Oermann et al., 2025). Teachers need to be aware of these when evaluating students' performance. For example, a teacher who prefers working with students who are outgoing and initiate conversation can be biased when assessing the performance of a beginning student who is quiet and needs guidance in interacting with patients. Issues with interactions can affect the communication competencies on the clinical evaluation tool, but they should not influence the assessment of other unrelated competencies. As students are learning, it is the teacher's responsibility to guide their development. In this situation, the teacher's goal should be to help this student develop skills and confidence in communication. The teacher's main role is teaching students to gain competencies for practice, not only to evaluate their performance.

Formative and Summative Clinical Evaluation

The teacher can evaluate students' performance to provide feedback for improving it (formative evaluation) or to indicate the outcomes met and competencies achieved in the clinical practicum (summative evaluation). In formative evaluation, the teacher provides feedback to students about their progress in the clinical practicum and how to improve performance. The goal of feedback is to help students learn and improve their clinical performance. This is good teaching: The nurse educator identifies gaps in learning and performance and provides specific and instructional feedback to resolve those gaps. Formative evaluation is diagnostic and should not be graded (Brookhart & Nitko, 2019).

At periodic intervals, the teacher summarizes the extent of learning achieved in the course. This is done in relation to the outcomes to be met, or the competencies to be developed, answering questions such as: What outcomes have been met by the student? What is the student's current level of performance? Summative clinical evaluation is typically done at midterm and the end of the clinical practicum to decide on the student's grade. Summative evaluation is for grading—it usually comes too late for students to have an opportunity to improve their performance (Oermann et al., 2025).

Importance of Feedback From the Educator

The teacher should focus on giving prompt and continuous feedback to students (formative evaluation) because the feedback will enable them to improve their performance. For feedback to guide student learning and improve performance, it should be:

1. *Precise, specific, and instructional.* Saying to a student, "Your organization needs to improve," or writing on a paper that the "content lacks depth" does not specify the problem with organization of care and the paper's content or how to improve. Instead, the teacher should indicate the specific skills and knowledge that are lacking and provide suggestions about what to do next to gain those missing skills. By incorporating guidance on how to improve, feedback is instructional and leads to improved performance.

2. *Delivered using varied and relevant modes.* With oral feedback, the teacher describes the observations made of performance, explains what to do differently, and shares other ways of thinking about the clinical situation. Some of the best learning occurs when students and teachers engage in dialogue about the feedback. For procedures and psychomotor skills, feedback should be verbal (explaining the errors in performance and *how* the skill should be performed) and visual (demonstrating the correct procedure). The student can then practice the skill under the guidance of the teacher or someone else with expertise. Written comments on students' papers and other assignments provide another mode of feedback and should meet the same criteria: precise, specific, and instructional.

3. *Prompt.* Feedback needs to be given at the time of learning or shortly thereafter. The longer the time between the performance and feedback, the less effective the feedback is because students cannot recall the specifics of their performance to be modified.

4. *Individualized.* Feedback should be based on the needs of the student. Students need varying degrees of feedback and positive reinforcement as they are learning, especially in the clinical setting. As they become more clinically competent, they are better able to assess their own performance, but with new experiences they still need feedback on their thinking and judgment as well as skills.

5. *Given in private.* No one likes to be told in public and for others to hear about improvements needed in their care. The teacher should be sensitive to the setting in which feedback is delivered: It should be communicated in a private setting, with the goal of guiding students in their learning.

Support of Students in the Evaluation Process

Being evaluated is stressful, especially in the clinical setting, where patients, family members, other nursing students, nurses, and others might observe the teacher assessing and sometimes correcting performance and giving feedback. Clinical practice in and of itself is stressful for students and being evaluated adds to that stress. Students need a supportive learning environment where they are comfortable asking for help and seeking feedback from the teacher. Both teachers and nursing staff need to support students in their learning and be cognizant of the stress students experience in clinical practice (Kaur et al., 2020; Ma et al., 2022; Mazalová et al., 2022).

CLINICAL EVALUATION METHODS
Selecting Appropriate Methods

Clinical evaluation should be based on the outcomes of the clinical course or practicum or the expected competencies to be developed by students. These indicate the expectations for performance and areas to be assessed. The learning activities planned for students, including patient assignments, should enable students to meet these outcomes and become proficient in the identified competencies—the teacher's observations and subsequent assessment should focus on whether these were achieved.

There are different clinical evaluation methods that can be used to assess performance. Using multiple methods takes into consideration individual student needs, abilities, and characteristics and avoids relying on one source of information about student learning (Oermann et al., 2025). Most often the methods provide data for assessing more than one outcome or objective. For example, an observation of the student completing a health history of an elderly patient would provide data related to assessment, interviewing, communication, developmental needs, and others. In deciding on the evaluation methods for a clinical course, the teacher should review the outcomes or competencies and select methods for assessing them. In this way the methods are geared to the learning expected of students.

The clinical evaluation methods planned for a course should be realistic, considering the types of experiences available in the clinical setting or through simulation, and both the student's and teacher's time. Planning for an evaluation method that depends on a certain type of patient in the clinical setting is not realistic; such an evaluation would be better done with simulation or standardized patients. Some methods are not feasible because they might not be available for all of the students or take too much time. Weekly writing assignments might provide data on a number of the course outcomes but require too much time for students considering other course and clinical requirements and demand too much of the teacher's time to review them and give prompt feedback. In such cases, an alternate assessment method might be used, such as a group project or discussions with students, or the teacher might use fewer papers but focus them on specific outcomes to be assessed.

Observation of Performance

Observations of students' performance provide data about their proficiency in the competencies to be demonstrated. These competencies guide the teacher on *what* to observe. Observations over a period of time in different clinical situations provide more reliable data on student performance than a one-time observation.

Teachers should share their observations with students and be willing to include student perceptions of their performance. The teacher might have had an incorrect impression, for example, deciding that a student lacked knowledge of a patient's problem, when in fact the student did not understand the teacher's question. Teachers should discuss their observations with students and be willing to modify their judgments about performance.

Observations of performance should be recorded because otherwise the educator cannot recall details about the performance and the clinical context. Some educators take notes that describe their observations of the student, with or without a judgment about how well the student performed; other educators record their observations using devices such as smartphones, tablets, or other types of portable devices. While notes serve as a way of documenting observations so the clinical teacher can remember them, the information should be shared frequently with students.

Checklists

Checklists are typically used for evaluating students' performance of procedures and skills. A checklist includes a list of specific actions or steps in a procedure to be observed and a place for marking if the student performed them correctly (Brookhart & Nitko, 2019). Checklists also allow learners to self-assess their performance before it is evaluated by the teacher. They are commonly used for assessing skills in learning laboratories and simulation. In using checklists, it is important to focus on the ability of students to perform the skill since there are often different ways of carrying out a procedure or skill.

Clinical Evaluation Tools (Rating Scales)

Clinical evaluation tools, which are types of rating scales, are more comprehensive than checklists. They typically list the outcomes to be met or competencies to be demonstrated at the end of the clinical practicum, with a scale for rating students' achievement or performance of them. Clinical evaluation tools are intended for summative evaluation. At midterm the teacher can rate how well the student is performing at that point in time, and then at the end of the clinical practicum can indicate the outcomes or competencies that were achieved.

Rating scales used for clinical evaluation can be pass–fail or satisfactory–unsatisfactory, or they can include multiple levels for rating performance, such as 1 to 4 or below average to exceptional. A pass–fail scale requires only two levels of judgment: Did the student achieve the outcome or perform the competency at a satisfactory level to indicate a pass?

With a rating form that has multiple levels, the teacher needs to judge the quality of the performance and decide which level it represents on the tool. Brookhart and Nitko (2019) suggested that for this type of instrument, a short description should be included with each number or level for each of the outcomes or competencies to improve consistency across teachers. For example, for the competency "Collects relevant data from patients," the descriptions for each level might be:

- 4: Collects significant data from patients and other sources, differentiates relevant from irrelevant data, analyzes data from multiple sources to identify additional information needed
- 3: Collects significant data from patients, uses multiple sources of data
- 2: Collects data from patients related to main problems
- 1: Does not collect significant data and misses important clues in data

Typically, students' performance is evaluated using the tool at midterm (documenting students' progress in developing the competencies) and at the end of the clinical practicum (documenting that they can safely and effectively perform them). Table 17.2 shows sample competencies from an evaluation tool used midway through a course and for the final evaluation.

TABLE 17.2 SAMPLE COMPETENCIES FROM CLINICAL EVALUATION TOOL

Competencies	Midterm			Final	
	S	NI	U	S	U
Patient-Centered Care					
Provides patient-centered care for residents in assisted living and long-term care settings					
Demonstrates caring behaviors with residents and family members . . .					
Teamwork and Collaboration					
Communicates effectively with patients, family members, staff, and others					
Uses ISBAR when giving report about patient . . .					
Evidence-Based Practice					
Identifies sources of evidence for patient care					
Implements evidence when planning care for residents . . .					

(continued)

TABLE 17.2 SAMPLE COMPETENCIES FROM CLINICAL EVALUATION TOOL (continued)

	Midterm			Final	
Competencies	S	NI	U	S	U
Quality Improvement					
Identifies areas of care needing improvement					
Describes ethical issues in long-term care . . .					
Safety					
Performs procedural skills safely					
Assesses patients for falls and use of interventions for fall prevention . . .					
Informatics					
Documents accurately in simulated electronic health record					
Protects confidentiality of patient information . . .					
Professionalism					
Demonstrates professional values					
Arrives at clinical site on time . . .					

ISBAR, identify, situation, background, assessment, and recommendation; NI, needs improvement; S, satisfactory; U, unsatisfactory.

Regardless of the outcomes or competencies on the tool, the areas rated and the rating scale must be understood by all involved in the process. Clinical nurse educators, students, preceptors, and others should understand what is meant by each competency to be rated and how to use the scale (Oermann et al., 2025). In addition, teachers should be able to identify examples of performance that reflect a pass or fail or at each level in the scale. For example, what is passing performance for "collects comprehensive data from patients?" If there are multiple levels in the scale, what is the difference in the collection of data at each level?

All educators involved in the course should discuss as a group the meaning of each outcome or competency on the tool and acceptable performance. These discussions enable educators to come to consensus about behaviors that demonstrate competency for each of the items on the instrument (Oermann et al., 2025). Faculty and other educators teaching in the clinical setting can practice using the tool to assess the performance of students in digitally recorded simulations or video clips. Discussing their ratings and rationale improves use of the tool and its reliability. In addition, teachers should review the instrument with students, explaining each outcome and competency and expected performance. Other important principles for using a clinical evaluation tool are listed in Exhibit 17.1.

EXHIBIT 17.1 Guidelines for Using Clinical Evaluation Tools (Rating Scales)

1. Be alert to the possible influence of your own values, attitudes, and biases in observing performance and making judgments about its quality.
2. Use the outcomes, objectives, or competencies to focus your observations. Give students feedback on other observations made about their performance.
3. Collect sufficient data on students' performance before arriving at conclusions and judgments about the quality of the performance.
4. Observe students more than one time before rating performance. Rating scales for clinical evaluation should represent a pattern of students' performance over a period of time.
5. Observe students' performance in different clinical situations or in simulation, or use additional methods for evaluation.
6. Do not rely on first impressions; these might not be accurate.
7. Always discuss observations with students, have students reflect on their performance and obtain their perceptions, and be willing to modify your own judgments and ratings when new data are presented.
8. Collect data on students' performance as it relates to the outcomes or competencies on the tool. These indicate the expectations for learning and performance and *what* should be evaluated in the clinical setting.
9. Avoid using the clinical evaluation tool as the only source of data about students' performance—use multiple methods for evaluating clinical practice.
10. Rate each outcome or competency on the tool separately based on your observations of performance and other data you have collected. If you have insufficient information to rate a particular outcome or competency, leave it blank.
11. Rate students' performance based on the data. Do not let your general impressions of students or personal biases influence the ratings.
12. If the clinical evaluation tool is not effective for judging students' performance in your clinical course, revise it. Consider these questions: Does use of the tool yield data for making valid decisions about students' competence? Does it yield reliable, stable data? Is it easy to use? Is it realistic for the types of learning activities students complete and that are available in clinical and simulation settings? Is there consistency across clinical educators in their use of the tool?
13. Discuss as a group (with other educators and preceptors involved in the evaluation) each competency on the clinical evaluation tool. Come to agreement as to the meaning of the competencies and what students' performance would look like for a pass or fail and at each rating level in your tool. Share examples of performance, how you would rate them, and your rationale. As a group exercise, observe a digital recording or simulation of a student's performance, rate it with the tool, and come to agreement as to the rating. Exercises and discussions such as these should be held before the course begins and periodically to ensure reliability across teachers and settings.
14. Review the clinical evaluation tool at least annually and modify as needed.

Source: Adapted from Oermann, M. H., Gaberson, K. B., & De Gagne, J. C. (2025). *Evaluation and testing in nursing education* (7th ed.). Springer Publishing Company. By permission of Springer Publishing Company.

EXHIBIT 17.2 Clinical Evaluation Methods

Observation	Case scenario
Notes on the student's performance	Unfolding case
Checklist	Case study
Clinical evaluation tool (rating form)	Media clip
Formal paper	Electronic portfolio
Short paper	Discussion and postclinical conference
Reflective journal and other types of journals	Group project
Nursing care plan	Objective structured clinical examination
Concept map	Self-evaluation

Other Clinical Evaluation Methods

Observations of students, summarizing observations in notes, using checklists to assess skills, and rating how well students performed the expected clinical competencies are not the only methods for evaluating clinical practice. Other methods are listed in Exhibit 17.2. These methods, which were presented in other chapters, provide additional data about student achievement of the outcomes of the clinical course and competencies to be developed.

GRADING CLINICAL COURSES

Clinical courses can be graded as pass–fail or satisfactory–unsatisfactory, or with letter grades such as A through F. When using pass–fail grading, faculty can specify that the student must pass all of the competencies to pass the course or can identify critical behaviors for passing. When letter grades are used, the grade can be determined according to the number of outcomes or competencies achieved by the student. For example, an A might be assigned if all of the competencies were met and a B if the essential ones and half of the others were achieved (Oermann et al., 2025). The grade can also incorporate other evaluation methods used in the course. For example, the rating on the clinical evaluation tool can count for 50% of the clinical grade, with the other 50% determined by grades on written assignments, a portfolio, and a conference presentation. Or the grade might be computed based only on the grades on assignments and other clinical evaluation methods used in the course, with the requirement that students receive a pass on the evaluation tool. In some schools, the clinical assignments and other evaluation methods provide data for determining whether students achieved the outcomes and competencies, but they are not evaluated and graded separately.

There are important principles related to grading clinical practice:

1. The teacher should understand the outcomes and competencies to be achieved in the course, expectations of performance, and specific evaluation methods used in the course.
2. Students need to know what competencies need to be developed in the course and how and when they are evaluated. This information should be communicated in writing to students and reviewed with them.

3. Students should understand how the course is graded. For example, if students must pass the clinical course to progress in the program, no matter what grade they have in the course overall, this information should be in the course syllabus and school policies and also should be reviewed with students.
4. Students need to receive prompt and specific feedback on their performance. Providing this feedback is the most important role of the educator in clinical practice. If the teacher identifies problems with performance, it is critical to discuss these with students early in the practicum.
5. Students should sign any evaluation documents and summaries of performance. Signing does not mean they agree with the evaluation, but it confirms that they had an opportunity to read what was written about their performance.

For students who are not performing at the expected level, a learning plan can be developed with specific learning activities and other strategies mapped out for the student to correct performance problems. Exhibit 17.3 is an example of a template that can be used to develop a learning plan. If the student is failing the clinical practicum, however, the learning plan serves as a contract with the student indicating the competencies not being met and what the student needs to do to pass the practicum. In that case the plan should include (a) due dates, (b) a statement that completing the learning plan does not guarantee passing the course, and (c) a statement that improvement in performance needs to continue throughout the practicum. Students have the full length of the clinical practicum to meet the outcomes and develop their competencies: Those statements represent the performance expected at the end of the course. In situations where the student exhibits unsafe clinical performance, then the teacher should follow the policy in the nursing program about unsafe clinical practice.

EXHIBIT 17.3 Learning Plan Template

Student Information: Name, Course, Contact Information
Teacher Information: Name, Course, Contact Information

Competencies	Learning Activities (With Due Date for Completion)	Evaluation and Who Is Responsible	Due Date for Achievement of Competencies
1.			
2.			
3.			
4.			

SUMMARY

Clinical evaluation is a process in which the teacher collects data through observations of performance and other assessment methods and, based on those data, makes judgments about the quality of the student's performance in practice. These judgments indicate whether the student is meeting or has met the outcomes of the course and can perform the competencies expected in the course. Through formative evaluation, the teacher provides feedback to the student about their progress in the clinical practicum and specifically how to improve their performance. Feedback should be prompt, specific, and instructional; continuous during the learning process; and given in private. Formative evaluation is diagnostic and is not graded. At periodic intervals, such as at midterm and at the end of the clinical practicum, the teacher summarizes the extent of learning and performance. This process is referred to as summative evaluation.

Clinical evaluation methods should be selected based on the outcomes or competencies of the clinical course. These indicate the expectations for performance and areas to be assessed. Observations of performance provide data about student achievement of the outcomes and their proficiency in the clinical competencies to be demonstrated. Observations over a period of time in different clinical situations provide more reliable data on student performance than a one-time observation. When assessing a skill or procedure, the teacher might use a checklist, which includes the specific steps to perform the skill or carry out the procedure and a place for marking if the student performed each step correctly and in the right order. Clinical evaluation tools, which are rating scales, are more comprehensive than checklists. They typically list the outcomes or competencies to be demonstrated at the end of the clinical practicum with a scale for rating their performance. Clinical evaluation tools are intended for summative evaluation. There are many evaluation methods that can be used in a course in addition to rating forms. These were listed in Exhibit 17.2.

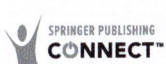

A robust set of instructor resources designed to supplement this text is located at http://connect.springerpub.com/content/book/978-0-8261-8892-2. Qualifying instructors may request access by emailing textbook@springerpub.com.

REFERENCES

Altmiller, G., & Hopkins-Pepe, L. (2019). Why quality and safety education for nurses (QSEN) matters in practice. *Journal of Continuing Education in Nursing, 50*(5), 199–200. https://doi.org/10.3928/00220124-20190416-04

American Association of Colleges of Nursing. (2021). *The essentials: Core competencies for professional nursing education.* AACN.

Betts, J., Muntean, W., & Dickison, P. (2024). Evaluating the importance of clinical judgment in entry-level nursing. *Journal of Nursing education, 63*(3), 156–162. https://doi.org/10.3928/01484834-20240108-06

Brookhart, S. M., & Nitko, A. J. (2019). *Educational assessment of students* (8th ed.). Pearson Education.

Cengiz, A., & Yoder, L. H. (2020). Assessing nursing students' perceptions of the QSEN competencies: A systematic review of the literature with implications for academic programs. *Worldviews on Evidence-based Nursing, 17*(4), 275–282. https://doi.org/10.1111/wvn.12458

Charania, N. A. M. A., & Patel, R. (2022). Diversity, equity, and inclusion in nursing education: Strategies and processes to support inclusive teaching. *Journal of Professional Nursing, 42*, 67–72. https://doi.org/10.1016/j.profnurs.2022.05.013

Dolansky, M. A., Dick, T., Byrd, E., Miltner, R. S., & Layton, S. S. (2024). The QSEN competency legacy threaded through the entry-level AACN Essentials: Shaping the future. *Nurse Educator, 49*(2), 73–79. https://doi.org/10.1097/NNE.0000000000001511

Foronda, C., Prather, S., Baptiste, D. L., & Luctkar-Flude, M. (2022). Cultural humility toolkit. *Nurse Educator, 47*(5), 267–271. https://doi.org/10.1097/NNE.0000000000001182

Interprofessional Education Collaborative Expert Panel. (2016). *Core competencies for interprofessional collaborative practice: 2016 update*. https://ipec.memberclicks.net/assets/2016-Update.pdf

Kaur, G., Chernomas, W. M., & Scanlan, J. M. (2020). Nursing students' perceptions of and experiences coping with stress in clinical practice. *International Journal of Nursing Education Scholarship, 17*(1). https://doi.org/10.1515/ijnes-2020-0005

Ma, H., Zou, J. M., Zhong, Y., Li, J., & He, J. Q. (2022). Perceived stress, coping style and burnout of Chinese nursing students in late-stage clinical practice: A cross-sectional study. *Nurse Education in Practice, 62*, 103385. https://doi.org/10.1016/j.nepr.2022.103385

Manetti, W. (2019). Sound clinical judgment in nursing: A concept analysis. *Nursing Forum, 54*(1), 102–110. https://doi.org/10.1111/nuf.12303

Manetti, W. (2022). A clinical preparation tool to foster clinical judgment. *Nurse Educator, 48*(2), 112–113. https://doi.org/10.1097/NNE.0000000000001290

Mazalová, L., Gurková, E., & Štureková, L. (2022). Nursing students' perceived stress and clinical learning experience. *Nurse Education in Practice, 64*, 103457. https://doi.org/10.1016/j.nepr.2022.103457

Murray, T. A., & Noone, J. (2022). Advancing diversity in nursing education: A groundwater approach. *Journal of Professional Nursing, 41*, 140–148. https://doi.org/10.1016/j.profnurs.2022.05.002

Oermann, M. H., Gaberson, K. B., & De Gagne, J. C. (2025). *Evaluation and testing in nursing education* (7th ed.). Springer Publishing Company.

Quality and Safety Education for Nurses. (2022). *QSEN home*. http://qsen.org

Shorten, A., Cruz Walma, D. A., Bosworth, P., Shorten, B., Chang, B., Moore, M. D., Vogtle, L., & Watts, P. I. (2023). Development and implementation of a virtual "collaborator" to foster interprofessional team-based learning using a novel faculty-student partnership. *Journal of Professional Nursing, 46*, 155–162. https://doi.org/10.1016/j.profnurs.2023.03.008

Sommer, S. K., Johnson, J. D., Clark, C. M., & Mills, C. M. (2021). Assisting learners to understand and incorporate functions of clinical judgment into nursing practice. *Nurse Educator, 46*(6), 372–375. https://doi.org/10.1097/NNE.0000000000001020

Tarhan, M., & Yıldırım, A. (2023). Effect of repeated multipatient simulations on professional readiness among senior nursing students. *Nurse Educator, 48*(4), 197–203. https://doi.org/10.1097/NNE.0000000000001373

Young, C., Ball, S., Flott, E., Goodman, J., & Hercinger, M. (2021). Threading QSEN competencies across a baccalaureate nursing program: The development of dedicated QSEN labs. *Journal of Nursing Education, 60*(9), 526–528. https://doi.org/10.3928/01484834-20210719-02

Program Evaluation and Accreditation

18

Marilyn H. Oermann

OBJECTIVES

1. Compare selected program evaluation models
2. Describe accreditation in nursing, types of accreditation, differences between regulation and accreditation, and standards for distance education programs
3. Identify the parts of a systematic program evaluation plan
4. Describe important principles of course and teacher evaluation

INTRODUCTION

Program evaluation provides data to judge the quality of a nursing program and evidence on its outcomes. Through program evaluation, faculty, administrators, and others involved in the evaluation process collect the data needed to make informed decisions and determine the effectiveness of the program in meeting its goals and achieving important outcomes. This chapter describes program evaluation in nursing and the development of a systematic program evaluation plan for a school of nursing. Discussion is included on accreditation of nursing programs, types of and standards for accreditation, differences between regulation and accreditation, and student evaluation of courses and teachers.

PROGRAM EVALUATION MODELS

There are various models of program evaluation that faculty can use to guide their evaluation in a school of nursing. Some models are goal oriented, evaluating the extent to which the curriculum improves student learning and performance. These models help faculty determine if the outcomes were achieved by students. Goal-oriented models are useful for measuring change within courses and programs.

Another type of model is decision oriented. The intent of these models is to provide information to decision-makers to improve the program. Decision models focus on collecting and using the evaluation data for quality improvement (QI). Stufflebeam's context, input, process, product (CIPP) model is an example of a decision-oriented model (Stufflebeam & Zhang, 2017). In this model *context* evaluations assess the current situation to identify the goals of the evaluation. This type of evaluation is typically done when a new program is being planned (Frye & Hemmer, 2012). Evaluation of *inputs* collects data on the resources needed for planning a new program including costs and alternative approaches that might be used. *Process* evaluations assess the implementation of a program and provide feedback for revisions. The final type of evaluation, *product*, measures the outcomes of the program (Oermann, 2023).

A logic model is used frequently when planning a program but also can guide evaluation of a program. A logic model includes:

- Inputs: What are the expected or actual resources of the program.
- Activities: The innovations, strategies, or changes planned for the educational program.
- Outputs: The tangible products and deliverables from the activities being implemented or completed. For example, an output might be the number of face-to-face courses transitioned to online or number of learners who completed a new course or continuing education program.
- Outcomes: Changes in learners and programs; for example, gain in knowledge and ability to perform new competencies. Outcomes may relate to the individual learner or faculty member, school as a whole, or community. Outcomes are short-, intermediate-, and long-term. (Idzik et al., 2021; Oermann, 2023)

When using the logic model, the educator starts with the outcomes and works backwards-from outcomes to inputs. Figure 18.1 is a visual of the logic model. The educator identifies the tangible products and deliverables needed to meet these outcomes, the activities that have to be done, and the resources needed for implementing those activities (Oermann, 2023).

Whatever model is selected for the program evaluation, it should provide the information needed to answer the questions raised by educators, administrators, and other stakeholders about the program. Stakeholders are the individuals and groups who are affected by the evaluation, directly or indirectly, and who are invested in the evaluation. For nursing programs, key stakeholders typically include students, faculty, administrators, staff, healthcare system and community partners, employers, and consumers. Stakeholders vary depending on the focus of the evaluation. When the goal is to obtain data for improving a course, key stakeholders might be

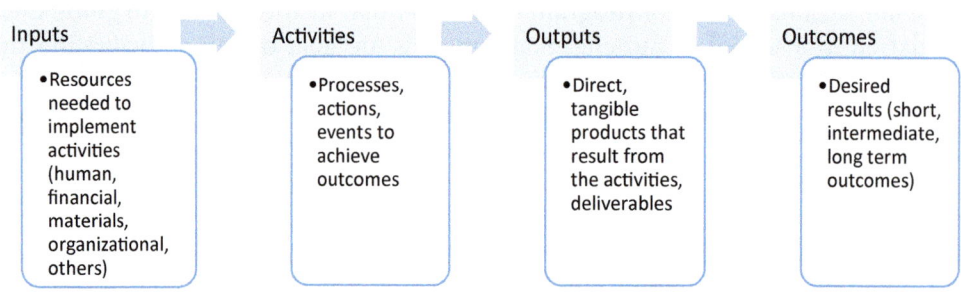

Figure 18.1 Logic model.

Source: Oermann M. H., Gaberson, K. B., & De Gagne, J. C. (2025). *Evaluation and testing in nursing education* (7th ed., p. 332). Springer Publishing Company. Reprinted by permission, Springer Publishing.

students in the course and ones who completed the course, course faculty, clinical nurse educators and preceptors, and skills or simulation laboratory personnel. For an evaluation to be used to decide if a program with low enrollment should be closed, the stakeholders might be similar but also would include alumni, employers of graduates of that program, healthcare and community agencies, consumers, and others who might be impacted by the decision to close the program.

ACCREDITATION

Accreditation is the process of evaluating the quality of a nursing education program based on the standards set by the accrediting agency, the school of nursing and institution, and professional nursing and healthcare organizations. By evaluating if a program meets these standards, the process serves as a way of assuring the public that the institution, school of nursing, and programs offered by the school provide a quality education. Accreditation is a QI process: The evaluation of different components of the program done continuously provides data to identify areas that might need to be revised and the information to make changes. With the focus on QI, it also documents processes that are effective and outcomes being met.

The accreditation process includes an internal and external review of the nursing program based on the program evaluation plan and accreditation standards. For the internal review, faculty, administrators, and others in the school systematically assess their own program and identify areas for improvement with actions to be taken and time frame for completion. Prior to the external review, faculty complete a self-study in which they document the outcomes of their assessment and provide evidence to indicate how the school and programs offered by the school are meeting the accreditation standards. This self-study is a narrative report that is reflective and comprehensive (Shellenbarger, 2023). The self-study prepares faculty for the external review done by the accrediting agency. The external review includes a site visit from the accrediting agency to verify the data provided in the self-study and collect additional information. The data from the program evaluation and site visit are subsequently reviewed by the accrediting agency to assess if standards were met and identify areas for improvement. Exhibit 18.1 indicates the steps in the accreditation process.

EXHIBIT 18.1 Steps in the Accreditation Process

1. Self-study: Faculty and administrators conduct a review of the nursing program and other components of the school of nursing based on the standards of the accrediting agency.
2. Site visit: Peers (volunteers who are prepared by the accrediting agency) make a site visit to the school of nursing (or healthcare agency) to verify information in the self-study and collect additional data.
3. Decision by accrediting agency: The accrediting agency (volunteer faculty and administrators from schools of nursing and public members) decide on the accreditation status and length of time for the accreditation.
4. Progress report for continuing accreditation: Schools conduct a self-study midpoint in the accreditation or as designated by the accrediting agency and submit a progress report. This is also required when there is a new program in the school or major change in the curriculum.

Institutional Versus Programmatic (Specialized) Accreditation

There are two types of accreditation: institutional (at the university, college, and community college level) and programmatic or specialized (at the program or field of study level). Institutional accreditation is performed by regional accrediting agencies such as the Middle States Commission on Higher Education. The United States is divided into regions, and each region has its own organization for institutional accreditation. There also are accrediting agencies for faith-based colleges and career-related or vocational schools.

Programmatic or specialized accreditation is for a discipline or field of study; for example, nursing, engineering, and medicine. There are three organizations that accredit nursing education programs in the United States: Accreditation Commission for Education in Nursing (ACEN), Commission on Collegiate Nursing Education (CCNE), and Commission for Nursing Education Accreditation (CNEA). Both ACEN and CNEA accredit practical, diploma, associate, baccalaureate, master's, and doctor of nursing practice programs, thus serving as an accrediting agency for all levels of nursing education. CCNE, in contrast, accredits baccalaureate, master's, and doctor of nursing practice programs; postgraduate advanced practice RN certificate programs; and entry-to-practice residency programs. The standards for evaluating nursing programs across these three accrediting agencies reflect the same broad areas although they are organized and labeled differently (ACEN, 2023; CCNE, 2024). Table 18.1 compares the standards for nursing's three agencies.

In nursing, there also are specialty accrediting agencies such as the Council on Accreditation of Nurse Anesthesia that accredits nurse anesthesia programs (postmaster's and postdoctoral certificate, master's, and doctoral). Nurse anesthetists need to graduate from an accredited nurse anesthesia program to be eligible for certification (Council on Accreditation of Nurse Anesthesia Educational Programs [CANAEP], 2024). In Canada, the accrediting agency for RN education is the Canadian Association of Schools of Nursing (CASN). Similar to the United States, the accreditation standards are broad and allow schools flexibility in how they implement the standards in their own settings and programs (CASN, 2024).

Accreditation of nursing programs extends from prelicensure through the doctor of nursing practice and other practice doctoral degrees. However, PhD and other research doctoral programs are not accredited by these agencies; these programs are offered by the graduate school of the university and evaluated through their processes.

Accreditation of Distance Education Programs

The standards from the nursing accrediting agencies incorporate distance education and online courses within their standards. For ACEN accreditation, nursing programs that are offered for distance education need to meet 10 criteria in addition to the overall standards for the program (Exhibit 18.2).

TABLE 18.1 AREAS OF ACCREDITATION STANDARDS FOR NURSING EDUCATION PROGRAMS

Areas	ACEN	CCNE	CNEA
Mission and governance	1. Administrative capacity and resources	I. Program quality: Mission and governance	II. Mission, governance, resources
Faculty	2. Faculty	II. Program quality: Institutional commitment and resources (includes faculty)	III. Faculty
Students	3. Students	In multiple standards	IV. Students
Curriculum	4. Curriculum	III. Program quality: Curriculum and teaching–learning practices	V. Curriculum and evaluation processes
Resources	1. Administrative capacity and resources	II. Program quality: Institutional commitment and resources	II. Mission, governance, resources
Outcomes	5. Outcomes	IV. Program effectiveness: Assessment and achievement of program outcome	I. Program outcomes
Available at	https://resources.acenursing.org/space/SAC/1824227333/2023+Standards+and+Criteria	https://www.aacnnursing.org/Portals/0/PDFs/CCNE/CCNE-Education-Standards-2024.pdf	https://cnea.nln.org/standards-of-accreditation

Note: Numbers indicate the number of the standard.

ACEN, Accreditation Commission for Education in Nursing; CCNE, Commission on Collegiate Nursing Education; CNEA, Commission for Nursing Education Accreditation.

Source: Oermann M. H., Gaberson, K. B., & De Gagne, J. C. (2025). *Evaluation and testing in nursing education* (7th ed., p. 329). Springer Publishing Company. Reprinted by permission, Springer Publishing.

> **EXHIBIT 18.2 Criteria for Accreditation of Distance Education Nursing Programs (ACEN)**
>
> 1. Congruence with the institutional mission
> 2. Instructional design and course delivery methods
> 3. Competence and preparation of faculty
> 4. Quality and accessibility of support services for students
> 5. Quality and accessibility of support services for faculty members
> 6. Current, relevant, and accessible learning resources
> 7. Current, appropriate offerings relative to the delivery method
> 8. Provision of opportunities for regular faculty–student and student–student interactions
> 9. Ongoing evaluation of student learning
> 10. Processes established for verifying student identity in courses

Source: Adapted from Accreditation Commission for Education in Nursing. (2020). *Policy #15 distance education.* https://resources.acenursing.org/space/AP/1827700861/POLICY+%2315%0ADISTANCE+EDUCATION

For CCNE accreditation, distance education is integrated in the accreditation standards. For example, Standard III on Curriculum and Teaching–Learning Practices indicates that teaching practices including distance education need to support student achievement of expected learning outcomes, and clinical practice is provided for all students including students in distance education offerings (CCNE, 2024). CNEA uses the same approach, weaving in distance education within the accreditation standards. As an example, under Standard II on Mission, Governance, and Resources, the guidelines include the need for the technological infrastructure to support student learning needs for on-campus and distance education environments (CNEA, 2021, p. 5).

In addition to the nursing accreditation standards, the National Council for State Authorization Reciprocity Agreements (NC-SARA); provides guidelines for ensuring quality in distance education programs, the *21st Century Distance Education Guidelines*, that can be used for evaluating online education programs in nursing (NC-SARA, 2021). The 2021 guidelines have six areas with standards to be met in each area:

1. Institutional capacity
2. Institutional transparency and disclosures
3. Academic programs
4. Support for students
5. Program review
6. Academic and institutional integrity

SYSTEMATIC PROGRAM EVALUATION PLAN

Program evaluation in a school of nursing is guided by the systematic program evaluation plan. This plan maps out the evaluation to be done and the timeframe with a feedback loop to ensure that the evaluation data are reviewed and used for program improvement and the school is in compliance with accreditation and regulatory standards. A systematic evaluation plan is required for accreditation, but the plan should be *used* by faculty and administrators to make decisions about the school and the programs it offers and to continually improve them. Many nursing programs use the accreditation standards, from the agency they select for their accreditation, as the framework for their evaluation plan and to guide their process although other areas for evaluation specific to the school of nursing should be added to plan.

The program evaluation plan is usually prepared as a table with these components:

1. Areas to be evaluated: The areas for the evaluation include the accreditation standards, additional criteria to be met (e.g., related to offering a nurse anesthesia program), regulatory standards, and other areas important to the school of nursing. The accreditation standards include mission and governance (administration), faculty, students, curriculum, resources, and program outcomes. The standards of the three nursing accrediting agencies reflect the same broad areas but are organized and labeled differently. This was shown in Table 18.1.

2. Expected levels of achievement: The expected levels of achievement are benchmarks that the school needs to meet. Some of these are set by the accrediting or regulatory bodies. For example, the CCNE accreditation standard specifies that the NCLEX-RN® pass rate is 80% or higher for first-time test takers. Schools of nursing can set higher benchmarks and might set 90% as its benchmark for the NCLEX-RN first-time pass rate. For other areas, such as research and scholarly productivity of faculty, the school determines its own benchmarks based on its mission and resources. Often more than one benchmark is set; for example, benchmarks for student readiness for the NCLEX-RN might be standardized test scores, mean score on the readiness test, percent of students who completed a review course, and extent of other preparation for the NCLEX-RN.

3. Responsible individuals and groups: To ensure that data are collected, analyzed, and used, the responsible individuals or roles in the school (e.g., associate dean for academic affairs) and groups (e.g., program evaluation committee) should be specified in the evaluation plan.

4. Assessment methods and time frame: These areas of the evaluation plan map out the methods used for collecting the data (e.g., surveys and interviews) and when the information is collected (e.g., end of the course), analyzed, and reported. Both quantitative and qualitative methods are used in program evaluation.

5. Results: Some evaluation plans include a column for reporting the results. For example, the mean scores on the NCLEX-RN readiness test might be recorded on the plan with dates. Other schools report the evaluation findings in minutes of meetings where they were discussed or upload these data at a school website for this purpose. Whatever mechanism is used, the date and other details should be included so the information can be tracked over time.

6. Actions taken: The results of the evaluation need to be reviewed by faculty, administrators, and other stakeholders; discussed by the evaluation committee and other relevant committees and groups in the school; and acted on if indicated. The evaluation plan should include a column for recording the decisions made and actions taken with dates for reassessment. If no action is needed, this should be indicated (Lewallen, 2023).

A sample format for a systematic evaluation plan is provided in Table 18.2. The names of the components are usually consistent with the standards of the accrediting agency selected by the school.

TABLE 18.2 SAMPLE FORMAT FOR A SYSTEMATIC EVALUATION PLAN

Areas for Evaluation or Criteria	Expected Level of Achievement (Benchmark)	Person or Group Responsible	Assessment Methods	Time Frame	Results	Actions Taken
Mission and Governance						
Mission, goals, outcomes congruent with parent institution …	■ Congruence of mission, goals, outcomes, and vision of school of nursing and university ■ 100% of evaluation committee members agree or strongly agree that these are clearly stated and are congruent with one another	■ Program evaluation committee	■ Review of documents including strategic plans	■ Every 2 years (May) unless there are university, school, or program changes	■ Congruent ■ 100% agreement among faculty on committee	■ None needed
Institutional Commitment and Resources						
Faculty are sufficient in number, academically and experientially prepared for areas teaching …	■ New faculty meet qualifications for position ■ At least 90% of full-time faculty are doctorally prepared ■ 100% of faculty teaching clinical courses have prior or current experience in clinical area or related specialty ■ 100% of faculty teaching NPs courses have current, relevant certification	■ Search committee review using checklist on hire ■ Department chairs	■ Review of CVs ■ Annual evaluation dossier ■ Credential check	■ Annually (May)	■ All faculty have necessary educational degrees, requirements to teach in assigned courses ■ Compliant with SACS standards for faculty qualifications to teach	■ Combine annual evaluation dossier with credential check (into one document)

Curriculum and Teaching–Learning Practices

Teaching–learning practices support achievement of student outcomes ...	- Mean scores are ≥3.0 on course evaluations - Mean scores are ≥4.5 on exit surveys (related factors, items) - e-portfolios document achievement of student learning outcomes (ratings ≥4.5)	- Course faculty (review course evaluations) - Program directors and committees - Program evaluation committee (score e-portfolios)	- Course evaluations - Exit surveys - e-portfolios	- End of each course Program directors and committees annual review of course evaluations and exit surveys (end of program, each cohort; May) e-portfolios mid-, end of program (January, May)	- 90% of course evaluations above 3.0 benchmark Exit survey scores (see report) Mean rating of e-portfolios 4.8 (see summary report)	- Review 2 areas on exit survey for MSN program with mean scores < 4.5

Assessment and Achievement of Program Outcomes

Licensure pass rates (standard is 80%)	- First-time NCLEX-RN® pass rate for BSN graduates is ≥90%	- BSN program director	- NCLEX-RN pass rate reports	- Every August and March - Report due dates: - October and June	- > 90% (see report)	- None

CV, curriculum vitae; NP, nurse practitioner; SACS, Southern Association of Colleges and Schools.

REGULATION OF NURSING PROGRAMS

Accreditation is not the same as regulation of nursing education programs. The regulation of programs is a responsibility of the state boards of nursing: They ensure that nursing programs provide the knowledge and skills that students need to practice safely and competently (National Council of State Boards of Nursing [NCSBN], 2024). Boards are charged with protecting the public; one of the ways they do this is by setting standards for nursing education and practice in the state. Nursing programs must be approved by the state board of nursing to operate, and only graduates of state board approved schools can take the NCLEX (NCSBN, 2024).

While a school of nursing must be approved by the state board of nursing, accreditation is voluntary. However, schools that are not accredited create impediments for students: Federal and state government financial aid is available only for students in an accredited nursing program, and most higher education institutions require applicants to have graduated from an accredited program.

EVALUATION OF TEACHING

At the end of a course and clinical practicum, students have an opportunity to evaluate the quality of and their satisfaction with the course and the teacher's effectiveness as an educator. Expert teaching includes five qualities: (a) knowledge of the content area in which teaching, (b) clinical competence, (c) teaching skills and competencies as an educator, (d) positive relationships with learners and others, and (e) personal characteristics such as enthusiasm for teaching, patience with students, integrity, perseverance, and willingness to admit mistakes among others (Oermann et al., 2025). These areas are typically reflected in the form used for student evaluations.

These evaluations serve as a way for learners to provide anonymous feedback to the teacher about the course and instruction and an overall rating. There are limitations, however, to the use of student evaluations. Students' ratings are affected by class size, for example: Larger classes are often rated lower than courses with a small number of students, and students often rate electives higher than required courses (Oermann et al., 2018). Other variables that affect student ratings also have been identified, and both faculty and administrators should understand these because they are important when interpreting scores.

Many colleges and universities have a standard form for course evaluations that is used in all courses in the institution including nursing. These forms generally ask students to rate the organization of the course, effectiveness of the teaching methods, value of the assignments, tests and other methods for assessment, grading, workload in and difficulty of the course, effectiveness of the teacher in helping students learn, communication and interactions with students, and enthusiasm of the teacher (Bush et al., 2018; Oermann et al., 2018). A sample course evaluation form is provided in Table 18.3. Course evaluation forms should include a question at the end for students to provide an overall rating of the course and teacher (Bush et al., 2018). Considering the importance of these student ratings in a school of nursing, forms should be piloted before use (Powell et al., 2014).

TABLE 18.3 SAMPLE COURSE AND TEACHER EVALUATION FORM

	Responses				
	SA	A	Neither A or D	D	SD
Course Evaluation					
The course expectations and requirements were clear.					
The content was well organized.					
The course was intellectually stimulating and made me think.					
The course assignments (papers, projects, etc.) helped me learn.					
The grading criteria were clear.					
The course workload was appropriate.					
Overall, this was an excellent course.					
Teacher Evaluation					
The teacher was well prepared for class.					
The teacher was enthusiastic about the content and teaching in the course.					
The teacher gave clear explanations.					
The teacher encouraged student participation and discussion.					
The teacher showed respect for students' views and opinions.					
The teacher provided prompt feedback.					
The teacher was available to students.					
Overall, this teacher was an effective teacher.					

SA, strongly agree; A, agree; D, disagree; SD, strongly disagree.

Most forms provide open-ended questions and other options for student comments in addition to ratings using Likert scales. It is recommended that these open-ended questions focus on aspects of the course that impacted students' learning versus asking for general comments about the course. For example, the open-ended questions about the course might be:

- What was the most valuable aspect of this course in terms of your learning?
- What would you change in this course to enhance learning?

For evaluating the teacher's effectiveness, the questions might be:

- What were the strengths of this teacher?
- What are areas for improvement for this teacher?

Faculty need a strategy for reviewing and making sense of the narrative feedback from students especially with large classes. One strategy is to categorize the comments, placing all the comments on a particular assignment together and all the comments on grading together. To better understand this feedback, an additional strategy is to develop groups based on the overall ratings of the course and teaching. Two groups might include students who rated the course overall at a high level and a second group with lower ratings (Oermann, 2017). With a large class, three groups might be formed based on the overall ratings (high, middle, and low). Narrative feedback from students who rated the course high on the Likert scale might differ from students who rated it low, which would be important to know when reading student comments.

McGhee and Morrison-Beedy (2024) recommend using data visualization techniques for examining course evaluation data. Data visualization software such as Tableau© can be used to create diagrams and visuals of data from course evaluations to show patterns and highlight areas for revision across courses.

Course evaluation forms for courses do not include areas of teaching that are important in the clinical setting and when teaching in simulation and skills laboratories. Questions on clinical teaching and guiding students in other practice settings can be added to the course evaluation forms, or a separate tool can be used. Sample questions for evaluating the effectiveness of the clinical teacher are found in Table 18.4.

PEER REVIEW

While student evaluations are important, they should not be the only source of information about a faculty member's performance. Peers can evaluate the quality of a course and teaching materials; review an online course and student–teacher interactions in it; and observe the teacher in the classroom, clinical setting, or laboratory and provide feedback. Observations of teaching performance are most appropriate for formative evaluation and should be supported by resources for faculty development and mentoring.

Peer observation should begin with a meeting to discuss the outcomes for the class and areas on which the teacher wants feedback. A debriefing following the observation provides an opportunity to discuss the observation, areas of strength, and areas to be improved. If the peer review is done for promotion and tenure, a specific form is often required for this process. For online courses, a peer can review

TABLE 18.4 SAMPLE CLINICAL INSTRUCTOR EVALUATION FORM

	Responses				
The clinical instructor:	SA	A	Neither A or D	D	SD
Provided clear guidelines on expectations and requirements for the clinical practicum.					
Helped me apply theoretical learning to clinical practice.					
Facilitated my learning.					
Communicated effectively with students, preceptors, and others in the clinical setting.					
Was a positive role model.					
Provided timely feedback on my performance.					
Overall, this clinical instructor was an effective teacher.					

SA, strongly agree; A, agree; D, disagree; SD, strongly disagree.

course materials and websites as guest users, quality and promptness of feedback given to students, and the extent to which the course engages students in learning.

SUMMARY

Program evaluation is the process of judging the quality of an educational program and evaluating its outcomes. Through program evaluation, faculty, administrators, and other stakeholders gather the data they need for making program and course decisions. Stakeholders are the individuals and groups who are affected by the evaluation, directly or indirectly. For nursing programs, key stakeholders often include students, faculty, administrators, staff, employers, and others. There are a number of models that can be used to guide program evaluation although many schools structure their evaluation plan based on the accreditation standards.

Accreditation is the process of evaluating the quality of a nursing education program based on the standards set by the accrediting agency, the school of nursing and institution, and professional nursing and healthcare organizations. Accreditation is a QI process: Evaluation of different components of the program are done continuously to identify areas that might need revision. There are two types of accreditation: institutional (at the university, college, or community college level) and programmatic or specialized (at the program or field of study level).

There are three organizations that accredit nursing education programs in the United States: ACEN, CCNE, and CNEA. Both ACEN and CNEA accredit practical, diploma, associate, baccalaureate, master's, and doctor of nursing practice programs, thus serving as an accrediting agency for all levels of nursing education. CCNE accredits baccalaureate, master's, and DNP programs; postgraduate advanced practice RN certificate programs; and entry-to-practice residency programs. The chapter also identified standards for distance education programs. Accreditation is not the same as regulation of nursing programs, also discussed in the chapter.

Program evaluation in a school of nursing is guided by the systematic program evaluation plan. This plan maps out the evaluation to be done and timeframe with a feedback loop to ensure the evaluation data are reviewed and used for program improvement and to document compliance with accreditation standards.

Students evaluate the quality of and their satisfaction with their courses and with the quality of teaching in their courses and clinical practicum. The chapter discussed teacher evaluation and provided an example of a sample form for course and teacher evaluation and also for clinical instructor evaluation. Peers can evaluate the quality of a course and teaching materials; review an online course; and observe the teacher in the classroom, clinical setting, or laboratory. Peer observations are most appropriate for formative evaluation.

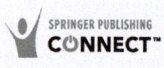 A robust set of instructor resources designed to supplement this text is located at http://connect.springerpub.com/content/book/978-0-8261-8892-2. Qualifying instructors may request access by emailing textbook@springerpub.com.

REFERENCES

Accreditation Commission for Education in Nursing. (2023). *Standards & criteria.* https://resources.acenursing.org/space/SAC/1824227333/2023+Standards+and+Criteria

Bush, M. A., Rushton, S., Conklin, J. L., & Oermann, M. H. (2018). Considerations for developing a student evaluation of teaching form. *Teaching and Learning in Nursing, 13*(2), 125–128. https://doi.org/10.1016/j.teln.2017.10.002

Canadian Association of Schools of Nursing. (2024). *CASN accreditation.* About us. https://accred.casn.ca/about-us/

Commission on Collegiate Nursing Education. (2024). *Standards for accreditation of baccalaureate and graduate degree nursing programs.* American Association of Colleges of Nursing. https://www.aacnnursing.org/Portals/0/PDFs/CCNE/CCNE-Education-Standards-2024.pdf

Commission on Collegiate Nursing Education. (2024). *CCNE accreditation.* American Association of Colleges of Nursing. https://www.aacnnursing.org/ccne-accreditation

Council on Accreditation of Nurse Anesthesia Educational Programs. (2024). *Accreditation policies and procedures manual, revised April 2024-1.* https://www.coacrna.org/wp-content/uploads/2024/03/Accreditation-Policies-and-Procedures-Manual-editorial-rev-Feb-2024-1.pdf

Frye, A. W., & Hemmer, P. A. (2012). Program evaluation models and related theories: AMEE guide no. 67. *Medical Teacher, 34*(5), e288–299. https://doi.org/10.3109/0142159x.2012.668637

Idzik, S., Buckley, K., Bindon, S., Gorschboth, S., Hammersla, M., Windemuth, B., & Bingham, D. (2021). Lessons learned using logic models to design and guide DNP projects. *Nurse Educator, 46*(5), E127–E131. https://doi.org/10.1097/nne.0000000000001025

Lewallen, L. P. (2023). Developing a systematic program evaluation plan for a school of nursing. In M. H. Oermann (Ed.), *A systematic approach to evaluation of nursing programs* (2nd ed., pp. 81–94). National League for Nursing.

McGhee, S., & Morrison-Beedy, D. (2024). A picture speaks a thousand words: Handling course evaluation data. *Nurse Educator, 49*(4), 205. https://doi.org/10.1097/NNE.0000000000001624

National Council for State Authorization Reciprocal Agreements. (2021). *Information and FAQs about the 21st century distance education guidelines, April 6, 2021*. https://nc-sara.org/sites/default/files/files/2021-04/21st_Century_Distance_Ed_Guidelines_Information_from_NC-SARA_06Apr21.pdf

National Council of State Boards of Nursing. (2024). *About U.S. nursing regulatory bodies*. https://www.ncsbn.org/nursing-regulation/about-nursing-regulatory-bodies.page

National League for Nursing Commission for Nursing Education Accreditation. (2021). *Accreditation standards for nursing education programs*. Accessed September 15, 2024. https://irp.cdn-website.com/cc12ee87/files/uploaded/CNEA%20Standards%20October%202021-4b271cb2.pdf

Oermann, M. H. (2017). Student evaluations of teaching: There is more to course evaluations than student ratings. *Nurse Educator, 42*(2), 55–56. https://doi.org/10.1097/nne.0000000000000366

Oermann, M. H. (2023). Program evaluation: What is it? In M. H. Oermann (Ed.), *A systematic approach to evaluation of nursing programs* (2nd ed., pp. 1–9). National League for Nursing/Wolters Kluwer.Oermann, M. H., Conklin, J. L., Rushton, S., & Bush, M. A. (2018). Student evaluations of teaching (SET): Guidelines for their use. *Nursing Forum, 53*(3), 280–285. https://doi.org/10.1111/nuf.12249

Oermann, M. H., Gaberson, K. B., & De Gagne, J. C. (2025). *Evaluation and testing in nursing education* (7th ed.). Springer Publishing Company.

Powell, N. J., Rubenstein, C., Sawin, E. M., & Annan, S. (2014). Student evaluations of teaching tools: A qualitative examination of student perceptions. *Nurse Educator, 39*(6), 274–279. https://doi.org/10.1097/NNE.0000000000000066

Shellenbarger, T. (2023). The accreditation process in nursing education. In M. H. Oermann (Ed.), *A systematic approach to evaluation of nursing programs* (2nd ed., pp. 66–80). National League for Nursing.

Stufflebeam, D. L., & Zhang, G. (2017). *The CIPP evaluation model: How to evaluate for improvement and accountability*. Guilford Press.

Scholarship, Service, and Leadership   VI

Evidence-Based Teaching in Nursing

19

Marilyn H. Oermann

OBJECTIVES

1. Describe evidence-based teaching in nursing, including each of its phases
2. Compare different types of evidence and the use of evidence in making educational decisions
3. Search for evidence about a teaching method

INTRODUCTION

Evidence-based teaching is the use of research findings and other evidence to guide educational decisions and practices. Available evidence should be used when developing the curriculum and courses, selecting teaching methods and approaches to use with students, planning clinical learning activities, and assessing students' learning and performance. Yet many nurse educators rarely search for evidence when they make educational decisions. They update their courses by incorporating new evidence about the content, but they might not seek evidence on how those courses are best designed, taught, and evaluated. How much practice do students need to retain their motor skills? What are best practices for debriefing? What characteristics of online courses are critical to learning and retention? These are the types of questions that every educator should be raising no matter what course or level of learner they are teaching.

Teachers can then search the literature for research studies and other evidence to answer these questions and guide their educational practices. By reviewing the literature, the teacher can also learn about the experiences of other educators to build on those rather than to start anew. This chapter describes evidence-based teaching in nursing, the need for more rigorous research in nursing education, and a process for engaging in evidence-based teaching.

EVIDENCE-BASED TEACHING IN NURSING: WHAT IS IT?

Evidence-based teaching is the use of research findings and other knowledge to guide educational practices in nursing. When making decisions about courses and teaching methods, including how to implement them, evidence generated from research in nursing and healthcare professions education informs those decisions. Nursing, medicine, education, and other fields have a body of knowledge that can be used to inform practice as a nurse, physician, or teacher: This knowledge provides the evidence to guide what we do. In evidence-based teaching, nurse educators use knowledge about how students learn, how best to promote their learning and performance, effective teaching and assessment methods, and other practices to guide what they do as educators.

Definitions of evidence-based nursing provide a framework for conceptualizing evidence-based teaching in nursing. Many of these definitions view evidence-based nursing as the integration of research evidence with clinical expertise and the values and preferences of the patient, resulting in better patient outcomes (Connor et al., 2023; Melnyk & Fineout-Overholt, 2019). Evidence-based teaching is the integration of the best research evidence with theories and concepts about learning, teaching, teaching strategies, assessment, and other areas related to nursing education with the teacher's own expertise and judgment and the learner's preferences and goals. Similar to evidence-based nursing, in evidence-based teaching, the goal is to use evidence to improve student learning outcomes.

NURSING EDUCATION RESEARCH AND EVIDENCE-BASED TEACHING

We need rigorous research in nursing education to generate evidence that can be used to guide teaching. Early on, many researchers explored nursing education topics, but over the years the focus of research has shifted to the study of clinical problems, with limited funding available for nursing education. Although the emphasis of nursing research is no longer on education, many nurse educators are conducting studies to build an evidence base for teaching. Some of these studies, however, involve small samples of students with investigator-developed tools that have not been validated. Educators should search for valid and reliable instruments to measure outcomes and if not available, should evaluate tools they developed before using them in a study. The lack of funding has made it difficult to conduct large, multisite educational studies in nursing and medicine (Gisondi et al., 2022; Oermann & Kardong-Edgren, 2018) and remains a barrier to implementing research with varied and diverse learners. However, evidence from rigorous studies done in one setting only using validated measurement tools can be accumulated similar to evidence-based practice. Studies can be replicated with different cohorts of students in a nursing program and by researchers in other schools to examine outcomes with varied learners (Oermann, 2020).

A critical need is for researchers in nursing education to measure learning outcomes and changes in performance rather than only student and faculty satisfaction with a new teaching practice or approach. Although important, satisfaction and what students perceive they have learned cannot be the only outcomes examined. Addressing these shortcomings is important to generalize the findings and determine whether the educational intervention or practice can be used with different students and settings.

Nurse educators develop many educational innovations and new initiatives, but without research to document their effectiveness and outcomes, it is not known whether the new approaches are better than the prior ones. Providing an evidence base for nursing education is not only important to advance the science of nursing education; faculty need evidence to make sound decisions about their teaching methods, considering the limited time available for student learning and extent of knowledge and skills students need to develop.

PHASES OF EVIDENCE-BASED TEACHING

Evidence-based teaching includes four phases: (a) questioning educational practices and identifying the need for evidence to guide teaching, (b) searching for research studies and other evidence on educational practices, (c) evaluating the quality of the evidence, and (d) deciding whether the findings are applicable to one's own program, courses, students, and context in which one is teaching. Similar to evidence-based practice in nursing and other fields, the teacher also considers theories and concepts about learning and teaching, and the teacher's own philosophy of nursing education and expertise as an educator. Students need to have input as to their preferences for learning and their personal goals to be met in the course. The evidence alone does not dictate what methods and practices to use. It is up to the teacher to integrate the evidence with these other considerations, as the teacher understands the students and context in which the education takes place.

Question Educational Practices and Identify Need for Evidence

The first phase in evidence-based teaching is for nurse educators to recognize that it is their responsibility to reflect on their educational practices and question whether there is a better way of teaching students. Reflection and questioning our practices as teachers are defining characteristics of a professional, and they are critical to thinking about changes in education that could lead to improved learning and performance.

The questions can be general questions about an educational practice or intervention being considered. These are descriptive questions that guide a search of the literature for information about the practice or intervention, but not necessarily about whether it is superior to others in terms of outcomes. Examples of these general questions are: How can team-based learning be used in online nursing courses? What are best practices in debriefing in simulation-based learning? These general questions are valuable too because they allow the teacher to learn about the experiences of other nurse educators.

Another type of question leads to a search for studies on the outcomes of various practices or interventions to make a decision on the best approach to use. Examples of this type of question include: Is there a difference in knowledge retention between online courses that use team-based learning and online courses with video recordings of lectures? Does the use of one specific debriefing or feedback intervention, compared to other types of debriefing or feedback interventions, improve educational and clinical outcomes in simulation-based education (Duff et al., 2024)? In nursing education, this type of question may be difficult to answer if sufficient research has not been done, or if the studies are of poor quality affecting the value of the findings for making educational decisions.

Search for Evidence on Educational Practices

In the second phase, teachers search the literature for studies on the topic and for other articles and resources to answer their questions. This research requires knowledge of bibliographic databases, search skills, and awareness of other resources, such as websites that report evidence on educational practices. Librarians are critical to locating and evaluating evidence. They can help with identifying questions to guide a search, have expertise in databases to search, and can develop an appropriate and a comprehensive search strategy. Nurse educators are advised to collaborate with librarians when searching for evidence for teaching.

Although there are many bibliographic databases that contain reports of studies that might be relevant to teaching in nursing, three databases are recommended for a search in nursing education:

1. MEDLINE, which has more than 36 million references to journal articles in biomedical and life sciences, including nursing education (U.S. National Library of Medicine [NLM], 2023). The MEDLINE database can be searched through PubMed, available at https://pubmed.ncbi.nlm.nih.gov/.

2. Cumulative Index to Nursing and Allied Health Literature (CINAHL), the database covering nursing and allied health literature (EBSCO, 2024).

3. Education Resources Information Center, from the Institute of Education Sciences, which indexes education research and also conference proceedings and other reports that might provide evidence about a teaching practice (Institute of Education Sciences, U.S. Department of Education [IES, USDE], n.d.).

For some questions, other bibliographic databases such as PsycINFO®, which covers research and other peer-reviewed literature in the behavioral and social sciences (American Psychological Association [APA], 2024), might be relevant, depending on the topic. It is important to search multiple databases because different journals are indexed in them, and thus a broad search of the literature provides a better evidence base.

The questions guide the search for studies. Nurse educators need to be proficient in *searching the literature*. They should be knowledgeable about the databases and the literature in them, as well as how they are organized. Educators should develop skills in selecting keywords, using controlled vocabularies (e.g., Medical Subject Headings [MeSH] terms in PubMed and subject headings in CINAHL), and combining search terms. Exhibit 19.1 lists strategies nurse educators can use to prepare themselves to conduct a search for evidence on teaching.

Evidence Synthesis

For areas of education that have been well studied, the teacher should begin by searching for an evidence synthesis in which experts critically appraise and synthesize the findings of multiple studies. While an individual study may suggest a teaching approach to use, that same approach may not be supported when multiple studies are considered as a whole. An evidence synthesis is a method that combines and analyzes findings of published studies with the aim of answering a research question (Gough et al., 2020). An evidence synthesis describes what is known and not known about an educational practice or intervention. One of the benefits of using a review of existing evidence is that it synthesizes multiple individual studies to arrive at a sound conclusion about the practice or intervention.

There are many types of evidence syntheses. One type is a systematic review in which researchers use an organized method of searching for studies, decide which studies to include in the review based on specific criteria, appraise the quality of

> **EXHIBIT 19.1 Strategies to Prepare for a Search**
>
> **Ask the Question**
>
> Learn how to ask clear and focused questions to guide a search.
>
> Develop a PICO(TS) question as applicable (P = population or problem, I = intervention, C = comparison, O = outcomes, T = timing [if relevant], and S = setting [if relevant]).
>
> If a PICO(TS) question is not appropriate, write a focused question you can use to guide your search.
>
> Collaborate with a librarian.
>
> Identify MeSH terms, subject headings, and text word terms for your topic or to answer your question.
>
> Find a few sample articles and confirm or alter the search terms.
>
> **Select and Search Appropriate Databases**
>
> Select relevant databases to search and use multiple databases.
>
> Become familiar with different bibliographic databases, including PubMed/MEDLINE, CINAHL, ERIC, PsycINFO, and others, depending on the subject.
>
> Review the types of literature indexed in each of the databases.
>
> Learn to use the databases through tutorials, help guides, and practice.
>
> Learn how to broaden and narrow a search, use filters, combine searches, conduct advanced searches, and use other search strategies in each database. (This skill is needed as you work with the librarian.)
>
> **Critically Evaluate the Search Terms and Process Based on Citations Returned**
>
> Be prepared to adjust or change search terms or strategies and/or databases used to match needs.
>
> Refer to Exhibit 19.2 for specifics on evaluating the nursing education studies retrieved in the search.
>
> **Organize Citations and Information Returned**
>
> Learn how to save searches, create collections, and manage citations as appropriate.
>
> Learn how to save and manage references in bibliographic management software.
>
> Review available resources such as the PRISMA (Preferred Reporting Items for Systematic Reviews and Meta-Analyses) checklist and flow diagram (http://www.prisma-statement.org/).
>
> Use the PRISMA checklist and flow diagram if conducting a systematic review or meta-analysis, and for recording search strategy for manuscripts.

each study, and synthesize the findings. As one example of a systematic review, Duff et al. (2024) analyzed 70 studies on debriefing in healthcare simulation to identify if a specific debriefing or feedback intervention, compared to other types of debriefing or feedback interventions, improved educational and clinical outcomes. There was insufficient evidence to support one debriefing strategy, framework, or technique over others.

When there are a sufficient number of systematic reviews done on a topic, an umbrella review might be conducted. An umbrella review is an analysis of systematic reviews, combining a large amount of evidence to reach conclusions about an educational practice or intervention. Metaverse is a virtual environment in which learners interact as avatars. With the aim of synthesizing evidence about the outcomes of metaverse in nursing education, De Gagne et al. (2023) analyzed

15 systematic reviews and found that metaverse interventions increased students' knowledge, self-confidence, and performance, and students found these virtual learning environments engaging.

Another type of evidence synthesis is a scoping review. The goal of a scoping review is to answer broad questions such as "What do we know about this topic or approach in nursing education?" by mapping all of the published research and other literature on the topic or practice to provide a comprehensive overview. Scoping reviews include evidence from any type of research method and may also include information from nonresearch publications (Peters et al., 2021). As an example, Poledna et al. (2022) conducted a scoping review on prelicensure nursing students' cue recognition during simulation to map the existing research and identify knowledge gaps. They analyzed 17 quantitative and qualitative studies using the Joanna Briggs Institute scoping review framework and found students often missed cues in simulations, such as not recognizing changes in respiratory rates, and in assessment as cues to patient deterioration (Poledna et al., 2022).

An integrative review summarizes empirical and theoretical literature to understand an educational topic or practice. These reviews include diverse types of literature and both experimental and nonexperimental studies (Whittemore & Knafl, 2005). For example, the aim of an integrative review, using the framework of Whittemore and Knafl, was to identify reasons for students' voluntary attrition from nursing programs. Ten studies were examined: Factors that influenced the decision to not continue in a nursing program were academic and emotional underpreparedness, financial challenges, and differences between the students' perceptions of nursing and their actual experiences in nursing practice, among others (Shaver & Viveiros, 2023).

A traditional literature review (a narrative review) is an examination of the literature from the author's perspective. The benefits of systematic reviews and other evidence syntheses are that only studies that meet certain criteria are included, the quality of individual studies is critiqued, and the reviews follow an established protocol. An issue with literature reviews is that they are frequently summaries of the findings of studies, with little analysis of their quality and the impact of that quality on the results. However, for some areas of nursing education, not enough research has been done to conduct a systematic or other type of review. A good example is a of a needed literature review is on policies in schools of nursing related to body art (tattoos and piercings; Pittman et al., 2022).

There are many other types of evidence syntheses that can be done to better understand the research in an area and generate evidence for teaching. Sutton et al. (2019) identified 48 types of reviews and grouped them in seven categories. Nurse educators should become familiar with varied types of reviews to select the most appropriate type to answer their questions and provide the evidence they are seeking for use in their teaching.

Individual Studies

When evidence syntheses and literature reviews are not available, the educator needs to review individual studies and critique their quality to determine whether the findings are valid, whether they answer the educational questions raised earlier in the process, and whether they will be useful considering the educator's own students and context; for example, were students randomly assigned to the teaching intervention and control groups, and were valid and reliable tools used to measure outcomes?

Flaws in the study design, the lack of a control or comparison group, use of measurement tools without established validity and reliability, issues with the procedures used for data collection (e.g., the teacher distributing surveys to their own students), errors in the statistical analysis, and so forth weaken the findings and limit their use.

Nurse educators also need to evaluate whether the results answer the questions identified for the review, support the educational practice or intervention, and are applicable to their own students and setting. The study might have been well designed, but a small sample in one school of nursing limits generalizing the findings to other groups of learners and settings. Exhibit 19.2 provides a general guide for analyzing nursing education research literature.

EXHIBIT 19.2 Guide for Analyzing Nursing Education Research Literature

Title
  Does it clearly describe the educational study reported in the paper? Is it informative?

Abstract
  Does it emphasize the study's purpose, method, major findings, and conclusions?
  Is this a quantitative, qualitative, or mixed-methods study in nursing education?

Introduction
  Does it state the problem in nursing education and why it is important to learn more about it?
  Does the introduction provide the background and rationale for the study?
  What is the purpose of the study, and is it clear and understandable?
  If a conceptual or theoretical framework is presented, does it relate to the purpose and describe the concepts underlying the study and their relationships?

Literature Review
  Is the literature critically reviewed?
  Are strengths and weaknesses of prior studies included in the review?
  Does the review support the reason for conducting the study and identify gaps in our understanding of how best to promote student learning, teach students, develop nursing programs, and so forth?
  Is the literature review up to date?
  Are key studies included in the literature review? What is missing?
  Are primary sources used?

Research Questions
  Are the research questions clear, specific, and stated appropriately?
  Are variables defined if appropriate?

Design
  Is the design consistent with the questions?
  What type of design is used?
  What are strengths and weaknesses of the design?

Sample
  What criteria were used to select the sample?
  Is the sample size adequate?
  Is the sample representative of learners, teachers, nursing programs, and so forth?

(continued)

> **EXHIBIT 19.2 Guide for Analyzing Nursing Education Research Literature** (*continued*)
>
> **Instruments**
> - Are the instruments and other measures described, and are they appropriate?
> - Are they valid and reliable?
>
> **Data Collection Procedure**
> - Is the procedure clearly described?
> - Are methods for collecting and analyzing qualitative data appropriate for the type of study?
>
> **Findings**
> - Are the findings interpreted correctly, including any statistical analyses?
> - Are the statistics appropriate for analyzing the data?
> - Are the findings presented clearly and in relation to the study questions or hypotheses?
> - Are the findings presented logically?
> - Are tables and figures easy to read, and do they support the text?
> - Are the statistics in the tables and figures and the statistics in the text consistent?
>
> **Discussion**
> - Is the discussion related to the literature, and does it include how the study builds on earlier research in nursing education (and higher education if relevant)?
> - Are the limitations identified, and could they have been resolved?
> - Can the findings be generalized and, if so, to what populations?
> - Are there implications for teaching, assessment, program development, and so forth, and are they relevant?
> - Are the conclusions based on the study results and are they accurate?
>
> **Strengths and Weaknesses**
> - Overall, what are the study's major strengths and weaknesses?

Source: Adapted from Oermann, M. H. (2024). *Writing for publication in nursing* (5th ed.). Springer Publishing Company.

Evaluate the Quality of the Evidence

There are many systems for rating the quality of the evidence that can be applied to nursing education. In traditional rating systems, evidence from systematic reviews and meta-analyses is at the highest level. These are followed by randomized controlled trials, then cohort studies (e.g., two groups or cohorts of students, one receives the educational intervention and the other does not); case control and descriptive studies; and last, expert opinion, the lowest level (Figure 19.1). The stronger the evidence, the more likely that it is valid and relevant for a particular educational situation.

As an example, a systematic review examined the effectiveness of peer video feedback on healthcare students' learning outcomes compared to other types of feedback, such as feedback from experts. The researchers reviewed 22 studies and concluded that peer video feedback was valuable for learning and had a positive effect on skill performance. Although students were satisfied with feedback from peers, they were concerned about its accuracy (Zhang et al., 2022).

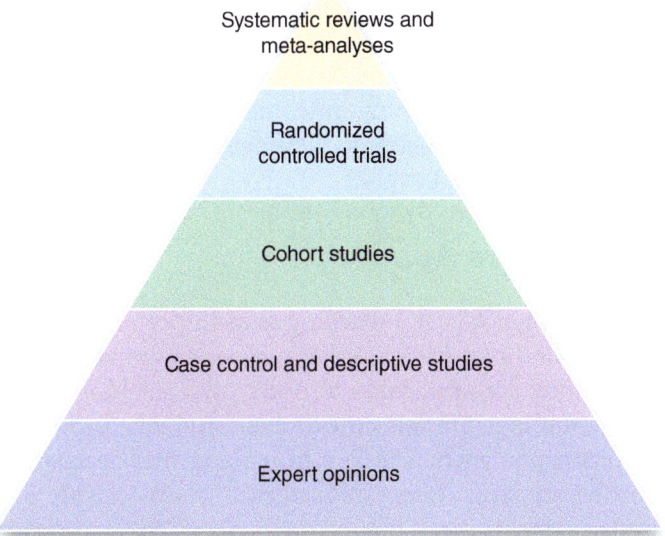

Figure 19.1 Levels of evidence.

In a qualitative study, Yoong et al. (2023) explored the accuracy and quality of peer feedback provided to first-year nursing students after simulated practice and the discrepancies in how skills were taught by faculty, peer tutors, and clinical staff. They concluded that with training, senior nursing students could provide detailed feedback to juniors, but they also found that expectations relating to each nursing skill differed among peer tutors, faculty members, and clinical staff. These two studies both address peer feedback. However, the systematic review of 22 studies provides stronger evidence on the outcomes than does the single qualitative study.

Another model that can be used to appraise educational evidence is Kirkpatrick's Four-Level Evaluation Model; the four levels for evaluation are:

1. Learners' reaction: How well did the students like the learning process? Were they actively involved? Will they have the opportunity to use the information in their practice?

2. Learning: What did they learn (e.g., the extent to which the learners gained knowledge, skills, attitudes, confidence, and commitment as a result of their education)?

3. Changes in behavior: What changes in behavior resulted from the learning process (e.g., changes in the learner's ability to perform newly learned skills)?

4. Results: What are the tangible results or outcomes of learning (Kirkpatrick & Kirkpatrick, 2016; Kirkpatrick Partners, 2022)?

Nursing education studies that examine learners' perceptions of and satisfaction with an educational practice or intervention, curriculum, course, teaching or assessment method, learning activity, and so forth, are at the lowest level (Level 1: Reactions). At the next level are studies that measure changes in the learners' knowledge, skills, attitudes, and confidence as a result of the education (Level 2: Learning). The next level of studies evaluates changes in performance and behaviors, such as ability to perform a new skill and transfer learning to the clinical setting (Level 3: Changes in Behavior). At Level 4: Results, outcomes of the educational practice or intervention are measured. As an example, Griffiths et al. (2022) conducted a scoping review of 56 studies to map educational strategies used in master's and doctoral nursing programs and categorized the learning outcomes based on the Kirkpatrick model. Most of the research assessed reactions of students (their satisfaction, Level 1) or their learning (knowledge gain, Level 2).

Decide if Findings Are Applicable

The fourth phase of evidence-based teaching is as important as the earlier phases: deciding whether the findings are ready for implementation based on the evidence and, if so, whether they are applicable to one's own teaching situation. Teachers should assess if the findings are relevant to their students, program, courses, and the context in which they teach. The key in making this decision is whether the characteristics of the students, nurse educators, and other aspects of the nursing program are similar to the research that has been done. The findings from a systematic review of studies with students in prelicensure nursing programs might not be applicable for teaching nurses and other staff. Studies done in a small school of nursing might not be transferable to a large school with a diverse student population.

Studies of the processes used by nurse educators to adopt evidence in their own courses and teaching are needed (Oermann, 2022; Oermann, Reynolds, & Granger, 2022). How do faculty and nurse educators in other settings implement new educational approaches? As a next step, if a new approach or educational intervention is adopted, studies should be planned to evaluate its effectiveness. Is the new method better than the previous one? Did it improve learning and performance? What outcomes changed as a result of this new approach? The goal is to design studies that measure outcomes other than satisfaction and student and faculty perceptions. Study designs and methods need to generate strong evidence that can be used to guide future decisions about teaching in nursing.

SUMMARY

Evidence-based teaching is the use of research findings and other evidence to guide educational decisions and practices. Available evidence should be used when developing the curriculum and courses, selecting teaching methods and approaches to use with students, planning clinical learning activities, and assessing students' learning and performance. This evidence is generated from rigorous pedagogical research; for findings to be useful to nurse educators, they must be valid and the result of well-designed studies. Studies in nursing education need to be replicated and include diverse samples of learners, teachers, and programs to determine whether the educational practice or method is applicable across settings and with varied student groups.

Evidence-based teaching includes four phases: (a) questioning educational practices and identifying the need for evidence to guide teaching, (b) searching for research studies and other evidence on educational practices, (c) evaluating the quality of the evidence, and (d) deciding whether the findings are applicable to one's own program, courses, students, and the context in which one is teaching.

Teachers also consider theories and concepts about learning and teaching, their own philosophy of nursing education, and their expertise as educators. The learner needs to have input and consideration as to preferences for learning and personal goals to be met in the course. The evidence alone does not dictate the educational practices to use. It is up to the teacher to integrate the evidence with these other considerations.

The first phase in evidence-based teaching is for nurse educators to reflect on their educational practices and to question whether there is a better way of teaching students. In the second phase, teachers search the literature for studies done on the topic and other articles and resources to answer their questions. This phase requires knowledge of databases to search, ability to conduct a search, and knowledge of other resources that might be relevant.

For areas of education that have been well studied, the teacher should begin by searching for an evidence synthesis such as a systematic review in which experts appraise and synthesize the findings of multiple studies on a particular educational topic to arrive at conclusions about best practices. When evidence syntheses are not available, the teacher should search for literature reviews or locate individual studies and critique their quality. Typically, a few studies on an educational practice will not be sufficient to make a major educational change.

There are many systems for rating the quality of the evidence that can be applied to nursing education, such as traditional rating systems (from systematic reviews and meta-analyses as the highest levels to expert opinion as the lowest level) and Kirkpatrick's Four-Level Evaluation Model. The fourth phase of evidence-based teaching involves deciding if the findings are ready for implementation and, if so, if they are relevant for the nurse educator's own students, program, courses, and context.

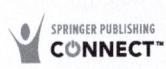 A robust set of instructor resources designed to supplement this text is located at http://connect.springerpub.com/content/book/978-0-8261-8892-2. Qualifying instructors may request access by emailing textbook@springerpub.com.

REFERENCES

American Psychological Association. (2024). *PsycINFO®*. https://www.apa.org/pubs/databases/psycinfo

Connor, L., Dean, J., McNett, M., Tydings, D. M., Shrout, A., Gorsuch, P. F., Hole, A., Moore, L., Brown, R., Melnyk, B. M., & Gallagher-Ford, L. (2023). Evidence-based practice improves patient outcomes and healthcare system return on investment: Findings from a scoping review. *Worldviews on Evidence-Based Nursing, 20*(1), 6–15. https://doi.org/https://doi.org/10.1111/wvn.12621

De Gagne, J. C., Randall, P. S., Rushton, S., Park, H. K., Cho, E., Yamane, S. S., & Jung, D. (2023). The use of metaverse in nursing education: An umbrella review. *Nurse Educator, 48*(3), E73–e78. https://doi.org/10.1097/nne.0000000000001327

Duff, J. P., Morse, K. J., Seelandt, J., Gross, I. T., Lydston, M., Sargeant, J., Dieckmann, P., Allen, J. A., Rudolph, J. W., & Kolbe, M. (2024). Debriefing methods for simulation in healthcare: A systematic review. *Simulation in Healthcare, 19*(1s), S112–S121. https://doi.org/10.1097/sih.0000000000000765

EBSCO. (2024). *CINAHL database*. https://www.ebsco.com/products/research-databases/cinahl-database

Gisondi, M. A., Michael, S., Li-Sauerwine, S., Brazil, V., Caretta-Weyer, H. A., Issenberg, B., Giordano, J., Lineberry, M., Olson, A. S., Burkhardt, J. C., & Chan, T. M. (2022). The purpose, design, and promise of medical education research labs. *Academic Medicine, 97*(9), 1281–1288. https://doi.org/10.1097/acm.0000000000004746

Gough, D., Davies, P., Jamtvedt, G., Langlois, E., Littell, J., Lotfi, T., Masset, E., Merlin, T., Pullin, A. S., Ritskes-Hoitinga, M., Røttingen, J. A., Sena, E., Stewart, R., Tovey, D., White, H., Yost, J., Lund, H., & Grimshaw, J. (2020). Evidence Synthesis International (ESI): Position statement. *Systematic Reviews, 9*(1), 155. https://doi.org/10.1186/s13643-020-01415-5

Griffiths, M., Creedy, D., Carter, A., & Donnellan-Fernandez, R. (2022). Systematic review of interventions to enhance preceptors' role in undergraduate health student clinical learning. *Nurse Education in Practice, 62*, 103349. https://doi.org/10.1016/j.nepr.2022.103349

Institute of Education Sciences. (n.d.). *ERIC: Educational Resources Information Center*. U.S. Department of Education. Accessed September 15, 2024. https://ies.ed.gov/ncee/projects/eric.asp#:~:text=ERIC%20is%20an%20internet%2Dbased,from%201966%20to%20the%20present

Kirkpatrick, J. D., & Kirkpatrick, W. K. (2016). *Kirkpatrick's four levels of training evaluation*. ATD Press.

Kirkpatrick Partners. (2022). *An introduction to The New World Kirkpatrick® Model*. Accessed September 15, 2024. https://www.kirkpatrickpartners.com/wp-content/uploads/2021/11/Introduction-to-The-New-World-Kirkpatrick%C2%AE-Model.pdf

Melnyk, B. M., & Fineout-Overholt, E. (2019). *Evidence-based practice in nursing and healthcare: A guide to best practice* (4th ed.). Wolters Kluwer Health.

Oermann, M. H. (2020). Nursing education research: A new era. *Nurse Educator, 45*(3), 115. https://doi.org/10.1097/NNE.0000000000000830

Oermann, M. H. (2022). Adopting evidence-based educational approaches in nursing: Using implementation science. *Nurse Educator, 47*(5), 259–260. https://doi.org/10.1097/nne.0000000000001257

Oermann, M. H. (2024). *Writing for publication in nursing* (5th ed.). Springer Publishing.

Oermann, M. H., & Kardong-Edgren, S. K. (2018). Changing the conversation about doctoral education in nursing: What about research in nursing education? *Nursing Outlook, 66*(6), 523–525. https://doi.org/10.1016/j.outlook.2018.10.001

Oermann, M. H., Reynolds, S. S., & Granger, B. B. (2022). Using an implementation science framework to advance the science of nursing education. *Journal of Professional Nursing, 39*, 139–145. https://doi.org/10.1016/j.profnurs.2022.01.014

Peters, M. D. J., Marnie, C., Tricco, A. C., Pollock, D., Munn, Z., Alexander, L., McInerney, P., Godfrey, C. M., & Khalil, H. (2021). Updated methodological guidance for the conduct of scoping reviews. *JBI Evidence Implementation, 19*(1), 3–10. https://doi.org/10.1097/xeb.0000000000000277

Pittman, A., Gary, J., & Pepper, C. (2022). An integrative review of body art in nursing. *Nurse Educator, 47*(4), 197–201. https://doi.org/10.1097/nne.0000000000001168

Poledna, M., Gómez-Morales, A., & Hagler, D. (2022). Nursing students' cue recognition in educational simulation: A scoping review. *Nurse Educator, 47*(5), 283–287. https://doi.org/10.1097/nne.0000000000001198

Shaver, D. E., & Viveiros, J. D. (2023). Voluntary attrition among traditional baccalaureate nursing students: An integrative review. *Nursing Education Perspectives, 45*(3), 150–154. https://doi.org/10.1097/01.Nep.0000000000001215

Sutton, A., Clowes, M., Preston, L., & Booth, A. (2019). Meeting the review family: exploring review types and associated information retrieval requirements. *Health Information and Libraries Journal, 36*(3), 202–222. https://doi.org/10.1111/hir.12276

United States National Library of Medicine. (2023). *PubMed overview*. https://pubmed.ncbi.nlm.nih.gov/about/

Whittemore, R., & Knafl, K. (2005). The integrative review: Updated methodology. *Journal of Advanced Nursing, 52*(5), 546–553. https://doi.org/10.1111/j.1365-2648.2005.03621.x

Yoong, S. Q., Wang, W., Seah, A. C. W., & Zhang, H. (2023). The quality of verbal feedback given by nursing near-peer tutors: A qualitative study. *Nurse Education Today, 130*, 105944. https://doi.org/10.1016/j.nedt.2023.105944

Zhang, H., Liao, A. W. X., Goh, S. H. L., Yoong, S. Q., Lim, A. X. M., & Wang, W. (2022). Effectiveness and quality of peer video feedback in health professions education: A systematic review. *Nurse Education Today, 109*, 105203. https://doi.org/10.1016/j.nedt.2021.105203

Becoming a Scholar in Nursing Education

Marilyn H. Oermann

20

OBJECTIVES

1. Discuss scholarship of teaching in nursing and various forms of scholarship
2. Examine the process of becoming a scholar in nursing education
3. Describe the process of and guidelines for writing for publication
4. Identify strategies for the assessment of scholarship including a teaching portfolio

INTRODUCTION

The role of the nurse educator includes more than teaching, assessing learning, and developing courses: It also includes scholarship and contributing to the development of nursing education as a science. Research in nursing education is essential, but scholarship is more than studies about students, teachers, and programs: Scholarship can be conceptualized broadly as inquiry about learning and teaching. Scholars in nursing education question and search for new ideas; they debate and think beyond how it has "always been done." For the teacher's work to be considered as scholarship, it needs to be public, peer-reviewed and critiqued, and shared with others so they can build on that work. This chapter examines scholarship in nursing education and developing one's role as a scholar. Because of the importance of dissemination to scholarship, the chapter includes a brief description of the process of writing for publication and other strategies for dissemination. The development of a teaching portfolio to document teaching excellence and scholarship is also discussed. This chapter builds on Chapter 1, which examined career development as a nurse educator.

SCHOLARSHIP OF TEACHING IN NURSING

Scholarship is essential to nursing education because without it our educational practices cannot develop further. It is through research and other forms of scholarship that teachers make contributions to the science, the body of knowledge, of nursing education. There are many different views about the scholarship of teaching. Scholarship in nursing education can be conceptualized broadly as inquiry about learning and teaching. That inquiry can involve developing new concepts about learning, systematic reflection on learning and teaching that becomes public, the discovery of new knowledge and evidence on educational practices, and translating and using research findings to guide teaching. Through scholarship about teaching and learning, teachers provide evidence to guide educational practices and disseminate that evidence widely through various methods such as articles in peer-reviewed journals.

Nurse educators engage in a wide range of teaching activities. These activities include developing the curriculum and courses, teaching innovations, learning activities for students, and assessment methods and implementing them: These are the practices of teaching in nursing. Sharing these practices through articles, presentations at conferences, and social media enables other educators to adopt these strategies in their own courses and to evaluate outcomes with their students, building evidence for teaching. Activities in which nurse educators engage when teaching others, however, may not reflect scholarly teaching. Scholarly teaching involves using research findings and evidence to guide teaching, assessment, and other educational practices. Scholarship of teaching is inquiry about student learning and development, and about teaching innovations (Oermann, 2017). To be considered scholarship, the work needs to be disseminated.

Boyer's Forms of Scholarship

Views about the scholarship of teaching in nursing education have been influenced significantly by Boyer (1990) and Glassick et al. (1997), who provided a broader view of scholarship than only formal research. Boyer's forms of scholarship were introduced earlier in Chapter 1 and Table 1.4, with examples of evidence of each type. Boyer believed that scholarship also involves searching for connections, building bridges between theory and practice, and communicating one's knowledge to learners. He identified four separate but overlapping forms of scholarship:

1. Scholarship of discovery: conducting original research that expands current knowledge and understanding in a field
2. Scholarship of integration: developing connections across disciplines and synthesizing research done by others, essential for evidence-based teaching
3. Scholarship of application: applying knowledge to practice and translating research findings into practical interventions that solve problems
4. Scholarship of teaching: engaging in inquiry that focuses on student learning resulting from our educational practices (Boyer, 1990)

Scholarship of Teaching in Nursing

The scholarship of teaching in nursing needs to embrace the many forms that scholarship can take. This includes:

- Original research that uncovers how students learn best and how to promote learning
- Evaluation studies of educational practices, methods, and approaches
- Reviews of research that synthesize knowledge and provide evidence for educational practices and decisions

- Development and application of concepts and theories to guide teaching and assessment, which lead to dissemination
- Development of educational innovations, initiatives, new programs, courses, teaching methods, and assessment methods, among others, that are systematically evaluated (Oermann, 2017)

The scholarship of teaching in nursing can take any of these forms, but it is not the same as excellence in teaching, evidenced by outstanding student evaluations. It also is not the same as scholarly teaching, which is teaching grounded in sound principles and reflecting well-designed strategies of course design, transmission, interaction with learners, and assessment (Shulman, 2000). Scholarship involves inquiry and reflection, the development of products as a result of the scholarly work, and their dissemination. By disseminating one's scholarship, peers can critique its quality and use the information in their own teaching if relevant. The most common product of teachers' scholarship is a published article about education in a peer-reviewed journal, but examples of other products are book chapters; books; instructional manuals; editorials; descriptions of teaching methods and materials, learning activities of students, educational innovations, a program or course, assessment strategies, new instruments and tools, and simulations; and development of media and technology for teaching (American Association of Colleges of Nursing [AACN], 2018; Oermann, 2017; Pinto et al., 2021; Smith & Walker, 2024).

BECOMING A SCHOLAR IN NURSING EDUCATION

To be considered scholarship, the work needs to be public, open to peer review and critique, and shared with other nurse educators, so they, in turn, can build on that work. Educational studies disseminated beyond a school of nursing can be replicated, and findings can be accumulated. Dissemination is critical to build evidence for teaching in nursing.

Meeting these three criteria transforms the teacher's work as an educator into scholarship. Nurse educators can begin this process by reflecting on their educational practices and experiences, which may lead to the development of new teaching methods or approaches to use with students. As a second phase in this process, educators can discuss their ideas, reflections, new teaching methods and approaches, and other aspects of teaching with colleagues in their school of nursing or other settings. This sharing helps educators refine ideas and provides an opportunity for feedback before disseminating scholarly work more widely. However, at some point, to be considered scholarship, the work needs to be disseminated. Table 20.1 summarizes the phases in the process of becoming a scholar in nursing education.

DISSEMINATING YOUR SCHOLARSHIP

One of the issues related to the scholarship of teaching in nursing is that too few nurse educators share their work. There are many lost opportunities to spread new ideas and innovations: Nurse educators in one setting develop an educational innovation and evaluate its effectiveness, but they never share that work

TABLE 20.1 PROCESS OF BECOMING A SCHOLAR IN NURSING EDUCATION

Phase 1: Reflect on Own Educational Practices	Phase 2: Share With Colleagues	Phase 3: Develop Own Scholarship of Teaching
Reflect on own teaching practices: Are students learning?	Engage in conversations about teaching and learning with others	Integrate nursing education research and evidence in teaching
Gather data about own educational practices and quality of teaching (e.g., review student evaluations of teaching, ask for peer evaluations)	Develop expertise in an area of nursing education and be recognized for that in your school or other setting	Conduct studies, evaluate teaching innovations and practices, and develop products of own scholarship of teaching
Read nursing education literature	Attend nursing education conferences and discuss ideas about teaching and possible approaches with colleagues	Publish articles in peer-reviewed journals, present scholarly work at conferences, and disseminate work through other venues
Develop expertise as a nurse educator	Expand knowledge base about teaching and learning	Become an expert in an area of nursing education and know the research done on that topic
Seek guidance and mentoring from nursing educator researchers and scholars	Mentor novice teachers	Mentor others on research and developing their scholarship of teaching

with others. There are many venues for teachers to disseminate the products of their scholarship to make them public and accessible for critique and use by others. They can present their scholarship at conferences, both nursing education and others; describe their work in newsletters; post summaries of their studies, projects, and innovations on relevant websites; report at faculty meetings, which provide an opportunity for critique; and disseminate their scholarly work through publications. Articles published in peer-reviewed journals provide the widest dissemination, spreading the ideas to other educators for consideration and use in their own teaching. When research findings are published, these results can be synthesized to generate evidence for teaching, as discussed in Chapter 19.

Writing for Publication

Publications in peer-reviewed journals are a requirement for promotion and tenure in many schools of nursing; this is another reason for teachers to disseminate their scholarship through publications. Even if not required for promotion and tenure, writing for publication is important for career development in any setting and is essential for disseminating new ideas for use by others. Nurse educators need to understand the criteria for contract renewal, promotion, and tenure in their school of nursing and the importance given to journal publications. In some settings, databased articles (papers that report the findings of research studies) published in peer-reviewed journals (also called refereed journals) are considered more important in these decisions than descriptive articles, chapters, and books about teaching and other educational topics. Peer-reviewed journals—for example, *Nurse Educator, Journal of Nursing Education, Journal of Professional Nursing, Nursing Education Perspectives, Nurse Education Today, Nurse Education in Practice,* and *Journal of Continuing Education in Nursing,* among others—have experts (peers) who critically evaluate manuscripts submitted to the journal, ensuring their quality.

Identify the Purpose of the Manuscript

In planning the dissemination of the teacher's scholarship, the first step is to identify the purpose of the manuscript (Oermann, 2024). The term *manuscript* is the unpublished paper; once published, it is referred to as an article. The purpose of the manuscript might be to share new ideas and concepts about learning and teaching in nursing; describe a nursing program or course; present a research study and findings or the results of an evaluation of an educational innovation; or report other educational topics. The purpose guides the development of the manuscript, and it should be stated early in the paper.

As part of the planning phase, the educator should do a quick review of the literature to assess what has already been published on the topic. A manuscript should present new information for readers. The literature review might reveal that the teacher's ideas and topic for dissemination have been reported by others. Then the key is to identify how the scholarly work builds on those ideas and provides new knowledge for readers.

Identify Possible Journals

Prior to beginning to write the paper, the teacher selects possible journals for submission of the manuscript. One consideration is whether readers of the journal would be interested in the topic. For example, if the manuscript reports the findings of a study on concept maps, potential readers would be nursing faculty members, and a journal intended for academic nurse educators would be more appropriate than one for nurse educators in professional development. In contrast, a manuscript on a virtual simulation to improve interprofessional collaboration would be of interest to nurse educators in schools of nursing and clinical settings, and to other healthcare professions educators, expanding the number of possible journals. It is also important to determine whether the journal publishes the type of manuscript being planned. Some journals publish mainly research in nursing education, whereas others do not.

There are hundreds of possible journals in which nurse educators can publish their scholarship. To search for appropriate journals, educators can use directories of journals available on the web. One of these directories is the Directory of Nursing Journals, maintained by the International Academy of Nursing Editors at https://nursingeditors.com/journals-directory/.

Another way to locate possible journals is to search in the Journal/Author Name Estimator (JANE) at https://jane.biosemantics.org/. With this website a search can be done using the title and/or abstract of a paper, or by keywords. For example, an abstract of a paper or poster presented at a nursing education conference can be pasted into the search box, or the educator could enter some keywords that reflect the topic of the intended manuscript. By clicking "find journals," a list of journals that publish those topics is provided for the educator to review. JANE searches for journals in PubMed (the search engine for accessing MEDLINE, the database of references in the life sciences and biomedical literature) and indicates if the journal is only in PubMed or if it is indexed in MEDLINE. To be in MEDLINE, the Literature Selection Technical Review Committee reviews and recommends biomedical and health-related journals for inclusion (National Library of Medicine [NLM], 2024). Journals also are reviewed before they are included in the Cumulative Index to Nursing and Allied Health Literature (CINAHL), Scopus, and Web of Science to ensure they meet quality standards. Nurse educators are advised to submit their manuscripts to journals indexed in one of these bibliographic databases—MEDLINE, CINAHL, Scopus, or Web of Science—to avoid submitting to a predatory (not reputable) journal. Predatory journals are not in those databases because journals are evaluated first for inclusion (Oermann et al., 2021, 2022).

Educators should select about five possible journals for submission, rank-order them, and prepare their manuscript consistent with the selected journal's author guidelines, which are available at the journal's website. A short query e-mail can be sent to the editors of the potential journals to determine their interest, although doing so is not essential. Although a manuscript can be submitted to only one journal at a time, query e-mails can be sent to multiple editors. If the manuscript is rejected by a journal, the nurse educator at that point can revise the paper and submit it to the next journal on the rank-order list.

Develop Skill in Using Reference Management Software

Accuracy in citations in the manuscript and in reference lists at the end is critical. Nurse educators need to develop their skill in using reference management software such as EndNote™ (Clarivate; https://endnote.com/), PaperPile (https://paperpile.com/), Zotero (https://www.zotero.org/), or other programs. EndNote and PaperPile have a fee, but Zotero is available for download at no cost. This software allows the educator to create citations and reference lists formatted in the reference style used by the journal. Most nurse educators are familiar with the reference style of the American Psychological Association (APA, 2020), but not all journals use the APA style. Some journals use a numbered citation format, such as the *AMA Manual of Style* (American Medical Association [AMA], 2020). The journal's author guidelines specify the style to use when preparing references.

Write a Draft

Prior to writing the first draft, the author should develop an outline of the content. The outline is a guide to writing the first draft and ensuring that essential content is included in the paper. The outline also allows the teacher to plan the approximate number of pages to write for each content area and to avoid preparing a manuscript that is too short or too long. Although journals have different limits on the number of pages for a manuscript, the allowed length is typically between 15 and 18 double-spaced pages, using 12 pt. font and 1-inch margins.

The goal of the first draft is to write quickly and without concern about grammar and writing style (Oermann, 2024). It is critical in this phase to include the citations as the content is developed. When the content is drafted sufficiently, the grammar, punctuation, writing style, and format can be revised. In preparing the final version of the paper, the teacher should explicitly follow the author guidelines in terms of format.

Submit the Paper for Peer Review

When the manuscript is submitted to the journal, it is then peer reviewed. Peer review is conducted by content experts who serve as reviewers for the journal. These experts evaluate the manuscript, identifying its strengths and weaknesses, and suggest revisions. The peer-review process ensures that articles published in the journal are of high quality and have accurate and up-to-date content; peers also critique the research methods if the paper reports a nursing education study (Oermann, 2024). In most nursing journals, peer review is a double-blind review: The author does not know who reviewed the paper, and the reviewers are unaware of the author's identity, removing potential bias.

Typically, reviewers rate the quality of the manuscript on a web-based form and provide a narrative summary of their critique of the paper. An example of a review form is in Table 20.2. The narrative summary is usually provided to the author with the editor's comments and decision about acceptance. Authors submit their manuscript at the journal website, and communication with the author, including the results of the peer review comments, are done electronically.

The editor may accept the manuscript without or with revisions, ask the author to revise and resubmit the paper for another review, or reject it. In revising the manuscript, the author should make the suggested revisions or provide a rationale for not making them (Oermann, 2024). A summary of the revisions proposed and made in the manuscript (addressing each suggested change) needs to be submitted with the revised paper. For rejected manuscripts, the author should consider the feedback from the reviewers, modify the paper as appropriate, and submit it to the next journal on the list established earlier.

PRESENTATIONS AT CONFERENCES AND OTHER DISSEMINATION METHODS

For scholarship not ready for dissemination in peer-reviewed journals, nurse educators should plan to disseminate their scholarship via other venues, such as presenting it at nursing education and other conferences. The educator can begin by presenting a paper at local, state, and regional conferences and then progress to national and international ones. Organizations such as the National League for Nursing (NLN), Sigma, and the regional nursing research societies (e.g., Midwest Nursing Research Society) sponsor education summits and conferences at which teachers can present their work. These venues also provide an opportunity to engage in discussions about teaching and scholarship, critical to developing as a scholar in nursing education.

TABLE 20.2 EXAMPLE OF FORM FOR PEER REVIEW OF MANUSCRIPT

Yes	No	Comments
–	–	Does the paper present new findings or ideas about nursing education?
		Is the content:
–	–	Timely/relevant?
–	–	Logically and clearly developed?
–	–	Sophisticated enough for our readers?
–	–	Innovative?
–	–	Introduction: Is the purpose of the paper clear?
		Methods (*research paper*):
–	–	Are the sample and sampling method adequate?
–	–	Are the instruments reliable and valid?
–	–	Are statistical tests appropriate?
		Methods (*other types of papers*):
–	–	Were the objectives clearly identified?
–	–	Were the outcomes evaluated adequately?
–	–	Do conclusions and implications go beyond what findings support?
–	–	Are the references current (the majority are within the past 3–5 years)?
–	–	Does the content include implications for teaching in nursing? Other implications for nursing education?
–	–	Was the paper interesting to read?
Recommendation: Accept for publication without revision Accept for publication after satisfactory revision Review again after major revision Reject		
Confidential Comments to Editor:		
Comments to Author:		

ASSESSMENT OF SCHOLARSHIP

In most settings in which nurse educators work, the quality of their teaching; scholarship; service to the nursing program and university, community, and profession; and clinical practice, if relevant, is assessed to provide feedback to the teacher (formative evaluation) and for annual performance reviews and personnel decisions (summative evaluation). These personnel decisions include contract renewal, promotion, and tenure. Students contribute to the assessment of teaching through their evaluations at the end of a course or clinical practicum and through other feedback they provide the faculty member during the course. Faculty may ask a colleague for feedback on their course, teaching methods, assignments, and other components, and peers may complete a formal observation of the faculty member's teaching (peer review). These were discussed in Chapter 18.

Peers also evaluate a faculty member's scholarship. This is done formatively when colleagues review the educator's accomplishments in terms of scholarship (research, grants submitted and received, publications, presentations, and evaluations of teaching approaches, among others) and provide feedback, suggestions, and mentoring. Peers also evaluate scholarship through reviews by formal committees such as the appointment, promotion, and tenure committee. Those reviews, however, are summative, documenting what has been accomplished to date. It is important for the educator's career development to get feedback and mentoring prior to these formal reviews. The administrator to whom the faculty member reports (e.g., the chair, assistant or associate dean, director, or dean depending on the organization of the school of nursing) also conducts an evaluation of a faculty member's scholarship. This is done for annual reviews, contract renewals, and promotion and tenure decisions. Most important is that teachers periodically reflect on and assess the quality of their own teaching and scholarship.

Teaching Portfolio

A teaching portfolio or dossier is a collection of materials selected by nurse educators to document the quality of their teaching, illustrate their creativity in teaching, present innovative teaching and assessment methods they have developed for their courses, and provide documentation of their overall teaching effectiveness. Teaching portfolios can be used to improve teaching (formative evaluation), providing an organized collection of documents for review and critique by others. Or, they may be submitted to the administrator to whom the faculty member reports and to committees such as the appointment, promotion, and review committee for formal peer review (summative evaluation). Types of documents typically included in the portfolio are listed in Exhibit 20.1. These provide a source of data for assessment by others of the nurse educator's expertise in teaching.

CAREER DEVELOPMENT

Chapter 1 explored the nurse educator role and career development in that role. In developing as a scholar, the teacher might need additional preparation and mentoring. Nurse educators need to set short- and long-term career goals for their scholarship and identify areas in which they need further learning and skills development. For some educators, additional course work might be required; for others,

> **EXHIBIT 20.1 Types of Documents Included in Teaching Portfolios**
>
> Philosophy of teaching and goals for teaching
>
> Syllabi
>
> Sample teaching methods and materials, student learning activities and assignments, assessment methods, evaluation tools, among others
>
> Innovations in teaching and descriptions of their success
>
> Descriptions of technologies developed for teaching
>
> Descriptions of and documents related to new courses and programs developed in school of nursing (with individual contributions described if work was done by a team)
>
> Publications of educational studies, teaching and assessment methods, innovations, new initiatives, and other types of scholarship of teaching
>
> Presentations related to education
>
> Educational grants
>
> Teaching awards and other recognition of teaching effectiveness
>
> Peer evaluations of teaching

continuing education programs and workshops such as those offered by the NLN, the AACN, other organizations, and schools of nursing will be adequate to meet their learning needs and advance their scholarship.

SUMMARY

Scholarship in nursing education can be conceptualized broadly as inquiry about learning and teaching. That inquiry can involve the discovery of new knowledge and evidence on educational practices, translating and using research findings to guide teaching, and developing new concepts about teaching and learning in nursing.

The scholarship of teaching in nursing needs to embrace the many forms that scholarship can take. These include conducting original research about teaching and learning; evaluation studies; reviews that synthesize knowledge and provide evidence for teaching; development and application of concepts and theories to guide teaching; and development of educational innovations, initiatives, new programs, courses, teaching methods, and assessment methods, among others, that are systematically evaluated and disseminated.

To transform the teacher's work as an educator into scholarship, all forms of scholarship need to be public, peer-reviewed and critiqued, and shared with other educators so they, in turn, can build on that work. There are many venues for teachers to disseminate the products of their scholarship to make them public and accessible for critique and use by others. They can present their scholarship at conferences, at faculty meetings, and through other venues. Articles published in peer-reviewed journals, however, provide the widest dissemination. A section in the chapter presented the phases of writing for publication and important principles for disseminating scholarship through publications.

In most settings in which nurse educators work, the quality of their teaching, scholarship, service, and clinical practice, if relevant, is assessed by students, peers, administrators, and formal committees. This evaluation, including the use of teaching portfolios, was discussed in the chapter. However, the most important evaluation is that done by teachers themselves: Nurse educators need to periodically reflect on and assess the quality of their own teaching and scholarship. With this self-assessment, combined with feedback from others, teachers can identify areas in which they need further development and mentoring, set short- and long-term career goals, find resources to help them with their career development, expand their teaching competencies, and advance their scholarship of teaching.

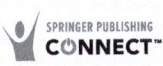

A robust set of instructor resources designed to supplement this text is located at http://connect.springerpub.com/content/book/978-0-8261-8892-2. Qualifying instructors may request access by emailing textbook@springerpub.com.

REFERENCES

American Association of Colleges of Nursing. (2018). *Defining scholarship for academic nursing: Task force consensus position statement*. https://www.aacnnursing.org/Portals/42/News/Position-Statements/Defining-Scholarship.pdf

American Medical Association. (2020). *AMA manual of style: A guide for authors and editors* (11th ed.). Oxford University Press.

American Psychological Association. (2020). *Publication manual of the American Psychological Association* (7th ed.). Author.

Boyer, E. L. (1990). *Scholarship reconsidered: Priorities of the professoriate*. Jossey-Bass.

Glassick, C. E., Huber, M. T., & Maeroff, G. I. (1997). *Scholarship assessed: Evaluation of the professoriate*. Jossey-Bass.

National Library of Medicine. (2024). *Journal selection for MEDLINE*. https://www.nlm.nih.gov/medline/medline_journal_selection.html

Oermann, M. H. (2017). Building your scholarship from your teaching: Plan now. *Nurse Educator, 42*(5), 217. https://doi.org/10.1097/NNE.0000000000000417

Oermann, M. H. (2024). *Writing for publication in nursing* (5th ed.). Springer Publishing Company.

Oermann, M. H., Nicoll, L. H., Carter-Templeton, H., Owens, J. K., Wrigley, J., Ledbetter, L. S., & Chinn, P. L. (2022). How to identify predatory journals in a search: Precautions for nurse clinicians. *Nursing, 52*(4), 41–45. https://doi.org/10.1097/01.NURSE.0000823280.93554.1a

Oermann, M. H., Wrigley, J., Nicoll, L. H., Ledbetter, L. S., Carter-Templeton, H., & Edie, A. H. (2021). Integrity of databases for literature searches in nursing: Avoiding predatory journals. *Advances in Nursing Science, 44*(2), 102–110. https://doi.org/10.1097/ANS.0000000000000349

Pinto, B. M., Dail, R. B., & Andrews, J. O. (2021). Strengthening collaborative research and scholarship in a College of Nursing. *Journal of Professional Nursing, 37*(2), 373–378. https://doi.org/10.1016/j.profnurs.2020.04.012

Shulman, L. S. (2000). From Minsk to Pinsk: Why a scholarship of teaching and learning? *Journal of Scholarship in Teaching and Learning, 1*(1), 48–53. https://scholarworks.iu.edu/journals/index.php/josotl/article/view/1582

Smith, S., & Walker, D. (2024). Scholarship and teaching-focused roles: An exploratory study of academics' experiences and perceptions of support. *Innovations in Education and Teaching International, 61*(1), 193–204, https://doi.org/10.1080/14703297.2022.2132981

Mentorship, Service, Leading, and Learner Success

21

Richard L. Pullen Jr.

OBJECTIVES

1. Describe the professional development of the nurse educator and its importance in terms of learner success
2. Explore opportunities for nurse educators to actively engage in service activities within their educational institutions and the broader community
3. Examine the role of the nurse educator as a leader
4. Describe strategies for effective advisement and support of learners, for fostering learner success, and for promoting the personal and professional growth of learners

INTRODUCTION

Nurse educators must be oriented and mentored in their academic roles as teachers, researchers, and clinicians to promote job satisfaction and learner success. Nurse educators engage in service and leadership activities to develop a scholarly persona and influence learners, colleagues, and the nursing profession. The convergence of competency-based education, the diverse ways students learn, the need for students to engage in active learning and develop a spirit of inquiry to lead change, the complexity of patient conditions, and the rapidly evolving technologies require nursing schools to provide academic support services and prepare learners for safe practice in dynamic healthcare environments.

This chapter discusses the professional development of the nurse educator to promote learner success. It emphasizes nurse educator orientation and mentorship and explores various opportunities for educators to actively engage in service activities within their educational institutions and the broader community. This includes active participation in committees, professional organizations, and community initiatives that significantly contribute to the advancement of nursing education. This chapter also addresses the role of the nurse educator as a leader. The chapter emphasizes strategies and effective advisement and supporting learners with guidance and mentorship. Strategies for fostering success, addressing challenges, and promoting personal and professional growth, including professional identity formation, are discussed.

ORIENTING NURSE EDUCATORS

The Association of Colleges of Nursing (AACN) emphasizes that comprehensive formalized onboarding orientation programs are vital for novice and experienced nurse educators to develop competencies for teaching and engaging in other educator roles and to promote job satisfaction, retention, and student outcomes (AACN, 2019). Novice nurse educators may be especially anxious to transition to an academic setting. It can be intimidating when they have yet to teach or develop a course syllabus, examination blueprint, and examination questions. Learning about the structure of an academic setting and the rules and regulations of professional organizations, such as the State Board of Nursing and accrediting bodies, can be overwhelming. Novice nurse educators must give themselves time to learn about the intricate details of nurse educator roles.

Orientation includes institution and school of nursing governance structure, policies, procedures, instructional technologies, curriculum, organizing and conceptual frameworks of the curriculum, job description, teaching competencies, and teaching assignments; advising students; student organizations; clinical facilities; service to the institution, school of nursing, community, and professional organizations; and peer evaluation, performance evaluation, and promotion and tenure (Cox et al., 2021; Groth et al., 2023; Rogers et al., 2020). Orientation should be completed over time based on the nurse educator's self-assessment of strengths and improvement areas.

MENTORING NURSE EDUCATORS

Mentoring in clinical practice, leadership, research, and education influences policymaking and standards of care globally (Gantz & Hafsteinsdorrir, 2023). A well-designed individualized mentoring program will help the nurse educator to acclimate and socialize to the academic culture (Groth et al., 2023; Knowles, 2020; Rogers et al., 2020; Vance, 2018). Mentoring is short-or long term and is personalized, guiding a nurse educator in their professional and personal development. Mentoring is a nurturing process where an experienced nurse educator guides, coaches, advises, and encourages a less-experienced educator in their professional and personal development.

Mentoring is a partnership that allows mentors and their mentees to experience giving and receiving each other's gifts within a safe environment. Clark (2022) describes the mentor–mentee partnership as nurturing, trusting, and conductive, and one that fosters the frank exchange of ideas and open communication. This collaborative partnership fosters accountability, trust, emotional intelligence, and integrity to strengthen the profession. Mentor–mentee partnerships promote professional identity and image development, creative expression, teaching efficacy, and scholarly productivity. Strong mentoring can promote a healthy work environment by creating a culture of civility, respect, and kindness. The National League for Nursing's (NLN) Mentoring Tool Kit (2022b) is a resource to help guide the mentor in the mentee's professional development. Mentees have diverse backgrounds and mentoring needs in the nurse educator role.

An effective mentor is trusted and respected by the mentee and has a reputation for positively influencing colleagues, learners, and nurses in clinical practice.

(Groth et al., 2023; Knowles, 2020; NLN, 2022b; Rogers et al., 2020; Vance, 2018). Trust and respect create open communication essential to a successful mentor–mentee partnership. The mentor must celebrate the mentee's strengths and be sensitive to areas needing further development. Mentors also should have a spirit of generosity to shape a nurse educator's professional persona, respect and embrace individuality and diversity, be authentic and compassionate, possess the knowledge and expertise to match the mentee's needs, have a record of scholarship, engage in lifelong learning, engage in mentoring workshops, and role-model building relationships.

Effective mentors are accessible; are fully present; listen attentively; pose thought-provoking questions; offer constructive criticism; provide informal advice on difficult situations, practice-related issues, clinical topics, and education; and regularly communicate with their mentees (Groth et al., 2023; Knowles, 2020; NLN, 2022b; Rogers et al., 2020; Vance, 2018). Mentees respect the mentor, have a spirit of curiosity and desire to learn, are goal oriented, ask questions, receive feedback, and implement success strategies. The partnership mentors and mentees share can identify the mentee's strengths and gaps in knowledge by goal setting. Exhibit 21.1 presents the mentor and mentee responsibilities (Rogers et al., 2020). Wells-Beede et al. (2023) conducted a scoping review to determine gaps in the preparation for nurse educator roles. One theme in the review is the need to amplify mentorship to help aspiring educators transition from clinical practice to the professoriate role. Forneris and Patterson (2024) state that ongoing mentorship is vital in the professional development of the nurse educator role.

EXHIBIT 21.1 Mentor and Mentee Responsibilities

Mentor Responsibilities
1. Agree to facilitate the transition of the mentee into the academic setting.
2. Set a regular schedule for meetings: at least weekly for the first month, biweekly for next 2 months, then monthly or more frequently as needed.
3. Develop and agree to ongoing communication methods with the mentee.
4. Review the Faculty Orientation Checklist with the mentee.
5. Assist the mentee in developing a plan for professional growth in teaching, scholarship, and service; provide feedback.
6. Help the mentee identify additional mentors in teaching and scholarship.
7. Coach mentees in developing a portfolio.
8. Support mentees in creating a promotion and tenure document.
9. Provide formal and informal networking or the mentee.
10. Set goals with the mentee about the mentor–mentee relationship.
11. Be available to answer mentee questions.

(continued)

EXHIBIT 21.1 Mentor and Mentee Responsibilities (*continued*)

Mentee Responsibilities
1. Agree to be mentored to facilitate the transition into the academic setting.
2. Attend regularly scheduled meetings.
3. Develop and agree to ongoing communication methods with the mentor.
4. Review all materials discussed by the mentor and incorporate the content into practice.
5. Draft a plan for professional growth in teaching, scholarship, and service; welcome feedback and input from the mentor.
6. Identify the need for additional mentoring in teaching and scholarship as needed.
7. Share portfolio with mentor and carefully consider mentor's input.
8. Share promotion and tenure document with mentor and carefully consider mentor's input.
9. Participate in formal and informal networking provided by the mentor.
10. Set goals with mentor for ongoing mentor–mentee relationship.
11. Maintain an ongoing list of questions to ask the mentor.

Source: Rogers, J., Ludwig-Beymer, P., & Baker, M. (2020). Nurse faculty orientation: An integrative review. *Nurse Educator, 45*(6), 343–346. https://doi.org/10.1097/NNE.0000000000000802. Reprinted by permission of Wolters Kluwer, 2024.

SERVICE AND LEADERSHIP OF THE NURSE EDUCATOR

The NLN core competencies of Function as a Change Agent and Leader and Pursue Continuous Quality Improvement in the Nurse Educator Role provide a framework for the nurse educator to engage in service and lead change (Halstead, 2019). Service and leadership promote professional development, contribute to the school of nursing and institution meeting outcomes, positively influence professional standards and requirements, promote safe patient care, and amplify the visibility of nursing as the most trusted profession. Newly appointed nurse educators should develop a plan for service and leadership activities but initially focus on being oriented and mentored for the teaching role.

Academic nurse educators serve on school of nursing and institutional committees and need to ensure currency, accuracy, validity, reliability, and rigor of school policies and procedures (Bednash, 2018; Ellis, 2024). Examples of committees in nursing include curriculum development, testing, admissions and progressions, program evaluation, scholarship, and student activities. Examples of committees in the institution include curriculum, technology, faculty senate, institutional effectiveness, instructional resources, professional development, and institutional review board. Special task forces also provide opportunities for nurse educators to serve.

Service also includes volunteer activities in local, state, national, and international communities. Professional service not only includes being a member of committees but also seeking leadership roles on committees, such as chair, chair-elect, secretary, and parliamentarian; mentoring nurse educator colleagues and learners; speaking at local, state, national, and international forums; serving on a community board; sponsoring a student organization; serving on an editorial board and as a manuscript reviewer for a peer-reviewed nursing journal; and leadership roles in nursing and nursing education professional organizations.

Nurse educators who assume leadership positions on committees and in professional organizations, and new roles in their school of nursing, institution, and community, communicate a desire to advance as leaders in the academic environment (Christensen & Simmons, 2020; Ellis, 2024; Neal-Boylan et al., 2018). Leadership shapes nursing education and the profession. Leadership is integral to the nurse educator role even when educators do not possess a formal leadership title. Formal leadership positions may include course leader, team coordinator, level coordinator, assistant director, director, and dean. The academic environment prioritizes the leader's personal and professional qualities to operationalize the mission and vision and achieve outcomes.

Leadership is a complex process whereby a nurse educator influences a group of individuals to achieve common goals. With influence, leadership is achieved. Leadership and management overlap to some degree. Leadership is proactive, based on influence and motivation, inspires people, inspires change, establishes direction, and aligns people. Management is reactive and focuses on planning, budgeting, organizing, staffing, controlling, problem-solving, and managing people. Leadership entails more of an emotional involvement with others than in management.

Foundational qualities of a leader include inspiring others through relationship building, letting others know they are valued, having strong interpersonal skills, and being able to communicate effectively (Boothe & Watson, 2023; Neal-Boylan et al., 2018). Leaders also must have emotional intelligence; show evidence of integrity; demonstrate conflict resolution; be problem-solvers; be motivated; facilitate an active learning and engaging environment for nurse educators, staff, and learners; and encourage shared decision-making among all team members. Leaders lead by example. Experienced academic nurse leaders can mentor aspiring nurse educators desiring to develop leadership skills. Aspiring leaders can perform a leadership self-assessment, and both the nurse educator and mentor can use this assessment to guide leadership growth. Table 21.1 presents leadership types. Malone and Davis (2023) emphasize that nurse educators as leaders must amplify teaching learners about social determinants of health (SDOH). The NLN's vision for nursing education leaders to integrate the SDOH in curricula (NLN, 2019) is in Exhibit 21.2.

Developing leaders is vital for succession planning to ensure leadership continuity (Phillips, 2021). Succession planning is an intentional and strategic process of identifying nurse educators with leadership potential and implementing strategies to guide them in developing the skill set required of an academic nurse leader. Succession planning preserves the first-hand experience of leaders in the mission, goals, vision, values, structure, and process of the school of nursing and institution. Succession planning establishes a healthy work environment by decreasing anxiety and improving morale. Succession planning requires sufficient funding from human resources and support from institutional administration.

TABLE 21.1. EXAMPLES OF LEADERSHIP APPROACHES

Leadership Approach	Main Theme
Trait	Some theorists believe that some people are born with leadership potential while other theorists believe leadership skills can be nurtured over time.
Skills	Achievement of skills and competencies, not personality traits.
Behavioral	Actions, behaviors, and decisions of the leader.
Situational	Adapts leadership style to unique situations or events. Leadership that assesses a situation and uses various leadership approaches to problem-solve.
Path/Goal	Establishes a supportive plan for goal achievement.
Leader–Member Exchange	Leaders and members develop unique relationships.
Transformational	Inspires, motivates, and stimulates problem-solving to effect change. Transformational leaders focus on transforming people and the organizational culture through energy, creativity, and vision. Transformational leaders are responsive to customer needs. For example, redesigning the curriculum to thread social determinants of health in all courses to prepare learners to care for diverse populations or writing a grant on an innovative model to attract learners to the nursing profession.
Authentic	Self-awareness, builds relationships, is disciplined, inspires change, leads by example, understands strengths and areas needing improvement, welcomes feedback from everyone before decision-making, is an effective communicator, and knows and implements the right thing to do.
Servant	Addresses the needs of others before their own (greater good). Celebrates and empowers their followers to help them reach their full potential to meet organizational outcomes.
Followership	Effective followers take direction well and motivate others to operationalize processes and embrace the leadership culture. Another term for follower is informal leader. Leaders may also place themselves into the role of follower to empower others to develop leadership skills.
Team	Aligning people in a group ensuring all have a voice in common goals.

Sources: Boothe, A., & Watson, J. (2023). Gaining personal insight: Being an effective follower and leader. In P. S. Yoder-Wise & S. Sportsman (Eds.), *Leading and managing in nursing* (8th ed., pp. 163–178). Elsevier Publishing Company; Greta, G., Lee, S., Tate, K., Penconek, T., Micaroni, S. P. M., Paananen, T., & Chatterjee, G. E. (2020). The essentials of nursing leadership: A systematic review of factors and educational interventions influencing nursing leadership. *International Journal of Nursing Studies, 115*, 103842. https://doi.org/10.1016/j.ijnurstu.2020.103842; Northouse, P. G. (2019). *Leadership: Theory and practice* (8th ed.). Sage Publishing.

> **EXHIBIT 21.2 National League for Nursing Leadership Strategies to Integrate Social Determinants of Health in Curricula**
>
> 1. Engage all nurse educators and staff in discussions about implicit and explicit biases about SDOH to nurture the development of an inclusive culture that affects health and wellness.
> 2. Encourage nurse educators to have discussions about the link among health, housing, income, equity, and access to resources and how they impact learning.
> 3. Provide professional development tools for nurse educators to help learners assess, plan, implement, and evaluate SDOH scenarios to reduce the impact of health disparities.
> 4. Establish partnerships with practice colleagues in the community to develop innovative initiatives addressing SDOH.
> 5. Support nurse educator and institutional research, teaching, and clinical projects and initiatives in SDOH to improve patient outcomes.

SDOH, social determinants of health.
Source: National League for Nursing. (2019). *Vision for the integration of social determinants of health in nursing curricula*. https://www.nln.org/docs/default-source/uploadedfiles/default-document-library/social-determinants-of-health.pdf?sfvrsn=aa66a50d_0

FACTORS AFFECTING LEARNER SUCCESS

Gaps in Diversity

The AACN (2021a) and Murray (2024) broadly define diversity, equity, and inclusion. Diversity is defined as being mindful of human differences. Diversity includes sex, gender identity, sexual orientation, race, ethnicity, age, language, religion, family structure, refugees, immigrants, learning, physical and functional ability, veterans, and socioeconomic status. Inclusive cultures embrace the unique characteristics of people. Equitable cultures provide fair opportunities for all people. *The Future of Nursing 2020–2030 Consensus Study Report* emphasizes that schools of nursing must build a diverse nursing workforce by recruiting, supporting, and providing diverse learners with educational experiences that address the SDOH, impacting health and health equity (National Academies of Sciences, Engineering, and Medicine, 2021). The National Council of State Boards of Nursing (NCSBN) and Forum for State Nursing Workforce Centers conducted a study in 2022 to evaluate the scope of the gender, racial, and ethnic landscape of the RN workforce in the United States (Smiley et al., 2023). Table 21.2 presents the demographics of RNs.

The Brookings Institution analysis of data from the U.S. Census Bureau (2020) projects that 48% of the population will be people of color by 2045. The NLN Annual Survey of Nursing Schools (ASNS, 2022) parallels the proportion of underrepresentation of minority learners (Table 21.3) and nurse educators (Table 21.4). Demographics of licensed practical and vocational nurses (LPNs/LVNs) parallel demographics in practice and nursing schools. Diversifying the workforce is vital to advance the health of all people globally (Fields & Wharton, 2023; NLN, 2016).

Diverse nurse educators are vital to promote learning, scholarship, school of nursing outcomes, and community healthcare outcomes. Diverse nurse educators can serve as role models and mentors to recruit underrepresented learners to the nursing profession. Nursing schools should establish a strategic approach to diversifying faculty and amplify teaching learners about diverse populations.

TABLE 21.2 DEMOGRAPHICS OF RNs 2022

Demographic Variable	Percentage
Female	88.5
Male	11.2
Nonbinary	0.3
Caucasian	80
Asian	7.4
African American	6.4
Hispanic or Latinx origin	6.9
American Indian—Alaskan Native	0.4
Native Hawaiian—Pacific Islander	0.4
Two or more races	2.5
Unknown	3
Total non-Hispanic or Latinx origin	93.1
Total Hispanic or Latinx origin	6.9

Source: Smiley, R. A., Allgeyer, R. L., Shobo, Y., Lyons, K. C., Letourneau, R., Zhong, E., Kaminski-Ozturk, N., & Alexander, M. (2023). The 2022 national nursing workforce survey. *The Journal of Nursing Regulation, 14*(Suppl), S12, S14. https://doi.org/10.1016/S2155-8256(23)00047-9 Reprinted by permission of Elsevier, 2024.

Community-based learning experiences are one strategy to help learners understand the impact of SDOH on diverse populations. Frazer et al. (2021) report that nurse educators can provide various patient care activities to help learners embrace diversity and inclusivity. The process begins with nurse educators having a deep understanding of diversity and inclusivity through self-reflection. Through self-reflection, nurse educators can intentionally support the needs of diverse learners.

Learning Styles

Learners have a variety of learning styles characteristic of a person's generation and are categorized into Baby Boomers (1946–1964), generation X (1965–1980), Generation Y (1981–1996), or Generation Z (1997–present; Lowell & Morris, 2019; Moore et al., 2021; Shatto & Erwin, 2017). Learners may have a preferred learning style that also overlaps with other ones. Baby Boomers are motivated by recognition, self-direction, and career goals and enjoy lectures and small group discussions. Generation X learners are motivated by the relevance of the topic to goals and enjoy active learning and immediate feedback in-person or electronically from

TABLE 21.3 DEMOGRAPHICS OF LEARNERS IN UNDERGRADUATE RN PROGRAMS 2022

Demographic Variable	Percentage
Female	86.4
Male	13.3
Transgender, genderqueer, or nonbinary	0.1
Gender unknown	0.2
Caucasian	58.5
Hispanic	13
African American	14.6
Asian	9
Native American	0.5
Unknown	4.4

Source: National League for Nursing. (2022a). *Annual survey of nursing schools.* https://www.nln.org/docs/default-source/research-statistics/nln-annual-survey-2022/headlineseditedgfm_8_15_2023_publication-.pdf?sfvrsn=2c6f050a_3

TABLE 21.4 DEMOGRAPHICS OF NURSE EDUCATORS

Demographic Variable	Percentage
Female	91.2
Male	8.1
Transgender	0.3
Gender unknown	0.4
Caucasian	76.4
Hispanic	11
African American	4.2
Asian	4.2
Multiracial	1.1
Native American	0.3
Unknown	2.8

Source: National League for Nursing. (2022a). *Annual survey of nursing schools.* https://www.nln.org/docs/default-source/research-statistics/nln-annual-survey-2022/headlineseditedgfm_8_15_2023_publication-.pdf?sfvrsn=2c6f050a_3

nurse educators. eneration Y learners are pragmatic and confident and frequently use social networking. Hands-on learning, mobile devices, and podcasts are strategies for these learners. Generation Z learners are ethnically savvy, digitally savvy, globally aware, and conservative. Generation Z learners dislike in-person learning, use technology in learning, and enjoy learning when it is fun.

The learning environment is comprised of learners with a mix of backgrounds, preferences, and values, requiring nurse educators to incorporate a variety of strategies for multigenerational learners, such as lectures, mobile devices, active engagement in small groups, and immediate feedback in one setting. Nurse educators can use the Myers-Briggs Type Indicator (MBTI) to identify a learner's personality preference (Childs-Kean et al., 2020; Diller, 2024). The Kolb Experiential Learning Profile helps learners identify learning preferences from life experiences (Diller, 2024; Ezzeddine et al., 2023). The integration of visual, aural, read/write, and kinesthetic (VARK) strategies (Diller, 2024) can promote engagement, critical thinking, and problem-solving in multigenerational learners and individuals with various learning preferences (Table 21.5).

Recruitment

Nursing schools have made progress in recruiting diverse learners. Nursing education must develop more strategies. The AACN has identified the recruitment of diverse learners as a high priority in underrepresented populations, including African American, Hispanic, Asian, American Indian, Alaskan Native, and males (AACN, 2023). The recruitment of diverse learners must start through amplified K–12 science education and outreach mentoring programs in middle and senior high schools (DeWitty & Byrd, 2021; National Academies of Sciences, Engineering, and Medicine [NASEM], 2021; Williams, 2018). Nursing schools should establish an educational pathway for diverse learners before enrolling in a prelicensure program. Many states permit dual credit, where learners can earn college credit while in high school to prepare them for nursing school success. Mentoring programs between nursing schools and K–12 are vital in attracting future nurses.

TABLE 21.5 VARK (VISUAL, AURAL, READ/WRITE, KINESTHETIC)–LEARNING STRATEGIES

Visual	Aural	Read/Write	Kinesthetic
Diagrams Maps and charts Posters Worksheets Student presentations Computer tutorials Games Simulations	Discussion Debates Student presentations Videos (Audio) Computer tutorials (Audio) Simulations	Reading Note-taking Case studies Creating maps and charts Developing worksheets NCLEX questions Simulations	Mobile devices Online learning Skills in clinical Operating technology Simulations

A fully funded nursing school or institutional recruitment department would reach diverse global populations and reduce the nurse educator workload for solely identifying, implementing, and evaluating recruitment and marketing strategies and outcomes.

Admissions

A strategic recruitment plan must be integral to the nursing school structure and directed toward holistic admission criteria to create a culture of inclusivity (AACN, 2024; Morrow, 2021). Nursing schools use cognitive and non–cognitive factors to admit learners. Cognitive factors include grade point average, individual course grades, admissions, and aptitude tests. Cognitive ability is vital in achieving knowledge, skills, and attitudes for safe practice. Still, it is only one factor when evaluating a learner's potential for success in nursing. Noncognitive factors include motivation, perseverance, compassion, resilience, personality, personal and professional experiences, service activities, leadership, problem-solving abilities, and age.

Holistic admissions processes evaluate a learner's unique attributes, experiences, and academic readiness to begin nursing school. These admissions processes add to the depth, breadth, and richness of the learning environment and increase the diversity of the nursing workforce. Nursing schools using holistic admissions report that academic metrics have remained constant or improved, and student engagement, openness, and teamwork have increased. The components of a holistic admissions process can vary according to the needs of a nursing school. The AACN has identified strategies nursing schools can consider (Exhibit 21.3).

Exhibit 21.3 AMERICAN ASSOCIATION OF COLLEGES OF NURSING HOLISTIC ADMISSIONS STRATEGIES

1. The mission statement for the Admissions Committee addresses diversity.
2. The Admissions Committee receives education about the nursing school's mission.
3. The Admissions Committee receives education on diversity and unconscious bias.
4. The Admissions Committee comprises diverse members in the nursing school and community.
5. Nonacademic admissions criteria are integral to metrics in the initial admissions screening process.
6. Applicants are required to submit a short essay or personal statement.
7. Several applicants are interviewed in person, over the phone, or by teleconferencing.
8. Applicants are obtained from a waitlist per the admissions criteria related to diversity.
9. There are specific admission criteria relevant to the mission and goals of the nursing school, such as a global health mission statement.

Source: Adapted from American Association of Colleges of Nursing. (2024). *Holistic admissions tool kit.* https://www.aacnnursing.org/our-initiatives/diversity-equity-inclusion/holistic admissions/holistic-admissions-tool-kit

Mentoring the Learner

Mentoring enhances academic success, socialization, self-efficacy, and self-confidence.

Triad mentor models, consisting of a partnership among representatives from nursing schools, clinical practice, and K–12, can be developed to prepare for the future nursing workforce. Nurse educators serving as mentors and role models help shape a learner's career trajectory in nursing (Vance, 2018). They create a nurturing environment where they feel supported. They are known for relationship building and the ability to stimulate intellectual curiosity in mentees. They also inform mentees about academic rigor to help them think critically to provide safe patient care.

The Robert Wood Johnson Foundation (RWJF) Mentoring Program (2017) amplifies the need for mentoring programs to promote positive academic outcomes. Gillespie et al. (2023) conducted a study to determine the characteristics of faculty mentoring in the RWJF Future of Nursing Scholars Program. In this program, faculty mentored PhD learners. An important finding was that faculty spent more time engaging with PhD learners in the Scholars Program than other PhD learners. A follow-up study by Kelley et al. (2023) indicated that PhD learners in the Scholars Program were confident in meeting the demand for rigorous doctoral studies, working collaboratively, and preparing for professional transitions and post-doctoral studies. Mentoring in the Scholars Program resulted in PhD learners meeting program rigor, having increased confidence, and embracing continued education, which are concepts applicable to all levels of nursing education.

Academic Advising

Academic preparation for nursing school rigor involves the learner, parents and other family members, middle and high school counselors, mentors, college recruiters, advisors, and nurse educators. Academic advising is vital to ensure learners engage in frequent educational activities and utilize the college support resources to help them succeed. Advising is integral to the nurse educator role (Flowers et al., 2022; NASEM, 2021; Saeedi & Parvizy, 2019). Learners should have college-level mathematics, vocabulary, reading, and grammar skills. Combined with nursing concepts, these foundational skills will enable learners to think critically and problem-solve at the application, analysis, evaluation, and synthesis cognitive levels. Many colleges provide courses and programs to prepare learners to achieve these skills, including programs for learners with English as a second language.

Grades in prerequisite science courses, particularly anatomy, physiology, microbiology, and chemistry, may be used as cognitive admission criteria and are reliable indicators for learner success. Nurse educators conducting advising sessions for potential learners should emphasize the importance of science grades in high school and prerequisite college courses. Connecting potential learners with the nurse educator and peer mentors, tutors, and academic advisors can prepare them for academic achievement in science courses and any standardized admission tests in nursing schools. A desire to have a career helping others and life experiences are noncognitive factors that are also reliable predictors of learner success. Learners from first-generation and underrepresented minority populations may have unique challenges. First-generation learners are individuals whose parents achieved no higher than a high school education and are more likely to be nonsuccessful in college than non-first-generation learners. Learners may have financial, environmental, and health disparities limiting academic achievement.

Self-Care and Socialization

Professional socialization begins with learners identifying self-care strategies before caring for others. The AACN *Essentials* Domain 10 calls for a curriculum promoting self-care behaviors and resiliency in learners and diverse populations (AACN, 2021b). The stress learners experience from the rigor of school and personal and professional obligations can be overwhelming and harmful to mental and physical health. Sleep, rest, exercise, nutrition, mindfulness strategies, and accessing college wellness programs are vital in meeting basic needs. Learners must also connect with others to help them be healthy physically, mentally, and socially (Monforto & Mancini, 2023).

Social support means having a social support network, academic support of a nurse educator mentor or role model, peer mentor, and emotional, positive appraisal, and self-esteem support (Choi et al., 2024; Kim & Lee, 2022; NASEM, 2021; Pai et al., 2021). Some nursing schools require newly admitted learners to attend a short immersion experience to introduce them to study, test taking, and socialization skills before the first semester of studies. The nurse educator creates active and engaging learning environments focused on diverse learners' socialization to the roles of the nurse (Halstead, 2019). Nurse educators in leadership positions in nursing schools, community agencies, and professional organizations role model the importance of service and socialization to advance the nursing profession (Christensen & Simmons, 2020). Learners emulating nurse educators' leadership service will facilitate socialization to the profession, shaping leadership paths, promoting health advocacy, influencing policymaking, and elevating standards of professional practice.

Learners can serve in professional organizations in school and continue service after graduation. Learners can join their school's student nurses association, the National Student Nurses Association, and the American Nurses Association free of charge. Learners can join other organizations at a reduced charge, including AACN, NLN, Society of Pediatric Nurses, American Association for Men in Nursing, Emergency Nurses Association, Academy of Medical-Surgical Nurses, American Association of Critical-Care Nurses, National Black Nurses Association, Transcultural Nursing Society, and the National Organization for Nurses with Disabilities. Many colleges have LGBTQ+, minority, and faith-based clubs to embrace these learners' unique attributes, life experiences, and contributions. These student organizations can serve in community activities to enhance their leadership and socialization skills, such as wellness fairs, homeless shelters, mentorship, and guest speakers at middle and high schools, the American Red Cross, nursing homes, hospices, hospitals, clinics, and animal shelters. Local, state, national, and international global health trips enable learners to serve diverse populations.

Financial

Cost is a significant concern for learners, particularly the impoverished or those with lowincome, compared to those with a higher income (National Academies of Sciences, NASEM, 2021). Nursing schools must ensure that learners' basic needs are met because many struggle with housing, food insecurities, childcare, and transportation. Advisors and recruitment coordinators must communicate educational costs and the availability of loans, scholarships, grants, and resources to secure housing, food, childcare, and healthcare. Learners must have financial assistance for tuition, books, fees, and supplies. Learners initiate financial assistance by completing the Free Application for Federal Student Aid (FAFSA) and other nursing school forms. The eligibility for financial assistance is usually based on holistic criteria such as grade point average, financial need, community service, professional goals, and a short essay on why financial assistance will help the learner achieve their goals. Most colleges have foundations with endowed and nonendowed scholarships and emergency funds for learners. Active military and veterans are eligible for up to 100% of tuition reimbursement through the GI Bill. Many employers provide learners with tuition reimbursement.

There are multiple examples of loan programs and scholarships available for nursing students. For example, the Public Service Loan Forgiveness Program offers complete forgiveness of loans after a person has made the equivalent of 120 payments (10 years; https://studentaid.gov/sites/default/files/public-service-application-for-forgiveness.pdf).

The Health Resources and Services Administration (HRSA) has scholarships and grants to increase the diversity of the nursing workforce. One HRSA scholarship is available to disadvantaged students (https://bhw.hrsa.gov/funding/apply-grant/faq-scholarships-disadvantaged-students). The HRSA also offers grants through the National Diversity Workforce Program to increase the number of minority nurses (https://www.hrsa.gov/grants/find-funding/HRSA-21-020). The AACN provides a listing of available scholarships, grants, fellowships, and loan forgiveness programs (https://www.aacnnursing.org/students/scholarships-financial-aid) for diverse learners. The NLN offers various scholarships for nurses and graduate learners (https://www.nln.org/nln-foundation/foundationoverview/nursing-education-scholarship-awards). Learners in a graduate program aspiring to be nurse educators may apply for the low-interest HRSA Nurse Faculty Loan Program to increase the number of nurse educators nationwide (https://bhw.hrsa.gov/funding/apply-loan-repayment/faculty-lrp). Loans and scholarships for nursing students change over time: Nurse educators are advised to refer students to the financial aid office of their school of nursing or institution for up-to-date information about these.

Equity-Focused Teaching

Inclusive learning environments embrace the differences of others and invite, welcome, and respect their perspectives to thrive and achieve their goals (Center for Research on Teaching and Learning [CRTL], n.d.; Charania & Patel, 2022; Murray, 2024). Equitable learning environments provide learners the resources to transcend barriers, fully participate, and ensure fairness. Equity-focused teaching recognizes that the social marginalization of underrepresented populations negatively impacts identity formation, confidence, relationships, and learning. Nurse educators should strategically create learning environments that foster mutual trust, respect, and collaboration, and provide engaging learning activities where learners are responsible for embracing diversity and have equal access to resources. Educators should understand the unique obstacles that learners from historically excluded backgrounds, such as underrepresented minorities, experience in society that impact learning and professional growth in nursing.

Nurse educators can create an equity-focused learning experience while holding the learner accountable for meeting the rigor of a course. The five principles of equity-focused teaching are: (a) critical engagement of difference, (b) structured interactions, (c) academic belonging, (d) transparency, and (e) flexibility. These principles and selected strategies are provided in Table 21.6.

TABLE 21.6 EQUITY-FOCUSED TEACHING STRATEGIES

Principles	Strategies
Critical engagement of difference Embrace learners' differences and experiences as an asset for learning.	Ask learners to introduce themselves and share information they want others to know. Acknowledge the uniqueness of learners and how diversity contributes to rich learning environments. Integrate diversity in learning activities.
Structured interactions Create policies, protocols, and procedures that support equity-focused teaching.	Integrate diversity, equity, and inclusion statements in the course syllabus to guide learning. Engage learners in group activities to embrace the diversity of ideas and problem-solving. Invite learners to share what they have learned in the course.
Academic belonging Cultivate learners' sense of connection to others and the nursing profession.	Call learners by their preferred name with correct pronunciation and pronouns. Ask learners to reflect on how their uniqueness shapes their identity as a nurse on a course discussion board for other learners to respond to. Integrate diverse learning activities related to gender, sociocultural contexts, and social determinants of health.
Transparency Communicate clear expectations of components of a course.	Communicate the course description, objectives, outcomes, assignments, and grading criteria. Let learners know how they can communicate with you, such as course e-mail, text messaging, or phone. Evaluate assignments promptly and provide meaningful feedback.
Flexibility Respond empathetically and adapt to learners' diverse circumstances.	Design courses with synchronous, asynchronous, and technology components for diverse learners. Provide special accommodations for learners with special needs. Provide formative and summative feedback.

Source: Center for Research on Teaching and Learning, University of Michigan. (2021). *Equity focused teaching.* https://crlt.umich.edu/equity-focused-teaching. Reprinted by permission of the Center for Research on Teaching and Learning.

Trauma-Informed Teaching

Nurse educators should understand how trauma and stress affect the brain and a person's ability to regulate emotions and learn. The Substance Abuse and Mental Health Services Administration (SAMHSA, 2014) defines trauma as harmful circumstances having a lasting effect on a person's physical, emotional, social, and spiritual health. Relationship strain, financial problems, chronic stress, substance misuse and abuse, chronic physical and mental illnesses, and post traumatic stress are examples adults may be coping with. Adverse childhood events, such as parental discord and physical, emotional or sexual abuse, poverty, and discrimination, may negatively impact a person's self-confidence and learning abilities.

Trauma-informed teaching practices (TITP) embrace diversity, including the varied backgrounds learners bring to the learning environment and an understanding that traumatic events may be a part of learners' life experiences (Clark, 2023; CRTL, n.d.; Mayer et al., 2023; Najjar et al., 2022). TITP are relationship-oriented, where trauma awareness and resilience-building wellness programs and resources create a safe environment for learners and nurse educators to flourish. Nursing leadership must ensure that TITP is a part of the structure and culture of a school. Nurse educators can include trauma-related scenarios in didactic instruction, case studies, simulations, and clinical learning.

Structure, culture, and learning activities in a nursing program can be framed using principles of TITP:

- Fostering a sense of safety
- Building open and trusting relationships
- Cultivating community and belonging
- Recognizing power imbalances to enhance collaboration and mutuality
- Empowering through voice and choice
- Being attuned to the cultural, historical, and gendered contexts (Clark, 2023; Mayer et al., 2023; Najjar et al., 2022)

Nurse educators can transform their pain from trauma into healing and be role models to learners and colleagues. When learners and nurse educators do not transcend their traumas, they may carry unresolved issues to the workplace, compromising relationships, productivity, and safety.

Nurse Educator Characteristics

Nurse educators must possess clinical expertise, a graduate degree in nursing, and engage in professional development with the NLN Core Competencies for Nurse Educators as a framework (Halstead, 2019). Effective teaching includes having a passion for nursing and teaching, being innovative, actively listening, showing compassion, having emotional intelligence, demonstrating leadership skills, being organized, being a role model, having adaptability, being a lifelong learner, being culturally competent, embracing diversity and inclusivity, integrating technology, and having a sense of humor (Collier, 2018; Labrague et al., 2020; Wanchai et al., 2022). The qualities of a nurse educator that students find most important are people skills, motivation, the ability to teach in a way they can understand, and having a professional persona.

Diversification of learners in nursing programs continues to broaden while nurse educator diversity shows only incremental growth. Diverse nurse educators are needed to expand the perspectives of learners, prepare learners for caring for diverse populations, and serve as role models. There needs to be an amplification of recruitment efforts to attract nurse educators from all backgrounds (Fields & Warton, 2023; Malone & Davis, 2023; NLN, 2016).

PROFESSIONAL IDENTITY FORMATION IN NURSE EDUCATORS AND LEARNERS

Professional identity formation is an evolving process and begins with a nurse having the knowledge, skills, and attitudes for safe practice (Godfrey & Young, 2020). There are multiple definitions of professional identify formation that are relevant for nurse educators and learners. The AACN *The Essentials: Core Competencies for Professional Nursing Education* views professional identity as a process occurring in stages where a nurse deeply internalizes the values of nursing in thinking, acting, and feeling like a member of an esteemed profession (AACN, 2021b). The International Society for Professional Identity in Nursing (ISPIN) defines a professional identity as "a sense of oneself, and others, that is influenced by characteristics, norms, values of nursing, resulting in a person thinking, acting, and feeling like a nurse" (University of Kansas, 2024).

Landis et al. (2022) conducted a national study to determine nurse educators' perception of a professional identity in nursing. A cohort of 50 leaders in academia, practice, and regulation developed the Professional Identity in Nursing Survey (PINS). A total of 1107 nurse educators rated the importance of each item on the survey. Nurse educators represented various program types: practical nursing (14.4%), associate degree (30%), diploma (3.6%), bachelor in nursing (47.6%), master in nursing (3.6%), and doctoral nursing (2.1%) programs.

The study identified four domains of professional identity:

1. Values and ethics: a set of core values and principles that guide conduct
2. Knowledge: analysis and application of information derived from nursing and other disciplines, experiences, critical reflection, and scientific discovery
3. Leadership: inspiring self and others to transform a shared vision into a reality
4. Professional comportment: a nurse's professional behavior demonstrated through words, actions, and presence. (Landis et al., 2022)

Each domain consists of attributes that nurse educators rated moderately important or very important. For example, more than 98% of nurse educators reported that being respectful, patient-centered, self-aware, collaborative, confident, engaged, motivated, and resilient were moderately to very important in the professional comportment. The most vital attributes in this study were being an effective communicator, being trustworthy, and having integrity.

Nursing schools must establish a culture that supports professional identity formation in learners. The curriculum should include professional identity language, the domains of professional identity, learning activities, nurse educator and peer mentors for promoting the development of professional identity, and exemplars of

TABLE 21.7 PROFESSIONAL IDENTITY FORMATION STRATEGIES

Domain	Strategies
Values and Ethics	Ensure patient privacy and role model ethical behavior. Engage in ethical committees and forums. Demonstrate caring relationships and alleviate patient fears. Create supportive and healing environments.
Knowledge	Seek educational activities to ensure currency in professional standards related to education and practice. Respect the need for lifelong learning and integration of interprofessional evidence-based literature and standards in education and practice.
Nurse as a Leader	Advocate for safe patient care and equity in access to care. Demonstrate leadership skills, including relationship building, compassion, being approachable, effective communication, collaboration, teamwork, conflict management, problem-solving, role modeling, and mentoring.
Professional Comportment	Support a "no tolerance" of incivility. Role model civil behaviors in all settings. Respect, value, acknowledge, and celebrate others. Use the power of presence, intentional caring, and caring in the moment to inspire others. Demonstrate a professional work ethic by arriving on time, acting and dressing as a professional, and greeting all in attendance.

professional identity in nursing (Godfrey & Young, 2020; Landis et al., 2022; University of Kansas, 2024). Learners should embrace the value of service as one attribute of their professional identity. Learners also can (a) develop a personal statement about what nursing means to them, (b) be active in school clubs, (c) join a professional nursing organization at a reduced charge as a learner, (d) engage in community activities, and (e) plan for lifelong learning and formal education. Godfrey and Young (2020) report that integrity, compassion, courage, humility, advocacy, and human flourishing are integral to having a professional identity. Table 21.7 presents selected additional strategies for professional identity formation (University of Kansas, 2024).

SUMMARY

This chapter focuses on the role of nurse educators in impacting learner success. Orientation and mentorship are vital to the professional development of the nurse educator as a teacher, leader, advisor, and mentor. Leaders shape a flourishing workplace culture, serve as role models, and value service. Respecting, valuing, inspiring, motivating, and relationship building are leadership characteristics that are essential in managing processes to achieve an organization's mission, vision, and outcomes. The diversity of learner demographics and the impact on SDOH in health disparities and equity require nursing schools to recruit diverse learners and nurse educators and to amplify learning experiences to promote safe care in diverse populations. Learners are coping with various stressors, including caring for their family, work, health, and meeting the demands of a rigorous nursing curriculum. Nursing schools should identify the barriers to learner success and evaluate learners' potential for success in nursing from a holistic perspective. Strategies must be in place to promote learner success and professional identity development from recruitment to graduation.

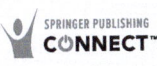

A robust set of instructor resources designed to supplement this text is located at http://connect.springerpub.com/content/book/978-0-8261-8892-2. Qualifying instructors may request access by emailing textbook@springerpub.com.

REFERENCES

American Association of Colleges of Nursing. (2019). *AACN's vision for academic nursing*. https://www.aacnnursing.org/Portals/0/PDFs/White-Papers/Vision-Academic-Nursing.pdf

American Association of Colleges of Nursing. (2021a). *Diversity, equity, and inclusion faculty tool kit*. https://www.aacnnursing.org/Portals/42/Diversity/Diversity-Tool-Kit.pdf

American Association of Colleges of Nursing. (2021b). *The essentials: Core competencies for professional nursing education*. https://www.aacnnursing.org/Portals/0/PDFs/Publications/Essentials-2021.pdf

American Association of Colleges of Nursing. (2023). *Fact sheet: Enhancing diversity in the workforce*. https://www.aacnnursing.org/Portals/0/PDFs/Fact-Sheets/Enhancing-Diversity-Factsheet.pdf

American Association of Colleges of Nursing. (2024). *Holistic admissions tool kit*. https://www.aacnnursing.org/our-initiatives/diversity-equity-inclusion/holistic-admissions/holistic-admissions-tool-kit

Bednash, G. (2018). Collegiality, service, and leadership roles of the nurse educator. In D. D. Hunt (Ed.), *The new nurse educator: Mastering academe* (2nd ed., pp. 225–234). Springer Publishing Company.

Boothe, A., & Watson, J. (2023). Gaining personal insight: Being an effective follower and leader. In P. S. Yoder-Wise & S. Sportsman (Eds.), *Leading and managing in nursing* (8th ed., pp. 163–178). Elsevier Publishing Company.

Brookings. Census 2020. (2020). Brookings Institution. Accessed October 16, 2024. https://www.brookings.edu/collection/census-2020/

Center for Research on Teaching and Learning. (n.d.). *Equity focused teaching*. University of Michigan. Accessed October 16, 2024. https://crlt.umich.edu/equity-focused-teaching

Charania, N. A. M. A., & Patel, R. (2022). Diversity, equity, and inclusion in nursing education: Strategies and processes to support inclusive teaching. *Journal of Professional Nursing, 42*, 67–72. https://doi.org/10.1016/j.profnurs.2022.05.013

Childs-Kean, L., Edwards, M., & Smith, M. D. (2020). Use of learning style frameworks in health science education. *American Journal of Pharmaceutical Education, 84*(7), 7885, 919–929. https://doi.org/10.5688/ajpe7885

Choi, M. Y., Park S., & Noh, G. O. (2024). Social support for nursing students: A concept analysis study. *Nursing Education Today, 132*, 106038. https://doi.org/10.1016/j.nedt.2023.106038

Christensen, L. S., & Simmons, L. E. (2020). *The scope of practice for academic nurse educators and academic clinical nurse educators* (3rd ed.). National League for Nursing. Wolters Kluwer.

Clark, C. M. (2022). *Core competencies of civility in nursing and healthcare.* Sigma.

Clark, C. M. (2023). Integrating trauma-informed teaching and learning principles into nursing education. *Journal of Nursing Education, 62*(3), 133–138. https://doi:10.3928/01484834-20230109-02

Collier, A. D. (2018). Characteristics of an effective nursing clinical instructor: The state of the science. *Journal of Clinical Nursing, 27*(1–2), 363–374. https://doi.org/10.1111/jocn.13931

Cox, C. W., Jordan, E. T., Valiga, T. M., & Zhou, Q. (2021). New faculty orientation for nurse educators: Offerings and needs. *Journal of Nursing Education, 60*(5), 273–276. https://doi.org/10.3928/01484834-20210420-06

DeWitty, V. P., & Byrd, D. A. (2021). Recruiting underrepresented students for nursing schools. *Creative Nursing, 27*(1), 40–45. https://doi.org/10.1891/crnr-d-20-00069

Diller, J. K. (2024). Strategies to support diverse learning needs of students. In D. M. Billings & J. A. Halstead (Eds.), *Teaching in nursing: A guide for faculty* (7th ed., pp. 610–614). Elsevier.

Ellis, P. (2024). Systematic program evaluation. In D. M. Billings & J. A. Halstead (Eds.), *Teaching in nursing: A guide for faculty* (7th ed., pp. 21–50). Elsevier.

Ezzeddine, N., Hughes, J., Kaulback, S., Houk, S., Mikhael, J., & Vickery, A. (2023). Implications of understanding the undergraduate nursing students' learning styles: A discussion paper. *Journal of Professional Nursing, 49*, 95–101. https://doi.org/10.1016/j.profnurs.2023.09.006

Fields, S. D., & Wharton, M. J. (2023). Diversifying the nursing workforce. In S. Hassmiller, A. D. Mahoney, & K. Beard (Eds.), *Future of nursing 2020–2030: Global applications to advance health equity* (pp. 23–38). Springer Publishing Company.

Flowers, M., Olenick, M., Maltseva, T., Simon, S., Diez-Sampedro, A., & Allen, L. A. (2022). Academic factors predicting NCLEX-RN success. *Nursing Education Perspectives, 43*(2), 112–114. https://doi.org/10.1097/01.NEP.0000000000000788

Forneris, S. G., & Patterson, B. J. (2024). Faculty development: Preparing to teach. In J. Noone & P. Gubrud (Eds.), *Best practices in teaching nursing* (pp. 67–84). National League for Nursing. Wolters Kluwer.

Frazer, C., Reilly, C. A., & Squellati, R. E. (2021). Instructional strategies: Teaching nursing in today's diverse and inclusive landscape. *Teaching and Learning in Nursing, 16*(3), 276–280. https://doi.org/10.1016/j.teln.2021.01.005

Gantz, N. R., & Hafsteinsdottir, T. B. (2023). *Mentoring in nursing through narrative stories across the world.* Springer Publishing Company.

Gillespie, G. L., Vallerand, A. P., & Fairman, J. (2023). Characteristics of faculty mentoring in the Robert Wood Johnson Foundation Future of Nursing Scholars Program. *Nursing Outlook, 71*(2), 101912, 1–11. doi: 10.1016/j.outlook.2022.101912

Godfrey, N., & Young, E. (2020). Professional identity. In J. F. Giddens (Ed.), *Concepts for nursing practice* (3rd ed., pp. 363–370). Elsevier.

Greta, G., Lee, S., Tate, K., Penconek, T., Micaroni, S. P. M., Paananen, T., & Chatterjee, G. E. (2020). The essentials of nursing leadership: A systematic review of factors and educational interventions influencing nursing leadership. *International Journal of Nursing Studies, 115*, 103842. https://doi.org/10.1016/j.ijnurstu.2020.103842

Groth, S. M., Duncan, R., Lassiter, J., & Madler, B. J. (2023). Onboarding orientation for novice nurse faculty: A quality improvement pilot project. *Teaching and Learning in Nursing, 18*(1), 212–218. https://doi.org/10.1016/j.teln.2022.07.010

Halstead, J. A. (2019). *NLN core competencies for nurse educators: A decade of influence.* Wolters Kluwer.

Kelley, H. J., Giordano, N., Boschitsch, M., Bastelica, A., Ladden, M. J., Wicks, M., McCarthye, M., & Fairman, J. (2023). The Robert Wood Johnson Foundation Future of Nursing Scholars Program: The scholar experience. *Nursing Outlook, 71*(2), 101902. https://doi.org/10.1016/j.outlook.2022.11.006

Kim, H. O., & Lee, L. (2022). The mediating effects of social support on the influencing relationship between grit and academic burnout of the nursing students. *Nursing Open, 9*(5), 2314–2324. https://doi.org/10.1002/nop2.1241

Knowles, S. (2020). Initiation of a mentoring program: Mentoring invisible nurse faculty. *Teaching and Learning in Nursing, 15*(3), 190–194. https://doi.org/10.1016/j.teln.2020.02.001

Labrague, L. J., McEnroe-Petitte, D. M., D'Souza, M. S., Hammad, K. S., & Hayudini, J. N. L. (2020). Nurse faculty teaching characteristics as perceived by nursing students: An integrative review. *Scandinavian Journal of Caring Sciences, 34*(1), 23–33. https://doi.org/10.1111/scs.12711

Landis, T., Godfrey, N., Barbosa-Leiker, C., Brewington, J. G., Luparell, S., & Priddy, K. D. (2022). National study of nursing faculty and administrators' perceptions of professional identity in nursing. *Nurse Educator, 47*(1), 13–18. https://doi.org/10.1097/NNE.0000000000001124Lowell, V. L., & Morris, J. M., Jr. (2019). Multigenerational classrooms in higher education: Equity and learning with technology. *The International Journal of Information and Learning Technology, 36*(2), 78–93. https://doi.org/10.1108/IJILT-06-2018-0068

Malone, B., & Davis, S. (2023). Strengthening nursing education to address social determinants of health: Systems leadership. In S. Hassmiller, A. D. Mahoney & K. Beard (Eds.), *Future of Nursing 2020–2030: Global applications to advance health equity* (pp. 67–83). Springer Publishing.

Mayer, K., Rothacker-Peyton, S., & Wilson-Anderson, K. (2023). Trauma-informed educational practices within the undergraduate nursing classroom: A pilot study. *Trauma Care, 3*(3), 114–125. https://doi:10.3390/traumacare3030012

Monforto, K., & Mancini, E. (2023). *Nursing student stress, role-modeling self-care.* American Nurse. https://www.myamericannurse.com/nursing-student-stress-role-modeling-self-care/

Moore, G., Parker, S., & Baksh, L. (2021). *Generational learning preferences.* American Nurse. https://www.myamericannurse.com/generational-learning-preferences/

Morrow, M. A. (2021). Holistic admission: What is it? How successful has it been nursing, and what are the possibilities? *Nursing Science Quarterly, 34*(3), 256–262. https://doi.org/10.1177/08943184211010431

Murray, T. A. (2024). Creating inclusive learning environments. In J. Noone & P. Gubrud (Eds.), *Best practices in teaching nursing* (pp.87–108). National League for Nursing/Wolters Kluwer.

Najjar, R., Jacobs, S., Keeney, S., Vidal, G., & Noone, J. (2022). Reflections on the process of implementing trauma-informed education lunch and learns. *Nurse Educator, 48*(4), E126–E130. https://doi.org/10.1097/nne.0000000000001338

National Academies of Sciences, Engineering, and Medicine. (2021). *The future of nursing 2020–2030: Charting a path to achieve health equity.* The National Academies Press. https://doi.org/10.17226/25982

National League for Nursing. (2016). *Achieving diversity and meaningful inclusion in nursing education: A living document.* https://www.nln.org/docs/default-source/uploadedfiles/professional-development-programs/vision-statement-achieving-diversity.pdf

National League for Nursing. (2019). *Vision for the integration of social determinants of health in nursing curricula.* https://www.nln.org/docs/default-source/uploadedfiles/default-document-library/social-determinants-of-health.pdf?sfvrsn=aa66a50d_0

National League for Nursing. (2022a). *Annual survey of nursing schools.* https://www.nln.org/docs/default-source/research-statistics/nln-annual-survey-2022/headlinesedit edgfm_8_15_2023_publication-.pdf?sfvrsn=2c6f050a_3

National League for Nursing. (2022b). *Mentoring tool kit.* https://www.nln.org/docs/default-source/default-document-library/nln-mentoring-toolkit-2022.pdfNeal-Boylan, L., Guillett, S. E., & Chappy, S. (2018). *Academic leadership in nursing: Effective strategies for aspiring faculty and leaders.* Springer Publishing Company.

Northouse, P. G. (2019). *Leadership: Theory and practice* (8th ed.). Sage Publishing.

Pai, H. S., Cheng, H. H., & Huang, Y. L. (2021). Factors that influence professional socialization in nursing students: A multigroup analysis. *Open Journal of Nursing, 11*, 104–120. https://doi.org/10.4236/ojn.2021.113010

Phillips, L. K. (2021). Succession planning in nursing education. *Nursing Outlook, 69*(1), 32–42. https://doi.org/10.1016/j.outlook.2020.08.004

Robert Wood Johnson Foundation. (2017). *Mentorship: A student success strategy mentoring program toolkit.* https://campaignforaction.org/wp-content/uploads/2020/04/Mentoring-Toolkit-2017.pdf

Rogers, J., Ludwig-Beymer, P., & Baker, M. (2020). Nurse faculty orientation: An integrative review. *Nurse Educator, 45*(6), 343–346. https://doi.org/10.1097/NNE.0000000000000802

Saeedi, M., & Parvizy, S. (2019). Strategies to promote academic motivation in nursing students: A qualitative study. *Journal of Education and Health Promotion, 8*, 86. http://doi.org10.4103/jehp.jehp_436_18

Shatto, B., & Erwin, K. (2017). Teaching millennials and generation z: Bridging the generational divide. *Creative Nursing, 23*(1), 24–28. https://doi.org/10.1891/1078-4535.23.1.24

Smiley, R. A., Allgeyer, R. L., Shobo, Y., Lyons, K. C., Letourneau, R., Zhong, E., Kaminski-Ozturk, N., & Alexander, M. (2023). The 2022 national nursing workforce survey. *The Journal of Nursing Regulation, 14*(1), Supplement 2, S1–S90. https://www.journalofnursingregulation.com/article/S2155-8256(23)00047-9/pdf

Substance Abuse and Mental Health Services Administration. (2014). *SAMSHAs concept of trauma and guidance for a trauma-informed approach.* https://store.samhsa.gov/sites/default/files/sma14-4884.pdf

University of Kansas. (2024). *What is professional identity in nursing?* https://www.kumc.edu/school-of-nursing/outreach/consulting/professional-identity/about/what-is-professional-identity-in-nursing.html

Vance, C. (2018). Reflection on the mentoring role. In D. D. Hunt (Ed.), *The new nurse educator: Mastering academe* (2nd ed., pp. 239–248). Springer Publishing Company.

Wanchai, A., Sangkhamkul, C., & Nakamadee, B. (2022). Characteristics of effective nurse educators from Thai nursing students' perspectives. *Belitung Nursing Journal, 8*(3), 245–250. https://doi.org/10.33546%2Fbnj.2085

Wells-Beede, E., Sharpnack, P., Gruben, D., Klenke-Borgmann, L., Goliat, L., & Yeager, C. (2023). Scoping review of nurse educator competencies: Mind the gap. *Nurse Educator, 48*(5), 234–239. https://doi.org/10.1097/NNE.0000000000001376

Williams, C. (2018). Recruiting middle school students into nursing. An integrative review. *Nursing Forum, 53*(2), 142–147. https://doi.org/10.1111/nuf.12235

Nursing Professional Development Practitioner in a Clinical Practice Setting

22

Joan Such Lockhart and Denise M. Petras

OBJECTIVES

1. Describe the roles and responsibilities of nursing professional development (NPD) practitioners employed in healthcare settings
2. Examine the relevance of NPD and its contribution to the practice setting
3. Explore pathways to prepare for, transition to, and develop in the NPD practitioner role

INTRODUCTION

Chapter 1 introduced readers to various nurse educator opportunities that exist in both academic and clinical practice settings. While both roles are considered nurse educators, it is important to compare these two roles, academic faculty and nursing professional development (NPD) practitioners.

First, nurse educators who assume the academic faculty role are employed by universities, colleges, community colleges, and/or hospital-based diploma schools of nursing. Excellence in practice for novice faculty is guided by the National League for Nursing (NLN) Core Competencies for Nursing Education (NLN, 2022). Learners in these academic settings vary by program level. For example, learners in schools that offer prelicensure RN curricula are often comprised of high school graduates or college graduates and practicing RNs pursuing nursing degrees. Learners progress through a curriculum designed by faculty and based on national standards framed by a local/regional needs assessment. Learning occurs in various settings, such as classrooms (face-to-face and/or virtual), skills and simulation laboratories, and diverse clinical practice settings. Assessment of learning outcomes occurs using a variety of evaluation methods, including formal examinations and assessment of clinical performance. Academic faculty may also teach graduate nursing students who are pursuing an advanced nursing role in an MSN program or a doctoral degree, such as the PhD in nursing or doctor of nursing practice (DNP).

Conversely, nurse educators employed in clinical practice settings, like hospitals and healthcare systems, are referred to as NPD practitioners (Harper & Maloney, 2022a) or by similar titles. These nurse educators are charged with helping employees to become competent in their roles, to provide patients with safe, equitable, and quality care that result in positive health outcomes. Similar to academic educators, NPD practitioners follow a set of core competencies that are published in the *Nursing Professional Development: Scope and Standards of Practice* (Harper & Maloney, 2022a); however, individual NPD roles may vary depending on specific position descriptions within an organization.

Their targeted learners often vary depending on the NPD role in each organization and NPD department. Most often, learners are nursing professionals such as newly graduated RNs beginning their first professional role, newly hired experienced nurses, or experienced nurses who are being deployed to a new clinical specialty unit or who are assuming a new leadership role within the organization. Learners may also be assistive/ancillary healthcare staff, such as unlicensed assistive personnel and healthcare workers from other professions. Learning environments are similar to those that faculty experience, but with emphasis on clinical practice work settings. Learning needs are assessed by an "analysis of a practice gap to differentiate a deficit in knowledge, skills, or practice implementation from system/process issues" (Harper & Maloney, 2022a, p. 122). Outcomes of educational offerings are systematically evaluated based on factors such as learner satisfaction, knowledge, behavior change, and impact on clinical practice and patient outcomes.

This chapter describes the role of NPD practitioners. Their scope and standards of practice, the importance of their role in clinical practice settings, and suggested pathways to prepare for, transition to, and develop in the NPD practitioner role are explained in the chapter.

NURSING PROFESSIONAL DEVELOPMENT AS A NURSING PRACTICE SPECIALTY

NPD is a "nursing practice specialty that improves the professional practice and role competence of nurses and other healthcare personnel by facilitating ongoing learning change, and role competence and growth with the intention of improving population health through indirect care" (Harper & Maloney, 2022a, p. 16). Since the 1970s, nurses employed in healthcare settings functioned in various educator roles supporting healthcare employees who provided patient-care services. Historically, NPD practitioners have assumed various titles such as staff development educator, in-service instructor, and/or clinical educator. Today, the titles and associated roles and responsibilities of NPD practitioners still vary depending on their professional qualifications, positions, and practice settings.

Over the past several decades, the NPD role has continually evolved and transitioned with support from various national professional nursing organizations such as the American Nurses Association (ANA), American Nurses Credentialing Center (ANCC), and Association for Nurses in Professional Development (ANPD). The ANPD, formerly known as National Nurses Staff Development Organization, serves as the national professional nursing organization for NPD practice and offers resources and support for nurses in this nursing specialty (ANPD, 2024). NPD practice has a defined scope and standards of practice that outlines specific competencies; national certification in NPD exists through the ANCC (n.d.).

Educators in Nursing Professional Development Roles

The NPD practitioner is an RN "with NPD practice judgment and expertise who influences professional role competence and growth of learners in a variety of settings with a desired outcome of improved population health" (Harper & Maloney, 2022a, p. 16). Specific standards of professional development are outlined in the most current *Nursing Professional Development: Scope and Standards of Practice* (Harper & Maloney, 2022a). The general format of these standards mirrors those standards for all nurses published by the ANA in *Nursing: Scope and Standards of Practice* (ANA, 2021), delineating standards of practice and professional performance.

Each of these 18 standards includes a set of expected competencies organized by two different NPD roles that build on expectations based on professional qualifications and experience (Harper & Maloney, 2022a). For example, an *NPD practitioner* (formerly called an *NPD generalist*) is usually a novice in NPD practice who is expected to perform at a beginning level. Conversely, a more advanced *NPD specialist* possesses higher credentials and experience in the specialty and "develops tools, theories, skills, and knowledge to advance the practice of the NPD specialty" (Harper & Maloney, 2022a, p. 16). Table 22.1 illustrates the professional qualifications required for each role.

For each standard, the first set of competencies applies to both levels of NPD practitioners. The NPD specialist, however, is expected to demonstrate an additional set of higher-level competencies. For example, in Standard of Practice 4 related to Planning, all NPD practitioners are expected to develop a "collaborative plan encompassing strategies to achieve expected outcomes" (Harper & Maloney, 2022a, p. 74). Along with other competencies, both practitioners and specialists are expected to "develop a plan that reflects compliance with current statutes, rules and regulations, and standards" (p. 74). In addition to this competency, the NPD specialist is expected to perform at a higher level and "analyzes cost-effectiveness and anticipated return on investment (ROI) and/or expectations for NPD initiatives" (p. 76).

TABLE 22.1 NURSING PROFESSIONAL DEVELOPMENT ROLES AND PROFESSIONAL QUALIFICATIONS

NPD Role	Professional Qualifications
Practitioner	RN prepared at the bachelor's level in nursing (or international equivalent), with/without NPD certification **or** RN prepared at the graduate level, without NPD certification
Specialist	RN prepared at the graduate level in nursing or a related field and NPD certified

NPD, nursing professional development.
Source: Harper, M., & Maloney, P. (Eds.). (2022a). *Nursing professional development: Scope and standards of practice* (4th ed.). Association for Nursing Professional Development.

UNDERSTANDING THE SCOPE OF NURSING PROFESSIONAL DEVELOPMENT PRACTICE USING A MODEL

The ANPD, in collaboration the ANA, revised a visual model that illustrates NPD practice aimed to help nurses understand the full scope of the specialty (Harper & Maloney, 2022a) This model uses a systems approach to provide a "big picture" perspective about the specialty. The NPD practice model outlines inputs, throughputs, and outputs that occur in a cyclic and fluid manner with feedback loop. A brief video overview of the model is available for viewing (ANPD Headquarters, 2023).

Inputs are assets, such as supplies and human resources, that are needed in NPD practice to attain expected outcomes. In this model, key inputs include NPD practitioners themselves along with the targeted learners they support based on interprofessional practice gaps and NPD standards.

Throughputs comprise the "processes that occur within the system to transform the input" (Harper & Maloney, 2022a, p. 22). Primary throughputs in the model include NPD responsibilities aligned with the organization's mission and vision. These standards mirror those for all RNs described in the ANA's *Nursing: Scope and Standards of Practice* (ANA, 2021).

Finally, outputs are "products that are exported into the environment" such as learning, change, and role competence and growth that foster outcomes such as "optimal care" and "population health" within an interprofessional perspective (Harper & Maloney, 2022a, pp. 22–23). Outputs also provide evidence for NPD practitioners to consider throughout the feedback cycle.

NURSING PROFESSIONAL DEVELOPMENT ROLES

As illustrated in Table 22.2, seven roles comprise the NPD practitioner's function, which support the NPD standards of practice. These standards drive how the roles are realized or powered in practice (Harper & Maloney, 2022a).

TABLE 22.2 NURSING PROFESSIONAL DEVELOPMENT PRACTITIONER ROLES AND RESPONSIBILITIES

Roles	Responsibilities
Learning facilitator	Onboarding/orientation
Change agent	Competency management
Mentor	Education
Leader	Role development
Champion for inquiry	Inquiry
Advocate for NPD specialty	Collaborative partnerships
Partner for practice transitions	

NPD, nursing professional development.
Source: Harper, M., & Maloney, P. (Eds.). (2022a). *Nursing professional development: Scope and standards of practice* (4th ed.). Association for Nursing Professional Development.

Learning Facilitator

As a learning facilitator, the NPD practitioner "uses the educational design process and adult learning principles to bridge the knowledge, skills and/or practice gaps identified through a needs assessment and evaluation of outcomes" (Harper & Maloney, 2022a, p. 3). The NPD practitioner role is often interchanged with the title of educator, which typically is used to describe one who is in the academic setting. The differentiating feature between the roles is the NPD practitioner specializes in imparting new knowledge to learners directly related to practice gaps (Woolforde, 2019). NPD practitioners facilitate learning by using active teaching strategies in their practice; to successfully influence behavior change, they must create an optimum learning environment, employ adult learning principles, and use varied teaching–learning techniques that best match learners' needs (Harper & Maloney, 2022a; Johnson & Smith, 2019). Creative teaching–learning strategies are the mark of a resourceful NPD practitioner.

An example of this is gamification, a teaching strategy that incorporates the use of games or game like activities to engage learners in more active learning experiences, such as an escape rooms aimed to help clinical nurses learn about quality improvement (QI; Bonn et al., 2022) or prepare nurses for the preceptor role (Coughlin et al., 2023). In another example, Foley and colleagues (2024) implemented an innovative "NPD practitioner at night program" aimed to help new graduate nurses transition to their clinical roles while they worked the night shift on critical care and medical-surgical units, foster socialization, and minimize new graduate attrition (p. 21).

The NPD practitioner also facilitates learning through precepting. Harper (2020) defines a preceptor as one who "guides, assesses, and validates the knowledge, skills, and attitudes needed to transition to a new role, specialty or environment in the healthcare setting" (p. 1). Preceptor roles and responsibilities mirror those of the NPD practitioner, so it is not unusual that they naturally assume preceptor duties. A typical example includes precepting undergraduate and graduate nursing students during their clinical practice experiences. In addition, they prepare and mentor other nurses who serve as preceptors as well as support graduate nurses during their transition to practice, helping them to build confidence in practice while meeting requisite orientation objectives (Liu et al., 2019; Nelson et al., 2019).

Change Agent

In the change agent role, the NPD practitioner "uses change management strategies and theories to drive desired outcomes" (Harper & Maloney, 2022a, p. 31). For example, practitioners can actively influence change within their healthcare organizations by facilitating the realization of the National Academies of Sciences, Engineering, and Medicine recommendations for change (NASEM, 2021) discussed more later in this chapter. NPD practitioners as change agent role models can create an environment within the healthcare setting to provide education across disciplines to ensure competence and for students to experience real-world learning in the clinical setting.

As healthcare continues to evolve, the NPD practitioner must keep pace and demonstrate flexibility as a change agent, which means serving as a "key driver for the specialty and will determine whether [practitioners] get out in front of the curve or even keep pace with change" (Maloney & Woolforde, 2019, p. 60). NPD practitioners have consistently been at the forefront of change, leading the charge by assessing readiness, identifying and influencing stakeholders, establishing a conducive work climate, leading and role modeling best practices, and ensuring that change is sustained. Adapting to and role modeling change is a requisite behavior for the NPD practitioner's success. During the pandemic, they led change in transforming traditional practices using creative strategies to meet staff onboarding and learning needs. Examples included a plethora of just-in-time education for managing the dynamics of infection prevention requirements for safe care; onboarding; and nurse residency programs (NRPs; Fox & Richter, 2021; Joseph et al., 2023; Pate et al., 2023; Weiss et al., 2021).

Mentor

As a mentor, the NPD practitioner "advances the profession of nursing and the NPD specialty by contributing to the professional development of others and supporting ongoing professional learning as individuals develop across practice, professional, and educational settings" (Harper & Maloney, 2022a, p. 31). For example, they not only mentor nursing students but "the professional growth of nurses and other healthcare personnel in various settings and encourage interprofessional education and collaboration" (Brunt & Bogdan, 2023, p. 1). Dickerson (2019) supports the NPD practitioner's importance in mentoring staff and leaders alike by developing their roles through education. In fact, they mentor beyond education to include engagement in committee work and career coaching as well as guidance using evidence-based practice (EBP) and research. In using their informal power, NPD practitioners have the ability to influence others (Harper, 2023).

Leader

The NPD practitioner "influences the interprofessional practice and learning environments, the NPD specialty, the profession of nursing, and healthcare" (Harper & Maloney, 2022a, p. 31). Given this charge, the NPD role is inherently a leadership role, even if not formally recognized as such in practice settings. Brunt and Bogdan (2023) identified the leadership skills required for success that include: excellent communication ethical and legal knowledge regulatory acumen; awareness of standard health laws (e.g. Health Insurance Portability and Accountability Act [HIPAA]); the ability to align education goals with that of the healthcare organization strategic planning and a transformational leadership style to influence others. NPD practitioners lead by role modeling, initiating practice changes, thinking strategically, aligning professional development work with organizational goals, and demonstrating expertise in data analysis and quantifying the return on investment (ROI) of their work (Chappell, 2020).

As formal and/or informal leaders, NPD practitioners represent the value of their work to the organization by positively impacting patient outcomes. In aligning their work with organizational objectives and strategic initiatives, they can influence culture and practice change through interprofessional teams, shared decision-making, and the application of QI practices (Harper & Maloney, 2022a).

The functions of formal NPD leaders are not unlike those of other leaders related to human resource management, fiscal accountability, and ensuring the impact of department work on organizational outcomes. In addition, the NPD leader has the challenge of demonstrating the value of professional development to senior leadership. Furthermore, they are accountable for advancing the profession through the development of others (Brunt & Bogdan, 2023).

Like other system leadership roles, NPD leaders who serve in top positions within a healthcare system are charged with "speaking with one voice for nursing, which requires a cohesiveness and alignment that begins with nursing leadership" (Boerger, 2020, p. 242). Key skills required at this level include strong communication, the ability to empower others, and the development of relationships across the system. As the NPD multisite leader role expanded, a study commissioned by the ANPD to determine the requisite competencies for the role yielded valuable evidence. In addition to competent NPD practice and nurse executive skills, the competencies of "communication, relationship building, business acumen, and organizational alignment" were identified as keys to success (Harper & Maloney, 2022b, p. 188).

Champion for Inquiry

As a champion for scientific inquiry, the NPD practitioner "promotes a spirit of inquiry, the generation and dissemination of new knowledge, and the use of evidence to advance NPD practice, guide clinical practice, and improve the quality of care for the healthcare consumer/partner" (Harper & Maloney, 2022a, p. 31). The NPD practitioner can fulfill this role by actively engaging in research or evaluating existing research for application in clinical practice. They are charged with ensuring that the work environment is conducive to supporting research and EBP and "engage in inquiry activities that align with the organizational mission, vision, and strategic plan" (Harper & Maloney, 2022a, p. 105).

Advocate

The NPD practitioner is expected to serve as an advocate who "actively supports, promotes, and demonstrates NPD as a nursing practice specialty" (Harper & Maloney, 2022a, p. 31). Advocacy for NPD was forged by visionary staff educators in the mid to late 1980s who foresaw this work as a specialty. Hospital-based education took on a new dimension as the first journal and national nursing organization for staff development formed and were well received. The early leaders in NPD set a standard that quickly evolved into a currently recognized specialty with a subsequent certification.

Today, and in the future, NPD practitioners must continue to support the pioneered work of the specialty, as many of the same challenges from the past linger in the present. Persistence in communicating and demonstrating the value of NPD to executives is critical, especially when budget cuts threaten positions. Professional development work that aligns with organizational strategic goals embeds the relevance of the work in relation to safe practice, quality patient-care outcomes, and reduced nursing turnover (Johnson & Smith, 2019).

Advocacy for the specialty can take a variety of forms. For example, the NPD practitioner can advocate for the specialty by joining and becoming active in the ANPD, which serves as a voice for the specialty, forum for learning, and vehicle for policy change. ANPD's mission, "to advance the quality of healthcare by defining and promoting NPD practice," is realized through its core values of leadership, practice excellence, and inquiry (ANPD, 2024). Woolforde (2020) offers the ANPD as an "investment" in professional development that serves practitioners in the present and prepares them for the future through the organization's plentiful resources. Local ANPD chapters offer opportunities for practitioners to engage in learning, leadership, and networking with peers as well as to recruit new practitioners to become active members. Advocating for the NPD specialty can be realized when practitioners showcase the specialty through their actions. Examples of such efforts include disseminating information and knowledge through podium presentations; publishing; engagement in committee and council work at a hospital, system, or community level; and maintaining active involvement in professional organizations and boards (Harper & Maloney, 2022a).

Finally, the NPD role includes advocacy beyond the specialty. In addition to advocating for peers, NPD practitioners are called to create a safe and respectable environment for learners; as change agents and leaders they ensure a culture of safety for patients and help to close practice gaps related to healthcare disparities. Furthermore, they accomplish such only when they practice self-reflection to identify and manage bias (Harper & Maloney, 2022a).

Partner for Practice Transitions

In this critical role, the NPD practitioner "supports the transition of nurses and other healthcare team members across learning and practice environments, roles and professional stages" (Harper & Maloney, 2022a, p. 31). The impetus for transition to practice programs, also known as nurse residency programs (NRPs), evolved over a decade ago to help nurses bridge the move from academia to professional practice with the intent of facilitating a smoother entrance into the work world as well as to improve retention rates over the first 2 years of practice (Institute of Medicine, 2011). These programs arose from both grassroots efforts within hospitals as well as structured, evidence-based offerings with the intent of improving the new graduates' job satisfaction.

In a review of the nurse residency literature, wide variations in the implementation of the programs were found. However, consistent themes emerged validating the value of a structured program in improving job satisfaction, competence, confidence, and retention in addition to facilitating new graduates' enculturation to the practice setting (Chant & Westendorf, 2019; Durkin, 2019; Suter & Painter, 2020). In addition to leadership, quality, decision-making, and EBP skills, a prime component of the NRPs focuses on the support of the residents and the development of relationships among nurse residents. The success of the NRPs depends on solid leadership, a well-planned curriculum, creative content delivery, trained facilitators, and strong mentorship (Chant & Westendorf, 2019). Based on the NPD practitioner's required skill set, they are likely candidates to assume leadership of NRP programs. Facilitating transition to practice is also consistent with the roles of facilitator and mentor.

In addition to NRPs, NPD practitioners often facilitate the transition of other healthcare professionals and unlicensed staff to new roles and/or additional duties in times of change and crisis. Such transitions may include helping nursing assistants assume unit secretary duties; preparing patient transport technicians as transport monitor technicians; and/or supporting clinical RNs in new preceptor or charge nurse roles. During the 2020 COVID-19 pandemic, redeployment of staff from a variety of disciplines and roles to areas of need required the successful assessment and training by NPD practitioners to ensure ready resources for maintaining patient care.

NURSING PROFESSIONAL DEVELOPMENT PRACTITIONERS' RESPONSIBILITIES

In addition to fulfilling multiple roles, NPD practitioners assume several responsibilities, action-oriented duties that define the performance expectations of the position (Table 22.2). These responsibilities, as identified in the NPD practice model, impact both practice and learning environments.

Onboarding/Orientation

Harper and Maloney (2022a) define onboarding as "the fluid process of hiring, orienting, socializing, and integrating an employee to the organization with a focus on retention and growth" (p. 34). Orientation, as an important component of the onboarding process, consists of an "individualized program to guide the new hire towards job competency" (p. 34). Orientation has been one of the primary NPD practitioner responsibilities and is a function in which they spend a large portion of time. This assumption was validated by Bauer et al. (2023) in their study of NPD practitioner workload that determined 25.2% of NPD time was devoted to onboarding and orientation.

Today, the focus is more than orienting new hires to their roles. The entire onboarding experience is critical to ensure that both professional and unlicensed new hires not only receive the preparation they need to function safely in their roles but are also supported in becoming engaged in their new organization. The transition from candidate to hire is heavily influenced through the successful collaboration with talent acquisition followed by an orientation experience that meets the needs of the new hires. The NPD practitioner plays an important role in the retention of orientees based on the success of the onboarding process; this function ultimately yields cost savings to the organization by positively influencing turnover. Orientation is not limited to new hires, but also for individuals who change roles and may include non nursing staff.

The orientation of new staff typically includes a didactic component that covers relevant information they need to function safely in the clinical environment, electronic medical record training, and mandatory learning, followed by a skills review and precepted clinical orientation on the orientees' home units. NPD practitioners are challenged with keeping content delivery fresh and contemporary to capture the attention of diverse learners, as well as being flexible in accommodating volume-based hiring trends.

Competency Management

The ANA states that competence implies an individual is "performing successfully at an expected level" (ANA, 2021, p. 145). Competence can also be defined as the ability to perform a job; competencies are typically described as a set of skills that assess performance in the critical thinking, psychomotor skills, or interpersonal skills domains. Competency management is "a dynamic process designed to support ongoing assessment and evaluation of performance" (Harper & Maloney, 2022a, p. 34). NPD practitioners collaborate with learners and organizational leadership to determine the competencies that require validation on a periodic schedule based on factors such as quality data, high risk/low volume activities, regulatory requirements, and acquisition of new skills. Ensuring an effective competency program impacts healthcare workers' abilities to provide quality, safe care. To plan and deliver an effective competency program, the NPD practitioners must possess knowledge and skill in competency assessment (Harper & Maloney, 2022a).

A widely popular competency option is the Wright competency model, which shifts the focus for developing competence to the healthcare worker and the assessment of competence in real time (Durkin, 2019). The tenets Wright's model of ownership, empowerment, and accountability rely on the commitment of employees to the competency process that has been coestablished with educators and leaders (Wright, 2021). An example of a more traditional competency assessment program is one often referred to as a "competency blitz," during which time all levels of staff present to a central location, offered on several days, to visit stations where they perform specific skills for validation. While this is a time-consuming and labor-intensive process, it gives the NPD practitioner control over the competence assessment process, creates an environment for comradery between/among staff, and ensures consistent evaluation. In the future, NPD practitioners will need to demonstrate flexibility by discovering and implementing additional methods to assess competence in practice.

Education

Education is designed to "improve professional practice and the provision of quality patient care" (Harper & Maloney, 2022a, p. 35). To provide relevant educational offerings for both licensed and unlicensed nursing staff, the NPD practitioner must be able to effectively assess learning needs and subsequently identify practice gaps. Education is a core function of the NPD role, as all work centers around this activity. Providing educational experiences for learners includes the most basic of tasks (e.g., nursing assistant preparation), complex clinical skills to prepare nurses to work in specialty areas (e.g., critical care, trauma, transplant, emergency or flight nursing), interpersonal relationship and communication skills, preceptor training, and leadership development. In the practice setting, continuing education also includes interprofessional education. NPD practitioners are responsible for "increasing rigor around continuing education that adds value and meets the needs of learners" (Cipriano, 2020, p. 114).

The delivery of education is based on the content and learner. Savvy NPD practitioners carefully plan teaching strategies best suited to the skill to be taught and the nature of the audience, including experience level, generational or cultural characteristics, and level of readiness. Traditional methods such as live lectures and discussions are still valid and often preferred by learners. However, many of the teaching strategies discussed in this book such as blended learning, flipped classrooms, independent computer modules, virtual reality, gaming, escape rooms, and asynchronous strategies are important to consider and often are necessary to ensure flexible content delivery. Access to learning must be nimble so learners can suit their needs relative to time and motivation (Weinschreider et al., 2019). Simulation, an effective tool for teaching and validating psychomotor skills, also has been successfully used as a cognitive tool for developing critical thinking or clinical judgment (Fogg et al., 2020; Norwood et al., 2023). Technologies such as mobile apps, webinars, podcasts, learning management systems, and even artificial intelligence are current and emerging delivery mechanisms that support creative education endeavors (Weinschreider et al., 2019).

DelMonte (2020) also suggests that NPD practitioners conserve resources by "standardizing education and broadening audiences to avoid duplication of resources" (p. 180). The opportunity for them to create educational offerings that move from being instructor-led to learner-directed can positively influence learning objectives and outcomes (Johnson & Smith, 2019). Effective delivery of education contributes to increased learner satisfaction and, ultimately, positively impacts the care of patients.

Role Development

Harper and Maloney (2022a) define professional role development as the "identification and application of strategies to facilitate continuous growth through ongoing professional learning" (p. 36). NPD practitioners often drive role development through both formal and informal processes. In an informal coaching role, they influence staff and their peers to continue their professional development in the pursuit of a promotion by providing access to academic programs, sharing personal exemplars, or fostering shadowing experiences with leaders. NPD practitioners also coordinate activities for gaining advanced knowledge to become proficient in a current role. Brunt and Bogdan (2023) believe NPD specialists are key in advancing the development of nurses through education.

Providing staff with experiences that foster their professional role development also, in turn, supports national recommendations discussed later in this chapter. Activities that support this effort include advising staff seeking advanced degrees, mentoring staff to prepare for successive roles, developing programs that will impact staff role development, non traditional approaches to orientation or transition to practice programs, charge role, and leadership training (Harper & Maloney, 2022a). Additionally, NPD practitioners help staff to advance in clinical ladders and facilitate staff lead/co lead of teams, committees, and councils.

Inquiry

Nursing research focuses on creating new knowledge. The implementation of EBP and QI projects integrates evidence into practice and provides a continuous process to improve the quality in healthcare. NPD practitioners promote research, EBP, and QI. The degree of involvement in any of these activities is based on the practitioner's academic preparation, experience, and competence as well as the environment in which they work (Harper & Maloney, 2022a). The NPD practitioner's responsibility of scholarly inquiry aligns with each of the NPD roles. Activities include literature reviews, policy changes, staff mentorship in the research or EBP process, implementing clinical initiatives based on evidence, providing evidence to support the work and value of NPD as related to organization goals, and incorporating EBP into the NRP program (Harper & Maloney, 2022a). Opperman et al. (2022) highlight the significance or the NPD practitioner's engagement in research that demonstrates the ROI of professional development in the clinical setting.

NPD practitioners are expected to track and trend evidence that has an impact on quality. Seeing situations from a different perspective enables them to foster interprofessional collaboration to identify innovative strategies that engage QI activities (Harper & Bindon, 2019; Park & Holschneider, 2020). In addition, NPD practitioners often lead QI teams that drive change. Many hospitals have teams that focus on managing nurse-sensitive indicators such as hospital-acquired pressure injuries, catheter-associated urinary tract infections, and patient falls. These teams are opportunities for front-line staff to engage in the identification of patient-related problems and to generate innovative, but realistic, solutions to mitigate problems. As a champion for this work, the NPD practitioner possesses the skill set to "guide data collection, data analysis, and development of measurable quality outcomes that align with the organization's strategic initiatives and priorities" (Smith & Johnson, 2019, p. 222). Finally, they use proven, evidence-based methods as a structure for leading QI work.

Collaborative Partnerships

Partnerships were discussed in Chapter 12. One of the strongest collaborative partnerships in which the NPD practitioner engages is with academic colleagues (Kiss et al., 2020). In this important role, they coordinate student placements, identify, and prepare staff nurses to precept students, ensure the orientation of students and clinical faculty to the organization, participate in scholarly work with the affiliating academic institution, and engage faculty and students in key clinical experiences such as rounding and patient-care conferences. The benefits of collaborative partnerships between service and academia include strengthening transition to practice programs and promoting enhanced sharing of resources (American Association of Colleges of Nursing [AACN], 2019). Faculty can provide education to staff as well as facilitate onsite cohorts for advanced degrees or act as NRP facilitators which may fulfill their faculty practice requirement. Often, NPD practitioners have dual roles as clinical instructors for nursing students.

The dedicated education unit (DEU) is a partnership between the academic and service settings that continues to realize positive outcomes and is a program typically coordinated and facilitated by the NPD practitioner. Despite challenges in clinical teaching models over the years, the DEU results in a "positive clinical learning environment where future nurses are supported with the development of necessary competencies, thus easing the transition from student to professional nurse" (Dimino et al., 2020, p. 127). The DEU is a model whereby staff nurses, after receiving training, function as clinical educators for one or two students with the faculty member onsite (or communicating via other means) to support the staff nurse who is teaching the students. Implementation of a DEU is a way for students to receive a rich, real-world clinical experience with the staff nurse as mentor. The DEU can create a win–win situation for both the academic partners and staff; it is a strategy to mitigate faculty shortages as well as provide the staff nurse an opportunity to be an educator, which is an enriching developmental experience. DEUs have a positive impact on students' learning outcomes and self confidence (Musallam et al., 2021) and on the hospital's onboarding of students as new RN hires after graduation.

ROLE IN PROMOTING SAFE, QUALITY, AND EQUITABLE HEALTHCARE

NPD practitioners have a central role in supporting equitable patient-centered care, patient safety, and quality health outcomes within healthcare organizations. In addition, NPD practitioners contribute to the organization's mission, vision, and strategic goals that address current healthcare trends. Nurses strengthen healthcare by developing a "culture of health by reducing disparities in individuals' ability to achieve their full health potential" (Johnson, 2022, p. 123). Results gleaned from *The Future of Nursing 2020–2023: Charting a Path to Achieve Health Equity,* a 2021 landmark study conducted by NASEM, provide nine recommendations for change (NASEM, 2021). As depicted in their current practice model, NPD practitioners are capable of supporting health equity and protecting consumers within their practice settings (Harper & Maloney, 2022a). More specifically, Johnson (2022) describes how NPD practitioners, functioning through their seven roles previously mentioned in this chapter, are prepared to address three of the nine recommendations (3, 6, 7).

Healthcare Organization Accreditation and Compliance

NPD practitioners help healthcare organizations attain and maintain their accreditation and compliance by ensuring that clinical practice performance standards are met (Dickerson & Durkin, 2022). This charge is managed through NPD standards of practice by providing ongoing staff development and support that helps workers attain/maintain their core competencies, conducting continuous QI initiatives, and tracking/monitoring available evidence against best practices. For example, NPD practitioners are instrumental in ensuring that healthcare professionals employed at their organizations comply with the most current Hospital National Patient Safety Goals established by The Joint Commission (TJC, 2024). Each year, TJC publishes standards that support patient safety in various healthcare settings. The 2024 standards for hospital settings include several goals related to patient safety: identify patients correctly; improve staff communication; use medicines safely; use alarms safely; prevent infection; identify patient safety risks; improve healthcare equity; and prevent mistakes in surgery (TJC, 2024). Supportive strategies that accompany these goals help NPD practitioners prioritize their efforts in assessing and analyzing practice gaps, designing and implementing learner-centered interventions aimed to address these gaps, and providing ongoing monitoring of changes in actual practice compared to best practices.

Strategic Goals of the Healthcare Organization

Healthcare organizations develop strategic plans that communicate the direction of the organization to all stakeholders. Sharing this plan with employees enables them to make informed decisions regarding departmental goals and daily work, determine the allocation of available resources, and collectively move toward a common goal. Since healthcare organizations strive to attain an advantage over their competitors, employing a team of healthcare professionals who are not only competent in their role but who are also dependable, satisfied, and contribute to the organization is an asset.

NPD practitioners have an essential role in recruiting, preparing, supporting, and retaining a workforce of nursing professionals who are competent and demonstrate nursing excellence. As such, NPD practitioners often provide leadership in preparing for and seeking national recognition for nursing excellence in their organization through the Magnet Recognition Program® and other similar programs. NPD practitioners are often charged to collect relevant data from the practice environment and prepare written evidence supporting positive patient-care outcomes. In addition, they provide educational offerings and other initiatives aimed to foster success in attaining this prestigious recognition.

Organizational Alignment and Managing Challenges

While the departments in which NPD practitioners work may differ in structure and function within various healthcare settings, it is important for NPD leaders to align their departmental (and individual) efforts with those of their healthcare organizations—specifically the mission, vision, and strategic goals. Working together toward common goals not only directs the NPD department's workflow with limited resources, but also facilitates the attainment of these goals. As such, accomplishments reported by NPD leaders should include evidence that supports these outcomes, their impact, and their value on the organization. Similarly, individual NPD practitioners should also align their annual goals with those of their department and illustrate evidence-based outcomes of their efforts.

Working in an era of economic constraints and constantly changing healthcare environments challenges NPD practitioners to anticipate, recognize, and manage their work using system-wide, evidence-based strategies. As previously mentioned, NPD practitioners and specialists are charged with quantifying the value that their work has on organizational priorities. The utilization of various program evaluation resources can help them systematically measure outcomes and document the impact of their efforts at the organizational level (Dickerson & Durkin, 2022). In addition, program planning should include cost–benefit calculations and impact on practice changes. Department reports should reflect measurable outcomes that illustrate an ROI (Opperman et al., 2022)

Working within constantly evolving clinical environments, NPD practitioners are challenged to carefully analyze practice gaps, plan and develop innovative offerings that engage and motivate a diverse group of learners, and evaluate the impact of their efforts on not only learners' knowledge, skills, and values, but also on patient outcomes. NPD practitioners need to be flexible and understand that strategies that are effective for newly hired nurses often differ from those for experienced nurses, ancillary staff, and/or members of the interprofessional team. These factors illustrate the need to devote attention to logistical considerations in prioritizing and coordinating NPD activities.

Urgent healthcare issues, such as the COVID-19 pandemic, illustrated the need for NPD practitioners to be flexible in leading both planned and unplanned changes and in minimizing the impact of the issue on the safety and health outcomes of patients, employees, and the overall organization. Work priorities rapidly changed to preparing and deploying existing healthcare staff to meet the needs of the organization for patient-care services (Brown et al., 2020).

DEVELOPING THE NURSING PROFESSIONAL DEVELOPMENT PRACTITIONER ROLE

Perhaps you observed an NPD practitioner in your healthcare organization, read about this nursing specialty in the literature, or learned about this role in your nursing education. You may be asking these questions:

- How can you learn more about the NPD practitioner role to determine if this career path is something to which you might aspire in your future?
- How can you transition to the NPD practitioner role from a clinical practice role?
- What opportunities exist to help you maintain and advance in the NPD practitioner role once you started this position?

Determining Your Interest and Preparation for the Role

First, consider talking with NPD practitioners in your own healthcare organization and express your potential interest in the role. Try to gain their personal perspectives and advice regarding how to best prepare yourself. Ask if you can shadow them for a day to better understand the role. Get to know your NPD colleagues and staff. Consider gaining a first-hand understanding of the role by volunteering to help with unit-based educational initiatives, department committees or task forces, or shared governance groups that focus on nursing education at your workplace. Volunteer as a preceptor for newly graduated nurses during their onboarding or residency period or for an experienced RN who is being deployed to an unfamiliar clinical specialty unit. If you have already engaged in some of these activities, go a step further by volunteering as a leader in these various initiatives.

Second, read and learn as much as you can about being an NPD practitioner. Appendix C offers a few examples of resources such as organizations, journals, and conferences that focus on the NPD practice. In addition, search for available books and webinars that focus on the NPD role. Enroll in a graduate-level academic program that has a nursing education specialty option. As you progress through the program, try to frame your assignments and course projects to the NPD practitioner role and choose an NPD specialist as a preceptor for your clinical practicum. If you already have a graduate degree, consider enrolling in a postmaster's certificate or concentration in nursing education that will provide you with the information that you will need to help you develop in the NPD role.

Third, conduct a self-assessment of your personal and professional strengths to determine how they relate to the NPD practitioner roles and responsibilities. Begin by reviewing an advertisement for an NPD practitioner position or a position description for the role at your organization, paying attention to the required/

preferred qualifications and responsibilities at an NPD practitioner level. Continue to build upon your strengths in your clinical specialty and in the NPD role as you wait for an available opportunity.

Last, prepare for a future NPD practitioner role using the resources previously mentioned. Create a professional development plan with targeted short- and long-term goals that will help guide your career plans. Revisit your plan yearly, perhaps around your annual performance review date at work, to track your progress and revise it as needed. Also, update your resume (or curriculum vitae) each year and document accomplishments related to the NPD practitioner role. Continue to build upon your knowledge, skills, and values required for the role. For example, the chapters contained in this book can help you develop your teaching expertise. Continue to build your professional portfolio related to the NPD practitioner role by reviewing available resources, networking with nurses in the NPD role, and becoming an active member in NPD-related professional organizations.

Transitioning to the Nursing Professional Development Practitioner Role

Once hired in an NPD practitioner role, carefully review your position description and role expectations with your manager and ask for clarification, as needed. Reflect how your role expectations compare with those outlined in the *Nursing Professional Development: Scope and Standards of Practice* (Harper & Maloney, 2022a). Chapter 2 in this text describes phases that clinicians often experience as they transition from a clinician to an academic educator role. Your transition experience to the NPD practitioner role may be similar. Remember that it takes time and effort to feel and think like an educator. It is important to realize that, although you have been an expert nurse clinician, you are now a novice educator and need to give yourself permission to learn this new role and how to function in a different role in the same work setting. It often takes time for you to get accustomed to your new role and for your colleagues to get accustomed to you in a new role. Fortunately, you are familiar with the organization and can apply your role to support its initiatives.

Organizations often vary in what resources they provide to orient or onboard NPD practitioners to their new role. Outcomes of a 6-month guided, virtual NPD fellowship program targeted to clinical nurses transitioning to the NPD role revealed an increase in their perceived confidence, a better understanding of the NPD role, and experience in applying the core NPD roles in practice (DeVolt et al., 2023). If no formal, structured orientation exists at your workplace, consider creating your own orientation program guided by your personal assessment, current position description, available resources (Appendix C), and support from more experienced NPD colleagues. Identify a mentor who can help you navigate this career path and who can serve as a sounding board to help problem-solve transition challenges. The personal experiences of others who transitioned to the NPD role, like the journey shared by Weimer (2021), can provide valuable insight.

If you lack access to a mentor, consider asking an NPD practitioner at another organization whom you met at a professional meeting or ask a former faculty member. Expert educators suggest getting prepared for the NPD role by collecting information about the roles and responsibilities; analyzing, organizing, and planning your work; and developing approaches to continually evaluate your performance.

Opperman (2023) emphasizes the value of cultivating knowledge, skills, and behaviors related to the core NPD roles.

Maintaining and Advancing in the Nursing Professional Development Practitioner Role

Once you have attained an NPD practitioner position, revise your professional development plan to help you not only maintain but advance your clinical specialty and NPD competencies. Continue to review and revise your plan. If you currently hold an NPD practitioner role, consider developing competencies that will help you advance to the NPD specialist level, when that position becomes available.

If enrolled in a graduate nursing education program, apply concepts learned in class using an NPD perspective. Your preceptored clinical experience can provide you with an opportunity to showcase your strengths in another setting and advance your professional goals.

Join and actively engage in professional nursing organizations at the national, regional, and/or local levels. Be selective in choosing associations that align with your professional goals. Consider those related to your clinical practice specialty and NPD roles. As previously mentioned, consider membership in a professional organization that supports the NPD practice specialty, like the ANPD, that will provide you with resources, ongoing development, and networking with other practitioners across the nation. Similarly, join a professional nursing organization tailored to your clinical specialty to maintain or advance your clinical perspective. Both examples of professional organizations can provide you with leadership opportunities, scholarships, national conferences, and access to peer-reviewed journals. Learn more about these organizations by talking with representatives at professional meetings. Volunteer for a task force that builds upon your strengths and aligns with your professional goals. Regardless of the professional development strategies that you chose, it is important to realize that a life-long learning perspective is essential (Park & Holtschneider, 2022).

Develop a plan to obtain national certification in Nursing Professional Development offered by the ANCC and accredited by the Accreditation Board for Specialty Nursing Certification (ANCC, n.d.). While NPD practitioners are expected to encourage and support professional certification among nurses within their organization, becoming certified themselves is an expectation outlined in the NPD Scope and Standards of Practice (Harper & Maloney, 2022a).

Begin the certification process by reviewing the ANCC Nursing Professional Development Specialist certification website (www.nursingworld.org/our-certifications/nursing-professional-development/). Check the eligibility criteria required for certification, incorporate needed changes into your professional development plan, and prepare a timeline based on your target date. Exhibit 22.1 outlines the current eligibility for NPD certification. Nurses who successfully earn certification use awarded the credential Registered Nurse-Board Certified (NPD-BC^{TM}). Certification lasts for 5 years and can be renewed through continuing nursing education. Keep current in your specialty by reading NPD publications, attending continuing education offerings, and networking with other professionals. Collaborate with your hospital librarian who can help you search the literature for evidence to help problem-solve practice issues you may encounter in your role. The opportunity

EXHIBIT 22.1 Eligibility for Certification in Nursing Professional Development

Current, active RN license in the United States or territory (or professional equivalent in another country)

Bachelor's degree or higher in nursing

Minimum of 2 years full-time practice as an RN (or equivalent)

At least 2,000 hours clinical practice in NPD within past 3 years

At least 30 hours of continuing education in NPD within past 3 years

NPD, Nursing Professional Development
Source: American Nurses Credentialing Center. (n.d.). *Nursing Professional Development Certification (NPD-BC)*. https://www.nursingworld.org/our-certifications/nursing-professional-development

---

to obtain a portfolio-based advanced certification in NPD, awarded with the credential of NPDA-BC, was recently implemented in late 2021 (Harper et al., 2023).

Finally, share the expertise and insight that you have gained over the years by mentoring others who may express interest in pursuing the NPD practitioner role. Recognize nurses who have demonstrated a potential for becoming more involved in the role, especially at the unit-based level. Remember that your role as an NPD practitioner is to advocate for NPD practice and the value that it provides to the nursing profession, healthcare organization, and consumers of healthcare.

SUMMARY

Nurse educators who assume the NPD practitioner role are engaged in an evolving nursing practice specialty with a defined set of scope and standards and guided with a practice model that delineates the professional standards of practice and roles and responsibilities. NPD practitioners help protect the public by supporting the competency and growth of healthcare professionals who provide patient-care services within a healthcare setting. They function within a variety of clinical practice settings and provide services that align with the organization and trends. Advancing to the NPD practitioner role involves dedicated preparation for the role, continuous engagement in the specialty, and advocating for the specialty.

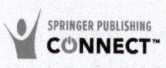 A robust set of instructor resources designed to supplement this text is located at http://connect.springerpub.com/content/book/978-0-8261-8892-2. Qualifying instructors may request access by emailing textbook@springerpub.com.

REFERENCES

American Association of Colleges of Nursing. (2019). *AACN's vision for academic nursing* [White paper]. https://www.aacnnursing.org/News-Information/Position-Statements-White-Papers/Vision-for-Nursing-Education

American Nurses Association. (2021). *Nursing: Scope and standards of practice* (4th ed.). Author.

American Nurses Credentialing Center. (n.d.). *Nursing Professional Development Certification* (NPD-BC). https://www.nursingworld.org/our-certifications/nursing-professional-development

ANPD Headquarters. (2023, August 24). *ANPD NPD model* [Video]. You Tube. https://www.youtube.com/watch?v=OchKI8W2UF8

Association for Nursing Professional Development. (2024). *About Us*. https://www.anpd.org/About/About-Us

Bauer, J., Pfeilsticker, A., Pearson, J., Hans Loesche, A., Grimsley, A., Peterson, K., Hamiel, M., & Dupre, C. (2023). Quantifying and qualifying nursing professional development practitioner workload. *Journal for Nurses in Professional Development, 40*(1), E21–E26. https://doi.org/10.1097/nnd.0000000000001004

Boerger, J. (2020). NPD practitioners in leadership roles: Leading systems. *Journal for Nurses in Professional Development, 36*(4), 241–242. https://doi.org/10.1097/nnd.0000000000000648

Bonn, J., Mulkey, D., & Goers, J. (2022). Using gamification to engage clinical nurses in quality improvement. *Journal for Nurses in Professional Development, 39*(5), E148–E153. https://doi.org/10.1097/NND.0000000000000898

Brown, H., Carerra, B., & Stanley, L. (2020). *Optimizing nursing staff during a pandemic.* Association for Nursing in Professional Development [ANPD Recorded Webinar]. https://anpd.mycrowdwisdom.com/diweb/catalog/item/id/5032242/sid/%2085111180/q/n=1&c=164

Brunt, B., & Bogdan, B. (2023, April 23). Nursing professional development leadership. In *StatPearls*. StatPearls Publishing. https://www.ncbi.nlm.nih.gov/books/NBK519064/

Chant, K., & Westendorf, D. (2019). Nurse residency programs: Key components for sustainability. *Journal for Nurses in Professional Development, 35*(4), 185–192. https://doi.org/10.1097/NND.0000000000000560

Chappell, K., & Burke, K. (2020). Leaders for learning and change. *Journal for Nurses in Professional Development, 36*(1), 52–53. https://doi.org/10.1097/NND.0000000000000603

Cipriano, P. (2020). NPD practitioners - Allies in achieving goals. *Journal for Nurses in Professional Development, 36*(2), 114–115. https://doi.org/10.1097/NND.0000000000000618

Coughlin, V., Ho, M. R., & Alvarez, G. (2023). Escape the room! Utilizing gamification in a preceptor training workshop. *Journal for Nurses in Professional Development, 40*(1), 41–44. https://doi.org/10.1097/nnd.0000000000000977

DelMonte, J. (2020). Saying "yes"! *Journal for Nurses in Professional Development, 36*(3), 180–181. https://doi.org/10.1097/NND.0000000000000640

DeVolt, M., Reid, R., Luttrell, J., & Robinson, E. (2023). Transition into practice for nursing professional development specialists. *Journal for Nurses in Professional Development, 39*(1), 5–11. https://doi.org/10.1097/NND.0000000000000783

Dickerson, P. S. (2019). Be present, be visible, be a leader. *Journal for Nurses in Professional Development, 35*(5), 300–301. https://doi.org/10.1097/nnd.0000000000000577

Dickerson, P. S., & Durkin, G. J. (2022). Nursing professional development standards of practice: Standards 1–6. *Journal for Nurses in Professional Development, 38*(4), 248–250. https://doi.org/10.1097/NND.0000000000000900

Dimino, K., Louie, K., Banks, J., & Mahon, E. (2020). Exploring the Impact of a Dedicated Education Unit on New Graduate Nurses' Transition to Practice. *Journal for Nurses in Professional Development, 36*(3), 121–128. https://doi.org/10.1097/NND.0000000000000622

Durkin, G. (2019). Implementation and evaluation of Wright's competency model. *Journal for Nurses in Professional Development, 35*(6), 305–315. https://doi.org/10.1097/NND.0000000000000575

Fogg, N., Kubin, L., Wilson, C., & Trinka, M. (2020). Using virtual simulation to develop clinical judgement in undergraduate nursing students. *Clinical Simulation in Nursing, 48*, 55–58. https://doi.org/10.1016/j.ecns.2020.08.010

Foley, J. A., Rosato, J. A., Monterio, T., Lincoln, N., & Zetlan, K. O. M. (2024). Nursing professional development at night. *American Nurse Journal, 19*(2), 21–25. https://doi.org/10.51256/ANJ022421

Fox, N., & Richter, S. (2021). The nursing professional development practitioner during a pandemic: Achieving the hat trick. *Journal for Nurses in Professional Development, 37*(3), 5–9. https://doi.org/10.1097/NND.0000000000000728

Harper, M. (2020). *ANPD position statement: Preceptors.* https://www.anpd.org/Portals/0/Docs/Resources/Preceptors%20Position%20Statement%202021_03_09_Approved.pdf

Harper, M. (2023). Informal power. *Journal for Nurses in Professional Development, 39*(2), 104–106. https://doi.org/10.1097/NND.0000000000000971

Harper, M., & Bindon, S. (2019). Envisioning the future of nursing professional development. *Journal for Nurses in Professional Development, 35*(1), 39–40. https://doi.org/10.1097/NND.0000000000000591

Harper, M., Brunt, B., & Holtschneider, M. E. (2023). Advanced certification in nursing professional development: An idea whose time has come. *Journal for Nurses in Professional Development, 39*(4), 201–206. https://doi.org/10.1097/NND.0000000000000932

Harper, M. G., & Maloney, P. (Eds.). (2022a). *Nursing professional development: Scope and standards of practice* (4th ed.). Association for Nursing Professional Development.

Harper, M. G., & Maloney, P. (2022b). The multisite NPD leader competency determination study. *Journal for Nurses in Professional Development, 38*(4), 185–195. https://doi.org/10.1097/NND.0000000000000836

Institute of Medicine. Committee on the Robert Wood Johnson Foundation Initiative on the Future of Nursing at the Institute of Medicine. (2011). *The future of nursing: Leading change, advancing health.* National Academies Press.

Johnson, C. S. (2022). Nursing professional development and the future of nursing 2020–2023: A winning combination. *Journal for Nurses in Professional Development, 38*(3), 123–126. https://doi.org/10.1097/NND.0000000000000879

Johnson, C. S., & Smith, C. (2019). The evolution from staff development to nursing professional development and continuing professional development. *Journal for Nurses in Professional Development, 35*(2), 104–106. http://doi.org/10.1097/NND.0000000000000506

Joseph, L., Therady, A., Rahman, A., & Varghese, R. (2023). "Just-in-time" COVID-19 education: The story of a nursing professional development unit. *Journal for Nurses in Professional Development, 39*(6)180–184. https://doi.org/10.1097/nnd.0000000000000905

Kiss, E., Simpson, A., & Smith, C. (2020). Nursing professional development practitioners in leadership roles: Leading academic-practice partnerships. *Journal for Nurses in Professional Development, 36*(2), 99–103. https://doi.org/10.1097/NND.0000000000000605

Liu, L., Fillipucci, D., & Mahajan, S. (2019). Quantitative analyses of the effectiveness of a newly designed preceptor workshop. *Journal for Nurses in Professional Development, 35*(3), 144–151. https://doi:10.1097/NND.0000000000000528

Maloney, P., & Woolforde, L. (2019). Ninety years and counting: The past, present, and future of the nursing professional development specialty. *Journal for Nurses in Professional Development, 35*(2), 56–65. https://doi.org/10.1097/NND.0000000000000532

Musallam, E., Ali, A. A., & Nicely, S. (2021). The impact of dedicated education model on nursing students' outcomes: An integrative review. *Nurse Educator, 46*(5), E113–E116. https://doi.org/10.1097/NNE.0000000000001022

National Academies of Sciences, Engineering, and Medicine. (2021). *The future of nursing 2020–2023: Charting a path to achieve health equity.* National Academies Press.

National League for Nursing. (2022). *Novice nurse educator core competencies with task statements.* https://www.nln.org/news/newsroomnln-position-documents/novice-nurse-educator-competencies-with-task-statements

Nelson, D., Joswiak, M., & Brake, K. (2019). "Just in time" training for novice preceptors. *Journal for Nurses in Professional Development, 35*(4), 228–231. https://doi.org/10.1097/NND.0000000000000562

Norwood, C., Zinkan, J., Perry, S., Tofil, N., Gaither, S., & Rutledge, C. (2023). Professional success: Utilizing simulation to remediate and retain nursing staff. *Journal for Nurses in Professional Development, 39*(6), 322–237. https://doi.org/10.1097/NND.0000000000000873

Opperman, C. (2023). Developing yourself! *Journal for Nurses in Professional Development, 39*(4), 234–235.

Opperman, C., Liebig, D., Bowling, J., Johnson, C., Stiesmeyer, J., & Miller, S. (2022). Measuring return on investment for professional development activities. *Journal for Nurses in Staff Development, 38*(6), 340–346. https://doi.10.1097/NND.0000000000000914

Park, C., & Holtschneider, M. (2020). Emerging opportunities for nursing professional development practitioners to impact our healthcare system. *Journal for Nurses in Professional Development, 36*(1), 44–45. https://doi.org/10.1097/NND.0000000000000604

Park, C., & Holtschneider, M. (2022). Building personal capabilities: Be a role model for lifelong learning. *Journal for Nurses in Professional Development, 38*(6), 367–368. https://doi.org/10.1097/NND.0000000000000940

Pate, K., Powers, K., Pagel, J., & Montegrico, J. (2023). Innovative strategies to facilitate newly licensed nurse transition to practice during the COVID-19 pandemic: A quality improvement project. *Journal for Nurses in Professional Development, 40*(1), 7–14. https://doi.org/10.1097/NND.0000000000000992

Smith, C., & Johnson, C. (2019). Preparing nurse leaders in nursing professional development: Quality improvement in nursing professional development. *Journal for Nurses in Professional Development, 35*(4), 222–224. https://doi.org/10.1097/NND.0000000000000540

Suter, A., & Painter, J. (2020). Nurse residency programs: Providing organization value. *Delaware Journal of Public Health, 6*(1), 58–61. https://doi.org/10.32481/djph.2020.04.013

The Joint Commission. (2024). *2024 Hospital national patient safety goals.* https://www.jointcommission.org/-/media/tjc/documents/standards/national-patient-safety-goals/2024/hap-npsg-simple-2024-v2.pdf

Weimer, N. (2021). My professional development journey. *Journal for Nurses in Professional Development, 38*(1), 47–48. https://doi.org/10.1097/NND.0000000000000832

Weinschreider, J., Sabourin, K., & Smith, C. (2019). Preparing nurse leaders in nursing professional development: Educational technology resources. *Journal for Nurses in Professional Development, 35*(5), 281–285. https://doi.org/10.1097/NND.0000000000000567

Weiss, R., Kennell, J., Lakadawala, L., Anzio, N., Klamut, K., Lucas, W., Antinori-Lent, Kellie, & Mininni, N. (2021). Nursing professional development specialists' role in adapting education, onboarding and just-tin-time education during the COVID-19 pandemic. *Journal for Nurses in Professional Development, 37*(3), 143–146. https://doi.org/10.1097/NND.0000000000000700

Woolforde, L. (2019). Nursing professional development practitioner or nurse educator: What's your response? *Journal for Nurses in Professional Development, 35*(3), 174–175. https://doi.org/10.1097/NND.0000000000000547

Woolforde, L. (2020). Invest in yourself through the association for nursing professional development! *Journal for Nurses in Professional Development, 36*(1), 50–51. https://doi.org/10.1097/NND.0000000000000597

Wright, D. (2021). *Competency assessment field guide: A real-world guide for implementation and application* (10th ed.). Creative Healthcare Management.

Appendices

Nursing and Higher Education Organizations

A

Organization	Mission	Website
American Academy of Nursing	Serves the public and nursing profession by advancing health policy and practice. Academy's members, known as Fellows, are nursing's most accomplished leaders in education, practice, administration, and research.	https://aannet.org
American Association of Colleges of Nursing	Represents baccalaureate and higher-degree nursing programs. Promotes quality nursing education. Offers faculty development programs and webinars. Collects data about nursing education programs, faculty, and students, and analyzes trends in nursing education. Publishes position papers.	https://aacnnursing.org
American Association of Community Colleges	Provides advocacy for community colleges at the national level. Works closely with states on policy.	https://aacc.nche.edu
American Association of University Professors	Focuses on advancing academic freedom and shared governance. Defines fundamental professional values and standards for higher education and faculty.	https://aaup.org

(continued)

Organization	Mission	Website
American Association of University Women	Promotes equity and education for women and girls. Advocates for fundamental educational, social, economic, and political issues.	https://aauw.org
American Council on Education	Represents presidents of accredited, degree-granting institutions (2- and 4-year colleges, private and public universities, and nonprofit schools) in the United States. Focuses on higher education challenges, with the goal to improve access and better prepare students.	https://acenet.edu
Association for Nursing Professional Development	Advances the specialty practice of nursing professional development. Includes resources for the nursing professional development practitioner.	https://anpd.org
Association of American Colleges and Universities	Focuses on promoting high-quality undergraduate liberal education. Website contains links to resources on liberal education, general education, curriculum, faculty work, assessment, diversity, and others.	https://aacu.org
Association of Black Nursing Faculty, Inc.	Provides a group for Black professional nurses with similar interests and concerns to promote health-related issues and nursing education. Assists members in professional development and provides continuing education.	https://abnf.net

(continued)

Organization	Mission	Website
Association of Community Health Nursing Educators	Focuses on promoting excellence in community and public health nursing education, research, and practice.	https://achne.org
EDUCAUSE	Advances higher education through use of information technology. Focuses on issues and emerging trends and technologies affecting higher education.	https://educause.edu
Interprofessional Education Collaborative (IPEC)	Collaborative of schools of health professions to promote efforts that advance interprofessional learning experiences to prepare future health professionals for team-based care and improved population health outcomes. These organizations that represent higher education in allopathic and osteopathic medicine, dentistry, nursing, pharmacy, and public health created core competencies for interprofessional collaborative practice to guide curricula development across health professions schools.	https://ipecollaborative.org
Multimedia Educational Resource for Learning and Online Teaching (MERLOT)	Includes repository of resources and information for faculty development and to download for use in teaching. Publishes *Journal of Online Learning and Teaching*.	https://merlot.org

(continued)

Organization	Mission	Website
National League for Nursing	Promotes excellence in nursing education at all levels. Offers faculty development programs, webinars, and annual educational conference. Sponsors certification programs for nurse educators (CNE®, CNE®cl, CNE®n). Publishes position papers on nursing education and has a grant program for nursing education research. The National League for Nursing (NLN) Commission for Nursing Education Accreditation (CNEA) accredits nursing programs.	https://nln.org
National Organization of Nurse Practitioner Faculties	Focuses on promoting quality nurse practitioner (NP) education at national and international levels. Leading organization for NP faculty in the United States and globally.	https://nonpf.org
National Student Nurses Association	Organization for nursing students with goal of enhancing their professional development and promoting transition into the profession.	https://nsna.org
Organization for Associate Degree Nursing (OADN)	Dedicated to enhancing the quality of associate degree (AD) nursing. Advocates for AD nursing and promotes academic progression of AD nursing graduates in furthering their education.	https://oadn.org

(continued)

APPENDIX A: NURSING AND HIGHER EDUCATION ORGANIZATIONS

Organization	Mission	Website
POD Network (Professional Organization Development)	Focuses on faculty, instructional, and organizational development in higher education.	https://podnetwork.org
Quality and Safety Education for Nurses (QSEN)	Collaborative of nurses and other healthcare professionals focused on education, practice, and scholarship to improve quality and safety of healthcare. Identifies knowledge, skills, and attitudes (KSAs) necessary to continuously improve quality and safety of healthcare. Website is a central repository of information on core QSEN competencies, KSAs, teaching strategies, and faculty development resources.	https://qsen.org
Sigma	Supports learning and professional development of nurses worldwide. Membership is by invitation to baccalaureate and graduate nursing students with excellence in scholarship and to nurse leaders with exceptional achievements in nursing. Offers conferences for sharing research and publishes *Journal of Nursing Scholarship*, among other resources.	https://sigmanursing.org

Worksheets to Align End-of-Program and Course Outcomes to AACN Essentials

B

END-OF-PROGRAM (EOP) OUTCOMES REVISION WORKSHEET

Comparison Table: Align current EOP outcome to domain it most closely represents

Current EOP Outcomes	Suggested Revision	AACN *Essentials* Domain
		Domain 1: Knowledge for Nursing Practice; Integration, translation, and application of established and evolving disciplinary nursing knowledge and ways of knowing, as well as knowledge from other disciplines, including a foundation in liberal arts and natural and social sciences.
		Domain 2: Person-Centered Care; Person-centered care focuses on the individual within multiple complicated contexts, including family and/or important others. Person-centered care is holistic, individualized, just, respectful, compassionate, coordinated, evidence-based, and developmentally appropriate. Person-centered care builds on a scientific body of knowledge that guides nursing practice regardless of specialty or functional area.
		Domain 3: Population Health; Population health spans the healthcare delivery continuum from public health prevention to disease management of populations and describes collaborative activities with both traditional and non traditional partnerships from affected communities, public health, industry, academia, health care, local government entities, and others for the improvement of equitable population health outcomes.

(continued)

Current EOP Outcomes	Suggested Revision	AACN *Essentials* Domain
		Domain 4: Scholarship for the Nursing Discipline; The generation, synthesis, translation, application, and dissemination of nursing knowledge to improve health and transform health care.
		Domain 5: Quality and Safety; Employment of established and emerging principles of safety and improvement science. Quality and safety, as core values of nursing practice, enhance quality and minimize risk of harm to patients and providers through both system effectiveness and individual performance.
		Domain 6: Interprofessional Partnerships; Intentional collaboration across professions and with care team members, patients, families, communities, and other stakeholders to optimize care, enhance the healthcare experience, and strengthen outcomes.
		Domain 7: Systems-Based Practice; Responding to and leading within complex systems of health care. Nurses effectively and proactively coordinate resources to provide safe, quality, and equitable care to diverse populations.
		Domain 8: Informatics and Healthcare Technologies; Information and communication technologies and informatics processes are used to provide care, gather data, form information to drive decision making, and support professionals as they expand knowledge and wisdom for practice. Informatics processes and technologies are used to manage and improve the delivery of safe, high-quality, and efficient healthcare services in accordance with best practice and professional and regulatory standards.
		Domain 9: Professionalism; Formation and cultivation of a sustainable professional identity, including accountability, perspective, collaborative disposition, and comportment, that reflects nursing's characteristics and values.

(continued)

APPENDIX B: WORKSHEETS TO ALIGN TO AACN *ESSENTIALS*

Current EOP Outcomes	Suggested Revision	AACN *Essentials* Domain
		Domain 10: Personal, Professional, and Leadership Development; Participation in activities and self-reflection that foster personal health, resilience, and well-being; contributes to lifelong learning; and support the acquisition of nursing expertise and the assertion of leadership.

AACN, American Association of Colleges of Nursing.

Source: Domains from American Association of College of Nursing. (AACN). (2021). *The essentials: Core competencies for professional nursing education.* AACN. https://www.aacnnursing.org/Portals/0/PDFs/Publications/Essentials-2021.pdf

Worksheet developed by Gerry Altmiller. Copyright Gerry Altmiller, 2024. Reprinted by permission, 2024.

COURSE OUTCOME DEVELOPMENT TEMPLATE

Name of Course:
Course Description:

Current learning outcomes/ objectives	What do you want students to be able to do at the end of this course?	Write competency statements that reflect what you want them to be able to do at the end of this course.	End-of-program outcome this course outcome aligns with

Copyright Gerry Altmiller, 2024. Reprinted by permission, 2024

Selected Organizations, Journals, and Educational Conferences of Interest for Nursing Professional Development Practitioners

C

ORGANIZATIONS

Organization and Website	Purpose
American Nurses Credentialing Center (ANCC) https://nursingworld.org/ancc Nursing Professional Development Certification https://nursingworld.org/our-certifications/nursing-professional-development Magnet Recognition Program® https://nursingworld.org/organizational-programs/magnet	The ANCC provides a variety of services for practitioners, including certification in nursing professional development and the Magnet Recognition Program for healthcare organizations.
Association for Nurses in Professional Development (ANPD) https://anpd.org	The ANPD "advances the specialty practice of nursing professional development for the enhancement of healthcare outcomes. The goal of ANPD is to be acknowledged as the expert voice, advocate, and leading resource for nursing professional development practice" (ANPD, 2024, para. 1).

(continued)

Organization and Website	Purpose
The Joint Commission (TJC) https://jointcommission.org	TJC "continually improves healthcare for the public, in collaboration with other stakeholders, by evaluating healthcare organizations and inspiring them to excel in providing safe and effective care of the highest quality and value" (TJC, 2024, para. 1). TJC provides a variety of services for healthcare providers including accreditation/certification, standards, measurement, performance improvement, and resources.
Vizient/AACN Nurse Residency Program™ https://aacnnursing.org/our-initiatives/education-practice/nurse-residency-program	Vizient and the American Association of Colleges of Nursing (AACN) connect "members with opportunities to learn, improve, and grow. The nurse residency program (NRP) focuses on new entry-level nurses as they transition into practice. The evidence-based curriculum incorporates seven key areas: Knowledge for Nursing Practice; Interprofessional Practice; Person-Centered Care; Leadership and Systems-Based Practice; Development of the Professional Nurse; Scholarship for Nursing Practice; and Foundations of Nursing: Quality and Safety" (AACN, 2024, para. 1).

American Association of Colleges of Nursing. (2024). *Vizient/AACN nurse residency program*. https://www.aacnnursing.org/our-initiatives/education-practice/nurse-residency-program; Association for Nursing Professional Development. (2024). *About us*. https://www.anpd.org/About/About-Us; The Joint Commission. (2024). *Joint Commission facts*. https://www.jointcommission.org/who-we-are/facts-about-the-joint-commission/joint-commission-faqs/

APPENDIX C: RESOURCES FOR NURSING PROFESSIONAL DEVELOPMENT

JOURNALS

Journal Name and URL	Mission
The Journal of Continuing Education in Nursing (JCEN) https://journals.healio.com/journal/jcen	Peer-reviewed journal publishing articles on continuing nursing education, directed toward continuing education and professional development educators, nurse administrators, and nurse educators in all healthcare settings
Journal for Nurses in Professional Development (JNPD) https://journals.lww.com/jnsdonline/pages/default.aspx	Official peer-reviewed journal of the ANPD; source of information for NPD specialists in all healthcare settings

ANPD, Association for Nursing Professional Development.
Source: Journal for Nurses in Professional Development. (2024). *About the journal.* https://journals.lww.com/jnsdonline/Pages/aboutthejournal.aspx; The Journal of Continuing Education in Nursing. (n.d.). *About the journal.* https://journals.healio.com/journal/jcen/about-the-journal

CONFERENCES

Conference and URL	Conference Description
Association for Nursing in Professional Development (ANPD) Aspire Convention https://anpd.org/aspire	Annual convention sponsored by ANPD and held in various locations across the United States; provides opportunities for professional presentations and networking with nursing professional development practitioners
Professional Nurse Educators Group (PNEG) https://uoflhealth.org/professional-nurse-educators-group Note: The PNEG home site is currently moving but information about the organization and future conferences can be accessed via https://pneg.wordpress.com	PNEG is a "virtual network of educators in the United States who are dedicated to lifelong learning of nurses." The group's aim is "to encourage, support and promote best practices in the delivery of nursing care among schools of nursing, hospitals, nursing leaders, entrepreneurs and continuing nursing education programs" (UofLHealth, 2024, para. 1). Annual PNEG conferences are sponsored at different locations across the United States and provides opportunities for professional presentations and networking with other educators from a variety of settings and academic and clinical practice. This 2023 conference provides information about the type of PNEG presentations

Source: University of Louisville Health, Inc. (UofLHealth). (2024). PNEG (Professional Nurse Educators Group).

Mapping Grids of Chapters and Certified Nurse Educator Examination Blueprints

These mapping grids indicate the chapters with content related to the competencies in each of the National League for Nursing Certified Nurse Educator Examination Blueprints:

> National League for Nursing. (2023). *Certified Nurse Educator (CNE®) 2023 Candidate Handbook.*
>
> National League for Nursing. (2023). *Certified Academic Clinical Nurse Educator (CNE®cl) 2023 Candidate Handbook.*
>
> National League for Nursing. (2023). *Certified Nurse Educator Novice (CNE®n) 2023 Candidate Handbook.*

The competencies in the mapping grids for the CNE® and CNE®cl are from Christensen, L.S., & Simmons, L.E. (2020). *The scope of practice for academic nurse educators and academic clinical nurse educators* (3rd ed.). National League for Nursing/Wolters Kluwer. The competencies in the mapping grid for the CNE®n are from the National League for Nursing. (2024). *Novice nurse educator competencies with task statements*. Available at https://www.nln.org/certification/Certification-for-Nurse-Educators/cne-n. Reprinted by permission, National League for Nursing, 2024. These competencies were used to develop the Certified Nurse Educator Examination Test Blueprints. Additional information about NLN Certification is available at https://www.nln.org/awards-recognition/certification-for-nurse-educators-overview

NATIONAL LEAGUE FOR NURSING CERTIFIED NURSE EDUCATOR (CNE®) EXAMINATION MAPPING GRID

Competencies[a]	Chapters[b]																					
	1 Role	2 Transition	3 Learning	4 Diverse Learner	5 Teaching Methods	6 Issues	7 Technology	8 Online	9 Simulation	10 Clinical Teaching	11 IPE	12 Partnerships	13 CBE	14 Curriculum	15 Assessment	16 Tests	17 Clinical Eval	18 Program Eval	19 EBT	20 Scholar	21 Service/Leader	22 Prof Develop
1: Facilitate Learning																						
A. Implements a variety of teaching strategies appropriate to learner needs, desired learner outcomes, content, and context	√		√	√	√		√	√	√	√			√									√
B. Grounds teaching strategies in educational theory and evidence-based teaching practices			√		√														√			√
C. Recognizes multicultural, gender, and experiential influences on teaching and learning				√	√																	
D. Engages in self-reflection and continued learning to improve teaching practices that facilitate learning					√				√	√												
E. Uses information technologies skillfully to support the teaching–learning process					√		√															√
F. Practices skilled oral, written, and electronic communication that reflects an awareness of self and others, along with an ability to convey ideas in a variety of contexts	√																			√		

(continued)

Competencies[a]	Chapters[b]																					
	1 Role	2 Transition	3 Learning	4 Diverse Learner	5 Teaching Methods	6 Issues	7 Technology	8 Online	9 Simulation	10 Clinical Teaching	11 IPE	12 Partnerships	13 CBE	14 Curriculum	15 Assessment	16 Tests	17 Clinical Eval	18 Program Eval	19 EBT	20 Scholar	21 Service/Leader	22 Prof Develop
G. Models critical and reflective thinking					√				√	√												
H. Creates opportunities for learners to develop their critical thinking and critical reasoning skills					√				√	√												
I. Shows enthusiasm for teaching, learning, and nursing that inspires and motivates students	√		√							√												√
J. Demonstrates interest in and respect for learners	√		√							√												√
K. Uses personal attributes (e.g., caring, confidence, patience, integrity, and flexibility) that facilitate learning	√		√							√												√
L. Develop collegial working relationships with students, faculty colleagues, and clinical agency personnel to promote positive learning environments										√	√	√										√
M. Maintains the professional practice knowledge base needed to help learners prepare for contemporary nursing practice																			√			
N. Serves as a role model of professional nursing	√									√												√

(continued)

Competencies[a]	Chapters[b]																					
	1 Role	2 Transition	3 Learning	4 Diverse Learner	5 Teaching Methods	6 Issues	7 Technology	8 Online	9 Simulation	10 Clinical Teaching	11 IPE	12 Partnerships	13 CBE	14 Curriculum	15 Assessment	16 Tests	17 Clinical Eval	18 Program Eval	19 EBT	20 Scholar	21 Service/Leader	22 Prof Develop
2: Facilitate Learner Development and Socialization																						
A. Identifies individual learning styles and unique learning needs of international, adult, multicultural, educationally disadvantaged, physically challenged, at-risk, and second-degree learners		√	√	√																		√
B. Provides resources to diverse learners that help meet their individual learning needs		√		√	√																	√
C. Engages in effective advisement and counseling strategies that help learners meet their professional goals																					√	√
D. Creates learning environments that are focused on socialization to the role of the nurse and facilitate learners' self-reflection and personal goal setting	√									√												√
E. Fosters the cognitive, psychomotor, and affective development of learners			√		√					√												√
F. Recognizes the influence of teaching styles and interpersonal interactions on learner outcomes					√																√	

(continued)

Competencies[a]	Chapters[b]																					
	1 Role	2 Transition	3 Learning	4 Diverse Learner	5 Teaching Methods	6 Issues	7 Technology	8 Online	9 Simulation	10 Clinical Teaching	11 IPE	12 Partnerships	13 CBE	14 Curriculum	15 Assessment	16 Tests	17 Clinical Eval	18 Program Eval	19 EBT	20 Scholar	21 Service/Leader	22 Prof Develop
G. Assists learners to develop the ability to engage in thoughtful and constructive self and peer evaluation															√		√					√
H. Models professional behaviors for learners including involvement in professional organizations, engagement in lifelong learning activities, dissemination of information through publications and presentations, and advocacy																					√	√
3: Use Assessment and Evaluation Strategies																						
A. Uses extant literature to develop evidence-based assessment and evaluation practices															√	√	√	√	√			
B. Uses a variety of strategies to assess and evaluate learning in the cognitive, psychomotor, and affective domains									√	√		√			√	√	√	√				
C. Implements evidence-based assessment and evaluation strategies that are appropriate to the learner and to learning goals									√	√		√			√	√	√		√			
D. Uses assessment and evaluation data to enhance the teaching-learning process									√			√			√	√	√	√				√
E. Provides timely, constructive, and thoughtful feedback to learners									√	√		√			√	√	√					

(continued)

Competencies[a]	Chapters[b]																					
	1 Role	2 Transition	3 Learning	4 Diverse Learner	5 Teaching Methods	6 Issues	7 Technology	8 Online	9 Simulation	10 Clinical Teaching	11 IPE	12 Partnerships	13 CBE	14 Curriculum	15 Assessment	16 Tests	17 Clinical Eval	18 Program Eval	19 EBT	20 Scholar	21 Service/Leader	22 Prof Develop
F. Demonstrates skill in the design and use of tools for assessing clinical practice										√							√					
4: Participate in Curriculum Design and Evaluation of Program Outcomes																						
A. Ensures that the curriculum reflects institutional philosophy and mission, current nursing and healthcare trends, and community and societal needs so as to prepare graduates for practice in a complex, dynamic, multicultural healthcare environment					√									√				√				√
B. Demonstrates knowledge of curriculum development, including identifying program outcomes, developing competency statements, writing learning objectives, and selecting appropriate learning activities and evaluation strategies													√	√				√				√
C. Bases curriculum design and implementation decisions on sound educational principles, theory, and research													√	√				√	√			√
D. Revises the curriculum based on assessment of program outcomes, learner needs, and societal and healthcare trends													√	√				√				√

(continued)

Competencies[a]	Chapters[b]																					
	1 Role	2 Transition	3 Learning	4 Diverse Learner	5 Teaching Methods	6 Issues	7 Technology	8 Online	9 Simulation	10 Clinical Teaching	11 IPE	12 Partnerships	13 CBE	14 Curriculum	15 Assessment	16 Tests	17 Clinical Eval	18 Program Eval	19 EBT	20 Scholar	21 Service/Leader	22 Prof Develop
E. Implements curricular revisions using appropriate change theories and strategies														√				√				
F. Creates and maintains community and clinical partnerships that support educational goals												√										
G. Collaborates with external constituencies throughout the process of curriculum revision												√		√				√				
H. Designs and implements program assessment models that promote continuous quality improvement of all aspects of the program														√				√				
5: Function as a Change Agent and Leader																						
A. Models cultural sensitivity when advocating for change														√							√	√
B. Integrates a long-term, innovative, and creative perspective into the nurse educator role	√																				√	√
C. Participates in interdisciplinary efforts to address healthcare and educational needs locally, regionally, nationally, or internationally											√	√										√
D. Evaluates organizational effectiveness in nursing education														√				√			√	√
E. Implements strategies for organizational change		√												√							√	√

(continued)

Competencies[a]	Chapters[b]																					
	1 Role	2 Transition	3 Learning	4 Diverse Learner	5 Teaching Methods	6 Issues	7 Technology	8 Online	9 Simulation	10 Clinical Teaching	11 IPE	12 Partnerships	13 CBE	14 Curriculum	15 Assessment	16 Tests	17 Clinical Eval	18 Program Eval	19 EBT	20 Scholar	21 Service/Leader	22 Prof Develop
F. Provides leadership in the parent institution as well as in the nursing program to enhance the visibility of nursing and its contributions to the academic community																				√	√	√
G. Promotes innovative practices in educational environments														√				√			√	√
H. Develops leadership skills to shape and implement change	√																				√	√
6: Pursue Continuous Quality Improvement in the Academic Nurse Educator Role																						
A. Demonstrates a commitment to lifelong learning	√	√																			√	√
B. Recognizes that career enhancement needs and activities change as experience is gained in the role	√																				√	√
C. Participates in professional development opportunities that increase one's effectiveness in the role	√																				√	√
D. Balances the teaching, scholarship, and service demands inherent in the role of educator and member of an academic institution																				√	√	
E. Uses feedback gained from self, peer, student, and administrative evaluation to improve role effectiveness		√																√				

(continued)

Competencies[a]	Chapters[b]																					
	1 Role	2 Transition	3 Learning	4 Diverse Learner	5 Teaching Methods	6 Issues	7 Technology	8 Online	9 Simulation	10 Clinical Teaching	11 IPE	12 Partnerships	13 CBE	14 Curriculum	15 Assessment	16 Tests	17 Clinical Eval	18 Program Eval	19 EBT	20 Scholar	21 Service/Leader	22 Prof Develop
F. Engages in activities that promote one's socialization to the role		√																				
G. Uses knowledge of legal and ethical issues relevant to higher education and nursing education as a basis for influencing, designing, and implementing policies and procedures related to students, faculty, and the educational environment						√																
H. Mentors and supports faculty colleagues		√																			√	
7: Engage in Scholarship																						
A. Draws on extant literature to design evidence-based teaching and evaluation practices																			√			
B. Exhibits a spirit of inquiry about teaching and learning, student development, evaluation methods, and other aspects of the role	√																		√	√		
C. Designs and implements scholarly activities in an established area of expertise																				√		
D. Disseminates nursing and teaching knowledge to a variety of audiences through various means																				√		

(continued)

Competencies[a]	Chapters[b]																					
	1 Role	2 Transition	3 Learning	4 Diverse Learner	5 Teaching Methods	6 Issues	7 Technology	8 Online	9 Simulation	10 Clinical Teaching	11 IPE	12 Partnerships	13 CBE	14 Curriculum	15 Assessment	16 Tests	17 Clinical Eval	18 Program Eval	19 EBT	20 Scholar	21 Service/Leader	22 Prof Develop
E. Demonstrates skill in proposal writing for initiatives that include research, resource acquisition, program development, and policy development																						
F. Demonstrates qualities of a scholar: integrity, courage, perseverance, vitality, and creativity																				√		
G. Draws on extant literature to design evidence-based teaching and evaluation practices																			√	√		
8: Function Within Organizational Environment and Academic Community																						
A. Uses knowledge of history and current trends and issues in higher education as a basis for making recommendations and decisions on educational issues	√				√	√	√					√						√				
B. Identifies how social, economic, political, and institutional forces influence higher education in general and nursing education in particular	√				√	√	√					√						√				
C. Develops networks, collaborations, and partnerships to enhance nursing's influence within the academic community											√	√										

(continued)

Competencies[a]	Chapters[b]																					
	1 Role	2 Transition	3 Learning	4 Diverse Learner	5 Teaching Methods	6 Issues	7 Technology	8 Online	9 Simulation	10 Clinical Teaching	11 IPE	12 Partnerships	13 CBE	14 Curriculum	15 Assessment	16 Tests	17 Clinical Eval	18 Program Eval	19 EBT	20 Scholar	21 Service/Leader	22 Prof Develop
D. Determines own professional goals within the context of academic nursing and the mission of the parent institution and nursing program	√																				√	√
E. Integrates the values of respect, collegiality, professionalism, and caring to build an organizational climate that fosters the development of students and teachers	√			√		√															√	
F. Incorporates the goals of the nursing program and the mission of the parent institution when proposing change or managing issues														√								
G. Assumes a leadership role in various levels of institutional governance																					√	√
H. Advocates for nursing and nursing education in the political arena	√																				√	

CBE, competency-based education; EBT, evidence-based teaching; IPE, interprofessional education

[a]Christensen, L.S., & Simmons, L.E. (2020). *The scope of practice for academic nurse educators and academic clinical nurse educators* (3rd ed.). National League for Nursing/Wolters Kluwer. Reprinted by permission, National League for Nursing, 2024. These competencies were used to develop the Certified Nurse Educator (CNE®) Examination Test Blueprint. Available at *Certified Nurse Educator (CNE®) 2023 Candidate Handbook*. https://www.nln.org/docs/default-source/default-document-library/cne-handbook-2023_11.15.2023.pdf?sfvrsn=2602b8b8_3

[b]Chapters:

1. Role of the Nurse Educator
2. The Transition From Clinician to Educator
3. Contemporary Learning Theories
4. Understanding the Diverse Learner

(continued)

5. Teaching Methods
6. Ethical, Legal, and Social Challenges in Academic Nursing
7. Integrating Technology in Education
8. Teaching in Online Learning Environments
9. Simulation in Nursing Education: Overview, Essentials, and the Evidence
10. Clinical Teaching in Nursing
11. Interprofessional Education
12. Academic–Practice Partnerships
13. Competency-Based Education in Nursing
14. Curriculum Development and Course Design in Nursing Education
15. Assessment Methods
16. Developing and Using Tests
17. Clinical Evaluation
18. Program Evaluation and Accreditation
19. Evidence-Based Teaching in Nursing
20. Becoming a Scholar in Nursing Education
21. Mentorship, Service, Leading, and Learner Success
22. Nursing Professional Development Practitioner in a Clinical Practice Setting

NATIONAL LEAGUE FOR NURSING CERTIFIED ACADEMIC CLINICAL NURSE EDUCATOR (CNE®CL) EXAMINATION MAPPING GRID

Competencies[a]	\multicolumn{22}{c}{Chapters[b]}
	1 Role	2 Transition	3 Learning	4 Diverse Learner	5 Teaching Methods	6 Issues	7 Technology	8 Online	9 Simulation	10 Clinical Teaching	11 IPE	12 Partnerships	13 CBE	14 Curriculum	15 Assessment	16 Tests	17 Clinical Eval	18 Program Eval	19 EBT	20 Scholar	21 Serviuce/Leader	22 Prof Develop
1. Function Within the Education and Healthcare Environments																						
A. Function in the Clinical Nurse Educator Role	√									√												√
1. Bridge the gap between theory and practice by helping learners apply classroom learning to the clinical setting					√					√												
2. Foster professional growth of learners																	√				√	√
3. Use technologies to enhance clinical teaching and learning							√		√	√												√
4. Value the contributions of others in the achievement of learner outcomes					√					√												
5. Act as a role model of professional nursing within the clinical learning environment	√									√											√	√
6. Demonstrate inclusive excellence			√							√											√	
B. Operationalize the Curriculum														√								
1. Assess congruence of the clinical agency to the curriculum, goals, and learner needs										√												
2. Plan meaningful and relevant clinical learning assignments and activities							√	√														√

(continued)

Competencies[a]	Chapters[b]																					
	1 Role	2 Transition	3 Learning	4 Diverse Learner	5 Teaching Methods	6 Issues	7 Technology	8 Online	9 Simulation	10 Clinical Teaching	11 IPE	12 Partnerships	13 CBE	14 Curriculum	15 Assessment	16 Tests	17 Clinical Eval	18 Program Eval	19 EBT	20 Scholar	21 Service/Leader	22 Prof Develop
3. Identify learners' goals and outcomes									√	√			√				√					√
4. Prepare learners for clinical experiences										√												√
5. Structure learner experiences within the learning environment to promote optimal learning									√	√												√
6. Implement clinical learning activities to help learners develop interprofessional collaboration and teamwork skills										√	√											√
7. Provide opportunities for learners to develop problem-solving and clinical reasoning skills related to learning outcomes				√					√	√					√		√					√
8. Implement assigned models for clinical teaching										√												
9. Engage in theory-based instruction				√						√												
10. Provide input to the nursing program for course development and review													√	√				√				
C. Abide by Legal Requirements, Ethical Guidelines, Agency Policies, and Guiding Framework						√			√	√												√

(continued)

MAPPING GRIDS

Competencies[a]	Chapters[b]																					
	1 Role	2 Transition	3 Learning	4 Diverse Learner	5 Teaching Methods	6 Issues	7 Technology	8 Online	9 Simulation	10 Clinical Teaching	11 IPE	12 Partnerships	13 CBE	14 Curriculum	15 Assessment	16 Tests	17 Clinical Eval	18 Program Eval	19 EBT	20 Scholar	21 Serviuce/Leader	22 Prof Develop
1. Apply ethical and legal principles to create a safe clinical learning environment						√																√
2. Assess learner abilities and needs prior to clinical learning experiences				√					√	√												
3. Facilitate learning activities that support the mission, goals, and values of the academic institution and the clinical agency										√		√										√
4. Inform others of program and clinical agency policies, procedures, and practices						√				√		√										√
5. Adhere to program and clinical agency policies, procedures and practices when implementing clinical experiences						√				√		√										√
6. Promote learner compliance with regulations and standards of practice										√		√										√
7. Demonstrate ethical behaviors						√				√											√	√
2. Facilitate Learning in the Healthcare Environment																						
A. Implement a variety of clinical teaching strategies congruent with learner needs, desired learner outcomes, content, and context	√		√	√	√				√	√		√										√

(continued)

Competencies[a]	\{ Chapters[b] \}																					
	1 Role	2 Transition	3 Learning	4 Diverse Learner	5 Teaching Methods	6 Issues	7 Technology	8 Online	9 Simulation	10 Clinical Teaching	11 IPE	12 Partnerships	13 CBE	14 Curriculum	15 Assessment	16 Tests	17 Clinical Eval	18 Program Eval	19 EBT	20 Scholar	21 Serviuce/Leader	22 Prof Develop
B. Ground teaching strategies in educational theory and evidence-based teaching practices			√		√				√	√									√			√
C. Use technology skillfully to support the teaching–learning process							√		√	√												√
D. Create opportunities for learners to develop critical thinking and clinical reasoning skills									√	√					√	√	√					
E. Promote a culture of safety and quality in the healthcare environment									√	√	√											√
F. Create a positive and caring learning environment		√							√	√							√					√
G. Develop collegial working relationships with learners, faculty, and clinical environment personnel										√	√	√										√
H. Demonstrate enthusiasm for teaching, learning, and nursing to inspire and motivate learners									√	√								√			√	

3. Demonstrate Effective Interpersonal Communication and Collaborative Interprofessional Relationships

A. Value collaboration and coordination of care									√	√	√	√										√

(continued)

Competencies[a]	Chapters[b]																					
	1 Role	2 Transition	3 Learning	4 Diverse Learner	5 Teaching Methods	6 Issues	7 Technology	8 Online	9 Simulation	10 Clinical Teaching	11 IPE	12 Partnerships	13 CBE	14 Curriculum	15 Assessment	16 Tests	17 Clinical Eval	18 Program Eval	19 EBT	20 Scholar	21 Serviuce/Leader	22 Prof Develop
B. Foster a shared learning community and cooperate with other members of the healthcare team									√	√	√	√					√					√
C. Support an environment of frequent, respectful, civil, and open communication with all members of the healthcare team									√	√	√	√					√					√
D. Act as a role model, showing respect for all members of the healthcare team, professional colleagues, clients, family members, as well as learners									√	√	√	√					√					√
E. Use clear and effective communication in all interactions										√							√					
F. Listen to learner concerns, needs, or questions in a nonthreatening way									√	√							√					√
G. Display a calm, empathetic, and supportive demeanor in all communications									√	√							√					
H. Manage emotions effectively when communicating in challenging situations										√											√	
I. Effectively manage conflict										√											√	
J. Maintain an approachable, nonjudgmental, and readily accessible demeanor									√	√	√	√										

(continued)

Competencies[a]	Chapters[b]																					
	1 Role	2 Transition	3 Learning	4 Diverse Learner	5 Teaching Methods	6 Issues	7 Technology	8 Online	9 Simulation	10 Clinical Teaching	11 IPE	12 Partnerships	13 CBE	14 Curriculum	15 Assessment	16 Tests	17 Clinical Eval	18 Program Eval	19 EBT	20 Scholar	21 Serviuce/Leader	22 Prof Develop
K. Recognize limitations in self and learners to provide opportunities for development										√							√					
L. Demonstrate effective communication in clinical learning environments with diverse colleagues, clients, cultures, healthcare professionals, and learners			√						√	√												
M. Communicate performance expectations to learners and agency staff									√	√		√					√					√
4. Apply Clinical Expertise in the Healthcare Environment																						
A. Maintain current professional competence relevant to the specialty area, practice setting, and clinical learning environment	√								√	√							√					
B. Translate theory into clinical practice by applying experiential knowledge, clinical reasoning, and using a client-centered approach to clinical instruction			√						√	√							√					
C. Use best evidence to address client-related problems									√	√							√		√			
D. Demonstrate effective leadership within the clinical learning environment	√								√	√							√				√	

(continued)

Competencies[a]	\multicolumn{22}{c	}{Chapters[b]}
	1 Role	2 Transition	3 Learning	4 Diverse Learner	5 Teaching Methods	6 Issues	7 Technology	8 Online	9 Simulation	10 Clinical Teaching	11 IPE	12 Partnerships	13 CBE	14 Curriculum	15 Assessment	16 Tests	17 Clinical Eval	18 Program Eval	19 EBT	20 Scholar	21 Service/Leader	22 Prof Develop
E. Demonstrate sound clinical reasoning					√				√	√						√						
F. Balance client care needs and student learning needs within a culture of safety									√													
G. Demonstrate competence with a range of technologies available in the clinical learning environment							√		√	√							√					
5. Facilitate Learner Development and Socialization																						
A. Mentor learners in the development of professional nursing behaviors, standards, and codes of ethics									√	√											√	
B. Promote a learning climate of respect for all									√	√	√						√					√
C. Promote professional integrity and accountability					√				√	√							√				√	
D. Maintain professional boundaries		√							√	√	√						√				√	
E. Encourage ongoing learner professional development									√	√											√	√
F. Assist learners in effective use of self-assessment and professional goal setting for ongoing self-improvement									√	√											√	√
G. Create learning environments that are focused on socialization to the role of the nurse		√							√												√	

(continued)

Competencies[a]	1 Role	2 Transition	3 Learning	4 Diverse Learner	5 Teaching Methods	6 Issues	7 Technology	8 Online	9 Simulation	10 Clinical Teaching	11 IPE	12 Partnerships	13 CBE	14 Curriculum	15 Assessment	16 Tests	17 Clinical Eval	18 Program Eval	19 EBT	20 Scholar	21 Serviuce/Leader	22 Prof Develop
H. Assist learners to develop the ability to engage in constructive peer feedback									√	√							√					
I. Inspire creativity and confidence									√	√											√	
J. Encourage various techniques to manage stress.										√											√	
K. Act as a role model for self-reflection, self-care, and coping skills										√											√	
L. Empower learners to achieve professional and educational goals									√	√											√	
M. Engage learners in applying best practices and quality improvement processes									√	√							√					
6. Implement Effective Clinical and Assessment Evaluation Strategies																						
A. Use a variety of strategies to determine achievement of learning outcomes				√					√	√		√			√	√	√					
B. Implement formative and summative evaluation that is appropriate to the learner and learning outcomes									√	√					√		√					
C. Engage in timely communication with course faculty regarding learners' clinical performance									√	√							√					

(continued)

Competencies[a]	Chapters[b]																					
	1 Role	2 Transition	3 Learning	4 Diverse Learner	5 Teaching Methods	6 Issues	7 Technology	8 Online	9 Simulation	10 Clinical Teaching	11 IPE	12 Partnerships	13 CBE	14 Curriculum	15 Assessment	16 Tests	17 Clinical Eval	18 Program Eval	19 EBT	20 Scholar	21 Serviuce/Leader	22 Prof Develop
D. Maintain integrity in the assessment and evaluation of learners															√		√					
E. Provide timely, objective, constructive, and fair feedback to learners								√	√						√		√					
F. Use learner data to enhance the teaching-learning process in the clinical learning environment									√								√					
G. Demonstrate skill in the use of best practices in the assessment and evaluation of clinical performance									√								√					

[a]Christensen, L.S., & Simmons, L.E. (2020). *The scope of practice for academic nurse educators and academic clinical nurse educators* (3rd ed.). National League for Nursing/Wolters Kluwer. Reprinted by permission, National League for Nursing, 2024. These competencies were used to develop the Certified Academic Clinical Nurse Educator (CNE®cl) Examination Test Blueprint. Available at *Certified Academic Clinical Nurse Educator (CNE®cl) 2023 Candidate Handbook*. https://www.nln.org/awards-recognition/certification-for-nurse-educators-overview/cne-cl/Certification-for-Nurse-Educatorscnecl/cne-cl-handbook

[b]Chapters:

1. Role of the Nurse Educator

2. The Transition From Clinician to Educator

3. Contemporary Learning Theories

4. Understanding the Diverse Learner

5. Teaching Methods

6. Ethical, Legal, and Social Challenges in Academic Nursing

7. Integrating Technology in Education

8. Teaching in Online Learning Environments

9. Simulation in Nursing Education: Overview, Essentials, and the Evidence

10. Clinical Teaching in Nursing

11. Interprofessional Education

(continued)

12. Academic–Practice Partnerships
13. Competency-Based Education in Nursing
14. Curriculum Development and Course Design in Nursing Education
15. Assessment Methods
16. Developing and Using Tests
17. Clinical Evaluation
18. Program Evaluation and Accreditation
19. Evidence-Based Teaching in Nursing
20. Becoming a Scholar in Nursing Education
21. Mentorship, Service, Leading, and Learner Success
22. Nursing Professional Development Practitioner in a Clinical Practice Setting

NATIONAL LEAGUE FOR NURSING CERTIFIED NURSE EDUCATOR NOVICE (CNE®N) EXAMINATION MAPPING GRID

Competencies[a]	Chapters[b]																					
	1 Role	2 Transition	3 Learning	4 Diverse Learner	5 Teaching Methods	6 Issues	7 Technology	8 Online	9 Simulation	10 Clinical Teaching	11 IPE	12 Partnerships	13 CBE	14 Curriculum	15 Assessment	16 Tests	17 Clinical Eval	18 Program Eval	19 EBT	20 Scholar	21 Serviuce/Leader	22 Prof Develop
1. Facilitate Learning																						
A. Implements a variety of teaching strategies appropriate to learner needs, desired outcomes, content, and context	√		√	√	√		√	√	√				√									√
B. Employs teaching strategies grounded in educational theories and evidence-based teaching practices			√		√														√			√
C. Engages in self-reflection and continued learning to improve teaching practices that facilitate learning		√						√	√											√		
D. Uses technologies skillfully to support the teaching-learning process					√		√	√	√	√												√
E. Uses oral, written, and electronic communication that reflects an awareness of self and others, along with an ability to convey ideas in a variety of contexts	√																		√			√
F. Engages in critical and reflective thinking, considering multiple perspectives		√			√			√	√	√			√		√	√	√					
G. Provides opportunities for learners to develop critical thinking and clinical judgment skills				√			√	√	√				√		√		√					√

(continued)

Competencies[a]	Chapters[b]																					
	1 Role	2 Transition	3 Learning	4 Diverse Learner	5 Teaching Methods	6 Issues	7 Technology	8 Online	9 Simulation	10 Clinical Teaching	11 IPE	12 Partnerships	13 CBE	14 Curriculum	15 Assessment	16 Tests	17 Clinical Eval	18 Program Eval	19 EBT	20 Scholar	21 Serviuce/Leader	22 Prof Develop
H. Shows enthusiasm for teaching, learning, and nursing that inspires and motivates learners	√	√	√					√	√	√									√		√	√
I. Demonstrates interest in and value for all learners	√	√		√				√	√												√	√
J. Uses personal attributes (e.g., caring, confidence, patience, integrity, flexibility) that facilitate learning		√		√				√	√									√				√
K. Participates positively in collegial working relationships with learners, faculty colleagues, and the interprofessional health-care team to promote learning		√							√	√	√	√										√
L. Maintains a professional practice knowledge base needed to assist learners to prepare for contemporary nursing practice		√							√	√			√								√	
M. Serves as a role model of professional nursing	√	√							√	√											√	√
N. Creates a physically, psychologically, emotionally safe learning environment		√	√						√	√											√	
O. Establishes professional boundaries		√								√	√	√										
2. Facilitate Learner Development and Socialization																						
A. Recognizes individual learning and professional socialization needs of diverse learner populations		√		√					√		√										√	√

(continued)

Competencies[a]	Chapters[b]																					
	1 Role	2 Transition	3 Learning	4 Diverse Learner	5 Teaching Methods	6 Issues	7 Technology	8 Online	9 Simulation	10 Clinical Teaching	11 IPE	12 Partnerships	13 CBE	14 Curriculum	15 Assessment	16 Tests	17 Clinical Eval	18 Program Eval	19 EBT	20 Scholar	21 Serviuce/Leader	22 Prof Develop
B. Identifies resources available for diverse learners that assist in meeting individual learning needs		√		√	√					√											√	√
C. Describes the advisement and counseling processes to support learners in the achievement of professional goals																					√	
D. Guides learner self-reflection and personal goal setting			√						√				√								√	√
E. Fosters the cognitive, psychomotor, and affective development of learners	√			√					√	√			√									
F. Recognizes the influence of teaching strategies and communication on learner outcomes					√								√									
G. Encourages learners to engage in thoughtful and constructive self-evaluation															√		√				√	√
H. Discusses the importance of involvement in professional organizations and a commitment to lifelong learning in pursuit of professional role development																					√	√
I. Communicates the value of interprofessional practice and collaboration among members of the healthcare team											√	√										√

(continued)

Competencies[a]	Chapters[b]																					
	1 Role	2 Transition	3 Learning	4 Diverse Learner	5 Teaching Methods	6 Issues	7 Technology	8 Online	9 Simulation	10 Clinical Teaching	11 IPE	12 Partnerships	13 CBE	14 Curriculum	15 Assessment	16 Tests	17 Clinical Eval	18 Program Eval	19 EBT	20 Scholar	21 Serviuce/Leader	22 Prof Develop
J. Recognizes the influences that social determinants of education have on teaching and learning			√	√																	√	√
3. Use Assessment and Evaluation Strategies																						
A. Uses extant literature to develop evidence-based assessment and evaluation practices												√			√	√	√		√			
B. Employs a variety of strategies to assess and evaluate learning in the cognitive, psychomotor, and affective					√							√			√	√	√					√
C. Implements formative and summative evidence-based assessment and evaluation strategies	√											√			√	√	√	√				√
D. Enhances the teaching–learning process based upon data															√	√	√	√				
E. Provides timely, constructive, and thoughtful feedback to learners	√											√			√	√	√					√
4. Participate in Curriculum Design and Evaluation of Program Outcomes																						
A. Identifies that the curriculum reflects institutional philosophy and mission, current nursing and healthcare trends, and community/social needs that prepare graduates for practice in a complex, dynamic, diverse healthcare environment	√													√				√				√

(continued)

Competencies[a]	Chapters[b]																					
	1 Role	2 Transition	3 Learning	4 Diverse Learner	5 Teaching Methods	6 Issues	7 Technology	8 Online	9 Simulation	10 Clinical Teaching	11 IPE	12 Partnerships	13 CBE	14 Curriculum	15 Assessment	16 Tests	17 Clinical Eval	18 Program Eval	19 EBT	20 Scholar	21 Service/Leader	22 Prof Develop
B. Recognizes the influences of accreditation and regulatory standards on curriculum development														√				√				√
C. Demonstrates knowledge of curriculum development including identification of program outcomes, developing competency statements, writing learning objectives, and selecting learning activities and evaluation strategies													√	√				√				√
D. Relates curriculum design and implementation decisions to sound educational principles, theory, and research													√	√					√			
E. Contributes to curriculum revision based on assessment of program outcomes, learner needs, and societal and health-care trends	√													√								√
F. Uses appropriate change theories and strategies when implementing curricular revisions														√								
G. Assists in maintaining community and clinical partnerships that support educational goals												√										
H. Collaborates with external constituencies regarding curriculum and evaluation of program outcomes														√				√				√

(continued)

Competencies[a]	Chapters[b]																					
	1 Role	2 Transition	3 Learning	4 Diverse Learner	5 Teaching Methods	6 Issues	7 Technology	8 Online	9 Simulation	10 Clinical Teaching	11 IPE	12 Partnerships	13 CBE	14 Curriculum	15 Assessment	16 Tests	17 Clinical Eval	18 Program Eval	19 EBT	20 Scholar	21 Serviuce/Leader	22 Prof Develop
I. Provides program assessment and evaluation data to promote continuous quality improvement of all aspects of the program																		√				√
5. Function as a Change Agent and Leader																						
A. Demonstrates cultural humility when advocating for change				√																	√	
B. Develops an inclusive, innovative, and creative perspective of the nurse educator role	√			√																	√	
C. Recognizes interprofessional efforts to address healthcare, health policy, and educational needs locally, regionally, nationally, and internationally	√										√			√								√
D. Describes the influence of organizational effectiveness in nursing education														√							√	
E. Identifies strategies for organizational change																					√	√
F. Explains the leadership structure in the nursing program and the parent institution	√																				√	√
G. Incorporates innovative practices in educational environments	√																					
H. Develops leadership behaviors for shaping and implementing change																					√	

(continued)

Competencies[a]	Chapters[b]																					
	1 Role	2 Transition	3 Learning	4 Diverse Learner	5 Teaching Methods	6 Issues	7 Technology	8 Online	9 Simulation	10 Clinical Teaching	11 IPE	12 Partnerships	13 CBE	14 Curriculum	15 Assessment	16 Tests	17 Clinical Eval	18 Program Eval	19 EBT	20 Scholar	21 Service/Leader	22 Prof Develop
6. Pursue Continuous Quality Improvement in the Role of Nurse Educator																						
A. Demonstrates a commitment to lifelong learning	√	√																			√	√
B. Recognizes that career enhancement needs and activities change as experience is gained in the role	√																				√	√
C. Engages in professional development opportunities that increase one's effectiveness in the role	√																				√	√
D. Describes the teaching, scholarship, and service demands inherent in the role of educator and member of the academic institution	√	√																√		√	√	
E. Uses feedback gained from self, peer, learner, and/or administrative evaluation to improve role effectiveness		√																			√	√
F. Engages in activities that promote socialization to the role		√																			√	√
G. Uses knowledge of legal and ethical issues relevant to higher education and nursing education	√	√			√																	
H. Seeks mentors to enhance development in the role		√																			√	√
7. Engage in Scholarship																						
A. Draws on extant literature to design evidence-based teaching practices																			√	√		

(continued)

Competencies[a]	Chapters[b]																					
	1 Role	2 Transition	3 Learning	4 Diverse Learner	5 Teaching Methods	6 Issues	7 Technology	8 Online	9 Simulation	10 Clinical Teaching	11 IPE	12 Partnerships	13 CBE	14 Curriculum	15 Assessment	16 Tests	17 Clinical Eval	18 Program Eval	19 EBT	20 Scholar	21 Serviice/Leader	22 Prof Develop
B. Exhibits a spirit of inquiry about teaching and learning, learner development, evaluation methods, and other aspects of the role	√	√																		√		
C. Designs and implements scholarly activities in an established area of expertise																				√		
D. Disseminates nursing and teaching knowledge to a variety of audiences through multiple means																				√		
E. Demonstrates qualities of a scholar of integrity, courage, perseverance, vitality, and creativity																				√		
8. Function within the Educational Environment																						
A. Identifies history, current trends, issues, roles, and boundaries in higher education	√	√			√																	√
B. Identifies how social, technological, economic, political, and institutional forces impact higher education in general and nursing education specifically	√				√							√										√
C. Engages in cross-mentorship (mentor–mentee), collaborations, and partnerships		√										√									√	
D. Participates in academic, professional, and community service	√	√																			√	

(continued)

Competencies[a]	Chapters[b]																					
	1 Role	2 Transition	3 Learning	4 Diverse Learner	5 Teaching Methods	6 Issues	7 Technology	8 Online	9 Simulation	10 Clinical Teaching	11 IPE	12 Partnerships	13 CBE	14 Curriculum	15 Assessment	16 Tests	17 Clinical Eval	18 Program Eval	19 EBT	20 Scholar	21 Serviuce/Leader	22 Prof Develop
E. Develops professional goals that align with the nursing program and the parent institution	√	√																			√	
F. Integrates the values of civility, collegiality, professionalism, and caring to build an organizational climate that fosters the development of learners and nurse educators		√		√		√				√											√	√
G. Supports the goals and mission of the nursing program and the parent institution when managing conflict	√																					√
H. Implements policies and procedures related to learners, faculty, and the educational environment					√				√	√												
I. Discusses the various levels of governance, including shared governance, within the nursing program and the parent institution	√																				√	
J. Uses social media in a manner consistent with professional and institutional guidelines							√															
K. Describes the role of faculty input into the budgetary processes of the program and parent institution														√								
L. Maintains professional role boundaries as an educator		√								√											√	

[a]National League for Nursing. (2024). *Novice nurse educator competencies with task statements*. Available at https://www.nln.org/news/newsroomnln-position-documents/novice-nurse-educator-competencies-with-task-statements. Reprinted by permission, National League for Nursing, 2024. These competencies were

(continued)

used to develop the *Certified Nurse Educator Novice (CNE®n) 2023 Candidate Handbook*. https://www.nln.org/certification/Certification-for-Nurse-Educatorscne-n/cne-n-handbook

[b]Chapters:

1. Role of the Nurse Educator
2. The Transition From Clinician to Educator
3. Contemporary Learning Theories
4. Understanding the Diverse Learner
5. Teaching Methods
6. Ethical, Legal, and Social Challenges in Academic Nursing
7. Integrating Technology in Education
8. Teaching in Online Learning Environments
9. Simulation in Nursing Education: Overview, Essentials, and the Evidence
10. Clinical Teaching in Nursing
11. Interprofessional Education
12. Academic–Practice Partnerships
13. Competency-Based Education in Nursing
14. Curriculum Development and Course Design in Nursing Education
15. Assessment Methods
16. Developing and Using Tests
17. Clinical Evaluation
18. Program Evaluation and Accreditation
19. Evidence-Based Teaching in Nursing
20. Becoming a Scholar in Nursing Education
21. Mentorship, Service, Leading, and Learner Success
22. Nursing Professional Development Practitioner in a Clinical Practice Setting

Index

AACN. *See* American Association of Colleges of Nursing
AANP. *See* American Association of Nurse Practitioners
A-B-C approach for facilitation of online discussions, 150
academic advising, 412–413
academic decisions, 118, 120
academic dishonesty, 112
academic integrity, 112, 113, 339
academic policies, 109, 113, 120, 270
academic-clinical partnership faculty practice model, 110, 249–250. *See also* faculty practice
academic–practice partnerships, 237
 Alliance for Clinical Education, 244–245
 and capacity management, 242–243
 clinical affiliation agreements, 243–244
 clinical scholar model, 247–248
 current status of, 238–239
 dedicated education units, 248–249
 evolution of, 237–238
 faculty practice model, 249–250
 formation and implementation of, 241
 future of, 251
 interprofessional education, 245–246
 meaningful, establishing, 239–241
 models of clinical education, 245–250
 role of NPD practitioners in, 434–435
 roles of participants in, 250–251
 service learning, 246–247
 sustaining, 251
accommodators (learning style), 65
accreditation, 4–5, 361–364, 368. *See also* program evaluation
 agencies, nursing. *See also* Accreditation Commission for Education in Nursing (ACEN); Commission for Nursing Education Accreditation (CNEA); Commission on Collegiate Nursing Education (CCNE)
 and course development, 281
 of distance education programs, 362, 364
 expenses, 289
 institutional, 362, 435
 process, steps in, 361
 programmatic (specialized), 362, 363
 standards, 274, 275, 281, 288, 291, 361, 362, 363, 364, 365
 systematic evaluation plan, 364–367
Accreditation Board for Specialty Nursing Certification, 439
Accreditation Commission for Education in Nursing (ACEN), 5, 281, 362, 363, 364
ACE. *See* Alliance for Clinical Education
ACEN. *See* Accreditation Commission for Education in Nursing
active learning, 25, 81–82, 90, 97, 408
 classrooms, 136
 and gamification, 427
 and online learning, 147, 152, 154
 strategies, 20, 25, 57, 82, 94, 128–129, 152, 154, 269
 strategies, for IPE didactic instruction, 227
 and technology, 128, 129, 133
adaptive learning systems, 131, 132
admissions, 53, 54, 411
adjunct faculty, 203. *See also* part-time faculty
adult learning/learners, 27, 45–46, 56–57, 87, 89, 148, 218–219, 427
advanced practice registered nurses (APRNs)
 clinical teaching considerations, 206–209
 growth rate of, 206
 orientation, 208
 programs, 194
 securing clinical sites for, 207
advocacy role of NPD practitioners, 429–430, 440
advocacy-inquiry debriefing, 175
affective domain of learning, 77, 79, 194, 199, 259–260, 298

age of students, 56–57
AI. *See* artificial intelligence
AIHC. *See* American Interprofessional Health Collaborative
AIIA. *See* Artificial Intelligence-enabled Intelligent Assistant framework
Alliance for Clinical Education (ACE), 244–245
alternatives (multiple-choice/multiple-response items), 325, 326–327
AMA Manual of Style, 394
American Academy of Nursing, 447
American Association of Colleges of Nursing (AACN), 14, 110, 274, 402, 410, 414, 447
   and academic–practice partnerships, 238, 239, 249, 251
   Digital Innovation Virtual Bootcamp, 137, 138
   Diversity, Equity, and Inclusion (DEI) Faculty Tool Kit, 69
   Essentials: Core Competencies for Professional Nursing Education, 20, 257, 258, 263, 264, 266, 267, 268, 281, 345–347, 413, 417, 453–455
   guiding principles for effective academic–practice partnerships, 239
   holistic admissions strategies of, 411
   Manatt Report, 238
   Practice Leadership Network, 250
American Association of Community Colleges, 447
American Association of Nurse Practitioners (AANP), 207
American Association of University Professors, 447
American Association of University Women, 448
American Council on Education, 448
American Interprofessional Health Collaborative (AIHC), 225
American Nurses Association (ANA), 109, 424, 426, 431
American Nurses Credentialing Center (ANCC), 16, 424, 439, 457
American Organization of Nurse Executives (AONE), 238, 239, 251
American Psychological Association (APA), 394
American University Game Lab, 128
Americans with Disabilities Act, 27. *See also* disabilities, students with

ANA. *See* American Nurses Association
analytic scoring, 333
ANCC. *See* American Nurses Credentialing Center
andragogy, 45, 56, 89, 219
ANPD. *See* Association for Nursing Professional Development
anticipation/expectation phase (NET model), 21
anxiety of students, 79, 206, 316, 341
AONE. *See* American Organization of Nurse Executives
APA. *See* American Psychological Association
Apple, 137, 138
APRNs. *See* advanced practice registered nurses
AR. *See* augmented reality
argument mapping, 90
ARS. *See* audience response system
artificial intelligence (AI), 124, 153, 269
   -enabled LMS, 132
   generative, 131–133
Artificial Intelligence-enabled Intelligent Assistant (AIIA) framework, 132
Ask Me 3®, 269
ASPE. *See* Association for Standardized Patient Educators
assessment, 27–28, 249, 283, 295–296. *See also* tests
   cases, 304, 306–307
   and CBE, 260, 262
   competencies and learning outcomes, 297–298
   concept mapping, 304, 305
   defined, 295
   discussions and conferences, 308
   electronic portfolios, 307
   group projects, 308–309
   media clips, 307
   methods, 297–312
   norm-referenced and criterion-referenced interpretation, 296
   objective structured clinical examinations, 310
   observations and rating scales, 310
   of online learning, 159–160
   paper and other written assignments, 300–304
   principles, 297
   self-, 91, 351, 402, 405, 437
   simulation, 163–181, 309
   standardized patients, 165–166, 309–310

assessment-criterion relationship, 316
assimilators (learning style), 65
associate degree in nursing (ADN), 4, 8, 21, 57, 179, 242
Association for Nursing Professional Development (ANPD), 14, 424, 426, 429–430, 439, 448, 457, 459
Association for Standardized Patient Educators (ASPE), 165–166
Association of American Colleges and Universities, 448
Association of Black Nursing Faculty, Inc., 448
Association of Community Health Nursing Educators, 448
audience response system (ARS), 93, 128
augmented reality (AR), 166, 167, 192
aural/auditory learning, 65–66, 410

Baby Boomers, 57, 58, 408
bachelor of science in nursing (BSN), 4, 8, 264
backward design framework, 76
  for competency-based education, 258, 260, 263, 267, 270
  for curriculum development, 274, 282, 283, 284–287
Bandura, Albert, 41
BCcampus, 132
behaviorism, 36–37, 39
best-work portfolios, 307
bibliographic databases, 380, 394
blended learning. *See* hybrid learning
Bloom's taxonomy, 40–41, 78, 259
blueprint, test, 320–321, 340
Board of Curators of the University of Missouri v. Horowitz, 118, 120
bow-tie items, 335, 337
Boyer's model of scholarship, 390
brain plasticity, 35–36, 45
brain-based learning, 44–45
brainstorming (problem-based learning), 94
Bring Your Own Device (BYOD), 130
Bring Your Own Everything (BTOE), 130
Bruner, Jerome, 40, 134
BSN. *See* bachelor of science in nursing
BTOE. *See* Bring Your Own Everything
budget, and curriculum development, 289–291
burnout, 14, 216
BYOD. *See* Bring Your Own Device

Campus Computing Survey, 153
Canadian Association of Schools of Nursing (CASN), 132, 362
Canadian Interprofessional Health Collaborative (CIHC), 217
Canvas, 153–154. *See also* learning management systems (LMSs)
capacity management, and academic–practice partnerships, 242–243
career ladder education programs, 4
career(s)
  development, and scholarship, 393, 397–398
  goals, 28, 29
  in nursing education, trends supporting, 3–4
Carnegie Classification, 7–8
Carnegie Foundation for the Advancement of Teaching, 20
case conferences, 231
case presentations, 208
case studies, 92–93, 137, 268, 306, 307, 335, 336
case-based learning (CBL), 225. *See also* cases
cases, 92–93, 137, 169, 228, 268, 304, 306–307, 335, 336
CASN. *See* Canadian Association of Schools of Nursing
CBE. *See* competency-based education
CBL. *See* case-based learning
CCEI. *See* Creighton Competency Evaluation Instrument
CCNE. *See* Commission on Collegiate Nursing Education
Center for Learning through Games and Simulations (CMU), 128
certification
  for nurse educators, 14–16
  in nursing professional development, 439–440
Certified Academic Clinical Nurse Educator (CNE®cl), 14–15, 473–482
Certified Novice Nurse Educator (CNE®n), 14, 15, 483–492
Certified Nurse Educator (CNE®), 14, 15, 462–472
change agents, 12, 13, 28, 427–428, 431
chat rooms, 137
ChatGPT, 131–132
cheating, 112, 113, 339
checklists, 351

CIHC. *See* Canadian Interprofessional Health Collaborative
CINAHL. *See* Cumulative Index to Nursing and Allied Health Literature
cinemeducation, 100
CIPP. *See* Context, Input, Process, Product model
class size
   and interprofessional education, 222
   and online learning, 146
   and student evaluations of teaching, 368, 370
classical conditioning, 37–38
classroom(s). *See also* didactic learning; learning environment
   design, and technology-integrated education, 135–136
   multicultural, 55
   multigenerational, 57, 59
   redesign, 135–137
clickers. *See* audience response system (ARS)
clinical activities, planning. *See also* clinical experiences
   clinical assignments, 197–198
   clinical orientation, 195–196
   creating effective learning environment, 194
   organization for faculty and students, 198
clinical affiliation agreements, 243–244
clinical assignments, 355
   selecting, 197–198
   written, 199
clinical competencies, 345–348
clinical conferences, 27, 198–199, 308, 395, 459
   postconferences, 198–199, 200–201, 231
   preconferences, 198
clinical evaluation, 345
   and bias of teachers, 348
   checklists, 351
   competencies developed and evaluated in clinical practice, 345–348, 350
   competency-based, 262
   formative and summative, 348–349
   grading clinical courses, 355–356
   importance of feedback, 349
   methods. *See* clinical evaluation methods
   observations, 348, 351
   process, 348–350
   support for students, 350
   tools, 351–354. *See also* rating scales
clinical evaluation methods
   checklists, 351
   clinical evaluation tools (rating scales), 351–354
   observation of performance, 351
   other methods, 355
   selection of, 350
clinical experiences, 25, 87, 93, 95, 189–191, 198, 206, 244, 245. *See also* clinical activities; simulation(s); standardized patients (SPs)
   of APRNs, 207, 208, 209
   global health, 192
   learning laboratories, 189–190, 192
   telehealth, 192
   virtual, 27, 126
clinical expertise, 13, 378, 416
clinical judgment, 27, 90, 92, 95, 178, 191, 198, 260–261, 262, 301, 304, 306, 308, 335–336, 337, 345, 433. *See also* NCSBN Clinical Judgment Measurement Model (NCJMM); Next Generation NCLEX®
clinical learning, 243, 346
   interprofessional, 230–231
   student expectations of, 192
clinical learning contracts, 89
clinical educators, clinical nurse educators, 10, 14–15, 23, 25, 27, 28, 29, 190–191, 194, 197, 198, 199, 203, 245, 310, 349, 353, 356, 423, 424, 434, 473–482
clinical orientation, 195–196. *See also* onboarding; orientation
clinical practice, 13–14, 22, 87, 110–111, 249–250. *See also* academic–practice partnerships; clinical activities; clinical experiences; nursing professional development practitioners; simulation(s)
   competencies developed and evaluated in, 345–348
   concept mapping, 304, 305
   criterion-referenced interpretation in, 297
   hours, for APRNs, 206
   norm-referenced interpretation in, 297
clinical reasoning, 28, 191, 192, 208, 259, 260, 304
clinical scholar model, 247–248
clinical site visits, 199, 201, 209

clinical teaching, 189, 250
  behaviors, 191
  clinical conferences, 198–199, 200–201
  clinical site visits for APRN
    students, 209
  clinical site visits for prelicensure
    students, 199, 201
  common challenges in, 202–206
  considerations, for APRNs, 206–209
  effective, principles of, 191–192
  evaluation of, 370, 371
  feedback, 201–202
  formal preparation for, 202–203
  identification of learning outcomes,
    193–194
  learner needs assessments, 194
  learning laboratories and clinical
    experiences, 189–191
  models of, 192–193
  planning clinical activities, 194–198
  positions, educational requirements for, 8
  principles of effective, 191–192
  process of, 193–202
  and student expectations, 192
  written clinical assignments, 199
cloud computing, 126
CMU. See Center for Learning through
  Games and Simulations
CNE®. See Certified Nurse Educator
CNEA. See Commission for Nursing
  Education Accreditation
CNE®cl. See Certified Academic Clinical
  Nurse Educator
CNE®n. See Certified Novice Nurse
  Educator
coaches, role of teachers as, 67
Code of Hammurabi, 35
cognitive constructivist theory of learning, 42
cognitive domain of learning, 77, 78, 193–
  194, 199, 259, 298. See also Bloom's
  taxonomy
cognitive growth theory, 40
cognitive presence, 47
cognitive psychology, 40
cognitivism, 37, 40–41
collaboration, 29, 133, 190, 192, 199,
  223, 238. See also academic–practice
  partnerships; interprofessional
  education (IPE)
  collaborative leadership, 217
  collaborative practice, 215, 216, 228
  group projects, 225–226, 308
  and online learning, 155
collaborative learning, 93–94, 148, 190, 218,
  220, 222
Commission for Nursing Education
  Accreditation (CNEA), 5, 281, 362,
  363, 364
Commission on Collegiate Nursing
  Education (CCNE), 4–5, 281, 362, 363,
  364, 365
communication, 78, 209, 269, 403
  and academic–practice partnerships, 251
  interprofessional, 229–230
  and online learning, 151
  oral, 308, 311
  strategies, in debriefing, 173
  and student stress, 203
  and teacher-student relationship, 67
  writing skills, 86–87
Communities of Practice Framework, 219
Community College Consortium for Open
  Educational Resources, 132
community colleges, 4, 9, 27
Community of Inquiry framework,
  47–48, 219
community-based learning, 192–193, 408
competency blitz, 432
competency management, role of NPD
  practitioners in, 431–432
competency-based education (CBE), 92,
  177, 257–271, 274, 282
  artificial intelligence, 269
  assessment of competency, 261–263
  backward design for, 258, 260, 263,
    267, 270
  course outcomes as competency
    statements, 265–266
  curriculum mapping, 265, 268
  definition of, 258
  development of competence, 259
  enhancement, strategies for, 267–269
  future directions in nursing
    education, 270
  infrastructure for, 263–267
  as a learning model, 258–261
  managing curricular drift, 267
  program outcomes aligned with
    standards as competency statements,
    263–264
  role of educators in, 269–270
  teacher-coach role in, 67
  and traditional nursing education,
    comparison, 258

completion items (test), 332
concept mapping, 89–90, 304, 305
conferences, 308, 459. *See also* postconferences; preconferences
   clinical, 27, 198–199, 200–201, 231
   presentations at, 395
confidentiality, 113
conflicts of interest, 108, 111
connectionism, 39
consequences of tests, 316
construct validation, 316
constructed response items (test), 318, 319
constructivism, 37, 42, 43, 47, 95, 134, 152, 219, 222, 281
contact between students and faculty in online learning, 146–147
contact hypothesis, 219
content validation, 316
Context, Input, Process, Product (CIPP) model, 359–360
context-dependent item sets, 323, 334–335
continuing education, 14, 143, 173, 432, 439
continuous quality improvement, 28–29, 280. *See also* quality improvement (QI)
contract learning, 88–89
conventional items (test), 318, 319
convergers (learning style), 65
cooperation among students, and online learning, 147. *See also* collaboration
cooperative learning, 93, 308, 312
Core Competencies for Academic Nurse Educators (NLN), 25, 416, 423
Council on Accreditation of Nurse Anesthesia, 362
course development, 281–282
course evaluations, 368–370
course learning contracts, 89
course management system, 158. *See also* learning management systems (LMSs)
course outcomes, 89, 270, 345. *See also* clinical evaluation; learning outcomes
   as competency statements, 265–266
   and competency-based education, 260, 261
   development template, 455
   and electronic portfolios, 307
   knowledge-based, 266
   and online learning, 159
course syllabus. *See* syllabus
Coursera®, 146
COVID-19 pandemic, 20, 126, 131, 154, 428, 431
   clinical simulation during, 226
   online learning during, 143, 144, 145, 206, 222
   and student stress, 206
CRAP (Contrast, Repetition, Alignment, Proximity) principles, 156
credentials/credentialing
   educational, of nursing faculty, 7
   of nurse educators, 4–5
   in simulation, 180
Creighton Competency Evaluation Instrument (CCEI), 178
criterion-referenced interpretation of data, 296
critical thinking, 82–83, 89, 90, 94, 98, 100, 126, 129, 136, 149, 191, 199, 208, 219, 248, 274, 301, 433
critical thinking ability, 82
critical thinking disposition, 82, 93
Cronbach's alpha, 316
culture, 24, 31, 41, 54–55, 115–116, 117, 134, 402, 407, 411, 416, 417
Cumulative Index to Nursing and Allied Health Literature (CINAHL), 380, 394
CUNY Games Network, 128
curriculum, 10, 13, 134, 260, 273
   competency-based education, 257–271, 274
   components of, 280–281
   curricular drift, 267
   design, 23, 28, 48
   integration of IPE into, 219, 220, 221–222
   integration of learning laboratory into, 190
   integration of SDOH into, 405, 407
   integration of simulation into, 168–171, 172
   LGBTQ+ health topics in, 59–60
   mapping, 265, 268, 288–289
   models, 83
   and professional identity formation, 417–418
   and technology, 133, 138
curriculum development, 10, 257, 273
   background, 274
   backward design framework for, 274, 282, 283, 284–287
   and budgets in academic setting, 289–290
   and budgets in healthcare setting, 290–291
   content considerations, 281, 282

course development, 281–282
curriculum/content mapping, 288–289
external frame factors, 275, 276–278
implementation plan, 283, 284–287
internal frame factors, 276, 278–280
managing curricular drift, 267
needs assessment, 274–276
review and approval process, 281
syllabus development, 283, 288
cybercivility, 151, 158
cyberethics, 151, 158

DASH. *See* Debriefing Assessment for Simulation in Healthcare©
data visualization, 370
debates, 100, 137
debriefing, 82, 96, 247, 381
   interprofessional education, 223, 228–229, 231
   methods, 174–176
   peer review of teaching performance, 370
   postconferences, 199
   role of debriefer, 173
   service learning, 247
   simulation, 169–170, 172–176, 228–229, 309
Debriefing Assessment for Simulation in Healthcare© (DASH), 175
Debriefing for Meaningful Learning© (DML), 174, 175
Debriefing for Meaningful Learning Evaluation Scale (DMLES), 175
Debriefing with Good Judgment, 174, 175
decision-oriented program evaluation models, 359
dedicated education units (DEUs), 248–249, 434–435
DEI. *See* diversity; equity; inclusion
desktop virtual reality, 166, 167
DEUs. *See* dedicated education units
Dewey, John, 42
dichotomous scoring, 319–320
didactic learning, 223–226, 227, 250
Digital Innovation Virtual Bootcamp, 137, 138
digital media, 101, 129
digital storytelling, 100
D-index. *See* discrimination index
Directory of Nursing Journals, 394
disabilities, students with, 27, 68–69
disciplinary distribution, and interprofessional education, 222

discovery learning, 96
discrimination index (D-index), 342
discussions, 91, 92, 147, 173, 308. *See also* debriefing
   discussion boards, 146–147, 226
   online, facilitation of, 149–151
   teacher responses for facilitation of, 92
disorientation phase (NET model), 21
dissemination of scholarship, 391–395
distance education/learning. *See also* online learning
   and COVID-19 pandemic, 144, 145
   programs, accreditation of, 362, 364
divergers (learning style), 65
diversity, 192, 407, 410, 411
   definition of, 407
   of learners. *See* learners
   of nurse educators, 407–408, 414, 417
Diversity, Equity, and Inclusion (DEI) Faculty Tool Kit, 69
DML. *See* Debriefing for Meaningful Learning©
DMLES. *See* Debriefing for Meaningful Learning Evaluation Scale
DNP. *See* Doctor of Nursing Practice
Doctor of Nursing Practice (DNP), 19, 251, 264
dossier. *See* teaching portfolios
double-blind peer review, 395
draft, writing, 394–395
drag-and-drop items, 329–330, 337
drama, 96
drop-down items, 329
dual credit, 410
Dweck, Carol, 45

EBP. *See* evidence-based practice
Education Resources Information Center, 380
educational games, 98, 100, 137
educational preparation for employment
   in academic settings, 4–8
   in healthcare settings, 8
EDUCAUSE, 153, 449
edX, 146
EHRs. *See* electronic health records
e-learning, 144
electronic books (e-books), 84
electronic health records (EHRs), 126, 137. *See also* electronic medical records (EMRs)
electronic medical records (EMRs), 196, 207, 208

electronic portfolios, 307
emotional intelligence, 203, 405, 416
emotional support to students, 67, 148
EMRs. *See* electronic medical records
EndNote, 394
end-of-program goals statement, 280
entrustable professional activities (EPAs), 262–263
EPAs. *See* entrustable professional activities
equity, 192, 407
   Diversity, Equity, and Inclusion (DEI) Faculty Tool Kit, 69
   -focused teaching, 414–415
error correction in online learning, 158
essay items, 332–334
Essentials: Core Competencies for Professional Nursing Education (AACN), 20, 257, 258, 263, 264, 266, 267, 268, 281, 345–347, 413, 417, 453–455
ethical behavior, 109–110, 151
evaluation, 27–28, 296. *See also* assessment; clinical evaluation; program evaluation
   of APRN student competencies, 209
   of clinical teaching, 368–370
   of interprofessional education, 232
   of clinical learning, learning, 295, 345
   of online learning, 159–160
   of program outcomes, 28
   self-, 309, 310–311
   student evaluations of teaching, 368–370, 397
   systematic evaluation plan, 28, 364–367
evidence-based nursing, 378
evidence-based practice (EBP), 345, 429, 433–434
evidence-based teaching, 191, 377–378
   applicability of findings, 386
   evaluation of evidence quality, 384–386
   evidence synthesis, 380–382
   levels of evidence, 385
   and nursing education research, 378
   questioning educational practices and identifying the need for evidence, 379
   review of individual studies, 382–383
   searching for evidence, 379–384
experiential learning, 42, 65, 91–92, 95, 96, 193, 219, 268
exposure learning, 220, 222, 223, 226
extended reality (XR), 166–168

facilitation
   facilitators of online learning, 148–151, 158
   of interprofessional education, 222–223, 226
   of simulation, 165, 172, 229
   of transition from clinician to educator, 23–24
faculty, 4, 5–10, 13–14, 24–31, 110–111, 114–115, 137–138, 155, 158–159, 198, 202–206, 222–223, 249–250, 423, 447. *See also* nurse educators; nursing faculty
faculty development, 14
faculty orientation, 24–31
faculty handbooks, 107, 111
faculty practice, 13–14, 110–111, 249–250. *See also* clinical practice
FAFSA. *See* Free Application for Federal Student Aid
Family Educational Rights and Privacy Act (FERPA), 29, 118, 119–120
feedback, 28, 191, 208, 209, 232, 262, 296, 356, 397
   and assessment, 295, 296, 299, 300, 301, 308, 309
   and CBE, 270
   clinical evaluation, 348–349
   in clinical settings, 201–202
   in clinical site visits, 199
   and discussions/conferences, 308
   and educational games, 98
   iSoBAR framework, 202
   modes, 349
   and online learning, 147, 155, 159
   in simulation debriefing, 173, 174, 309
   and written assignments, 301
feminist pedagogy, 37, 44
FERPA. *See* Family Educational Rights and Privacy Act
film as a teaching method, 100
financial assistance to students, 414
financial barriers of learners, 413–414
first-degree relatives, conflict of interest in employment of, 111
first-generation learners, 412–413
five-minute preceptor (FMP) approach, 209
fixed mindset, 63
flipped classroom, 136–137
FMP. *See* five-minute preceptor approach
formal papers, 300

formative assessments/evaluation, 262, 296, 308, 309, 310, 348–349
formative feedback, 98, 160, 173, 270. *See also* feedback
Four-Level Evaluation Model (Kirkpatrick), 160, 385–386
Free Application for Federal Student Aid (FAFSA), 414
Fry, Roger, 42
full-time clinical faculty, 10
funding
    for nursing education research, 378
    for nursing programs, 289–290

Gagne, Robert, 40
Game Studio (Boise State University), 128
Game-based Education and Advanced Research Studies (GEARS) Lab, 128
game-based learning (GBL), 127–128, 427
games, educational, 98, 100, 137
Gardner, Howard, 46
Garrison, D. R., 47
GAS. *See* Gather-Analyze-Summarize
Gather-Analyze-Summarize (GAS), 174, 175
GBL. *See* game-based learning
GEARS. *See* Game-based Education and Advanced Research Studies Lab
gender diversity of students, 57, 59–60
Generation X, 57, 58, 408
Generation Y. *See* Millennials
Generation Z, 57, 58, 410
generational differences
    between educators and students, 203
    in learning styles, 408
    in values, learning, and teaching methods, 57, 58
generative artificial intelligence, 131–133
Gilligan, C., 44
global health clinical experiences, 193
goal-oriented program evaluation models, 359
grading, 296–297, 301, 349
    of clinical courses, 355–356
    disputes, 118, 119–120
    of essay items, 333
    of group projects, 309
    of written assignments, 301–303
    rubrics, 159–160, 170, 303
grants, 290, 414
group discussion, 91, 308
group projects, 225–226, 308–309

growth mindset, 63–64, 208
growth portfolios, 307
guest speakers, cross-professional, 225
Guide to Effective Interprofessional Education Experiences in Nursing Education, 224
guided reflection, 82

head mounted displays (HMDs), 166, 167
Health Insurance Portability and Accountability Act (HIPAA), 113
Health Resources and Services Administration (HRSA), 414
healthcare organizations. *See also* academic–practice partnerships
    accreditation and compliance of, 435
    alignment of NPD practitioners with, 436
    strategic goals of, 435–436
Healthcare Simulation Standards Endorsement™ program, 180
Healthcare Simulation Standards of Best Practice™ (HSSOBP), 166, 180
heutagogy, 129
hierarchy of needs (Maslow), 42–43
high-frequency, low-impact simulations, 169
highlight items, 330–331
HIPAA. *See* Health Insurance Portability and Accountability Act
HMDs. *See* head mounted displays
holistic admissions approach, 53, 54, 411
holistic scoring, 333
Horizon Report, 153
Hospital National Patient Safety Goals, 435
hotspots. *See* highlight items
HPSs. *See* human patient simulators
HRSA. *See* Health Resources and Services Administration
HSSOBP. *See* Healthcare Simulation Standards of Best Practice™
human patient simulators (HPSs), 164. *See also* manikin-based simulation
humanism, 37, 42–44
hybrid learning, 144, 153

identity formation phase (NET model), 22
IHI. *See* Institute for Health Improvement
Illinois Online Network (ION), 148
immersion learning, 220–221, 230, 232
immersive virtual reality (IVR), 166–167, 168

incivility, 23, 59, 114–117, 119–120, 151
   critical elements to consider related to, 115
   faculty, 114–115, 203
   and grade disputes, 118, 119–120
   parent, 119–120
inclusion, 192
   definition of, 407
   Diversity, Equity, and Inclusion (DEI) Faculty Tool Kit, 69
   inclusive learning environment, 59, 60, 148, 153, 154, 414
   inclusive pedagogy, 48
   in multicultural classrooms, 55
Inclusive Excellence Ecosystem for Academic Nursing, 69
independent learning methods
   concept mapping, 89–90
   contract learning, 88–89
   reading, 83–85
   reflection, 86–88
   self-paced modules/reusable learning objects, 90–91
   writing, 86–87
individual learning contracts, 89
information processing theory, 40
information seeking phase (NET model), 21
infrastructure
   for competency-based education, 263–267
   for curriculum, 263–267
   technological, 124, 133, 155, 339
Institute for Connected Learning (UCL), 128
Institute for Health Improvement (IHI), 225
Institute of Education Sciences, 380
Institute of Medicine (IOM), 4, 215, 262
institutional accreditation, 362, 435. *See also* accreditation
instructor presence in online learning, 158
integrative reviews, 382
integrity, academic, 112, 113
Interactive Media & Games Division (USC), 128
internal consistency method, 316
International Academy of Nursing Editors, 394
International Society for Professional Identity in Nursing (ISPIN), 417
Internet, 124. *See also* online learning
interpretive exercise. *See* context-dependent item sets

interprofessional collaboration, 216–217, 434
Interprofessional Core Competencies for Collaborative Practice, 216
interprofessional education (IPE), 13, 215–216, 245–246
   clinical learning, 230–231
   definition of, 216
   didactic learning, 223–226, 227
   evaluation of, 232
   IPEC Core Competencies, 217–218, 220
   learner considerations, 221–222
   learning experiences, theories for designing, 218–220
   learning outcomes, 221
   process, models for conceptualizing, 220–221
   resources, 224–225
   role of faculty, 222–223
   simulation, 170, 226, 228–230
   student readiness, 221
   timing, 222
Interprofessional Education Collaborative (IPEC), 216, 217–218, 226, 227, 448
Interprofessional.Global, 225
IOM. *See* Institute of Medicine
ION. *See* Illinois Online Network
IPE. *See* interprofessional education
IPEC. *See* Interprofessional Education Collaborative
iSoBAR feedback, 202
ISPIN. *See* International Society for Professional Identity in Nursing
items, test. *See also* tests
   analysis, 341–342
   arranging in logical sequence, 337–338
   case studies, 336
   context-dependent item sets, 334–335
   drag-and-drop items, 329–330
   drop-down items, 329
   essay items, 332–334
   format of, 318–319
   highlight items, 330–331
   matching exercises, 324, 325
   matrix items, 327–328
   multiple-choice/multiple-response items, 324–327
   numbering of, 338
   short-answer items, 332
   stand-alone clinical judgment items, 337
   true-false items, 323–324
   writing, 321–325
IVR. *See* immersive virtual reality

JANE. *See* Journal/Author Name Estimator
JCEN. *See* Journal of Continuing Education in Nursing
Jensen, Eric, 44
JNPD. *See* Journal for Nurses in Professional Development
job shadowing, 9, 197, 230–231, 437
The Joint Commission (TJC), 435, 458
Josiah Macy Jr. Foundation, 226
Journal for Nurses in Professional Development (JNPD), 459
Journal of Continuing Education in Nursing (JCEN), 459
Journal/Author Name Estimator (JANE), 394
journaling, 193, 208, 247, 301
journals for publication, 392, 393–394, 459

K-12 education, 410, 412
Khan Academy, 146
kinesthetic learning, 65–66, 410
Knowles, Malcolm, 45, 56
Kolb, David, 42
Kolb Experiential Learning Profile, 410
KR. *See* Kuder-Richardson coefficient
Kuder-Richardson (KR) coefficient, 316

laboratories, 77, 189–190, 192, 267
language
   non-native speakers, 54, 203
   in tests, 322
large-class teaching methods
   debate, 100
   film, 100
   lecture, 97
   narrative pedagogy/storytelling, 100–101
   questioning, 98, 99
Lasater Clinical Judgment Rubric (LCJR), 178
Lave, Jean, 41
LCJR. *See* Lasater Clinical Judgment Rubric
leadership, 10, 13, 86, 243
   approaches, 406
   collaborative, 217
   qualities of leader, 405
   role, of NPD practitioners, 428, 436
   role, of nurse educators, 11, 12, 28, 30, 404, 405–407, 413
   toxic, 114–117

learner success, factors affecting
   academic advising, 412–413
   admissions, 411
   equity-focused teaching, 414–415
   financial barriers, 413–414
   gaps in diversity, 407–408
   learning styles, 408, 410
   mentoring, 412
   nurse educator characteristics, 416–417
   recruitment of diverse learners, 410–411
   self-care/socialization, 413
   trauma-informed teaching practices, 416
learners
   age of, 56–57
   attributes of, 53–63
   characteristics of, 78–79
   culture of, 54–55
   demographics, 55–60, 409
   development and socialization, 27
   with disabilities, 27, 68–69
   diversity of, 53
   expectations, in clinical teaching, 192
   gender and sexual diversity of, 57, 59–60
   and interprofessional education, 221–222
   membership in professional and student organizations, 413
   needs, assessment of, 194, 296
   professional identity formation in, 417–418
   race of, 55–56
   strategic, 63–64
   in undergraduate RN programs, demographics, 409
learning. *See also* online learning
   active, 25, 81–82, 90, 94, 97, 128, 129, 133, 136, 147, 152, 154, 227, 269, 408, 427
   adaptive learning systems, 131, 132
   adult, 27, 45–46, 56–57, 87, 89, 148, 218–219, 427
   affective, 77, 79, 194, 199, 259–260, 298. *See also* affective domain of learning
   and assessment, 27, 148, 159–160, 249, 260–263, 283, 295–296, 297–312, 423, 432
   aural/auditory, 65–66, 410
   brain-based, 44–45
   case-based, 225. *See also* case studies
   clinical, 192, 230–231, 243, 346
   cognitive, 77, 78, 193–194, 199, 259, 298
   collaborative, 93–94, 148, 190, 218, 220, 222

community-based, 192–193, 408
cooperative, 93, 308, 312
definition of, 36
didactic, 223–226, 227, 250
distance, 144, 145, 362, 364. *See also* online learning
domains of, 77–78, 79, 80, 177, 259–260, 298
effective clinical teaching behaviors for fostering, 191
e-learning, 144
experiential, 42, 65, 91–92, 95, 96, 193, 219, 268
facilitation, and new faculty orientation, 25, 27
game-based, 127–128, 427
generational differences in, 57, 58
hybrid, 144, 153
immersion, 220–221, 230, 232
kinesthetic, 65–66, 410
learning style preferences, 64–66, 67
mastery, 221
materials for, 81
microlearning, 129–130
motivational, 45
peer, 246
plan, 356
problem-based, 94–95
psychomotor, 77, 80, 190, 194, 259, 298
reading/writing, 65–66, 410
relational, 219
service, 96–97, 197, 231, 246–247
social determinates of learning model, 62–63
styles, 64–66, 408, 410
teaching elements that promote safety in, 76
team-based, 94, 137
and technology, 36, 46–47
visual, 65–66, 90, 410
Western and Eastern perspectives of, 54
learning analytics, 130–131
learning contract. *See* contract learning
learning environment, 54, 190, 350, 410
and academic–practice partnerships, 243, 244, 245
and admissions, 411
APRN clinical teaching, 208
clinical, 191, 194, 195, 424, 434
collaborative, 93, 94
development, 75–76
and discussions, 308
equitable, 414
gender-inclusive, 60
inclusive, 59, 60, 148, 153, 154, 414
and learner socialization, 413
and learning style preferences, 66
and lecturing, 97
and movies, 100
online, 144, 148, 151, 152, 155–159
and questioning, 98
and role-play, 95
and student stress, 203
and teacher-student relationship, 67
and technology-integrated education, 135–136
Learning Games Lab (University of North Carolina at Chapel Hill), 128
learning laboratories, 77, 189–190, 192
learning management systems (LMSs), 125, 132, 137, 153–154, 155, 339
learning outcomes, 82, 88, 203, 260, 423, 433. *See also* assessment; tests
and academic–practice partnerships, 244
and assessment, 295, 297–298
clinical teaching, 193–194
and contract learning, 89
and curriculum development, 274, 275, 281, 282
and debriefing, 173
and interprofessional education, 221
and learning styles, 64, 66
in online learning, 146, 149, 156, 160
of simulations, 166, 167, 168, 171, 226, 228, 229
and teaching methods, 76–77, 83
learning theories, 36
adult learning theory, 45–46
beginning of, 35–36
behaviorism, 36–37, 39
brain-based learning, 44–45
cognitivism, 37, 40–41
Community of Inquiry framework, 47–48
constructivism, 37, 42, 43
feminist pedagogy, 37, 44
foundational, 36–44
humanism, 37, 42–44
inclusive pedagogy, 48
motivational learning, 45
sociological, 41
and teaching philosophy, 49
technology-mediated learning, 46–47
theory of multiple intelligences, 46
transformative, 38, 44–48

lectures, 81, 97
legal counsel, 107–109
length of tests, 318
LGBTQ+ nursing students, 59–60
librarians, 81, 131, 380, 439
literature review, 380–382, 393
literature search, 377, 379–380, 439
Literature Selection Technical Review Committee, 394
LMSs. *See* learning management systems
loan programs, 414
lockdown browsers, 339
logic model, 360
low-frequency, high impact simulations, 168–169

Magnet Recognition Program®, 436, 457
male nurses, 57, 59
Manatt Report, 238
manikin-based simulation, 164–165
manuscript, purpose of, 393
mapping grids and certified nurse educator blueprints, 461–492
Maslow, Abraham, 42–43
Maslow's hierarchy of needs, 42–43
Massive Open Online Courses (MOOCs), 146
master of science in nursing (MSN), 8, 264
matching exercises, 324, 325
matrix items, 327–328
MBTI. *See* Myers-Briggs Type Indicator
media clips, 307
mediation, 109
medication administration, competency for, 260, 261
MEDLINE, 380, 394
Mentoring Tool Kit (NLN), 402
mentors/mentoring, 407, 438
    of faculty for development of competencies in technology, 137–138
    and learner success, 412
    mentor-mentee partnership, 402, 403
    NPD practitioners as, 428, 440
    and nurse educator transition, 23–24, 25, 27–28, 29, 30
    of nurse educators, 402–403
    peer, 23, 24, 68, 197
    and recruitment of diverse learners, 410
    responsibilities of mentors and mentees, 403–404

MERLOT. *See* Multimedia Educational Resource for Learning and Online Teaching
metaverse, 127, 381–382
microaffirmations, 55
microaggressions, 55, 56
microlearning, 129–130
Millennials, 57, 58, 410
mind mapping, 90
minority students, 192, 412, 414
mission statement, 280, 282
MIT Game Lab, 128
MIT OpenCourseWare (OCW), 132
mixed reality (MR), 166, 167
mobile computing, 130
mobile devices, 128, 130
MOOCs. *See* Massive Open Online Courses
Moodle, 153–154
motivational learning, 45
moulage, 165
movies as a teaching method, 100
MR. *See* mixed reality
MSN. *See* master of science in nursing
multicultural classrooms, 55
multigenerational classrooms, 57, 59
Multimedia Educational Resource for Learning and Online Teaching (MERLOT), 132, 449
multiple-choice (MC) items, 324–327
multiple-choice matrix, 327
multiple-choice questions, 94
multiple-response (MR) items, 324–327
multiple-response matrix, 327
Myers-Briggs Type Indicator (MBTI), 410

narrative pedagogy, 100–101
National Academies of Sciences, Engineering, and Medicine, 427, 435
National Center for Higher Education Management Systems (NCHEMS), 364
National Center for Interprofessional Practice and Education (NCIPE), 224, 232
National Council for State Authorization Reciprocity Agreements (NC-SARA), 364
National Council Licensure Exam (NCLEX®), 257, 299, 319, 335–337, 368
National Council of State Boards of Nursing (NCSBN), 179, 407

National Diversity Workforce Program, 414
National Institute of Standards and Technology (NIST), 126
National League for Nursing (NLN), 5, 14, 20, 25, 171, 257, 274, 395, 402, 405, 407, 414, 423, 450
National Organization of Nurse Practitioner Faculties (NONPF), 110, 207, 249, 250, 450
National Student Nurses Association, 450
NCHEMS. *See* National Center for Higher Education Management Systems
NCIPE. *See* National Center for Interprofessional Practice and Education
NCJMM. *See* NCSBN Clinical Judgment Measurement Model
NCLEX®. *See* National Council Licensure Exam
NC-SARA. *See* National Council for State Authorization Reciprocity Agreements
NCSBN. *See* National Council of State Boards of Nursing
NCSBN Clinical Judgment Measurement Model (NCJMM), 336, 337
needs assessment, 274–276, 427
negative reinforcement, 39
NET. *See* Nurse Educator Transition model
Next Generation NCLEX®, 335–336
  case studies, 336
  stand-alone clinical judgment items, 337
NIST. *See* National Institute of Standards and Technology
NLN. *See* National League for Nursing
NLN/Jeffries Simulation Theory, 95, 176
non-native students, 54, 203
NONPF. *See* National Organization of Nurse Practitioner Faculties
nontenure track, 5–6
norm-referenced interpretation of data, 296
NPD. *See* nursing professional development
NRPs. *See* nurse residency programs
NURS. *See* Nursing Universal Retention and Success model
nurse anesthetists, 362
Nurse Educator Transition (NET) model, 21–22

nurse educators, 3, 423–424. *See also* faculty; nursing faculty; nursing professional development practitioners
  and academic–practice partnerships, 250
  balancing role responsibilities, 13–14
  career development of, 397–398
  certification for, 14–16, 461–492
  characteristics, and learner success, 416–417
  demographics of, 409
  educational preparation for employment in academic settings, 4–8
  educational preparation for employment in healthcare settings, 8
  educational requirements for employment as, 9
  orientation of, 23, 24–31, 402
  preparation for teaching, 8–9
  professional identity formation in, 417–418
  questions to consider prior to seeking employment as, 31
  responsibilities of, 9–12
  role of, 9–12, 13–14, 25–30
  and students, generational differences between, 203
  teaching activities of, 390
  transition process, 19–32
Nurse Faculty Loan Program (HRSA), 414
nurse residency programs (NRPs), 430
nursing education. *See also* competency-based education (CBE); evidence-based teaching
  continuing education, 14, 143, 173, 432, 439
  inclusive environment in, 59
  integration of technology into, 133–137
  performance assessment in, 262
  preparation for, 19–20
  programs, accreditation of, 5. *See also* accreditation
  research, and evidence-based teaching, 378
  research literature, guide for analyzing, 383–384
  role of NPD practitioners in, 432–433
  studies, 380, 385–386
  trends supporting careers in, 3–4
nursing faculty, 110, 423. *See also* faculty; nurse educators

and academic–practice partnerships, 249–250
balancing role responsibilities, 13–14
competencies in technology, development of, 137–138
development, 14
faculty practice, 110–111, 249–250
incivility of, 114–115, 203
new faculty orientation, 24–31
organizations for, 198, 447
preparation for online instruction, 155
ranks, 5
role in interprofessional education, 222–223
salary of, 14
shortage of, 4, 202–203
stress, 204–205, 206
teaching and managing online learning environments, 158–159
tenure and nontenure tracks, 5–6
types of appointments and educational credentials, 7–8, 9
workforce, aging of, 4
nursing professional development (NPD), 29, 138, 423–424
certification in, 439–440
educators in, 8
and mentoring, 402–403
NPD Practice Model, 426
as a nursing practice specialty, 424–425
roles and professional qualifications, 425
Nursing Professional Development Certification, 457
nursing professional development practitioners, 4, 13, 423–424
as advocates, 429–430
balancing role responsibilities, 13–14
challenges of, 436–437
as change agents, 427–431
leadership role of, 428–429, 436
as learning facilitators, 427
membership in professional organizations, 439
as mentors, 428
and practice transitions, 430–431
promotion of safe, quality, and equitable health care, 435–437
resources for, 457–459
responsibilities of, 431–435
role, interest in and preparation for, 437–438
role, maintaining and advancing in, 439–440
role, transition to, 438–439
Nursing Professional Development: Scope and Standards of Practice, 424, 425, 438
nursing professional development specialists, 425, 439
Nursing: Scope and Standards of Practice (ANA), 425, 426
nursing shortages, 3, 203
Nursing Universal Retention and Success (NURS) model, 131

OADN. *See* Organization for Associate Degree Nursing
objective structured clinical examinations (OSCEs), 95, 165, 310
observation of students for assessment/ evaluation, 178, 310, 348, 351
OCW. *See* MIT OpenCourseWare
OER Commons, 132
OERs. *See* open educational resources
OLC. *See* Online Learning Consortium
ombudsperson, 109
OMP. *See* one-minute preceptor approach
onboarding. *See also* orientation
    definition of, 431
    of nurse educators, 402
    role of NPD practitioners in, 431
one-minute care plan, 200
one-minute preceptor (OMP) approach, 208–209
online learning, 27, 79, 80, 125, 143, 144, 206
    accessibility and usability of online materials in, 154–155
    advantages and disadvantages of, 144–145
    assessment and evaluation, 159–160
    assessment tools, 148
    cybercivility and cyberethics, 151
    facilitators, 148–151, 158
    and interprofessional education, 222, 226
    pedagogy, 152–153
    prevalence of online courses, 145–146
    principles of good practice in online teaching, 148
    role of technology in, 153–155
    rules and policies for, 147
    student success, 148, 149, 156
    successful online courses, 146–148
    technology reports, 153
Online Learning Consortium (OLC), 157

online learning environments, 148, 151
  designing online courses and modules, 156
  interactions in, 144, 156
  quality, 157–158
  stages and process of creating, 152
  teaching and managing, 158–159
Online Readiness Questionnaire (North Carolina Central University), 148
online tests, 339–340
open educational resources (OERs), 131, 132
Open SUNY Course Quality Review (OSCQR) scorecard, 157
open-ended questions, 98, 308, 370
OpenStax, 132
operant conditioning, 39
Organization for Associate Degree Nursing (OADN), 14, 450
organizations, nursing and higher education, 447–451
organizations, journals, educational conferences for NPD practitioners, 457–459
orientation
  and APRN clinical teaching, 208
  assessment and evaluation strategies, 27–28
  change agent and leadership roles, 28
  clinical, 195–196
  clinical nurse educators, 25
  components of, 26–31
  continuous quality improvement, 28–29
  of course management system, 158
  curriculum design and evaluation of program outcomes, 28
  engagement in scholarship, 29
  facilitation of learning, 25, 27
  faculty, 24–25
  functioning within the education environment, 29–30
  learner development and socialization, 27
  of NPD practitioners, 438
  of nurse educators, 23, 24–31, 402
  part-time faculty, 25
  programs, 23, 24, 25
  resources for novice educators, 30–31
  role of NPD practitioners in, 431
  time period, 25
OSCEs. *See* objective structured clinical examinations
OSCQR. *See* Open SUNY Course Quality Review scorecard

PaperPile, 394
papers, formal, 300
parent incivility, 119–120
partial scoring methods, 320
part-time clinical educators, orientation for, 25
part-time faculty, 21, 25, 110, 203
pass–fail grading, 351, 355
patient assignment form, 197
patient education, 276, 290–291
patient rounding, 231
patient safety
  and ethical behavior, 109, 112
  and simulation, 126
  TJC standards of, 435
patient stories, 226
Pavlov, Ivan, 37–38
PBL. *See* problem-based learning
PEARLS. *See* Promoting Excellence and Reflective Learning in Simulation
pedagogy
  feminist, 37, 44
  inclusive, 48
  narrative, 100–101
  online, 152–153
  relational, 219–220
peer(s), 76
  critique, of test items, 323
  encouragement, for nontraditional learners, 56
  feedback, 384–385
  mentoring, 23, 24, 68, 197
  peer-reviewed journals, 392, 393
  review, of scholarship, 391, 395, 396, 397
  review, of teaching performance, 370–371
  teaching and learning, 197, 246
Penn State Behrend eLearning Assessment, 148
performance evaluation. *See* clinical evaluation
physical spaces, and teaching method selection, 80
Piaget, Jean, 42
plagiarism, 112
Plus Delta, 174
PNEG. *See* Professional Nurse Educators Group
POD Network, 451
point biserial correlation coefficient, 342
polling, 128–129
+/− scoring method, 320

positive reinforcement, 39, 349
positive wording in tests, 322
postconferences, 198–199, 200–201, 231
posters, 226
practical nursing programs, 4
Practice Leadership Network, 250
pre-briefing (simulation), 172
preceptors/preceptorships, 193, 437
   for APRN students, 206–209
   definition of, 427
   NPD practitioners as, 427
   for prelicensure students, 199
   remote, 193
preconferences, 198
prelicensure nursing programs, 194, 423. *See also* associate degree in nursing (ADN); bachelor of science in nursing (BSN)
   clinical site visits, 199, 201
   nursing student assignment sheet for, 197
presentations, 96, 226, 395
privacy, 29, 113–114, 197
problem analysis (problem-based learning), 94
problem-based learning (PBL), 83, 94–95, 134
productive struggle, 226
professional development. *See* nursing professional development (NPD)
professional development plan of NPD practitioners, 438, 439
professional identity, 22, 112
   definition of, 417
   domains of, 417
   formation, 417–418
Professional Nurse Educators Group (PNEG), 459
professional role development, 433
program evaluation, 359, 436. *See also* accreditation
   of distance education programs, 362, 364
   models, 359–361
   peer review, 370–371
   plan, systematic, 364–367
   regulation of nursing programs, 368
   student evaluation of teaching, 368–370
program outcomes, 360. *See also* learning outcomes
   aligned with standards as competency statements, 263–264
   and curriculum development, 283
   evaluation of, 28. *See also* program evaluation
   revision worksheet, 453–455
programmatic (specialized) accreditation, 362, 363
progressive education, 42
Promoting Excellence and Reflective Learning in Simulation (PEARLS), 174, 175
proofreading of tests, 338
psychological safety, 217, 229
psychomotor domain of learning, 77, 80, 190, 194, 259, 298
PsycINFO®, 380
Public Service Loan Forgiveness Program, 414
publications, writing for, 393
   draft writing, 394–395
   identification of journals, 393–394
   peer review of manuscript, 395, 396
   process of, 393–395
   purpose of manuscript, 393
   reference management software, 394
   PubMed, 394
punishment (operant conditioning), 39
pyramid of competence (Miller), 259

QI. *See* quality improvement
QM. *See* Quality Matters
QSEN. *See* Quality and Safety Education for Nurses
Quality and Safety Education for Nurses (QSEN), 262, 263, 267, 346, 451
quality improvement (QI), 28–29, 238, 250, 251, 280, 359, 361, 427, 433–434. *See also* accreditation
Quality Matters (QM), 157–158
Qualtrics® report, 267
questioning, 82, 98, 99, 158, 198, 199, 208, 308

race of students, 55–56
ranks, nursing faculty, 5
rapid cycle evaluation, 232
rating scales, 310, 351–352, 353
Rcampus™, 160
reading, 83–85
reciprocity among students, and online learning, 147
recruitment of diverse learners, 410–411
reference management software, 394

reflection, 86–88, 96, 192, 379
  in active learning, 82, 101, 152
  questions for framing, 88
  self-, 44, 98, 168, 408, 430
  in service learning, 247
  in simulation debriefing, 174, 175, 229
reflective journaling, 193, 208, 301
Regents of the University of Michigan v. Ewing, 118, 120
registered nurses (RNs)
  average age of, 3, 57
  demographics of, 408
  educational preparation for academic employment, 4
  gender diversity of, 57
  racial diversity of, 55
  shortage of, 3
regulation
  of nursing programs, 368
  of simulation, 180
relational learning theory, 219
relational pedagogy, 219–220
reliability of test measurements, 317–318
remote preceptorships, 193
remote proctoring systems, 339
resource centers. *See* learning laboratories
responsibilities of nurse educators, 9–10
  balancing role responsibilities, 13–14
  scholarship, 11
  service, 11–12
  teaching, 10–11
reusable learning objects (RLOs), 90–91
RLOs. *See* reusable learning objects
RNs. *See* registered nurses
Robert Wood Johnson Foundation (RWJF) Mentoring Program, 412
Rogers, Carl, 42, 43
role development, 433
role models/role modeling, 12, 59, 60, 67, 223, 226, 407, 412, 413, 427, 428
role-play, 95–96, 137, 165, 268
roles of nurse educators/faculty, 9–12, 13–14, 25–30. *See also* responsibilities of nurse educators
rubrics
  clinical evaluation, 351–354
  for competency assessment, 262
  for evaluation of formal papers and written assignments, 301–304
  for group project assessment, 309
  scoring, 333

RWJF. *See* Robert Wood Johnson Foundation Mentoring Program

salary of nursing faculty, 14
sandwich method, 158
SBAR. *See* Situation, Background, Assessment, and Recommendation
scaffolding, 281, 282
scholarship, 389
  of application, 12, 390
  assessment of, 397
  Boyer's forms of, 390
  and career development, 397–398
  criteria for, 391
  definition of, 11
  of discovery, 12, 390
  dissemination of, 391–395, 396
  engagement of nurse educators in, 9, 29
  of integration, 12, 390
  presentations at conferences, 395
  process of becoming a scholar, 390, 392
  responsibilities of nurse educators, 11
  role of NPD practitioners in, 433–434
  of teaching, 12, 389–391
  writing for publication, 393–395
scholarship (financial aid), 414
scoping reviews, 382
Scopus, 394
scoring procedures (test), 319–320
screen-based simulation, 166
screencasting, 196
SDOH. *See* social determinants of health
SDOL. *See* social determinates of learning model
SECTIONS model, 134–135
selected response items (test), 318, 319
self-assessment/self-evaluation, 91, 309, 310–311, 351, 402, 405, 437
self-care, 413
self-directed learning (problem-based learning), 94. *See also* problem-based learning
self-paced modules, 90–91
self-reflection, 44, 98, 168, 408, 430
Serious Games Center (Purdue University), 128
serious gaming, 127. *See also* games, educational
service activities of nurse educators, 404–405
service learning, 96–97, 197, 231, 246–247

service responsibilities of nurse educators, 11–12
sexual diversity of students, 57, 59–60
short papers, 301
short-answer items, 332
Shrewsbury, C. M., 44
Sigma, 395, 451
Simulation Innovation Research Center, NLN, 171
simulation(s), 163, 190, 192, 223, 309, 350, 433
  as an evaluation tool, 170
  -based education, 95
  and competency-based education, 267–268
  credentialing, 180
  debriefing, 169–170, 172–176, 228–229, 309
  evaluation of, 177–179
  extended reality, 166–168
  fidelity, 164, 165, 229
  and generative artificial intelligence, 132
  high-frequency, low-impact simulations, 169
  high-stakes, 170
  implementation of, 171–172
  integration into curriculum, 168–171, 172
  interdisciplinary, 170
  interprofessional, 170, 226, 228–230
  and learner objectives, 164
  low-frequency, high impact simulations, 168–169
  manikin-based, 164–165
  and modified cases, 169–170
  pre-made/purchased, 171–172
  regulation, 180
  research, 179
  resources, 172
  scenarios, writing, 171
  simulation theory, 176
  standardized patients, 165–166
  standards, 177
  and time requirements, 172
  traditional, 163–166
  and unfolding cases, 169
  virtual, 126–127
situated learning theory, 41
Situation, Background, Assessment, and Recommendation (SBAR), 269
skills laboratories. *See* learning laboratories
Skinner, B. F., 39

small-group teaching methods
  case studies, 92–93
  collaborative learning, 93–94
  discussion, 91, 92
  experiential learning, 91–92, 95
  problem-based learning, 94–95
  service learning, 96–97
  simulation, standardized patients, role-play, and drama, 95–96
  teaching others and making presentations, 96
  team-based learning, 94
SNAPPS technique, 209
social cognitivism, 41
social determinants of health (SDOH), 61, 127, 193, 266, 405, 407, 408
social determinates of learning (SDOL) model, 61–63
social learning theory, 41
social media
  behavior, of students, 112–114
  and microlearning, 129–130
social presence, 47
social-cultural cognition, 41
socialization, 27, 190, 219, 413
Society for Simulation in Healthcare (SSH), 180
Socratic method, 35, 98, 99
split-length/split-half internal consistency method, 316
spouses, conflict of interest in employment of, 111
SPs. *See* standardized patients
SSH. *See* Society for Simulation in Healthcare
stakeholders of nursing programs, 360–361
stand-alone clinical judgment items, 337
standardized patients (SPs), 95, 165–166, 223, 309–310, 350
Standards for Quality Nurse Practitioner Education NTF, 206
stem (multiple-choice/multiple-response items), 325–326
storytelling, 100–101, 158
strategic learners, 63–64
strategic plans of healthcare organizations, 435–436
strategic technology plan, 133
stress
  of faculty, 204–205, 206
  of students, 75, 79, 203, 206, 350, 413

student engagement, 25, 42, 66, 68, 222
 and academic–practice partnerships, 250
 and active learning, 25, 81–82, 90, 94, 97, 128, 129, 133, 136, 147, 152, 154, 227, 269, 408, 427
 and audience response systems (ARS), 128, 129
 and clinical conferences, 198
 and clinical teaching, 203
 and game-based learning, 127
 and interprofessional education simulation, 228
 during lectures, 97
 and online learning, 147, 154, 156, 158
 and RLOs, 91
 and telehealth clinical experiences, 192
student evaluations of teaching, 368–370, 397
student handbooks, 107
student stress, 75, 79, 203, 206, 350, 413
student-initiated learning contracts, 89
student-led teaching, 137
succession planning, 405
summative assessments/evaluation, 262, 296, 301, 308, 309, 310, 348, 349, 351
support staff, and teaching method selection, 81
syllabus, 114, 147, 267
 development, 283, 288
 template, 288
systematic evaluation plan, 28, 364–367
systematic reviews, 380–382, 384

Tableau©, 370
TBL. *See* team-based learning
teacher-student relationship, 22, 66–67, 75, 192, 310–311
teaching methods, 75, 83, 125, 206
 case study, 92–93
 collaborative learning, 93–94
 concept mapping, 89–90
 contract learning, 88–89
 and curriculum models, 83
 debate, 100
 discussion, 91, 92
 and domains of learning, 77–78, 79, 80
 drama, 96
 educational games, 98, 100
 experiential learning, 91–92
 film, 100
 generational differences in, 57, 58
 independent learning methods, 83–91
 large-class methods, 97–101
 and learner characteristics, 78–79
 lecture, 97
 planning for active learning, 81–82
 for promotion of critical thinking, 83
 presentations, 96
 problem-based learning, 94–95
 questioning, 98, 99. *See also* Socratic method
 reading, 83–85
 reflection, 86, 87–88
 resources, 80–81
 role-play, 95–96
 selection of, 76–81
 self-paced modules/RLO, 90–91
 service learning, 96–97
 simulation, 95. *See also* simulation
 small-group methods, 91–97
 standardized patients, 95
 storytelling, 101–102
 team-based learning, 94
 time plan, 80
 writing, 86–87
teaching philosophy, 49, 398
teaching portfolios, 397, 398
teaching presence, 47
teaching responsibilities of nurse educators, 10–11, 13–14, 20, 75, 390. *See also* clinical teaching
team learning contracts, 88, 93–94
team-based learning (TBL), 94, 137
technology, 81, 123. *See also* online learning
 clickers and polling, 128–129. *See also* audience response systems
 cloud computing, 126
 development of faculty competencies and mentoring, 137–138
 and educational games, 98
 game-based learning, 127–128
 generative artificial intelligence, 131–133
 Internet, 124
 and learning, 36, 46–47
 learning analytics, 130–131
 learning management systems, 125
 metaverse, 127
 microlearning and social media, 129–130
 mobile devices, 130
 open educational resources, 131, 132
 reports, 153
 role in education, 123–124, 433
 role in online learning, 153–155
 virtual simulation, 126–127
 World Wide Web, 124, 125–126

technology, integration into education
　alignment with institutional mission and goals, 133–134
　classroom redesign, 135–136
　constructivism and technology-enhanced learning, 134
　decision-making framework for technology selection, 134–135
　infrastructure, 124, 133, 155, 339
　principles of good practice, 135
technology-enhanced items (TEI), 318, 319, 327–330
technology-mediated learning, 46–47
TEI. *See* technology-enhanced items
telehealth, 192, 230
tenure track, 5, 6, 29
test planning, 318
　characteristics of the students to be tested, 318
　item formats, 318–319
　length of test, 318
　purpose of test, 318
　scoring procedures, 319–320
tests, 299, 315
　answer key for, 339
　arranging items in logical sequence, 337–338
　assembling test, 337–339
　assessment reliability of, 317–318
　assessment validity of, 315–317
　avoiding crowding in, 338
　blueprint, 320–321, 340
　directions, writing, 338
　items, types of, 321–335
　keeping related material together, 338
　Next Generation NCLEX®, 335–337
　numbering of items, 338
　online, 339–340
　planning, 318–320
　preparation of students to take, 340–341
　principles for writing, 323–337
　proofreading of, 338
　scores, interpretation of, 297
　test anxiety, 341
　test statistics and item analysis, 341–342
　test-taking skills, 340–341
testwiseness, 340
theory of multiple intelligences, 46
Thorndike, Edward, 39
TJC. *See* The Joint Commission
toxic leadership, 114–117

transition from clinician to educator, 19, 438
　barriers to, 23, 24
　experience of, 20–21
　facilitators for, 23–24
　new faculty orientation, 24–31
　Nurse Educator Transition model, 21–22
　preparing nurse educators, 19–20
trauma-informed teaching practices (TTIP), 416
trend items, 335, 337
triad mentor models, 412
true–false items, 323–324
TTIP. *See* trauma-informed teaching practices
tuition reimbursement, 414

UBC. *See* University of British Columbia
Udemy, 146
UDL. *See* Universal Design for Learning
umbrella reviews, 381–382
UNESCO OER, 132
unfolding cases, 169, 228, 306
Unified Theory of Acceptance and Use of Technology (UTAUT), 138
Universal Design for Learning (UDL), 48, 153, 154
university legal counsel, 107–109
University of British Columbia (UBC), 220–221
university ombudsperson, 109
UTAUT. *See* Unified Theory of Acceptance and Use of Technology

validity of test measurements, 315–317
values (philosophy) statement, 280, 282
VARK learning model, 65–66, 410
video-recorded lectures, 97
virtual reality (VR), 192, 230
virtual simulation (VS), 126–127, 230
virtual site visits, 209
vision statement, 280, 282
visual learning, 65–66, 90, 410
Vizient/AACN Nurse Residency Program™, 458
vocational nursing programs. *See* practical nursing programs
VR. *See* virtual reality
VS. *See* virtual simulation
Vygotsky, Lev, 41

WCAG. *See* Web Content Accessibility Guidelines
WDL. *See* World Digital Library
Web. *See* World Wide Web
Web 1.0, 125
Web 2.0, 125, 129
Web 3.0, 125
Web 4.0, 125
Web Content Accessibility Guidelines (WCAG), 154
Web of Science, 394
Wenger, Etienne, 41
WHO. *See* World Health Organization
work environment, 243, 429. *See also* work-life balance
  healthy, 12, 117–118
  and mentoring, 402
  and succession planning, 405
  and toxic leadership, 115–117
workforce diversification, 407–408, 414, 417
work-life balance, 110–111
World Digital Library (WDL), 132
World Health Organization (WHO), 216
World Wide Web, 124, 125–126, 143
Wright competency model, 432
writing, 86–87
  assignments, 86–87, 199, 300–304, 350
  for publications, 393–395
  read/write (VARK), 65–66

XR. *See* extended reality

0/1 scoring, 320
zone of proximal development, 41
Zoom, 230
Zotero, 394